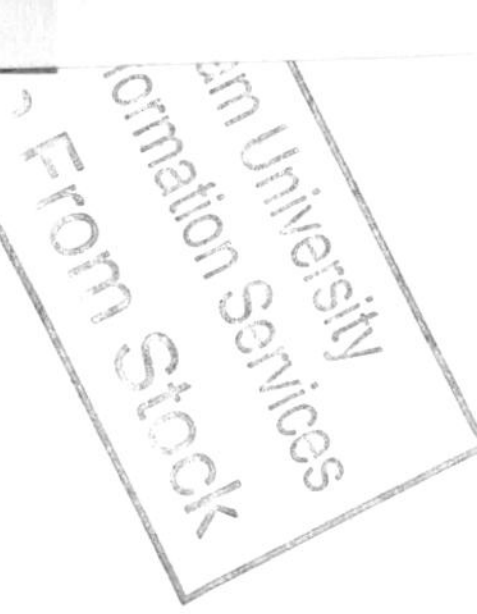

FENICHEL'S CLINICAL PEDIATRIC NEUROLOGY

Content Strategist: Charlotta Kryhl
Content Development Specialist: Alexandra Mortimer
Content coordinator: Humayra Rahman
Project Manager: Vinod Kumar Iyyappan
Marketing Manager: Carla Holloway

FENICHEL'S CLINICAL PEDIATRIC NEUROLOGY

A Signs and Symptoms Approach

Seventh Edition

J. Eric Piña-Garza, MD
Associate Professor of Neurology
Director, Pediatric Neurology
Director, Pediatric Epilepsy and EEG Lab
Monroe Carell, Jr. Children's Hospital at Vanderbilt
Nashville, Tennessee, USA

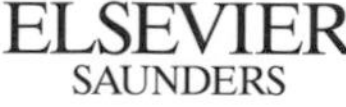

London, New York, Oxford, St Louis, Sydney, Toronto

ELSEVIER
SAUNDERS

SAUNDERS is an imprint of Elsevier Inc.

First edition 1988
Second edition 1993
Third edition 1997
Fourth edition 2001
Fifth edition 2005
Sixth edition 2009
Seventh edition 2013

ISBN: 978-1-4557-2376-8
Ebook ISBN: 978-1-4557-4812-9

Printed in China

Last digit is the print number: 9 8 7 6 5 4 3 2 1

CONTENTS

Foreword

I have had the great pleasure of writing this text through most of my academic career. It has been widely received, translated into five other languages, and served as my continuing medical education. Once retired, I expected to stop writing the text, which requires active patient experience. Dr. Piña-Garza served as my trainee, then long-term faculty associate and friend, and now as my successor as Division Chief of Pediatric Neurology in Children's Hospital at Vanderbilt. No one is better qualified to carry on the tradition. I thank my readers and publishers for making the book a success and assure them that the text will continue in the same spirit.

Gerald M. Fenichel, M.D.
Professor of Neurology, emeritus
Vanderbilt University School of Medicine
Nashville, Tennessee

PREFACE

In 1988, I read the first edition of *Clinical Pediatric Neurology* during my internship, and was struck by how different it was from other medical texts. The concept of organizing the book based on 'chief complaints' rather than 'disease categories' made intuitive sense to me, as this is how patients present to the clinician. That book proved to be an invaluable resource to me during my development as a pediatrician. Almost three years later I decided to do an elective with the author, Dr Gerald M. Fenichel, and this encounter confirmed my desire to pursue my child neurology training under his supervision. Dr Fenichel became not only a teacher, but a true mentor and a great friend. We practiced together for 16 years, and in 2010 he honored me with the continuation of this text.

This edition strives to maintain the goal of providing practical information for physicians who care for children and adolescents with neurological disease. Guidelines, standards of practice and evidence-based medicine are included whenever possible, and advice from our own experience and within our own biases is given when this information is not available.

Writing the new edition of this book has been a great learning experience for me. Reviewing the medical literature, organizing my thoughts and cataloguing my experiences have allowed me to gain a more comprehensive understanding of the field. I hope this translates into a benefit for our readers and, most importantly, for their patients.

J. Eric Piña-Garza, MD

DEDICATION

To my parents, Jose Piña Mendez and Maria Edelia Garza Gonzalez and all my family, who gave me so much love, guidance, emotional and spiritual nourishment. Thanks to their example, I was able to become who I am today.

To my beautiful wife Kaitlin C. James and my adorable daughter Josephine Anna Maria Piña-James, the loves of my life, who make me, appreciate every minute of my life.

Last but not least to my mentor, Gerald M. Fenichel, for the opportunity to continue his great work.

J. Eric Piña-Garza, MD

CHAPTER 1

PAROXYSMAL DISORDERS

Paroxysmal disorders are characterized by the sudden onset of neurological dysfunction and stereotyped recurrence. In children, such events often clear completely. Examples of paroxysmal disorders include epilepsy, migraine, periodic paralysis, and paroxysmal movement disorders.

APPROACH TO PAROXYSMAL DISORDERS

The diagnosing physician rarely witnesses the paroxysmal event. It is important to obtain the description of the event from the observer and not second hand. The information easily becomes distorted if transferred from the observer to the parent and then to you. Most *spells* are not seizures, and epilepsy is not a diagnosis of exclusion. Physicians often misdiagnose syncope as a seizure, as many people stiffen and tremble at the end of a faint. The critical distinction is that syncope is associated with pallor and preceded by dimming of vision, and a feeling of lightheadedness or clamminess, whereas seizures rarely are.

"Spells" seldom remain unexplained when viewed. Because observation of the spell is critical to diagnosis, ask the family to record the spell. Most families either own or can borrow a camera or a cell phone with video capability. Even when a purchase is required, a video is often more cost effective than brain imaging and the family has something useful to show for the expenditure. Always ask the following two questions: Has this happened before? Does anyone else in the family have similar episodes? Often, no one offers this important information until requested. Episodic symptoms that last only seconds and cause no abnormal signs usually remain unexplained and do not warrant laboratory investigation. The differential diagnosis of paroxysmal disorders is somewhat different in the neonate, infant, child, and adolescent, and presented best by age groups.

PAROXYSMAL DISORDERS OF NEWBORNS

Seizures are the main paroxysmal disorder of the newborn, occurring in 1.8–3.5 % of live births in the United States, and an important feature of neurological disease (Silverstein & Jensen, 2007). Uncontrolled seizures may contribute to further brain damage. Brain glucose decreases during prolonged seizures and excitatory amino acid release interferes with DNA synthesis. Therefore, seizures identified by electroencephalography (EEG) that occur without movement in newborns paralyzed for respiratory assistance are important to identify and treat. The challenge for the clinician is to differentiate seizure activity from normal neonatal movements and from pathological movements caused by other mechanisms (Box 1-1).

The long-term prognosis in children with neonatal seizures is better in term newborns than in premature newborns (Ronen et al, 2007). However, the etiology of the seizures is the primary determinant of prognosis.

Seizure Patterns

Seizures in newborns, especially in the premature, are poorly organized and difficult to distinguish from normal activity. Newborns with hydranencephaly or atelencephaly are capable of generating the full variety of neonatal seizure patterns. This supports the notion that seizures may arise from the brainstem as well as the hemispheres. The absence of myelinated pathways for seizure propagation may confine seizures arising in the brainstem. For the same reason, seizures originating in one hemisphere are less likely to spread beyond the contiguous cortex or to produce secondary bilateral synchrony.

Box 1-2 lists clinical patterns that have been associated with epileptiform discharges in newborns. This classification is useful but does not do justice to the rich variety of patterns actually

BOX 1-1 Movements That Resemble Neonatal Seizures

Benign nocturnal myoclonus*
Jitteriness*
Nonconvulsive apnea
Normal movement
Opisthotonos
Pathological myoclonus

*Denotes the most common conditions and the ones with disease modifying treatments

BOX 1-2 Seizure Patterns in Newborns

Apnea with tonic stiffening of body
Focal clonic movements of one limb or both limbs on one side*
Multifocal clonic limb movements*
Myoclonic jerking
Paroxysmal laughing
Tonic deviation of the eyes upward or to one side*
Tonic stiffening of the body

*Denotes the most common conditions and the ones with disease modifying treatments

observed. Nor does the classification account for the 50% of prolonged epileptiform discharges on the EEG without visible clinical changes. Generalized tonic-clonic seizures rarely occur. Many newborns suspected of having generalized tonic-clonic seizures are actually *jittery* (see Jitteriness, discussed later in this chapter). Newborns paralyzed to assist mechanical ventilation pose an additional problem in seizure identification. In this circumstance, the presence of rhythmic increases in systolic arterial blood pressure, heart rate, and oxygenation desaturation should alert physicians to the possibility of seizures.

The term *subtle seizures* encompass several different patterns in which tonic or clonic movements of the limbs are lacking. EEG monitoring often fails to show that such movements are associated with epileptiform activity. One exception is tonic deviation of the eyes, which is usually a seizure manifestation. One of the most common manifestations of seizures in the young infant is behavioral arrest and unresponsiveness. Behavioral arrest is only obvious when the child is very active, which is not common in a sick neonate and therefore often goes unnoticed.

The definitive diagnosis of neonatal seizures often requires EEG monitoring. A split-screen 16-channel video-EEG is the ideal means for monitoring. An aEEG (amplitude EEG) is also a useful monitoring technique. Seizures in the newborn may be widespread and electrographically detectable even when the newborn is not convulsing clinically.

Focal Clonic Seizures

Clinical Features. Repeated, irregular slow clonic movements (1 to 3 jerks/second) affecting one limb or both limbs on one side are characteristic of focal clonic seizures. Rarely do such movements sustain for long periods, and they do not "march" as though spreading along the motor cortex. *In an otherwise alert and responsive full-term newborn, unifocal clonic seizures always indicate a cerebral infarction or hemorrhage or focal brain dysgenesis.* In newborns with states of decreased consciousness, focal clonic seizures may indicate a focal infarction superimposed on a generalized encephalopathy.

Diagnosis. During the seizure, the EEG may show a unilateral focus of high-amplitude sharp waves adjacent to the central fissure. The discharge can spread to involve contiguous areas in the same hemisphere and can be associated with unilateral seizures of the limbs and adversive movements of the head and eyes. The interictal EEG may show focal slowing, sharp waves or amplitude attenuation.

Newborns with focal clonic seizures should be immediately evaluated using magnetic resonance imaging (MRI) with diffusion-weighted images. Computed tomography (CT) or ultrasound is acceptable for less stable neonates unable to make the trip to the MRI suite or tolerate the time needed for this procedure.

Multifocal Clonic Seizures

Clinical Features. In multifocal clonic seizures, migratory jerking movements are noted in first one limb and then another. Facial muscles may be involved as well. The migration appears random and does not follow expected patterns of epileptic spread. Sometimes, prolonged movements occur in one limb, suggesting a focal rather than a multifocal seizure. Detection of the multifocal nature comes later, when nursing notes appear contradictory concerning the side or the limb affected. Multifocal clonic seizures are a neonatal equivalent of generalized tonic-clonic seizures. They are ordinarily associated with severe, generalized cerebral disturbances such as hypoxic-ischemic encephalopathy, but may also represent benign neonatal convulsions when noted in an otherwise healthy neonate.

Diagnosis. Standard EEG usually detects multifocal epileptiform activity. If not, a 24-hour monitor is appropriate.

Myoclonic Seizures

Clinical Features. Brief, nonrhythmic extension and flexion movements of the arms, the legs, or all limbs characterize myoclonic seizures. They constitute an uncommon seizure pattern in the newborn, but their presence suggests severe, diffuse brain damage.

Diagnosis. No specific EEG pattern is associated with myoclonic seizures in the newborn. Myoclonic jerks often occur in babies born to drug-addicted mothers. Whether these movements are seizures, jitteriness, or myoclonus (discussed later) is uncertain.

Tonic Seizures

Clinical Features. The characteristic feature of tonic seizures are extension and stiffening of the body, usually associated with apnea and upward deviation of the eyes. Tonic posturing without the other features is rarely a seizure manifestation. Tonic seizures are more common in premature than in full-term newborns and usually indicate structural brain damage rather than a metabolic disturbance.

Diagnosis. Tonic seizures in premature newborns are often a symptom of intraventricular hemorrhage and an indication for ultrasound study. Tonic posturing also occurs in newborns with forebrain damage, not as a seizure manifestation but as a disinhibition of brainstem reflexes. Prolonged disinhibition results in *decerebrate posturing*, an extension of the body and limbs associated with internal rotation of the arms, dilation of the pupils, and downward deviation of the eyes. Decerebrate posturing is often a terminal sign in premature infants with intraventricular hemorrhage caused by pressure on the upper brainstem (see Chapter 4).

Tonic seizures and decerebrate posturing look similar to *opisthotonos*, a prolonged arching of the back not necessarily associated with eye movements. The cause of opisthotonos is probably meningeal irritation. It occurs in kernicterus, infantile Gaucher disease, and some aminoacidurias.

Seizure-Like Events

Apnea

Clinical Features. An irregular respiratory pattern with intermittent pauses of 3 to 6 seconds, often followed by 10 to 15 seconds of hyperpnea, is a common occurrence in premature infants. The pauses are not associated with significant alterations in heart rate, blood pressure, body temperature, or skin color. Immaturity of the brainstem respiratory centers causes this respiratory pattern, termed *periodic breathing*. The incidence of periodic breathing correlates directly with the degree of prematurity. Apneic spells are more common during active than quiet sleep.

Apneic spells of 10 to 15 seconds are detectable at some time in almost all premature and some full-term newborns. Apneic spells of 10 to 20 seconds are usually associated with a 20 % reduction in heart rate. Longer episodes of apnea are almost invariably associated with a 40 % or greater reduction in heart rate. The frequency of these apneic spells correlates with brainstem myelination. Even at 40 weeks conceptional age, premature newborns continue to have a higher incidence of apnea than do full-term newborns. The incidence of apnea sharply decreases in all infants at 52 weeks conceptional age. Apnea with bradycardia is unlikely to be a seizure. Apnea with tachycardia raises the possibility of seizure and should be evaluated with simultaneous EEG recording.

Diagnosis. Apneic spells in an otherwise normal-appearing newborn is typically a sign of brainstem immaturity and not a pathological condition. The sudden onset of apnea and states of decreased consciousness, especially in premature newborns, suggests an intracranial hemorrhage with brainstem compression. Immediate ultrasound examination is in order.

Apneic spells are almost never a seizure manifestation unless associated with tonic deviation of the eyes, tonic stiffening of the body, or characteristic limb movements. *However, prolonged apnea without bradycardia, and especially with tachycardia, is a seizure until proven otherwise.*

Management. Short episodes of apnea do not require intervention. The rare ictal apnea requires the use of anticonvulsant agents.

Benign Nocturnal Myoclonus

Clinical Features. Sudden jerking movements of the limbs during sleep occur in normal people of all ages (see Chapter 14). They appear primarily during the early stages of sleep as repeated flexion movements of the fingers, wrists, and elbows. The jerks do not localize consistently, stop with gentle restraint, and end abruptly with arousal. When prolonged, the usual misdiagnosis is focal clonic or myoclonic seizures.

Diagnosis. The distinction between nocturnal myoclonus and seizures or jitteriness is that benign nocturnal myoclonus occurs solely during sleep, is not activated by a stimulus, and the EEG is normal.

Management. Treatment is unnecessary, and education and reassurance are usually sufficient. Rarely a child with violent myoclonus experiences frequent arousals disruptive to sleep, and a small dose of clonazepam may be considered. Videos of children with this benign condition are very reassuring for the family to see and are available on the internet.

Jitteriness

Clinical Features. Jitteriness or tremulousness is an excessive response to stimulation.

BOX 1-3 Differential Diagnosis of Neonatal Seizures by Peak Time of Onset

24 HOURS

- Bacterial meningitis and sepsis* (see Chapter 4)
- Direct drug effect
- Hypoxic-ischemic encephalopathy*
- Intrauterine infection (see Chapter 5)
- Intraventricular hemorrhage at term* (see Chapter 4)
- Laceration of tentorium or falx
- Pyridoxine dependency*
- Subarachnoid hemorrhage*

24 TO 72 HOURS

- Bacterial meningitis and sepsis* (see Chapter 4)
- Cerebral contusion with subdural hemorrhage
- Cerebral dysgenesis* (see Chapter 18)
- Cerebral infarction* (see Chapter 11)
- Drug withdrawal
- Glycine encephalopathy
- Glycogen synthase deficiency
- Hypoparathyroidism-hypocalcemia
- Idiopathic cerebral venous thrombosis
- Incontinentia pigmenti
- Intracerebral hemorrhage (see Chapter 11)
- Intraventricular hemorrhage in premature newborns* (see Chapter 4)
- Pyridoxine dependency*
- Subarachnoid hemorrhage
- Tuberous sclerosis
- Urea cycle disturbances

72 HOURS TO 1 WEEK

- Cerebral dysgenesis (see Chapter 18)
- Cerebral infarction (see Chapter 11)*
- Familial neonatal seizures
- Hypoparathyroidism
- Idiopathic cerebral venous thrombosis*
- Intracerebral hemorrhage (see Chapter 11)
- Kernicterus
- Methylmalonic acidemia
- Nutritional hypocalcemia*
- Propionic acidemia
- Tuberous sclerosis
- Urea cycle disturbances

1 TO 4 WEEKS

- Adrenoleukodystrophy, neonatal (see Chapter 6)
- Cerebral dysgenesis (see Chapter 18)
- Fructose dysmetabolism
- Gaucher disease type 2 (see Chapter 5)
- GM_1 gangliosidosis type 1 (see Chapter 5)
- Herpes simplex encephalitis*
- Idiopathic cerebral venous thrombosis*
- Ketotic hyperglycinemias
- Maple syrup urine disease, neonatal*
- Tuberous sclerosis
- Urea cycle disturbances

*Denotes the most common conditions and the ones with disease modifying treatments

Touch, noise, or motion provokes a low-amplitude, high-frequency shaking of the limbs and jaw. Jitteriness is commonly associated with a low threshold for the Moro reflex, but it can occur in the absence of any apparent stimulation and be confused with myoclonic seizures.

Diagnosis. Jitteriness usually occurs in newborns with perinatal asphyxia that may have seizures as well. EEG monitoring, the absence of eye movements or alteration in respiratory pattern, and the presence of stimulus activation distinguishes jitteriness from seizures. Newborns of addicted mothers and newborns with metabolic disorders are often jittery.

Management. Reduced stimulation decreases jitteriness. However, newborns of addicted mothers require sedation to facilitate feeding and to decrease energy expenditure.

Differential Diagnosis of Seizures

Seizures are a feature of almost all brain disorders in the newborn. The time of onset of the first seizure indicates the probable cause (Box 1-3). Seizures occurring during the first 24 hours, and especially in the first 12 hours, are usually due to hypoxic-ischemic encephalopathy. Sepsis, meningitis, and subarachnoid hemorrhage are next in frequency, followed by intrauterine infection and trauma. Direct drug effects, intraventricular hemorrhage at term, and pyridoxine and folinic acid dependency are relatively rare causes of seizures.

The more common causes of seizures during the period from 24 to 72 hours after birth are intraventricular hemorrhage in premature newborns, subarachnoid hemorrhage, cerebral contusion in large full-term newborns, and sepsis and meningitis at all gestational ages. The cause of unifocal clonic seizures in full-term newborns is often cerebral infarction or intracerebral hemorrhage. Head CT is diagnostic. Cerebral dysgenesis causes seizures at this time and remains an important cause of seizures throughout infancy and childhood. All other conditions are relatively rare. *Newborns with metabolic disorders are usually lethargic and feed poorly before the onset of seizures.* Seizures are rarely the first clinical feature. After 72 hours, the initiation of protein and glucose feedings makes inborn errors of metabolism, especially aminoacidurias, a more important consideration. Box 1-4 outlines a battery of screening tests for metabolic disorders. Transmission of herpes simplex infection is during delivery and symptoms begin during

BOX 1-4 Screening for Inborn Errors of Metabolism that Cause Neonatal Seizures

Blood Glucose Low
- Fructose 1,6-diphosphatase deficiency
- Glycogen storage disease type 1
- Maple syrup urine disease

Blood Calcium Low
- Hypoparathyroidism
- Maternal hyperparathyroidism

Blood Ammonia High
- Argininosuccinic acidemia
- Carbamylphosphate synthetase deficiency
- Citrullinemia
- Methylmalonic acidemia (may be normal)
- Multiple carboxylase deficiency
- Ornithine transcarbamylase deficiency
- Propionic acidemia (may be normal)

Blood Lactate High
- Fructose 1,6-diphosphatase deficiency
- Glycogen storage disease type 1
- Mitochondrial disorders
- Multiple carboxylase deficiency

Metabolic Acidosis
- Fructose 1,6-diphosphatase deficiency
- Glycogen storage disease type 1
- Maple syrup urine disease
- Methylmalonic acidemia
- Multiple carboxylase deficiency
- Propionic acidemia

the second half of the first week. Conditions that cause early and late seizures include cerebral dysgenesis, cerebral infarction, intracerebral hemorrhage, and familial neonatal seizures.

Aminoacidopathies

Maple Syrup Urine Disease. An almost complete absence (less than 2 % of normal) of branched-chain ketoacid dehydrogenase (BCKD) causes the neonatal form of maple syrup urine disease (MSUD). BCKD is composed of six subunits, but the main abnormality in MSUD is deficiency of the E1 subunit on chromosome 19q13.1–q13.2. Leucine, isoleucine, and valine cannot be decarboxylated, and accumulate in blood, urine, and tissues (Figure 1-1). Descriptions of later-onset forms are in Chapters 5 and 10. Transmission of the defect is by autosomal recessive inheritance (Strauss et al, 2009).

Clinical Features. Affected newborns appear healthy at birth, but lethargy, feeding difficulty, and hypotonia develop after ingestion of protein. A progressive encephalopathy develops by 2 to 3 days postpartum. The encephalopathy includes lethargy, intermittent apnea, opisthotonos, and stereotyped movements such as "fencing" and "bicycling." Coma and central respiratory failure may occur by 7to10 days of age. Seizures begin in the second week and are associated with the development of cerebral edema. Once seizures begin, they continue with increasing frequency and severity. Without therapy, cerebral edema becomes progressively worse and results in coma and death within 1 month.

Diagnosis. Plasma amino acid concentrations show increased plasma concentrations of the three branch-chained amino acids. Measures of enzyme in lymphocytes or cultured fibroblasts serve as a confirmatory test. Heterozygotes have diminished levels of enzyme activity.

Management. Hemodialysis may be necessary to correct the life-threatening metabolic acidosis. A trial of thiamine (10–20 mg/kg/day) improves the condition in a *thiamine-responsive MSUD variant.* Stop the intake of all natural protein, and correct dehydration, electrolyte imbalance, and metabolic acidosis. A special diet, low in branched-chain amino acids, may prevent further encephalopathy if started immediately by nasogastric tube. Newborns diagnosed in the first 2 weeks and treated rigorously have the best prognosis.

Glycine Encephalopathy. A defect in the glycine cleaving system causes glycine encephalopathy (nonketotic hyperglycinemia). Inheritance is autosomal recessive (Hamosh, 2009).

Clinical Features. Affected newborns are normal at birth but become irritable and refuse feeding anytime from 6 hours to 8 days after delivery. The onset of symptoms is usually within 48 hours but delays by a few weeks occur in milder allelic forms. *Hiccupping* is an early and continuous feature; some mothers relate that the child hiccupped in utero as a prominent symptom. Progressive lethargy, hypotonia, respiratory disturbances, and myoclonic seizures follow. Some newborns survive the acute illness, but cognitive impairment, epilepsy, and spasticity characterize the subsequent course.

In the milder forms range, the onset of seizures is after the neonatal period. The developmental outcome is better, but does not exceed moderate cognitive impairment.

Diagnosis. During the acute encephalopathy, the EEG demonstrates a burst-suppression pattern, which evolves into hypsarrhythmia during infancy. The MRI may be normal or may show agenesis or thinning of the corpus callosum. Delayed myelination and atrophy are later findings. Hyperglycinemia and especially elevated concentrations of glycine in the cerebrospinal fluid (CSF), in the absence of hyperammonemia,

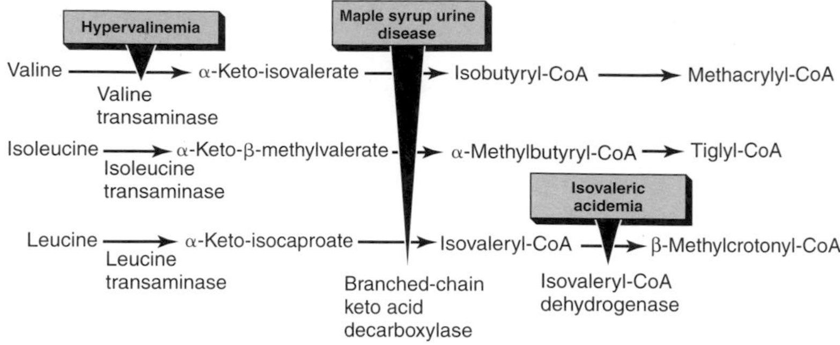

FIGURE 1-1 ■ Branched-chain amino acid metabolism. 1. Transaminase system; 2. branched-chain α-keto-acid dehydrogenase; 3. isovaleryl-CoA dehydrogenase; 4. α-methyl branched-chain acyl-CoA dehydrogenase; 5. propionyl-CoA carboxylase (biotin cofactor); 6. methylmalonyl-CoA racemase; 7. methylmalonyl-CoA mutase (adenosylcobalamin cofactor).

organic acidemia or valproic acid treatment establishes the diagnosis.

Management. No therapy has proven to be effective. Hemodialysis provides only temporary relief of the encephalopathy, and diet therapy has not proved successful in modifying the course. Diazepam, a competitor for glycine receptors, in combination with choline, folic acid, and sodium benzoate, may stop the seizures. Oral administration of sodium benzoate at doses of 250–750 mg/kg/day can reduce the plasma glycine concentration into the normal range. This substantially reduces but does not normalize CSF glycine concentration. Carnitine, 100 mg/kg/day, may increase the glycine conjugation with benzoate.

Urea Cycle Disturbances. Carbamyl phosphate synthetase (CPS) deficiency, ornithine transcarbamylase (OTC) deficiency, citrullinemia, argininosuccinic acidemia, and argininemia (arginase deficiency) are the disorders caused by defects in the enzyme systems responsible for urea synthesis. A similar syndrome results from deficiency of the cofactor producer N-acetyl glutamate synthetase (NAGS). Arginase deficiency does not cause symptoms in the newborn. OTC deficiency is an X-linked trait; transmission of all others is by autosomal recessive inheritance (Summar, 2011). The estimated prevalence of all urea cycle disturbances is 1:30 000 live births.

Clinical Features. The clinical features of urea cycle disorders are due to ammonia intoxication (Box 1-5). Progressive lethargy, vomiting, and hypotonia develop as early as the first day after delivery, even before the initiation of protein feeding. Progressive loss of consciousness and seizures follow on subsequent days. Vomiting and lethargy correlate well with plasma ammonia concentrations greater than 200 µg/dL (120 µmol/L). Coma correlates with concentrations greater than 300 µg/dL (180 µmol/L) and seizures with those greater than 500 µg/dL (300 µmol/L). Death follows quickly in untreated newborns. Newborns with partial deficiency of CPS and female carriers of OTC deficiency may become symptomatic after ingesting a large protein load.

BOX 1-5 Causes of Neonatal Hyperammonemia

LIVER FAILURE

PRIMARY ENZYME DEFECTS IN UREA SYNTHESIS

- Argininosuccinic acidemia
- Carbamyl phosphate synthetase deficiency
- Citrullinemia
- Ornithine transcarbamylase deficiency

OTHER DISORDERS OF AMINO ACID METABOLISM

- Glycine encephalopathy
- Isovaleric acidemia
- Methylmalonic acidemia
- Multiple carboxylase deficiency
- Propionic acidemia

TRANSITORY HYPERAMMONEMIA OF PREMATURITY

Diagnosis. Suspect the diagnosis of a urea cycle disturbance in every newborn with a compatible clinical syndrome and hyperammonemia without organic acidemia. Hyperammonemia can be life threatening, and diagnosis within 24 hours is essential. Determine the blood ammonia concentration and the plasma acid–base status. A plasma ammonia concentration of 150 mmol/L strongly suggests a urea cycle disorder. Quantitative plasma amino acid analysis helps differentiate the specific urea cycle disorder. Molecular genetic testing is available for some disorders, but others still require liver biopsy to determine the level of enzyme activity. The most common cause of hyperammonemia is difficult phlebotomy with improper sample processing. Accurate serum ammonia testing requires a good phlebotomist, sample placement on ice, and rapid processing.

Management. Treatment cannot await specific diagnosis in newborns with symptomatic hyperammonemia due to urea cycle disorders. The treatment measures include reduction of plasma ammonia concentration by limiting nitrogen intake to 1.2–2.0 g/kg/day and using essential amino acids for protein; allowing alternative pathway excretion of excess nitrogen with sodium benzoate and phenylacetic acid; reducing the amount of nitrogen in the diet; and reducing catabolism by introducing calories supplied by carbohydrates and fat. Arginine concentrations are low in all inborn errors of urea synthesis except for arginase deficiency and require supplementation.

Even with optimal supervision, episodes of hyperammonemia may occur and may lead to coma and death. In such cases, intravenous administration of sodium benzoate, sodium phenylacetate, and arginine, coupled with nitrogen-free alimentation, are appropriate. If response to drug therapy is poor, then peritoneal dialysis or hemodialysis is indicated.

Benign Familial Neonatal Seizures

In some families, several members have seizures in the first weeks of life but do not have epilepsy or other neurological abnormalities later on. Two genes, *KCNQ2* and *KCNQ3*, are associated with the disorder. In each, transmission of the trait is autosomal dominant and mutations affect the voltage gated potassium channel.

Clinical Features. Brief multifocal clonic seizures develop during the first week, sometimes associated with apnea. Delay of onset may be as long as 4 weeks. With or without treatment, the seizures usually stop spontaneously within the first months of life. Febrile seizures occur in up to one-third of affected children; some have febrile seizures without first having neonatal seizures. Epilepsy develops later in life in as many as a third of affected newborns. The seizure types include nocturnal generalized tonic-clonic seizures and simple focal orofacial seizures.

Diagnosis. Suspect the syndrome when seizures develop without apparent cause in a healthy newborn. Laboratory tests are normal. The EEG often demonstrates multifocal epileptiform discharges and may be normal interictally. A family history of neonatal seizures is critical to diagnosis but may await discovery until interviewing the grandparents; parents are frequently unaware that they had neonatal seizures.

Management. Treat with anticonvulsants. Oxcarbazepine at doses of 20 mg/kg/day for a couple of days and titrated to 40 mg/kg/day can be helpful. The duration of treatment needed is unclear. We often treat infants for about 9 months, after which we discontinue treatment if the child remains seizure-free and the EEG has normalized.

Bilirubin Encephalopathy

Unconjugated bilirubin is bound to albumin in the blood. *Kernicterus*, a yellow discoloration of the brain that is especially severe in the basal ganglia and hippocampus, occurs when the serum unbound or free fraction becomes excessive. An excessive level of the free fraction in an otherwise healthy newborn is approximately 20 mg/dL (340 µmol/L). Kernicterus was an important complication of hemolytic disease from maternal–fetal blood group incompatibility, but this condition is now almost unheard of in most countries. The management of other causes of hyperbilirubinemia in full-term newborns is not difficult. Critically ill premature infants with respiratory distress syndrome, acidosis, and sepsis are the group at greatest risk. In such newborns, lower concentrations of bilirubin may be sufficient to cause bilirubin encephalopathy, and even the albumin-bound fraction may pass the blood–brain barrier.

Clinical Features. Three distinct clinical phases of bilirubin encephalopathy occur in full-term newborns with untreated hemolytic disease. Hypotonia, lethargy, and a poor sucking reflex occur within 24 hours of delivery. Bilirubin staining of the brain is already evident in newborns during this first clinical phase. On the second or third day, the newborn becomes febrile and shows increasing tone and opisthotonic posturing. Seizures are not a constant feature but may occur at this time. Characteristic of the third phase is apparent improvement with normalization of tone. This may cause second thoughts about the accuracy of the diagnosis, but the improvement is short-lived. Evidence of neurological dysfunction begins to appear toward the end of the second month, and the symptoms become progressively worse throughout infancy.

In premature newborns, the clinical features are subtle and may lack the phases of increased tone and opisthotonos.

The typical clinical syndrome after the first year includes extrapyramidal dysfunction, usually athetosis, which occurs in virtually every case (see Chapter 14); disturbances of vertical gaze, upward more often than downward, in 90%; high-frequency hearing loss in 60%; and mental retardation in 25%. Survivors often develop a choreoathetoid form of cerebral palsy.

Diagnosis. In newborns with hemolytic disease, the basis for a presumed clinical diagnosis is a significant hyperbilirubinemia and a compatible evolution of symptoms. However, the diagnosis is difficult to establish in critically ill premature newborns, in which the cause of brain damage is more often asphyxia than kernicterus.

Management. Maintaining serum bilirubin concentrations below the toxic range, either by phototherapy or exchange transfusion, prevents kernicterus. Once kernicterus has occurred, further damage can be limited, but not reversed, by lowering serum bilirubin concentrations. Diazepam and baclofen are often needed for management of dystonic postures associated with the cerebral palsy.

Drug Withdrawal

Marijuana, alcohol, narcotic analgesics, and hypnotic sedatives are the nonprescribed drugs most commonly used during pregnancy. Marijuana and alcohol do not cause drug dependence in the fetus and are not associated with withdrawal symptoms, although ethanol can cause fetal alcohol syndrome. Hypnotic sedatives, such as barbiturates, do not ordinarily produce withdrawal symptoms unless the ingested doses are very large. Phenobarbital has a sufficiently long half-life in newborns that sudden withdrawal does not occur. The prototype of narcotic withdrawal in the newborn is with heroin or methadone, but a similar syndrome occurs with codeine and propoxyphene. Cocaine and methamphetamine also cause significant withdrawal syndromes.

Clinical Features. Symptoms of opiate withdrawal are more severe and tend to occur earlier in full-term (first 24 hours) than in premature (24 to 48 hours) newborns. The initial feature is a coarse tremor, present only during the waking state, which can shake an entire limb. Irritability, a shrill, high-pitched cry, and hyperactivity follow. The newborn seems hungry but has difficulty feeding and vomits afterward. Diarrhea and other symptoms of autonomic instability are common.

Myoclonic jerking is present in 10–25 % of newborns undergoing withdrawal. Whether these movements are seizures or jitteriness is not clear. Definite seizures occur in fewer than 5 %. Maternal use of cocaine during pregnancy is associated with premature delivery, growth retardation, and microcephaly. Newborns exposed to cocaine, in utero or after delivery through the breast milk, often show features of cocaine intoxication including tachycardia, tachypnea, hypertension, irritability, and tremulousness.

Diagnosis. Suspect and anticipate drug withdrawal in every newborn whose mother has a history of substance abuse. Even when such a history is not available, the combination of irritability, hyperactivity, and autonomic instability should provide a clue to the diagnosis. Careful questioning of the mother concerning her use of prescription and nonprescription drugs is imperative. Blood, urine, and meconium analyses identify specific drugs.

Management. Symptoms remit spontaneously in 3 to 5 days, but appreciable mortality occurs among untreated newborns. Benzodiazepines or chlorpromazine, 3 mg/kg/day, may relieve symptoms and reduce mortality. Consider phenobarbital 8 mg/kg/day for refractory cases. Secretion of morphine, meperidine, opium, and methadone in breast milk is insufficient to cause or relieve addiction in the newborn. Levetiracetam 40 mg/kg/day is a good option for seizures.

The occurrence of seizures, in itself, does not indicate a poor prognosis. The long-term outcome relates more closely to the other risk factors associated with substance abuse in the mother.

Hypocalcemia

The definition of hypocalcemia is a blood calcium concentration less than 7 mg/dL (1.75 mmol/L). The onset of hypocalcemia in the first 72 hours after delivery is associated with low birth weight, asphyxia, maternal diabetes, transitory neonatal hypoparathyroidism, maternal hyperparathyroidism, and the DiGeorge syndrome (DGS). Later-onset hypocalcemia occurs in children fed improper formulas, in maternal hyperparathyroidism, and in DGS.

Hypoparathyroidism in the newborn may result from maternal hyperparathyroidism or may be a transitory phenomenon of unknown cause. Hypocalcemia occurs in less than 10 % of stressed newborns and enhances their vulnerability to seizures, but it is rarely the primary cause.

DGS is associated with microdeletions of chromosome 22q11.2 (McDonald-McGinn et al, 2005). Disturbance of cervical neural crest migration into the derivatives of the pharyngeal arches and pouches explains the phenotype. Organs derived from the third and fourth pharyngeal pouches (thymus, parathyroid gland, and great vessels) are hypoplastic.

Clinical Features. The 22q11.2 syndrome encompasses several similar phenotypes: DGS, *velocardiofacial syndrome* (VCFS), and Shprintzen syndrome. The acronym CATCH is used to describe the phenotype of cardiac abnormality, T-cell deficit, clefting (multiple minor facial anomalies), and hypocalcemia. The identification of most children with DGS is in the neonatal period with a major heart defect, hypocalcemia, and immunodeficiency. Diagnosis of children with

VCFS comes later because of cleft palate or craniofacial deformities.

The initial symptoms of DGS may be due to congenital heart disease, hypocalcemia, or both. Jitteriness and tetany usually begin in the first 48 hours after delivery. The peak onset of seizures is on the third day but a 2-week delay may occur. Many affected newborns die of cardiac causes during the first month; survivors fail to thrive and have frequent infections secondary to the failure of cell-mediated immunity.

Diagnosis. Newborns with DGS come to medical attention because of seizures and heart disease. Seizures or a prolonged Q-T interval brings attention to hypocalcemia. Molecular genetic testing confirms the diagnosis.

Management. Management requires a multispecialty team including cardiology, immunology, medical genetics, and neurology. Plastic surgery, dentistry, and child development contribute later on. Hypocalcemia generally responds to parathyroid hormone or to oral calcium and vitamin D.

Hypoglycemia

A transitory, asymptomatic hypoglycemia is detectable in 10 % of newborns during the first hours after delivery and before initiating feeding. Asymptomatic, transient hypoglycemia is not associated with neurological impairment later in life. Symptomatic hypoglycemia may result from stress or inborn errors of metabolism (Box 1-6).

Clinical Features. The time of onset of symptoms depends upon the underlying disorder. Early onset is generally associated with perinatal asphyxia, maternal diabetes or intracranial hemorrhage, and late onset with inborn errors of metabolism. Hypoglycemia is rare and mild among newborns with classic MSUD, ethylmalonic aciduria, and isovaleric acidemia and is invariably severe in those with 3-methylglutaconic aciduria, glutaric aciduria type 2, and disorders of fructose metabolism.

The syndrome includes any of the following symptoms: apnea, cyanosis, tachypnea, jitteriness, high-pitched cry, poor feeding, vomiting, apathy, hypotonia, seizures, and coma. Symptomatic hypoglycemia is often associated with later neurological impairment.

Diagnosis. Neonatal hypoglycemia is defined as a whole blood glucose concentration of less than 20 mg/dL (1 mmol/L) in premature and low-birth-weight newborns, less than 30 mg/dL (1.5 mmol/L) in term newborns during the first 72 hours, and less than 40 mg/dL (2 mmol/L) in full-term newborns after 72 hours. Finding a low glucose concentration in a newborn with seizures prompts investigation into the cause of the hypoglycemia.

Management. Intravenous administration of glucose normalizes blood glucose concentrations, but the underlying cause must be determined before providing definitive treatment.

BOX 1-6 Causes of Neonatal Hypoglycemia

PRIMARY TRANSITIONAL HYPOGLYCEMIA*
- Complicated labor and delivery
- Intrauterine malnutrition
- Maternal diabetes
- Prematurity

SECONDARY TRANSITIONAL HYPOGLYCEMIA*
- Asphyxia
- Central nervous system disorders
- Cold injuries
- Sepsis

PERSISTENT HYPOGLYCEMIA
- Aminoacidurias
  - Maple syrup urine disease
  - Methylmalonic acidemia
  - Propionic acidemia
  - Tyrosinosis
- Congenital hypopituitarism
- Defects in carbohydrate metabolism
  - Fructose 1, 6-diphosphatase deficiency
  - Fructos e+ intolerance
  - Galactosemia
  - Glycogen storage disease type 1
  - Glycogen synthase deficiency
- Hyperinsulinism
- Organic acidurias
  - Glutaric aciduria type 2
  - 3-Methylglutaryl-CoA lyase deficiency

*Denotes the most common conditions and the ones with disease modifying treatments

Hypoxic-Ischemic Encephalopathy

Asphyxia at term is usually an intrauterine event, and hypoxia and ischemia occur together; the result is hypoxic-ischemic encephalopathy (HIE). *Acute total asphyxia* often leads to death from circulatory collapse. Survivors are born comatose. Lower cranial nerve dysfunction and severe neurological handicaps are the rule.

Partial, prolonged asphyxia is the usual mechanism of HIE in surviving full-term newborns (Miller et al, 2005). The fetal circulation accommodates to reductions in arterial oxygen by maximizing blood flow to the brain, and to a lesser extent the heart, at the expense of other organs.

Clinical experience indicates that fetuses may be subject to considerable hypoxia without the development of brain damage. The incidence of cerebral palsy among full-term newborns with a 5-minute Apgar score of 0 to 3 is only 1 % if the 10-minute score is 4 or higher. Any episode of hypoxia sufficiently severe to cause brain damage also causes derangements in other organs. Newborns with mild HIE always have a history of irregular heart rate and usually pass meconium. Those with severe HIE may have lactic acidosis, elevated serum concentrations of hepatic enzymes, enterocolitis, renal failure, and fatal myocardial damage.

Clinical Features. *Mild HIE* is relatively common. The newborn is lethargic but conscious immediately after birth. Other characteristic features are jitteriness and sympathetic over-activity (tachycardia, dilatation of pupils, and decreased bronchial and salivary secretions). Muscle tone is normal at rest, tendon reflexes are normoreactive or hyperactive, and ankle clonus is usually elicited. The Moro reflex is complete, and a single stimulus generates repetitive extension and flexion movements. Seizures are not an expected feature, and their occurrence suggests concurrent hypoglycemia, the presence of a second condition or a more significant HIE.

Symptoms diminish and disappear during the first few days, although some degree of over-responsiveness may persist. Newborns with mild HIE are believed to recover normal brain function completely. They are not at greater risk for later epilepsy or learning disabilities.

Newborns with *severe HIE* are stuporous or comatose immediately after birth, and respiratory effort is usually periodic and insufficient to sustain life. Seizures begin within the first 12 hours. Hypotonia is severe, and tendon reflexes, the Moro reflex, and the tonic neck reflex are absent as well. Sucking and swallowing are depressed or absent, but the pupillary and oculovestibular reflexes are present. Most of these newborns have frequent seizures, which may appear on EEG without clinical manifestations. They may progress to status epilepticus. The response to antiepileptic drugs is usually incomplete. Generalized increased intracranial pressure characterized by coma, bulging of the fontanelles, loss of pupillary and oculovestibular reflexes, and respiratory arrest often develops between 24 and 72 hours of age.

The newborn may die at this time or may remain stuporous for several weeks. The encephalopathy begins to subside after the third day, and seizures decrease in frequency and eventually stop. Jitteriness is common as the child becomes arousable. Tone increases in the limbs during the succeeding weeks. Neurological sequelae are expected in newborns with severe HIE.

Diagnosis. EEG and MRI are helpful in determining the severity and prognosis of HIE. In mild HIE, the EEG background rhythms are normal or lacking in variability. In severe HIE, the background is always abnormal and shows suppression of background amplitude. The degree of suppression correlates well with the severity of HIE. The worst case is a flat EEG or one with a burst-suppression pattern. A bad outcome is invariable if the amplitude remains suppressed for 2 weeks or a burst-suppression pattern is present at any time. Epileptiform activity may also be present but is less predictive of the outcome than is background suppression.

MRI with diffusion-weighted images are helpful to determine the full extent of injury. The basal ganglia and thalamus are often affected by HIE.

Management. The management of HIE in newborns requires immediate attention to derangements in several organs and correction of acidosis. Clinical experience indicates that control of seizures and maintenance of adequate ventilation and perfusion increases the chance of a favorable outcome. A treatment approach involves either whole body or selective head cooling (Gluckman et al, 2005).

A separate section details the treatment of seizures in newborns. The use of intravenous levetiracetam is promising (Furwentsches et al, 2010). Seizures often cease spontaneously during the second week, and long-term anticonvulsant therapy may not be necessary. The incidence of later epilepsy among infants who had neonatal seizures caused by HIE is 30–40 %. Continuing antiepileptic therapy after the initial seizures have stopped does not influence whether the child goes on to develop epilepsy as a lifelong condition.

Organic Acid Disorders

Characteristic of organic acid disorders is the accumulation of compounds, usually ketones, or lactic acid that causes acidosis in biological fluids (Seashore, 2009). Among the dozens of organic acid disorders are abnormalities in vitamin metabolism, lipid metabolism, glycolysis, the citric acid cycle, oxidative metabolism, glutathione metabolism, and 4-aminobutyric acid metabolism. The clinical presentations vary considerably and several chapters contain descriptions. Defects in the further metabolism of branched-chain amino acids are the organic acid disorders that most often cause neonatal seizures. Molecular genetic testing is clinically available for detection of several of these diseases, including MSUD, propionic acidemia, methylmalonic acidemia, biotin-unresponsive 3-methylcrotonyl-CoA carboxylase deficiency, isovaleric acidemia, and glutaric acidemia type 1.

Isovaleric Acidemia. Isovaleric acid is a fatty acid derived from leucine. The enzyme isovaleryl-CoA dehydrogenase converts isovaleric acid to 3-methylcrotonyl-CoA (see Figure 1-1). Genetic transmission is autosomal recessive inheritance. The heterozygote state is detectable in cultured fibroblasts.

Clinical Features. Two phenotypes are associated with the same enzyme defect. One is an acute, overwhelming disorder of the newborn; the other is a chronic infantile form. Newborns with the acute disorder are normal at birth but within a few days become lethargic, refuse to feed, and vomit. The clinical syndrome is similar to MSUD except that the urine smells like "sweaty feet" instead of maple syrup. Sixty per cent of affected newborns die within 3 weeks. The survivors have a clinical syndrome identical to the chronic infantile phenotype.

Diagnosis. The excretion of isovaleryl-lysine in the urine detects isovaleric acidosis. Assays of isovaleryl-CoA dehydrogenase activity utilize cultured fibroblasts, and molecular testing is available. The clinical phenotype correlates not with the percentage of residual enzyme activity, but with the ability to detoxify isovaleryl-CoA with glycine.

Management. Dietary restriction of protein, especially leucine, decreases the occurrence of later psychomotor retardation. L-Carnitine, 50 mg/kg/day, is a beneficial supplement to the diet of some children with isovaleric acidemia. In acutely ill newborns, oral glycine, 250–500 mg/day, in addition to protein restriction and carnitine, lowers mortality.

Methylmalonic Acidemia. D-Methylmalonyl-CoA is racemized to L-methylmalonyl-CoA by the enzyme D-methylmalonyl racemase and then isomerized to succinyl-CoA, which enters the tricarboxylic acid cycle. The enzyme D-methylmalonyl-CoA mutase catalyzes the isomerization. The cobalamin (vitamin B_{12}) coenzyme adenosylcobalamin is a required cofactor. Genetic transmission of the several defects in this pathway is by autosomal recessive inheritance. *Mutase deficiency* is the most common abnormality. Propionyl-CoA, propionic acid, and methylmalonic acid accumulate and cause hyperglycinemia and hyperammonemia.

Clinical Features. Affected children appear normal at birth. In 80 % of those with complete mutase deficiency, the symptoms appear during the first week after delivery; those with defects in the synthesis of adenosylcobalamin generally show symptoms after 1 month. Symptoms include lethargy, failure to thrive, recurrent vomiting, dehydration, respiratory distress, and hypotonia after the initiation of protein feeding. Leukopenia, thrombocytopenia, and anemia are present in more than one half of patients. Intracranial hemorrhage may result from a bleeding diathesis. The outcome for newborns with complete mutase deficiency is usually poor. Most die within 2 months of diagnosis; survivors have recurrent acidosis, growth retardation, and cognitive impairment.

Diagnosis. Suspect the diagnosis in any newborn with metabolic acidosis, especially if associated with ketosis, hyperammonemia, and hyperglycinemia. Demonstrating an increased concentration of methylmalonic acid in the urine and elevated plasma glycine levels helps confirm the diagnosis. The specific enzyme defect can be determined in fibroblasts. Techniques for prenatal detection are available.

Management. Some affected newborns are cobalamin responsive and others are not. Management of those with mutase deficiency is similar to propionic acidemia. The long-term results are poor. Vitamin B_{12} supplementation is useful in some defects of adenosylcobalamin synthesis, and hydroxocobalamin administration is reasonable while awaiting the definitive diagnosis. Maintain treatment with protein restriction (0.5–1.5 g/kg/day) and hydroxocobalamin (1 mg) weekly. As in propionic acidemia, oral supplementation of L-carnitine reduces ketogenesis in response to fasting.

Propionic Acidemia. Propionyl-CoA forms as a catabolite of methionine, threonine, and the branched-chain amino acids. Its further carboxylation to D-methylmalonyl-CoA requires the enzyme propionyl-CoA carboxylase and the coenzyme biotin (see Figure 1-1). Isolated deficiency of propionyl-CoA carboxylase causes propionic acidemia. Transmission of the defect is autosomal recessive.

Clinical Features. Most affected children appear normal at birth; symptoms may begin as early as the first day after delivery or delayed for months or years. In newborns, the symptoms are nonspecific: feeding difficulty, lethargy, hypotonia, and dehydration. Recurrent attacks of profound metabolic acidosis, often associated with hyperammonemia, which respond poorly to buffering is characteristic. Untreated newborns rapidly become dehydrated, have generalized or myoclonic seizures, and become comatose.

Hepatomegaly caused by a fatty infiltration occurs in approximately one-third of patients. Neutropenia, thrombocytopenia, and occasionally pancytopenia may be present. A bleeding diathesis accounts for massive intracranial hemorrhage in some newborns. Children who survive beyond infancy develop infarctions in the basal ganglia.

Diagnosis. Consider propionic acidemia in any newborn with ketoacidosis or with hyperammonemia without ketoacidosis. Propionic acidemia is the probable diagnosis when the plasma concentrations of glycine and propionate and the urinary concentrations of glycine, methylcitrate, and β-hydroxypropionate are increased. While the urinary concentration of propionate may be normal, the plasma concentration is always elevated, without a concurrent increase in the concentration of methylmalonate.

Deficiency of enzyme activity in peripheral blood leukocytes or in skin fibroblasts establishes the diagnosis. Molecular genetic testing is available. Detecting methylcitrate, a unique metabolite of propionate, in the amniotic fluid and by showing deficient enzyme activity in amniotic fluid cells provides prenatal diagnosis.

Management. The newborn in ketoacidosis requires dialysis to remove toxic metabolites, parenteral fluids to prevent dehydration, and protein-free nutrition. Restricting protein intake to 0.5–1.5 g/kg/day decreases the frequency and severity of subsequent attacks. Oral administration of L-carnitine reduces the ketogenic response to fasting and may be useful as a daily supplement. Intermittent administration of nonabsorbed antibiotics reduces the production of propionate by gut bacteria.

Herpes Simplex Encephalitis

Herpes simplex virus (HSV) is a large DNA virus separated into two serotypes, HSV-1 and HSV-2. HSV-2 is associated with 80 % of genital herpes and HSV-1 with 20 %. The overall prevalence of genital herpes is increasing and approximately 25 % of pregnant woman have serological evidence of past HSV-2 infection. Transmission of HSV to the newborn can occur in utero, peripartum, or postnatally. However, 85 % of neonatal cases are HSV-2 infections acquired during the time of delivery. The highest risk for perinatal transmission occurs when a mother with no prior HSV-1 or HSV-2 antibodies acquires either virus in the genital tract within 2 weeks prior to delivery (first-episode primary infection). Postnatal transmission can occur with HSV-1 through mouth or hand by the mother or other caregiver.

Clinical Features. The clinical spectrum of perinatal HSV infection is considerable. Among symptomatic newborns, one-third has disseminated disease, one-third has localized involvement of the brain, and one-third has localized involvement of the eyes, skin, or mouth. Whether infection is disseminated or localized, approximately half of infections involve the central nervous system. The overall mortality rate is over 60 %, and 50 % of survivors have permanent neurological impairment.

The onset of symptoms may be as early as the fifth day but is usually in the second week. A vesicular rash is present in 30 %, usually on the scalp after vertex presentation and on the buttocks after breech presentation. Conjunctivitis, jaundice, and a bleeding diathesis may be present. The first symptoms of encephalitis are irritability and seizures. Seizures may be focal or generalized and are frequently only partially responsive to therapy. Neurological deterioration is progressive and characterized by coma and quadriparesis.

Diagnosis. Culture specimens are collected from cutaneous vesicles, mouth, nasopharynx, rectum, or CSF. Polymerase chain reaction is the standard for diagnosis herpes encephalitis. The EEG is always abnormal and shows a periodic pattern of slow waves or spike discharges. The CSF examination shows a lymphocytic leukocytosis, red blood cells, and an elevated protein concentration.

Management. The best treatment is prevention. Cesarean section should be strongly considered in all women with active genital herpes infection at term whose membranes are intact or ruptured for less than 4 hours.

Intravenous acyclovir is the drug of choice for all forms of neonatal HSV disease. The dosage is 60 mg/kg per day divided in 3 doses, given intravenously for 14 days in skin/eye/mouth disease and for 21 days for disseminated disease. All patients with central nervous system (CNS) HSV involvement should undergo a repeat lumbar puncture at the end of intravenous acyclovir therapy to determine that the CSF is polymerase chain reaction (PCR) negative and normalized. Therapy continues until documenting a negative PCR. Acute renal failure is the most significant adverse effect of parenteral acyclovir. Mortality remains 50 % or greater in newborns with disseminated disease.

Trauma and Intracranial Hemorrhage

Neonatal head trauma occurs most often in large term newborns of primiparous mothers.

Prolonged labor and difficult extraction is usual because of fetal malpositioning or fetal-pelvic disproportion. A precipitous delivery may also lead to trauma or hemorrhage. Intracranial hemorrhage may be subarachnoid, subdural, or intraventricular. Discussion of intraventricular hemorrhage is in Chapter 4.

Idiopathic Cerebral Venous Thrombosis. The causes of cerebral venous thrombosis in newborns are coagulopathies, polycythemia and sepsis. Cerebral venous thrombosis, especially involving the superior sagittal sinus, also occurs without known predisposing factors, probably due to the trauma even in relatively normal deliveries.

Clinical Features. The initial symptom is focal seizures or lethargy beginning any time during the first month. Intracranial pressure remains normal, lethargy slowly resolves, and seizures tend to respond to anticonvulsants. The long-term outcome is uncertain and probably depends upon the extent of hemorrhagic infarction of the hemisphere.

Diagnosis. CT venogram or MR venogram are the standard tests for diagnosis. CT venogram is a more sensitive and accurate imaging modality.

Management. Anticoagulation may decrease the risk of thrombus progression, venous congestion leading to hemorrhage and stroke, and facilitate re-canalization of the venous sinus. Response to therapy varies widely, and dosages of low molecular weight heparin frequently require readjustment to maintain therapeutic anti-Xa levels of 0.5–1 U/mL. A starting dose of 1.7 mg/kg every 12 hours for term infants, or 2.0 mg/kg every 12 hours for preterm infants, may be beneficial (Yang et al, 2010). Ultimately, therapeutic decisions must incorporate treatment of the underlying cause of the thrombosis, if known.

Primary Subarachnoid Hemorrhage

Clinical Features. Blood in the subarachnoid space probably originates from tearing of the superficial veins by shearing forces during a prolonged delivery with the head molding. Mild HIE is often associated with subarachnoid hemorrhage (SAH), but the newborn is usually well when an unexpected seizure occurs on the first or second day of life. Lumbar puncture, performed because of suspected sepsis, reveals blood in the CSF. The physician may suspect a traumatic lumbar puncture; however, red blood cell counts in first and last tube typically show similar counts in subarachnoid hemorrhage and clearing numbers in traumatic taps. Most newborns with subarachnoid hemorrhages will not suffer long-term sequelae.

Diagnosis. CT is useful to document the extent of hemorrhage. Blood is present in the interhemispheric fissure and the supratentorial and infratentorial recesses. EEG may reveal epileptiform activity without background suppression. This suggests that HIE is not the cause of the seizures, and that the prognosis is more favorable. Clotting studies are needed to evaluate the possibility of a bleeding diathesis.

Management. Seizures usually respond to anticonvulsants. Specific therapy is not available for the hemorrhage, and posthemorrhagic hydrocephalus is uncommon.

Subdural Hemorrhage

Clinical Features. Subdural hemorrhage is usually the consequence of a tear in the tentorium near its junction with the falx. Causes of tear include excessive vertical molding of the head in vertex presentation, anteroposterior elongation of the head in face and brow presentations, or prolonged delivery of the aftercoming head in breech presentation. Blood collects in the posterior fossa and may produce brainstem compression. The initial features are those of mild to moderate HIE. Clinical evidence of brainstem compression begins 12 hours or longer after delivery. Characteristic features include irregular respiration, an abnormal cry, declining consciousness, hypotonia, seizures, and a tense fontanelle. Intracerebellar hemorrhage is sometimes present. Mortality is high, and neurological impairment among survivors is common.

Diagnosis. MRI, CT or ultrasound visualizes the subdural hemorrhages.

Management. Small hemorrhages do not require treatment, but surgical evacuation of large collections relieves brainstem compression.

Pyridoxine Dependency

Pyridoxine dependency is a rare disorder transmitted as an autosomal recessive trait (Gospe, 2012). The genetic locus is unknown but the presumed cause is impaired glutamic decarboxylase activity.

Clinical Features. Newborns experience seizures soon after birth. The seizures are usually multifocal clonic at onset and progress rapidly to status epilepticus. Although presentations consisting of prolonged seizures and recurrent episodes of status epilepticus are typical, recurrent self-limited events including partial seizures, generalized seizures, atonic seizures, myoclonic events, and infantile spasms also occur. The seizures only respond to pyridoxine. A seizure-free interval up to 3 weeks may occur after pyridoxine discontinuation. Outcome may be improved and cognitive deficits decreased with early diagnosis and treatment.

Atypical features include late-onset seizures (up to age 2 years); seizures that initially respond to antiepileptic drugs and then do not; seizures that do not initially respond to pyridoxine but then become controlled; and prolonged seizure-free intervals occurring after stopping pyridoxine. Intellectual disability is common.

Diagnosis. Suspect the diagnosis in newborns with an affected older sibling, or in newborns with daily seizures unresponsive to anticonvulsants, with progressive course and worsening EEGs. Characteristic of the infantile-onset variety is intermittent myoclonic seizures, focal clonic seizures, or generalized tonic-clonic seizures. The EEG is continuously abnormal because of generalized or multifocal spike discharges and tends to evolve into hypsarrhythmia. An intravenous injection of pyridoxine, 100 mg, stops the clinical seizure activity and often converts the EEG to normal in less than 10 minutes. However, sometimes 500 mg is required. When giving pyridoxine IV, arousals may look like improvement in EEG since hypsarrhythmia is a pattern seen initially during sleep. Comparing sleep EEG before and after pyridoxine is needed to confirm an EEG response. CSF neurotransmitter testing is available to confirm the diagnosis.

Management. A lifelong dietary supplement of pyridoxine, 50–100 mg/day, prevents further seizures. Subsequent psychomotor development is best with early treatment, but this does not ensure a normal outcome. The dose needed to prevent mental retardation may be higher than that needed to stop seizures.

Folinic Acid Dependency

Folinic acid dependent seizures present similarly to pyridoxine dependency.

Clinical Features. Infants develop seizures during the first week of life that are not responsive to anticonvulsants or pyridoxine.

Diagnosis. A characteristic peak on CSF electrophoresis confirms the diagnosis (Torres et al, 1999).

Management. Treat the disorder with folinic acid supplementation, 2.5–5 mg twice daily.

Incontinentia Pigmenti (Bloch–Sulzberger Syndrome)

Incontinentia pigmenti is a rare neurocutaneous syndrome involving the skin, teeth, eyes, and CNS. Genetic transmission is X-linked (Xq28) with lethality in the hemizygous male (Scheuerle, 2010).

Clinical Features. The female-to-male ratio is 20:1. An erythematous and vesicular rash resembling epidermolysis bullosa is present on the flexor surfaces of the limbs and lateral aspect of the trunk at birth or soon thereafter. The rash persists for the first few months and a verrucous eruption that lasts for weeks or months replaces the original rash. Between 6 and 12 months of age, deposits of pigment appear in the previous area of rash in bizarre polymorphic arrangements. The pigmentation later regresses and leaves a linear hypopigmentation. Alopecia, hypodontia, abnormal tooth shape, and dystrophic nails may be associated. Some have retinal vascular abnormalities that predispose to retinal detachment in early childhood.

Neurological disturbances occur in fewer than half of the cases. In newborns, the prominent feature is the onset of seizures on the second or third day, often confined to one side of the body. Residual neurological handicaps may include cognitive impairment, epilepsy, hemiparesis, and hydrocephalus.

Diagnosis. The clinical findings and biopsy of the skin rash are diagnostic. The basis for diagnosis is the clinical findings and the molecular testing of the *IKBKG* gene.

Management. Neonatal seizures caused by incontinentia pigmenti usually respond to standard anticonvulsant drugs. The blistering rash requires topical medication and oatmeal baths. Regular ophthalmological examinations are needed to diagnose and treat retinal detachment.

Treatment of Neonatal Seizures

Animal studies suggest that continuous seizure activity, even in the normoxemic brain, may cause brain damage by inhibiting protein synthesis, breaking down polyribosomes, and via neurotransmitter toxicity. In premature newborns, an additional concern is that the increased cerebral blood flow associated with seizures will increase the risk of intraventricular hemorrhage. Protein binding of anticonvulsant drugs may be impaired in premature newborns and the free fraction concentration may be toxic, whereas the measured protein-bound fraction appears therapeutic.

The initial steps in managing newborns with seizures are to maintain vital function, identify and correct the underlying cause, i.e., hypocalcemia or sepsis, when possible, and rapidly provide a therapeutic blood concentration of an anticonvulsant drug when needed.

In the past, treatment of neonatal seizures had little support based on evidence. Conventional treatments with phenobarbital and phenytoin seem to be equally effective or ineffective (Painter, 1999). Levetiracetam, oxcarbazepine, and lamotrigine have been studied in infants as young as 1 month of age, demonstrating safety and efficacy (Piña-Garza et al, 2005, 2008a,b, 2009).

When treating neonatal seizures we must first answer two questions: (1). Is the treatment effective? Neonates have a different chloride transporter in the first weeks of life, and opening the chloride pore by GABA activation may result in a hyperexcitable state rather than anticonvulsant effect. Furthermore, neuromotor dissociation has been documented when using phenobarbital in neonates, causing cessation of clinical convulsions while electrographic seizures continue. (2). Are the seizures worse than the possible unknown and known negative effect of medications in the developing brain, such as apoptosis? A few brief focal seizures may be acceptable in the setting of a resolving neonatal encephalopathy.

Antiepileptic Drugs

Levetiracetam. The introduction of intravenous levetiracetam (100 mg/mL) provides a new and safer option for the treatment of newborns. Because levetiracetam is not liver metabolized, but excreted unchanged in the urine, no drug–drug interactions exist. Use of the drug requires maintaining urinary output. We consider it an excellent treatment option and recommend it as initial therapy. The initial dose is 30–40 mg/kg; the maintenance dose is 40 mg/kg/day in the first 6 months of life, and up to 60 mg/kg/day between 6 months and 4 years (Piña-Garza, 2009). The maintenance dose is dependent on renal clearance. Reduce the dosage and dosing interval in neonates with hypoxic injury with associated lower renal function.

Oxcarbazepine. Oxcarbazepine suspension is a good option in neonates with functioning gastrointestinal tracts and a lower risk for necrotizing enterocolitis. Doses between 20 and 40 mg/kg/day for infants less than 6 months, and up to 60 mg/kg/day divided two or three times a day, are adequate for older infants and young children (Piña-Garza, 2005).

Phenobarbital. Intravenous phenobarbital is a widely used drug for the treatment of newborns with seizures. However, its efficacy and safety is under review. The chloride transporters in newborns may convert phenobarbital into a proconvulsant or at least a less effective anticonvulsant. A unitary relationship usually exists between the intravenous dose of phenobarbital in milligrams per kilogram of body weight and the blood concentration in micrograms per milliliter measured 24 hours after the load. A 20 µg/mL blood concentration is safely achievable with a single intravenous loading dose of 20 mg/kg injected at a rate of 5 mg/min. The usual maintenance dose is 4 mg/kg/day. Use additional boluses of 10 mg/kg, to a total of 40 mg/kg, for those who fail to respond to the initial load. In term newborns with intractable seizures from HIE the use of this drug to achieve a burst suppression pattern is an alternative. The half-life of phenobarbital in newborns varies from 50 to 200 hours.

Phenytoin. *Fosphenytoin sodium* is safer than phenytoin for intravenous administration. Oral doses of phenytoin are poorly absorbed in newborns. The efficacy of phenytoin in newborns is less than impressive and concerns exist regarding potential apoptosis. A single intravenous injection of 20 mg/kg at a rate of 0.5 mg/kg/min safely achieves a therapeutic blood concentration of 15–20 µg/mL (40–80 µmol/L). The half-life is long during the first week, and the basis for further administration is current knowledge of the blood concentration. Most newborns require a maintenance dosage of 5–10 mg/kg/day.

Duration of Therapy

Seizures caused by an acute, self-limited and resolved encephalopathy, such as mild HIE, do not ordinarily require prolonged maintenance therapy. In most newborns, seizures stop when the acute encephalopathy is over. Therefore, discontinuation of therapy after a period of complete seizure control is reasonable unless signs of permanent cortical injury are confirmed by EEG, imaging or clinical examination. If seizures recur, reinitiate antiepileptic therapy.

In contrast to newborns with seizures caused by acute resolved encephalopathy, treat seizures caused by cerebral dysgenesis or symptomatic epilepsies continuously as most of them are lifetime epileptic conditions.

PAROXYSMAL DISORDERS IN CHILDREN LESS THAN 2 YEARS OLD

The pathophysiology of paroxysmal disorders in infants is more variable than in newborns (Box 1-7). Seizures, especially febrile seizures,

BOX 1-7 Paroxysmal Disorders in Children Younger than 2 Years

APNEA AND BREATH-HOLDING
- Cyanotic*
- Pallid

DYSTONIA
- Glutaric aciduria (see Chapter 14)
- Transient paroxysmal dystonia of infancy

MIGRAINE
- Benign paroxysmal vertigo* (see Chapter 10)
- Cyclic vomiting*
- Paroxysmal torticollis* (see Chapter 14)

SEIZURES*
- Febrile seizures
  - Epilepsy triggered by fever
  - Infection of the nervous system
  - Simple febrile seizure
- Nonfebrile seizures
  - Generalized tonic-clonic seizures
  - Partial seizures
    - Benign familial infantile seizures
    - Ictal laughter
- Myoclonic seizures
- Infantile spasms
- Benign myoclonic epilepsy
- Severe myoclonic epilepsy
- Myoclonic status
- Lennox-Gastaut syndrome
- Stereotypies (see Chapter 14)

*Denotes the most common conditions and the ones with disease modifying treatments

are the main cause of paroxysmal disorders, but apnea and syncope (breath-holding spells) are relatively common as well. Often, the basis for requested neurological consultation in infants with paroxysmal disorders is the suspicion of seizures. The determination of which "spells" are seizures is often difficult and relies more on obtaining a complete description of the spell than any diagnostic tests. Ask the parents to provide a sequential history. If more than one spell occurred, they should first describe the one that was best observed or most recent. The following questions should be included: What was the child doing before the spell? Did anything provoke the spell? Did the child's color change? If so, when and to what color? Did the eyes move in any direction? Did the spell affect one body part more than other parts?

In addition to obtaining a home video of the spell, ambulatory or prolonged split-screen video-EEG monitoring is the only way to identify the nature of unusual spells. Seizures characterized by decreased motor activity with indeterminate changes in the level of consciousness arise from the temporal, temporoparietal, or parieto-occipital regions, while seizures with motor activity usually arise from the frontal, central, or frontoparietal regions.

Apnea and Syncope

The definition of infant apnea is cessation of breathing for 15 seconds or longer, or for less than 15 seconds if accompanied by bradycardia. Premature newborns with respiratory distress syndrome may continue to have apneic spells as infants, especially if they are neurologically abnormal.

Apneic Seizures

Apnea alone is rarely a seizure manifestation (Freed & Martinez, 2001). The frequency of apneic seizures relates inversely to age, more often in newborns than infants, and rare in children. Isolated apnea occurs as a seizure manifestation in infants and young children but, when reviewed on video, identification of other features becomes possible. Overall, reflux accounts for much more apnea than seizures in most infants and young children. Unfortunately, among infants with apneic seizures, EEG abnormalities only appear at the time of apnea. Therefore, monitoring is required for diagnosis.

Breath-Holding Spells

Breath-holding spells with loss of consciousness occur in almost 5% of infants and young children. The cause is a disturbance in central autonomic regulation probably transmitted by autosomal dominant inheritance with incomplete penetrance. Approximately 20–30% of parents of affected children have a history of the condition. The term *breath-holding* is a misnomer because breathing always stops in expiration. Both cyanotic and pallid breath-holding occurs; cyanotic spells are three times more common than pallid spells. Most children experience only one or the other, but 20% have both.

The spells are involuntary responses to adverse stimuli. In approximately 80% of affected children, the spells begin before 18 months of age, and in all cases they start before 3 years of age. The last episode usually occurs by age 4 years and no later than age 8 years.

Cyanotic Syncope

Clinical Features. The usual provoking stimulus for cyanotic spells is anger, pain, frustration, or fear. The infant's sibling takes away a toy, the child cries, and then stops breathing in expiration. Cyanosis develops rapidly, followed quickly by limpness and loss of consciousness. Crying may not precede cyanotic episodes provoked by pain.

If the attack lasts for only seconds, the infant may resume crying on awakening. Most spells, especially the ones referred for neurological evaluation, are longer and are associated with tonic posturing of the body and trembling movements of the hands or arms. The eyes may roll upward. These movements are mistaken for seizures by even experienced observers, but they are probably a brainstem release phenomenon. Concurrent EEG shows flattening of the record, not seizure activity.

After a short spell, the child rapidly recovers and seems normal immediately; after a prolonged spell, the child first arouses and then goes to sleep. Once an infant begins having breath-holding spells, the frequency increases for several months and then declines, and finally cease.

Diagnosis. The typical sequence of cyanosis, apnea, and loss of consciousness is critical for diagnosis. Cyanotic syncope and epilepsy are confused because of lack of attention to the precipitating event. It is not sufficient to ask, "Did the child hold his breath?" The question conjures up the image of breath-holding during inspiration. Instead, questioning should be focused on precipitating events, absence of breathing, facial color, and family history. The family often has a history of breath-holding spells or syncope.

Between attacks, the EEG is normal. During an episode, the EEG first shows diffuse slowing and then rhythmic slowing followed by background attenuation during the tonic-clonic, tonic, myoclonic or clonic activity.

Management. Education and reassurance. The family should be educated to leave the child in supine with airway protection until he or she recovers consciousness. Picking up the child, which is the natural act of the mother or observer, prolongs the spell. If the spells occur in response to discipline or denial of the child's wishes, I recommend caretakers comfort the child but remain firm in their decision, as otherwise children may learn that crying translates into getting their wish. This may in turn reinforce the spells.

Pallid Syncope

Clinical Features. The provocation of pallid syncope is usually a sudden, unexpected, painful event such as a bump on the head. The child rarely cries but instead becomes white and limp and loses consciousness. These episodes are truly terrifying to behold. Parents invariably believe the child is dead and begin mouth-to-mouth resuscitation. After the initial limpness, the body may stiffen, and clonic movements of the arms may occur. As in cyanotic syncope, these movements represent a brainstem release phenomenon, not seizure activity. The duration of the spell is difficult to determine because the observer is so frightened that seconds seem like hours. Afterward the child often falls asleep and is normal on awakening.

Diagnosis. Pallid syncope is the result of reflex asystole. Pressure on the eyeballs to initiate a vagal reflex provokes an attack. I do not recommend provoking an attack as an office procedure. The history alone is diagnostic.

Management. As with cyanotic spells, the major goal is to reassure the family that the child will not die during an attack. The physician must be very convincing.

Febrile Seizures

An infant's first seizure often occurs at the time of fever. Three explanations are possible: (1) an infection of the nervous system; (2) an underlying seizure disorder in which the stress of fever triggers the seizure, although subsequent seizures may be afebrile; or (3) a *simple febrile seizure*, a genetic age-limited epilepsy in which seizures occur only with fever. The discussion of nervous system infection is in Chapters 2 and 4. *Children who have seizures from encephalitis or meningitis do not wake up afterward; they are usually obtunded or comatose.* The distinction between epilepsy and simple febrile seizures is sometimes difficult and may require time rather than laboratory tests.

Epilepsy specialists who manage monitoring units have noted that a large proportion of adults with intractable seizures secondary to mesial temporal sclerosis have prior histories of febrile seizures as children. The reverse is not true. Among children with febrile seizures, mesial temporal sclerosis is a rare event (Tarkka et al, 2003).

Clinical Features. Febrile seizures not caused by infection or another definable cause occur in approximately 4 % of children. Only 2 % of children whose first seizure is associated with fever will have nonfebrile seizures (epilepsy) by age 7 years. The most important predictor of subsequent epilepsy is an abnormal neurological or developmental state. Complex seizures, defined as prolonged, focal, or multiple, and a family history of epilepsy slightly increase the probability of subsequent epilepsy.

A single, brief, generalized seizure occurring in association with fever is likely to be a simple febrile seizure. The seizure need not occur during the time when fever is rising. “Brief” and “fever” are difficult to define. Parents do not time seizures. When a child has a seizure, seconds seem like minutes. A prolonged seizure is one that is still in progress after the family has contacted the doctor or has left the house for the emergency room. Postictal sleep is not part of seizure time.

Simple febrile seizures are familial and probably transmitted by autosomal dominant inheritance with incomplete penetrance. One-third of infants who have a first simple febrile seizure will have a second one at the time of a subsequent febrile illness, and half of these will have a third febrile seizure. The risk of recurrence increases if the first febrile seizure occurs before 18 months of age or at a body temperature less than 40°C. More than three episodes of simple febrile seizures are unusual and suggest that the child may later have nonfebrile seizures.

Diagnosis. Any child thought to have an infection of the nervous system should undergo a lumbar puncture for examination of the CSF. Approximately one-quarter of children with bacterial or viral meningitis have seizures. After the seizure from CNS infection, prolonged obtundation is expected.

In contrast, infants who have simple febrile seizures usually look normal after the seizure. Lumbar puncture is unnecessary following a brief, generalized seizure from which the child recovers rapidly and completely, especially if the fever subsides spontaneously or is otherwise explained.

Blood cell counts, measurements of glucose, calcium, electrolytes, urinalysis, EEG, and cranial CT or MRI on a routine basis are not cost effective and discouraged. Individual decisions for laboratory testing depend upon the clinical circumstance. Obtain an EEG on every infant who is not neurologically normal or who has a family history of epilepsy. Infants with complex febrile seizures may benefit from an EEG or MRI.

Management. Because only one-third of children with an initial febrile seizure have a second seizure, treating every affected child is unreasonable. Treatment is unnecessary in the low-risk group with a single, brief, generalized seizure. No evidence has shown that a second or third simple febrile seizure, even if prolonged, causes epilepsy or brain damage. I always offer families the option to have diazepam gel available for prolonged or acute repetitive seizures.

I consider the use of anticonvulsant prophylaxis in the following situations:

1. Complex febrile seizures in children with neurological deficits.
2. Strong family history of epilepsy and recurrent simple or complex febrile seizures.
3. Febrile status epilepticus.
4. Febrile seizures with a frequency higher than once per quarter.

Nonfebrile Seizures

Disorders that produce nonfebrile seizures in infancy are not substantially different from those that cause nonfebrile seizures in childhood (see the following section). Major risk factors for the development of epilepsy in infancy and childhood are congenital malformations (especially migrational errors), neonatal seizures and insults, and a family history of epilepsy.

A complex partial seizure syndrome with onset during infancy, sometimes in the newborn period, is *ictal laughter* associated with hypothalamic hamartoma. The attacks are brief, occur several times each day, and may be characterized by odd laughter or giggling. The first thought is that the laughter appears normal, but then facial flushing and pupillary dilatation are noted. With time, the child develops drop attacks and generalized seizures. Personality change occurs and precocious puberty may be an associated condition.

A first partial motor seizure before the age of 2 years is associated with a recurrence rate of 87 %, whereas with a first seizure at a later age the rate is 51 %. The recurrence rate after a first nonfebrile, asymptomatic, generalized seizure is 60–70 % at all ages. The younger the age at onset of nonfebrile seizures of any type correlates with a higher incidence of symptomatic rather than idiopathic epilepsy.

Approximately 25 % of children who have recurrent seizures during the first year, excluding neonatal seizures and infantile spasms, are developmentally or neurologically abnormal at the time of the first seizure. The initial EEG has prognostic significance; normal EEG results are associated with a favorable neurological outcome.

Intractable seizures in children less than 2 years of age are often associated with later cognitive impairment. The seizure types with the greatest probability of cognitive impairment in descending order are myoclonic, tonic-clonic, complex partial, and simple partial.

Transmission of *benign familial infantile epilepsy* is by autosomal dominant inheritance. Onset is as early as 3 months. The gene locus, on chromosome 19, is different from the locus for benign familial neonatal seizures. Motion arrest, decreased responsiveness, staring or blank eyes, and mild focal convulsive movements of the limbs characterize the seizures. Anticonvulsant drugs provide easy control, and seizures usually stop spontaneously within 2–4 years.

Myoclonus and Myoclonic Seizures

Infantile Spasms. Infantile spasms are age-dependent myoclonic seizures that occur with an incidence of 25 per 100 000 live births in the United States and Western Europe. An underlying cause can be determined in approximately 75 % of patients; congenital malformations and perinatal asphyxia are common causes, and tuberous sclerosis accounts for 20 % of cases in some series (Box 1-8). Despite considerable concern in the past, immunization is not a cause of infantile spasms.

The combination of infantile spasms, agenesis of the corpus callosum (as well as other midline cerebral malformations), and retinal malformations is referred to as *Aicardi syndrome* (Sutton & Van den Veyver, 2010). Affected children are always females, and genetic transmission of the disorder is as an X-linked dominant trait with hemizygous lethality in males.

Clinical Features. The peak age at onset is between 4 and 7 months and onset always before 1 year of age. The spasm can be a flexor, extensor or mixed movement. Spasms generally occur in clusters during drowsiness, feedings and shortly after the infant awakens from sleep. A rapid flexor spasm involving the neck, trunk, and limbs followed by a tonic contraction sustained for 2–10 seconds is characteristic. Less severe flexor spasms consist of dropping of the head and abduction of the arms or by flexion at the waist. Extensor spasms resemble the second component of the Moro reflex: the head moves backward and the arms suddenly spread. Whether flexor or extensor, the movement is usually symmetrical and brief and tends to occur in clusters with similar intervals between spasms.

When the spasms are secondary to an identifiable cause (symptomatic), the infant is usually abnormal neurologically or developmentally at spasms onset. Microcephaly is common in this group. Prognosis depends on the cause, the interval between the onset of clinical spasm and hypsarrhythmia, and the rapidity of treatment and control of this abnormal EEG pattern.

Idiopathic spasms characteristically occur in children who had been developing normally at the onset of spasms and have no history of prenatal or perinatal disorders. Neurological findings, including head circumference, are normal. It had been thought that 40 % of children with idiopathic spasms would be neurologically normal or only mildly cognitively impaired subsequently. Some of these children may have had benign myoclonus. With improvement in diagnostic testing, idiopathic infantile spasms are less frequent.

BOX 1-8 Neurocutaneous Disorders Causing Seizures in Infancy

INCONTINENTIA PIGMENTI

- Seizure type
  - Neonatal seizures
  - Generalized tonic-clonic
- Cutaneous manifestations
  - Erythematous bullae (newborn)
  - Pigmentary whorls (infancy)
  - Depigmented areas (childhood)

LINEAR NEVUS SEBACEOUS SYNDROME

- Seizure type
  - Infantile spasms
  - Lennox-Gastaut syndrome
  - Generalized tonic-clonic
- Cutaneous manifestation
  - Linear facial sebaceous nevus

NEUROFIBROMATOSIS

- Seizure type
  - Generalized tonic-clonic
  - Partial complex
  - Partial simple motor
- Cutaneous manifestations
  - Café au lait spots
  - Axillary freckles
  - Neural tumors

STURGE-WEBER SYNDROME

- Seizure type
  - Epilepsia partialis continuans
  - Partial simple motor
  - Status epilepticus
- Cutaneous manifestation
  - Hemifacial hemangioma

TUBEROUS SCLEROSIS

- Seizure type
  - Neonatal seizures
  - Infantile spasms
  - Lennox-Gastaut syndrome
  - Generalized tonic-clonic
  - Partial simple motor
  - Partial complex
- Cutaneous manifestations
  - Abnormal hair pigmentation
  - Adenoma sebaceum
  - Café au lait spots
  - Depigmented areas
  - Shagreen patch

TABLE 1-1 Electroencephalographic (EEG) Appearance in Myoclonic Seizures of Infancy

Seizure Type	EEG Appearance
Infantile spasms	Hypsarrhythmia Slow spike and wave Burst suppression
Benign myoclonus	Normal
Benign myoclonic epilepsy	Spike and wave (3 cps) Polyspike and wave (3 cps)
Severe myoclonic epilepsy	Polyspike and wave (>3 cps)
Lennox-Gastaut syndrome	Spike and wave (2–2.5 cps) Polyspike and wave (2–2.5 cps)

cps, cycles per second.

Diagnosis. The delay from spasm onset to diagnosis is often considerable. Infantile spasms are so unlike the usual perception of seizures that even experienced pediatricians may be slow to realize the significance of the movements. Colic is often the first diagnosis because of the sudden flexor movements, and is treated several weeks before suspecting seizures.

EEG helps differentiate infantile spasms from benign myoclonus of early infancy (Table 1-1). The EEG is the single most important test for diagnosis. However, EEG findings vary with the duration of recording, sleep state, duration of illness and underlying disorder. *Hypsarrhythmia* is the usual pattern recorded during the early stages of infantile spasms. A chaotic and continuously abnormal background of very high voltage and random slow waves and spike discharges are characteristic. The spikes vary in location from moment to moment and are generalized but never repetitive. Typical hypsarrhythmia usually starts during active sleep, progresses to quiet sleep and finally wakefulness as a progressive epileptic encephalopathy. During quiet sleep, greater interhemispheric synchrony occurs and the background may have a burst-suppression appearance.

The EEG may normalize briefly upon arousal but, when spasms recur, an abrupt attenuation of the background or high-voltage slow waves appear. Within a few weeks, greater interhemispheric synchrony replaces the original chaotic pattern of hypsarrhythmia. The distribution of epileptiform discharges changes from multifocal to generalized, and background attenuation follows the generalized discharges.

Management. A practice parameter for the medical treatment of infantile spasms is available (Mackay et al, 2004). Adrenocorticotropic hormone (ACTH), the traditional treatment for infantile spasms, is effective for short-term treatment control of the spasms. ACTH has no effect on the underlying mechanism of the disease and is only a short-term symptomatic therapy. The ideal dosages and treatment duration is not established. ACTH gel is usually given as an intramuscular injection of 150 U/m^2/day with a gradual tapering at weekly intervals over 6 to 8 weeks. Oral prednisone, 2–4 mg/kg/day, with a tapering at weekly intervals over 6 to 8 weeks is an alternative therapy. Even when the response is favorable, one-third of patients have relapses during or after the course of treatment with ACTH or prednisone.

Several alternative treatments avoid the adverse effects of corticosteroids and may have a longer-lasting effect. Clonazepam, levetiracetam (Gümüs et al, 2007; Mikati et al, 2008), and zonisamide (Lotze and Wilfong, 2004) are probably the safest alternatives. Valproate monotherapy controls spasms in 70 % of infants with doses of 20–60 mg/kg/day, but due to concern for fatal hepatotoxicity has limited use in this age group. This concern is higher in idiopathic cases as an underlying inborn error of metabolism or mitochondrial disease may exist and increase the risk for liver failure even in the absence of valproate. Topiramate is an effective adjunctive treatment in doses up to 30 mg/kg/day (Glausser, 2000). It is typically well tolerated with few adverse effects; the most significant is a possible metabolic acidosis at high doses due to its carbonic anhydrase activity.

Vigabatrin is effective for treating spasms in children with tuberous sclerosis and perhaps cortical dysplasia (Parisi et al, 2007). This medication is also helpful in other etiologies. The main concern regarding vigabatrin is the loss of peripheral vision. Its use is justified in children with West syndrome (IS, developmental regression and hypsarrhythmia) as most of them have cortical visual impairment as part of the epileptic encephalopathy and may actually gain functional vision if vigabatrin is effective.

Monotherapy for infantile spasms often fails, which suggests that early polypharmacy may provide better chances of controlling the progressive epileptic encephalopathy. The authors often combine ACTH or prednisone with rapid titration of topiramate, vigabatrin or valproic acid. Close follow-up with serial EEGs is essential for evaluation of treatment efficacy, and to determine if adding additional anticonvulsants, is necessary. "Time is Brain."

Benign Myoclonus of Infancy

Clinical Features. Many series of patients with infantile spasms include a small number with normal EEG results. Such infants cannot be distinguished from others with infantile spasms by clinical features because the age at onset and the appearance of the movements are the same. The spasms occur in clusters, frequently at mealtime. Clusters increase in intensity and severity over a period of weeks or months and then abate spontaneously. After 3 months, the spasms usually stop altogether, and, although they may recur occasionally, no spasms occur after 2 years of age. Affected infants are normal neurologically and developmentally and remain so afterward. The term *benign myoclonus* indicates that the spasms are an involuntary movement rather than a seizure.

Diagnosis. A normal EEG during awake and sleep or while the myoclonus occurs distinguishes this group from other types of myoclonus in infancy. No other tests are required.

Management. Education and reassurance.

Benign Myoclonic Epilepsy. *Despite the designation "benign," the association of infantile myoclonus with an epileptiform EEG rarely yields a favorable outcome.*

Clinical Features. Benign myoclonic epilepsy is a rare disorder of uncertain cause. One-third of patients have family members with epilepsy suggesting a genetic etiology. Onset is between 4 months and 2 years of age. Affected infants are neurologically normal at the onset of seizures and remain so afterward. Brief myoclonic attacks characterize the seizures. These may be restricted to head nodding or may be so severe as to throw the child to the floor. The head drops to the chest, eyes roll upward, the arms move upward and outward, and legs flex. Myoclonic seizures may be single or repetitive, but consciousness is not lost. No other seizure types occur in infancy, but generalized tonic-clonic seizures may occur in adolescence.

Diagnosis. EEG during a seizure shows generalized spike-wave or polyspike-wave discharges. Sensory stimuli do not activate seizures. The pattern is consistent with primary generalized epilepsy.

Management. Valproate produces complete seizure control, but levetiracetam and zonisamide are safer options for initial treatment. Developmental outcome generally is good with early treatment, but cognitive impairment may develop in some children. If left untreated, seizures may persist for years.

Early Epileptic Encephalopathy with Burst Suppression. The term *epileptic encephalopathy* encompasses several syndromes in which an encephalopathy is associated with continuous epileptiform activity. The onset of two syndromes, early infantile epileptic encephalopathy (*Ohtahara syndrome*) and early myoclonic encephalopathy (Dulac, 2001), which may be the same disorder, is in the first 3 months of age. Tonic spasms and myoclonic seizures occur in each. Both are associated with serious underlying metabolic or structural abnormalities. Some cases are familial, indicating an underlying genetic disorder. Progression to infantile spasms and the Lennox-Gastaut syndrome is common as with all epilepsies refractory to medical treatment. On EEG, a suppression pattern alternating with bursts of diffuse, high-amplitude, spike-wave complexes is recorded. These seizures are refractory or only partially responsive to most anticonvulsants drugs. The drugs recommended for infantile spasms are used for these infants.

Severe Myoclonic Epilepsy of Infancy. Severe myoclonic epilepsy of infancy (*Dravet syndrome*) is an important but poorly understood syndrome (Korff & Nordli, 2006). Some patients show a mutation in the sodium-channel gene (*SCN1A*). A seemingly healthy infant has a seizure and then undergoes progressive neurological deterioration that ends in a chronic brain damage syndrome (Dravet, 1978).

Clinical Features. A family history of epilepsy is present in 25 % of cases. The first seizures are frequently febrile, are usually prolonged, and can be generalized or focal clonic in type. Febrile and nonfebrile seizures recur, sometimes as status epilepticus. Generalized myoclonic seizures appear after 1 year of age. At first mild and difficult to recognize as a seizure manifestation, they later become frequent and repetitive and disturb function. Partial complex seizures with secondary generalization may also occur. Coincident with the onset of myoclonic seizures are the slowing of development and the gradual appearance of ataxia and hyperreflexia.

Diagnosis. The initial differential diagnosis is febrile seizures. The prolonged and sometimes focal nature of the febrile seizures raises suspicion of symptomatic epilepsy. A specific diagnosis is not possible until the appearance of myoclonic seizures in the second year. Interictal EEG findings are normal at first. Paroxysmal abnormalities appear in the second year. These are characteristically generalized spike-wave and polyspike-wave complexes with a frequency greater than 3 cps. Photic stimulation, drowsiness, and quiet sleep activate the discharges.

Management. Dravet syndrome is quite difficult to treat and typically requires polypharmacy.

Sodium channel drugs such as phenytoin, carbamazepine, lamotrigine, and oxcarbazepine tend to exacerbate seizures. Medications such as levetiracetam (Striano et al, 2007), divalproex sodium, topiramate, zonisamide and rufinamide are good alternatives.

Biotinidase Deficiency. Genetic transmission of this relatively rare disorder is as an autosomal recessive trait (Wolf, 2011). The cause is defective biotin absorption or transport and was previously called *late-onset multiple (holo) carboxylase deficiency*.

Clinical Features. The initial features in untreated infants with profound deficiency are seizures and hypotonia. Later features include hypotonia, ataxia, developmental delay, hearing loss, and cutaneous abnormalities. In childhood, patients may also develop weakness, spastic paresis, and decreased visual acuity.

Diagnosis. Ketoacidosis, hyperammonemia, and organic aciduria are present. Showing biotinidase deficiency in serum, during newborn screening, establishes the diagnosis. In profound biotinidase deficiency, mean serum biotinidase activity is less than 10% of normal. In partial biotinidase deficiency, serum biotinidase activity is 10–30% of normal.

Management. Early treatment with biotin, 5–20 mg/day, successfully reverses most of the symptoms, and may prevent mental retardation.

Lennox-Gastaut Syndrome. The triad of seizures (atypical absence, atonic, and myoclonic), 1.5–2 Hz spike-wave complexes on EEG, and cognitive impairment characterize the Lennox-Gastaut syndrome (LGS). LGS is the description of one stage in the spectrum of a progressive epileptic encephalopathy. Nobody is born with LGS. LGS is the result of epilepsies refractory to medical management, evolving into symptomatic generalized epilepsies with the characteristics described above. The characteristics of the syndrome fade away in many survivors and the EEG may evolve into a multifocal pattern with variable seizure types. I often used the term Lennox-Gastaut spectrum (also LG little s) for the stages preceding and following the stage described by Lennox and Gastaut.

Clinical Features. The peak age at onset is 3 to 5 years; less than half of the cases begin before age 2 years. Approximately 60% have an identifiable underlying cause. Neurocutaneous disorders such as tuberous sclerosis, perinatal disturbances, and postnatal brain injuries are most common. Twenty percent of children with the LGS have a history of infantile spasms before development of the syndrome.

Most children are neurologically abnormal before seizure onset. Every seizure type exists in LGS, except for typical absences. Atypical absence seizures occur in almost every patient and drop attacks (atonic and tonic seizures) are essential for the diagnosis. Characteristic of atonic seizures is a sudden dropping of the head or body, at times throwing the child to the ground. Most children with the syndrome function in the cognitively impaired range by 5 years of age.

Diagnosis. An EEG is essential for diagnosis. The waking interictal EEG consists of an abnormally slow background with characteristic 1.5–2.5 Hz slow spike-and-wave interictal discharges, often with an anterior predominance. Tonic seizures are associated with 1 cps slow waves followed by generalized rapid discharges without postictal depression.

In addition to EEG, looking for the underlying cause requires a thorough evaluation with special attention to skin manifestations that suggest a neurocutaneous syndrome (see Box 1-8). MRI is useful for the diagnosis of brain dysgenesis, postnatal disorders, and neurocutaneous syndromes.

Management. Seizures are difficult to control with drugs, diet, and surgery. Rufinamide, valproate, lamotrigine, topiramate, felbamate, clobazam, and clonazepam are usually the most effective drugs. Consider the ketogenic diet and surgery when drugs fail. Vagal nerve stimulation (VNS) and corpus callosotomy are alternatives for drop attacks refractory to medications and diet.

Migraine

Clinical Features. Migraine attacks are uncommon in infancy, but, when they occur, the clinical features are often paroxysmal and suggest the possibility of seizures. Cyclic vomiting is probably the most common manifestation. Attacks of vertigo (see Chapter 10) or torticollis (see Chapter 14) may be especially perplexing, and some infants have attacks in which they rock back and forth and appear uncomfortable.

Diagnosis. The stereotypical presentation of *benign paroxysmal vertigo* is recognizable as a migraine variant. Other syndromes often remain undiagnosed until the episodes evolve into a typical migraine pattern. A history of migraine in one parent, usually the mother, is essential for diagnosis.

Management. There is little if any evidence on migraine prophylaxis or abortive treatment in this age group. I have used small doses of amitriptyline (5 mg) in cases requiring prophylaxis with some success and ibuprofen, acetaminophen, prochlorperazine or promethazine as abortive therapies.

PAROXYSMAL DISORDERS OF CHILDHOOD

Like infants, seizures are the usual first consideration for any paroxysmal disorder. Seizures are the most common paroxysmal disorder requiring medical consultation. Syncope, especially presyncope, is considerably more common but diagnosis and management usually occur at home unless associated symptoms suggest a seizure.

Migraine is probably the most common etiology of paroxysmal neurological disorders in childhood; its incidence is 10 times greater than that of epilepsy. Chapters 2, 3, 10, 11, 14, and 15 describe migraine syndromes that may suggest epilepsy. Several links exist between migraine and epilepsy (Minewar, 2007): (1) ion channel disorders cause both; (2) both are genetic, paroxysmal, and associated with transitory neurological disturbances; (3) migraine sufferers have an increased incidence of epilepsy and epileptics have an increased incidence of migraine; and (4) they are both disorders associated with a hyperexcitable brain cortex. In children who have epilepsy and migraine, both disorders may have a common aura and one may provoke the other. Basilar migraine (see Chapter 10) and benign occipital epilepsy best exemplify the fine line between epilepsy and migraine. Characteristic of both are seizures, headache, and epileptiform activity. Children who have both epilepsy and migraine require treatment for each condition but some drugs (valproate and topiramate) serve as prophylactic agents for both.

Paroxysmal Dyskinesias

Paroxysmal dyskinesia occurs in several different syndromes. The best delineated are familial paroxysmal (kinesiogenic) choreoathetosis (FPC), paroxysmal nonkinesiogenic dyskinesia (PNKD), supplementary sensorimotor seizures, and paroxysmal nocturnal dystonia. The clinical distinction between the first two depends upon whether or not movement provokes the dyskinesia. The second two are more clearly epilepsies and discussed elsewhere in this chapter. A familial syndrome of *exercise induced dystonia and migraine* does not show linkage to any of the known genes for paroxysmal dyskinesias (Munchau et al, 2000). Channelopathies account for all paroxysmal dyskinesias.

Familial Paroxysmal Choreoathetosis

Genetic transmission is as an autosomal dominant trait and the gene maps to chromosome 16p11.2. The disorder shares some clinical features with benign familial infantile convulsions and paroxysmal choreoathetosis. All three disorders map to the same region on chromosome 16, suggesting that they may be allelic disorders.

Clinical Features. FPC usually begins in childhood. Most cases are sporadic. Sudden movement, startle, or changes in position precipitate an attack, which last less than a minute. Several attacks occur each day. Each attack may include dystonia, choreoathetosis, or ballismus (see Chapter 14) and may affect one or both sides of the body. Some patients have an "aura" described as tightness or tingling of the face or limbs.

Diagnosis. The clinical features distinguish the diagnosis.

Treatment. Low dosages of carbamazepine or phenytoin are effective in stopping attacks. Other sodium channel drugs such as lamotrigine or oxcarbazepine may be beneficial. Lacosamide acts on the sodium channel differently, but is also helpful.

Familial Paroxysmal Nonkinesiogenic Dyskinesia

Genetic transmission of PNKD is as an autosomal dominant trait (Spacey & Adams, 2011). The *MR1* gene on chromosome 2 is responsible.

Clinical Features. PNKD usually begins in childhood or adolescence. Attacks of dystonia, chorea, and athetosis last from 5 minutes to several hours. Precipitants are alcohol, caffeine, hunger, fatigue, nicotine, and emotional stress. Preservation of consciousness is a constant during attacks and life expectancy is normal.

Diagnosis. Molecular diagnosis is available on a research basis. Ictal and interictal EEGs are normal. Consider children with EEG evidence of epileptiform activity to have epilepsy and not a paroxysmal dyskinesia.

Management. PNKD is difficult to treat, but clonazepam taken daily or at the first sign of an attack may reduce the frequency or severity of attacks. Gabapentin is effective in some children.

Hyperventilation Syndrome

Hyperventilation induces alkalosis by altering the proportion of blood gases. This is easier to accomplish in children than in adults.

Clinical Features. During times of emotional upset, the respiratory rate and depth may increase insidiously, first appearing like sighing and then as obvious hyperventilation. The occurrence of tingling of the fingers disturbs the patient further and may induce greater hyperventilation. Headache is an associated symptom. Allowing hyperventilation to continue may result in loss of consciousness.

Diagnosis. The observation of hyperventilation as a precipitating factor of syncope is essential to diagnosis. Often patients are unaware that they were hyperventilating, but probing questions elicit the history in the absence of a witness.

Management. Breathing into a paper bag aborts an attack in progress.

Sleep Disorders

Narcolepsy-Cataplexy

Narcolepsy-cataplexy is a sleep disorder characterized by an abnormally short latency from sleep onset to rapid eye movement (REM) sleep. A person with narcolepsy attains REM sleep in less than 20 minutes instead of the usual 90 minutes. Characteristic of normal REM sleep are dreaming and severe hypotonia. In narcolepsy-cataplexy, these phenomena occur during wakefulness.

Human narcolepsy, unlike animal narcolepsy, is not a simple genetic trait (Scammell, 2003). Evidence suggests an immunologically mediated destruction of hypocretin-containing cells in human narcolepsy. An alternate name for hypocretin is *orexin*. Most cases of human narcolepsy with cataplexy have decreased hypocretin 1 in the CSF (Nishino, 2007) and an 85–95 % reduction in the number of orexin/hypocretin-containing neurons.

Clinical Features. Onset may occur at any time from early childhood to middle adulthood, usually in the second or third decade and rarely before age 5 years. The syndrome has five components:

1. *Narcolepsy* refers to short sleep attacks. Three or four attacks occur each day, most often during monotonous activity, and are difficult to resist. Half of the patients are easy to arouse from a sleep attack, and 60 % feel refreshed afterward. Narcolepsy is usually a lifelong condition.
2. *Cataplexy* is a sudden loss of muscle tone induced by laughter, excitement, or startle. Almost all patients who have narcolepsy have cataplexy as well. The patient may collapse to the floor and then arise immediately. Partial paralysis, affecting just the face or hands, is more common than total paralysis. Two to four attacks occur daily, usually in the afternoon. They are embarrassing but usually do not cause physical harm.
3. *Sleep paralysis* occurs in the transition between sleep and wakefulness. The patient is mentally awake but unable to move because of generalized paralysis. Partial paralysis is less common. The attack may end spontaneously or when the patient is touched. Two-thirds of patients with narcolepsy-cataplexy also experience sleep paralysis once or twice each week. Occasional episodes of sleep paralysis may occur in people who do not have narcolepsy-cataplexy.
4. *Hypnagogic hallucinations* are vivid, usually frightening, visual, and auditory perceptions occurring at the transition between sleep and wakefulness: a sensation of dreaming while awake. These are an associated event by half of the patients with narcolepsy-cataplexy. Episodes occur less than once a week.
5. *Disturbed night sleep* occurs in 75 % of cases *and automatic behavior* in 30 %. Automatic behavior is characterized by repeated performance of a function such as speaking or writing in a meaningless manner or driving on the wrong side of the road or to a strange place without recalling the episode. These episodes of automatic behavior may result from partial sleep episodes.

Diagnosis. Syndrome recognition is by the clinical history. However, the symptoms are embarrassing or sound "crazy" and considerable prompting is required before patients divulge a full history. Narcolepsy can be difficult to distinguish from other causes of excessive daytime sleepiness. The multiple sleep latency test is the standard for diagnosis. Patients with narcolepsy enter REM sleep within a few minutes of falling asleep.

Management. Symptoms of narcolepsy tend to worsen during the first years and then stabilize while cataplexy tends to improve with time. Two scheduled 15-minute naps each day can reduce excessive sleepiness. Most patients also require pharmacological therapy.

Modafinil, a wake-promoting agent distinct from stimulants, has proven efficacy for narcolepsy and is the first drug of choice. The adult dose is 200 mg each morning, and, while not approved for children, reduced dosages, depending on the child's weight, are in common usage. If modafinil fails, methylphenidate or pemoline is usually prescribed for narcolepsy but should be given with some caution because of potential abuse. Use small dosages on schooldays or workdays and no medicine, if possible, on weekends and holidays. When not taking medicine, patients should be encouraged to schedule short naps.

Treatment for cataplexy includes selective serotonin reuptake inhibitors (SSRIs), clomipramine, and protriptyline.

Sleep (Night) Terrors and Sleepwalking

Sleep terrors and sleepwalking are partial arousals from nonrapid eye movement (non-REM) sleep. A positive family history is common.

Clinical Features. The onset usually occurs by 4 years of age and always by age 6 years. Two hours after falling asleep the child awakens in a terrified state, does not recognize people, and is inconsolable. An episode usually lasts for 5–15 minutes but can last for an hour. During this time the child screams incoherently, may run if not restrained, and then goes back to sleep. Afterward, the child has no memory of the event.

Most children with sleep terrors experience an average of one or more episodes each week. Night terrors stop by 8 years of age in one-half of affected children but continue into adolescence in one-third.

Diagnosis. Half of the children with night terrors are also sleepwalkers, and many have a family history of either sleepwalking or sleep terrors. The history alone is the basis for diagnosis. A sleep laboratory evaluation often shows that children with sleep terrors suffer from sleep-disordered breathing (Guilleminault et al, 2003).

Management. Correction of the breathing disturbance often ends sleep terrors and sleepwalking.

Stiff Infant Syndrome (Hyperekplexia)

Five different genes are associated with the syndrome. Both autosomal dominant and autosomal recessive forms exist (De Koning-Tijssen & Rees, 2009).

Clinical Features. The onset is at birth or early infancy. When the onset is at birth, the newborn may appear hypotonic during sleep and develop generalized stiffening on awakening. Apnea and an exaggerated startle response are associated signs. Hypertonia in the newborn is unusual. Rigidity diminishes but does not disappear during sleep. Tendon reflexes are brisk, and the response spreads to other muscles.

The stiffness resolves spontaneously during infancy, and by 3 years of age most children are normal; however, episodes of stiffness may recur during adolescence or early adult life in response to startle, cold exposure, or pregnancy. Throughout life, affected individuals show a pathologically exaggerated startle response to visual, auditory, or tactile stimuli that would not startle normal individuals. In some, the startle is associated with a transitory, generalized stiffness of the body that causes falling without protective reflexes, often leading to injury. The stiffening response is often confused with the stiff man syndrome (see Chapter 8).

Other findings include periodic limb movements in sleep (PLMS) and hypnagogic (occurring when falling asleep) myoclonus. Intellect is usually normal.

Diagnosis. A family history of startle disease helps the diagnosis, but often is lacking. In startle disease, unlike startle-provoked epilepsy, the EEG is always normal.

Management. Clonazepam is the most useful agent to reduce the attack frequency. Valproate or levetiracetam are also useful. Affected infants get better with time.

Syncope

Syncope is loss of consciousness because of a transitory decline in cerebral blood flow. The pathological causes include an irregular cardiac rate or rhythm, or alterations of blood volume or distribution. *However, syncope is a common event in otherwise healthy children, especially in the second decade affecting girls more than boys. Diagnostic testing is rarely necessary.*

Clinical Features. The mechanism is a vasovagal reflex by which an emotional experience produces peripheral pooling of blood. Other stimuli that provoke the reflex are overextension or sudden decompression of viscera, the Valsalva maneuver, and stretching with the neck hyperextended. Fainting in a hot, crowded church is especially common. Usually, the faint occurs as the worshipper rises after prolonged kneeling.

Healthy children do not faint while lying down and rarely while seated. Fainting from anything but standing or arising suggests a cardiac arrhythmia and requires further investigation. The child may first feel faint (described as "faint," "dizzy," or "light-headed") or may lose consciousness without warning. The face drains of color and the skin is cold and clammy. With loss of consciousness, the child falls to the floor. The body may stiffen and the limbs may *tremble.*

The latter is not a seizure and the trembling movements never appear as clonic movements. The stiffening and trembling are especially common when keeping the child upright, which prolongs the reduced cerebral blood flow. This is common in a crowded church where the pew has no room to fall and bystanders attempt to bring the child outside "for air." A short period of confusion may follow, but recovery is complete within minutes.

Diagnosis. The criteria for differentiating syncope from seizures are the precipitating factors and the child's appearance. Seizures are unlikely to produce pallor and cold, clammy skin. Always inquire about the child's facial color in all initial evaluations of seizures. Diagnostic tests are not cost effective when syncope occurs in expected circumstances and the results of the clinical examination are normal. Recurrent orthostatic syncope requires investigation of autonomic function, and any suspicion of cardiac abnormality deserves ECG monitoring. Always ask the child if irregular heart rate or beats occurred at the time of syncope or at other times.

Management. Infrequent syncopal episodes of obvious cause do not require treatment. Holding deep inspiration at the onset of symptoms may abort an attack (Norcliffe-Kauffman et al, 2008). Good hydration and avoiding sudden change from prolonged supine into standing position decreases orthostasis and orthostatic syncope.

Staring Spells

Daydreaming is a pleasant escape for people of all ages. Children feel the need for escape most acutely when in school and may stare vacantly out of the window to the place where they would rather be. Daydreams can be hard to break, and a child may not respond to verbal commands. Neurologists and pediatricians often recommend EEG studies for daydreamers. Sometimes, the EEG shows sleep-activated central spikes or another abnormality not related to staring, which may lead the physician to prescribe inappropriate antiepileptic drug therapy. The best test for unresponsiveness during a staring spell is applying a mild noxious stimulus, such as pressure on the nail bed. Children with behavioral staring will have an immediate response and children with absence or partial seizures will have a decreased or no response.

Staring spells are characteristic of absence epilepsies and complex partial seizures. They are usually distinguishable because absence is brief (5–15 seconds) and the child feels normal immediately afterward, while complex partial seizures usually last for more than 1 minute and are followed by fatigue and psychomotor slowing. The associated EEG patterns and the response to treatment are quite different, and the basis for appropriate treatment is precise diagnosis before initiating treatment.

Absence seizures occur in four epileptic syndromes: childhood absence epilepsy, juvenile absence epilepsy, juvenile myoclonic epilepsy, and epilepsy with grand mal on awakening. All four syndromes are genetic disorders transmitted as autosomal dominant traits. The phenotypes have considerable overlap. The most significant difference is the age at onset.

Absence Epilepsy

Childhood absence epilepsy usually begins between ages 5 and 8 years of age. As a rule, later onset is more likely to represent juvenile absence epilepsy, with a higher frequency of generalized tonic-clonic seizures, and persistence into adult life.

Clinical Features. The reported incidence of epilepsy in families of children with absence varies from 15% to 40%. Concurrence in monozygotic twins is 75% for seizures and 85% for the characteristic EEG abnormality.

Affected children are otherwise healthy. Typical attacks last for 5–10 seconds and occur up to 100 times each day. The child stops ongoing activity, stares vacantly, sometimes with rhythmic movements of the eyelids, and then resumes activity. Aura and postictal confusion never occur. Longer seizures may last for up to 1 minute and are indistinguishable by observation alone from complex partial seizures. Associated features may include myoclonus, increased or decreased postural tone, picking at clothes, turning of the head, and conjugate movements of the eyes. Occasionally, prolonged absence status causes confusional states in children and adults. These often require emergency department visits (see Chapter 2).

A small percent age of children with absence seizures also have generalized tonic-clonic seizures. The occurrence of a generalized tonic-clonic seizure in an untreated child does not change the diagnosis or prognosis, but changes medication selection for seizure control.

Diagnosis. The background rhythms in patients with typical absence seizures usually are normal. The interictal EEG pattern for typical absence seizures is a characteristic 3 Hz spike-and-wave pattern lasting less than 3 seconds that may cause no clinical changes (Figure 1-2). Longer paroxysms of 3 cps spike-wave complexes are concurrent with the clinical seizure (ictal

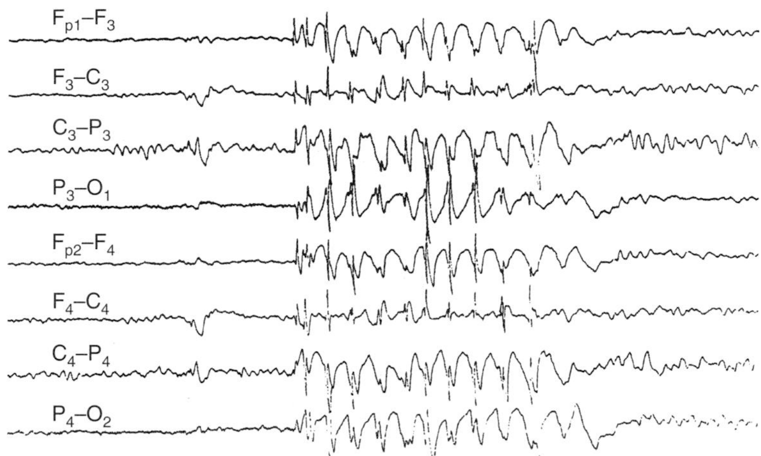

FIGURE 1-2 ■ Absence epilepsy. A generalized burst of 3 cps spike-wave complexes appears during hyperventilation.

pattern). The amplitude of discharge is greatest in the frontocentral regions, but variants with occipital predominance may occur. Although the discharge begins with a frequency of 3 cps, it may slow to 2 cps as it ends.

Hyperventilation usually activates the discharge. The interictal EEG is usually normal, but brief generalized discharges are often seen.

Although the EEG pattern of discharge is stereotyped, variations on the theme in the form of multiple spike and wave discharges and bi-frontal or bi-occipital 3 Hz delta waves are also acceptable. During sleep, the discharges often lose their stereotypy and become polymorphic and change in frequency but remain generalized. Once a correlation between clinical and EEG findings is made, looking for an underlying disease is unnecessary. The distinction between absence epilepsy and juvenile myoclonic epilepsy (see later discussion on Myoclonic Seizures) is the age at onset and absence of myoclonic seizures.

Management. Ethosuximide is the most effective drug with complete seizure control in about 80 %. Lamotrigine and valproate are equally effective with each providing complete relief of seizures in about 60 % of children. Ethosuximide is preferred because of its lower incidence of serious side effects. Levetiracetam and zonisamide seem to work in a smaller percentage of patients and topiramate is relatively ineffective for absence seizures. If neither drug alone provides seizure control, use them in combination at reduced dosages or substitute another drug. The EEG becomes normal if treatment is successful, and repeating the EEG is useful to confirm the seizure-free state.

Clonazepam is sometimes useful in the treatment of refractory absence. Carbamazepine may accentuate the seizures and cause absence status.

Complex Partial Seizures

Complex partial seizures arise in the cortex, most often the temporal lobe, but can originate from the frontal, occipital or parietal lobes as well. Complex partial seizures (discussed more fully in a later section) may be symptomatic of an underlying focal disorder.

Clinical Features. Impaired consciousness without generalized tonic-clonic activity characterizes complex partial seizures. Some altered mentation, lack of awareness or amnesia for the event are essential features. They either occur spontaneously or are sleep-activated. Most last 1–2 minutes and rarely less than 30 seconds. Less than 30 % of children report an aura. The aura is usually a nondescript unpleasant feeling, but may also be a stereotyped auditory or visual hallucination or abdominal discomfort. The first feature of the seizure can be staring, automatic behavior, tonic extension of one or both arms, or loss of body tone. Staring is associated with a change in facial expression and followed by automatic behavior.

Automatisms are more or less coordinated, involuntary motor activity occurring during a state of impaired consciousness either in the course of or after an epileptic seizure and usually followed by amnesia. They vary from facial grimacing and fumbling movements of the fingers to walking, running, and resisting restraint. Automatic behavior in a given patient tends to be similar from seizure to seizure.

The seizure usually terminates with a period of postictal confusion, disorientation, or lethargy. Transitory aphasia is sometimes present. Secondary generalization is likely if the child is not treated or if treatment is abruptly withdrawn.

Partial complex status epilepticus is a rare event characterized by impaired consciousness, staring alternating with wandering eye movements, and automatisms of the face and hands. Such children may arrive at the emergency department in a confused or delirious state (see Chapter 2).

Diagnosis. The etiology of complex partial seizures is heterogeneous, and a cause is often not determined. Contrast-enhanced MRI is an indicated study in all cases. It may reveal a low-grade glioma or dysplastic tissue, especially migrational defects.

Record an EEG in both the waking and sleeping states. Hyperventilation and photic stimulation are not useful as provocative measures. Results of a single EEG may be normal in the interictal period, but prolonged EEGs usually reveal either a spike or a slow wave focus in the epileptogenic area. During the seizure a discharge of evolving amplitude, frequency, and morphology occurs in the involved area of cortex.

Management. All seizure medications with the exception of ethosuximide have similar efficacy controlling partial seizures. I often select oxcarbazepine, levetiracetam or lamotrigine based on safety, tolerability and potential side effects. Topiramate and divalproex sodium are good alternatives for migraine sufferers with disability from this co-morbidity. Surgery should be offered to good surgical candidates with epilepsy refractory to treatment or unacceptable side effects. Consider ketogenic diet and vagal nerve stimulation for all other patients with partial response to treatments (see section on Surgical Approaches to Childhood Epilepsy).

Eyelid Myoclonia With or Without Absences (Jeavons Syndrome)

Jeavons syndrome is a distinct syndrome.

Clinical Features. Children present between age 2 and 14 years with eye closure induced seizures (*eyelid myoclonia*), photosensitivity, and EEG paroxysms, which may be associated with absence. Eyelid myoclonia, a jerky upward deviation of the eyeballs and retropulsion of the head, is the key feature. The seizures are brief but occur multiple times per day. In addition to eye closure, bright light, not just flickering light, may precipitate seizures. Jeavons syndrome appears to be a lifelong condition. The eyelid myoclonia is resistant to treatment. The absences are responsive to ethosuximide, divalproex sodium, and lamotrigine.

An apparently separate condition, *perioral myoclonia with absences*, also occurs in children. A rhythmic contraction of the orbicularis oris muscle causes protrusion of the lips and contractions of the corners of the mouth. Absence and generalized tonic-clonic seizures may occur. Such children are prone to develop absence status epilepticus.

Diagnosis. Reproduce the typical features with video/EEG.

Treatment. Treatment is similar to the other idiopathic generalized epilepsies: ethosuximide, lamotrigine, levetiracetam, divalproex sodium.

Myoclonic Seizures

Myoclonus is a brief, involuntary muscle contraction (jerk) that may represent: (1) a seizure manifestation, as in juvenile myoclonic epilepsy; (2) a physiological response to startle or to falling asleep; (3) an involuntary movement of sleep; or (4) an involuntary movement from disinhibition of the spinal cord (see Table 14-7). Myoclonic seizures are often difficult to distinguish from myoclonus (the movement disorder) on clinical grounds alone. Chapter 14 discusses *essential myoclonus* and other nonseizure causes of myoclonus.

Juvenile Myoclonic Epilepsy

Juvenile myoclonic epilepsy (JME) is an hereditary disorder, probably inherited as an autosomal dominant trait (Wheless & Kim, 2002). It accounts for up to 10 % of all cases of epilepsy. Many different genetic loci produce JME syndromes.

Clinical Features. JME occurs in both genders with equal frequency. Seizures in affected children and their affected relatives may be tonic-clonic, myoclonic, or absence. The usual age at onset of absence seizures is 7–13 years; of myoclonic jerks, 12–18 years; and of generalized tonic-clonic seizures, 13–20 years.

The myoclonic seizures are brief and bilateral, but not always symmetric, flexor jerks of the arms, which may be repetitive. The jerk sometimes affects the legs, causing the patient to fall. The highest frequency of myoclonic jerks is in the morning. Consciousness is not impaired so the patient is aware of the jerking movement. Seizures are precipitated by sleep deprivation, alcohol ingestion, and awakening from sleep.

Most patients also have generalized tonic-clonic seizures, and a third experience absence. All are otherwise normal neurologically. The potential for seizures of one type or another continues throughout adult life.

Diagnosis. Delays in diagnosis are common, often until a generalized tonic-clonic seizure brings the child to medical attention. Ignoring the myoclonic jerks is commonplace. *Suspect JME in any adolescent driver involved in a motor vehicle accident, when the driver has no memory of the event, but*

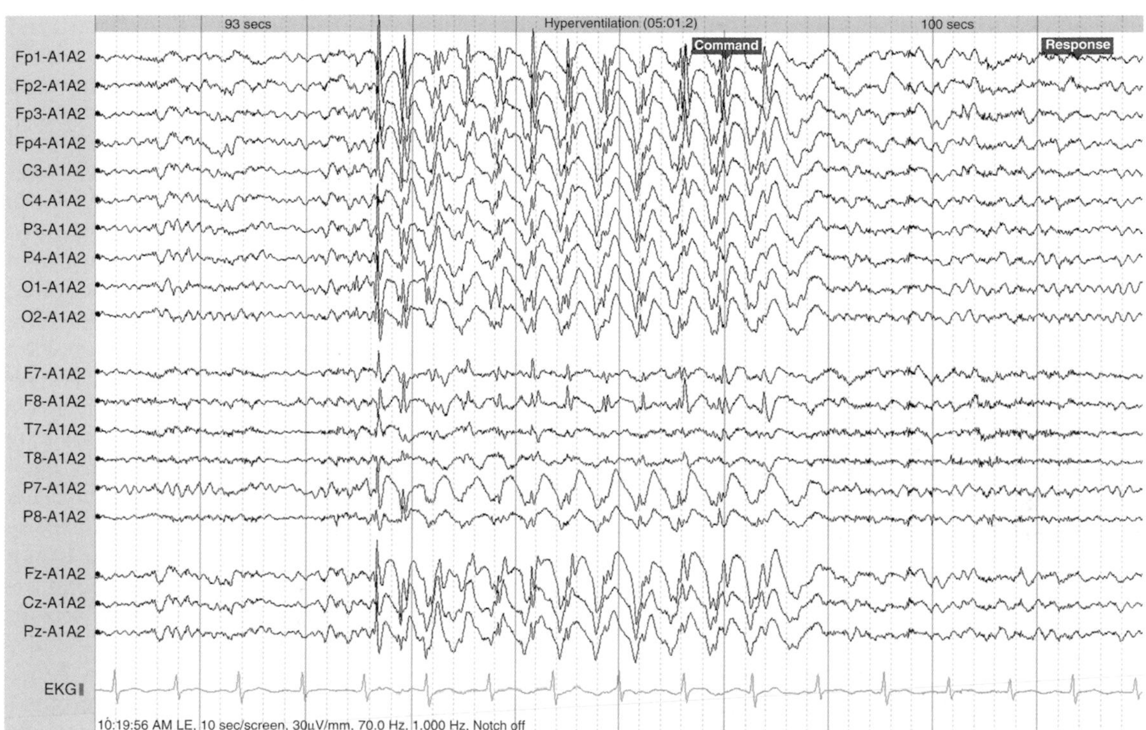

FIGURE 1-3 ■ Childhood absence epilepsy: 3.2 Hz generalized spike and slow wave discharge lasting 4.5 seconds during hyperventilation.

did not sustain a head injury. The interictal EEG in JME consists of bilateral, symmetrical spike and polyspike-and-wave discharges of 3.5–6 Hz, usually maximal in the frontocentral regions (Figure 1-3). Photic stimulation often provokes a discharge. Focal EEG abnormalities may occur.

Management. Levetiracetam is excellent therapy, stopping seizures in almost all cases (Sharpe et al, 2008). Other effective drugs include valproate, lamotrigine, and topiramate. Treatment is lifelong.

Progressive Myoclonus Epilepsies

The term *progressive myoclonus epilepsies* is used to cover several progressive disorders of the nervous system characterized by: (1) myoclonus; (2) seizures that may be tonic-clonic, tonic, or myoclonic; (3) progressive mental deterioration; and (4) cerebellar ataxia, involuntary movements, or both. Some of these disorders are due to specific lysosomal enzyme deficiencies, whereas others are probably mitochondrial disorders (Box 1-9).

BOX 1-9 Progressive Myoclonus Epilepsies

- Ceroid lipofuscinosis, juvenile form (see Chapter 5)
- Glucosylceramide lipidosis (Gaucher type 3) (see Chapter 5)
- Lafora disease
- Myoclonus epilepsy and ragged-red fibers (see Chapter 5)
- Ramsay-Hunt syndrome (see Chapter 10)
- Sialidoses (see Chapter 5)
- Unverricht-Lundborg syndrome

Lafora Disease. Lafora disease is a rare hereditary disease transmitted by autosomal recessive inheritance (Jansen & Andermann, 2011). A mutation in the *EPM2A* gene, encoding for laforin, a tyrosine kinase inhibitor, is responsible for 80 % of patients with Lafora disease. Laforin may play a role in the regulation of glycogen metabolism.

Clinical Features. Onset is between 11 and 18 years of age, with the mean at age 14 years. Tonic-clonic or myoclonic seizures are the initial feature in 80 % of cases. Hallucinations from occipital seizures are common. Myoclonus becomes progressively worse, may be segmental or massive, and increases with movement. Cognitive impairment begins early and is relentlessly progressive. Ataxia, spasticity, and involuntary movements occur late in the course. Death occurs 5 to 6 years after the onset of symptoms.

Diagnosis. The EEG is normal at first and later develops nonspecific generalized polyspike discharges during the waking state. The background becomes progressively disorganized and epileptiform activity more constant. Photosensitive discharges are a regular feature late in the course. The basis for diagnosis is the detection of one of the two known associated mutations.

Management. The seizures become refractory to most anticonvulsant drugs. Zonisamide, levetiracetam and divalproex sodium are the most effective drugs in myoclonic epilepsies. Divalproex is a good alternative when the diagnosis is known and mitochondrial disease is not suspected. Treatment of the underlying disease is not available.

Unverricht-Lundborg Syndrome. Unverricht-Lundborg syndrome is clinically similar to Lafora disease, except that inclusion bodies are not present. Genetic transmission is by autosomal recessive inheritance. Most reports of the syndrome are from Finland and other Baltic countries but distribution is worldwide. Mutations in the cystatin B gene cause defective function of a cysteine protease inhibitor (Lehesjoki & Koskiniemi, 2009).

Clinical Features. Onset is usually between 6 and 15 years of age. The main features are stimulus-sensitive myoclonus and tonic-clonic seizures. As the disease progresses, other neurological symptoms including cognitive impairment and coordination difficulties appear.

Diagnosis. EEG shows marked photosensitivity. Genetic molecular diagnosis is available.

Management. Zonisamide, levetiracetam (Crest et al, 2004) and divalproex sodium are the most effective drugs in myoclonic epilepsies. Divalproex is a good alternative when the diagnosis is known and mitochondrial disease is not suspected. Treatment of the underlying disease is not available.

Partial Seizures

This section discusses several different seizure types of focal cortical origin other than complex partial seizures. Such seizures may be purely motor or purely sensory or may affect higher cortical function. The *benign* childhood partial epilepsies are a common cause of partial seizures in children. Benign centrotemporal (rolandic) epilepsy and benign occipital epilepsy are the usual forms. The various benign partial epilepsy syndromes begin and cease at similar ages, have a similar course, and occur in the members of the same family. They may be different phenotypic expressions of the same genetic defect.

Partial seizures are also secondary to underlying diseases, which can be focal, multifocal, or generalized. Neuronal migrational disorders and gliomas often cause intractable partial seizures (Porter et al, 2003). MRI is a recommended study for all children with focal clinical seizures, seizures associated with an unexplained focal abnormality on EEG, or with a new or progressing neurological deficit.

Cerebral cysticercosis is an important cause of partial seizures in Mexico and Central America and is now common in the Southwestern United States (Carpio & Hauser, 2002) and becoming more common in contiguous regions. Ingestion of poorly cooked pork containing cystic larvae of the tapeworm *Taenia solium* causes the infection.

Any seizure that originates in the cortex may become a generalized tonic-clonic seizure (secondary generalization). If the discharge remains localized for a few seconds, the patient experiences a focal seizure or an aura before losing consciousness. Often the secondary generalization occurs so rapidly that a tonic-clonic seizure is the initial symptom. In such cases, cortical origin of the seizure may be detectable on EEG. However, normal EEG findings are common during a simple partial seizure and do not exclude the diagnosis.

Acquired Epileptiform Aphasia

Acquired aphasia in children associated with epileptiform activity on EEG is the *Landau-Kleffner syndrome*. The syndrome appears to be a disorder of auditory processing. The cause is unknown except for occasional cases associated with temporal lobe tumors.

Clinical Features. Age at onset ranges from 2 to 11 years, with 75 % beginning between 3 and 10 years. The first symptom may be aphasia or epilepsy. Auditory verbal agnosia is the initial characteristic of aphasia. The child has difficulty understanding speech and stops talking. "Deafness" or "autism" develops. Several seizure types occur, including generalized tonic-clonic, partial, and myoclonic seizures (Camfield & Camfield, 2002). Atypical absence is sometimes the initial feature and may be associated with continuous spike and slow waves during slow wave sleep. Hyperactivity and personality change occur in half of affected children, probably caused by aphasia. The neurological examination is otherwise normal.

Recovery of language is more likely to occur if the syndrome begins before 7 years of age. Seizures cease generally by age 10 and always by age 15.

Diagnosis. Acquired epileptiform aphasia, as the name implies, is different from autism and hearing loss because the diagnosis requires that the child have normal language and cognitive development prior to onset of symptoms and normal hearing. The EEG shows multifocal cortical spike discharges with a predilection for the temporal and parietal lobes. Involvement is bilateral in 88% of cases. An intravenous injection of diazepam may normalize the EEG and transiently improve speech, but this should not suggest that epileptiform activity causes the aphasia. Instead, both features reflect an underlying cerebral disorder.

Every child with the disorder requires cranial MRI to exclude the rare possibility of a temporal lobe tumor.

Management. Standard anticonvulsants usually control the seizures but do not improve speech. Corticosteroid therapy, especially early in the course, may normalize the EEG and provide long-lasting remission of aphasia and seizures. One 5-year-old girl showed improved language and control of seizures with levetiracetam monotherapy, 60 mg/kg/day (Kossoff et al, 2003a). Immunoglobulins 2 mg/kg over two consecutive days have also shown efficacy.

Acquired Epileptiform Opercular Syndrome

This syndrome and *autosomal dominant rolandic epilepsy and speech apraxia* are probably the same entity. They are probably different from acquired epileptiform aphasia but may represent a spectrum of the same underlying disease process.

Clinical Features. Onset is before age 10 years. Brief nocturnal seizures occur that mainly affect the face and mouth but may become secondarily generalized. Oral dysphasia, inability to initiate complex facial movements (blowing out a candle), speech dysphasia, and drooling develop concurrently with seizure onset. Cognitive dysfunction is associated. Genetic transmission is by autosomal dominant inheritance with anticipation.

Diagnosis. The EEG shows centrotemporal discharges or electrical status epilepticus during slow wave sleep.

Management. The dysphasia does not respond to anticonvulsant drugs.

Autosomal Dominant Nocturnal Frontal Lobe Epilepsy

Bizarre behavior and motor features during sleep are the characteristics of this epilepsy syndrome, often misdiagnosed as a sleep or psychiatric disorder. Several different gene loci are identifiable among families.

Clinical Features. Seizures begin in childhood and usually persist into adult life. The seizures occur in non-REM sleep and sudden awakenings with brief hyperkinetic or tonic manifestations are characteristic. Patients frequently remain conscious and often report auras of shivering, tingling, epigastric or thoracic sensations, as well as other sensory and psychic phenomena.

Clusters of seizures, each lasting less than a minute, occur in one night. Video-EEG recordings demonstrate partial seizures originating in the frontal lobe. A vocalization, usually a gasp or grunt that awakens the child, is common. Other auras include sensory sensations, psychic phenomena (fear, malaise, etc.), shivering, and difficulty breathing. Thrashing or tonic stiffening with superimposed clonic jerks follows. The eyes are open, and the individual is often aware of what is happening; many sit up and try to grab on to a bed part.

Diagnosis. The family history is important to the diagnosis, but many family members may not realize that their own attacks are seizures or want others to know that they experience such bizarre symptoms. The interictal EEG is usually normal, and concurrent video-EEG is often required to capture the event, which reveals rapidly generalized discharges with diffuse distribution. Often, movement artifact obscures the initial ictal EEG.

Children who have seizures when awake and no family history of epilepsy may have supplementary sensorimotor seizures (see later section on Supplementary Sensorimotor Seizures).

Management. Any of the anticonvulsant agents except for ethosuximide may be effective. Many of these patients get only partial control with monotherapy and multiple combinations are tried. I have many patients that ended up with a combination of oxcarbazepine and divalproex sodium to get their seizures under control.

Childhood Epilepsy With Occipital Paroxysms

Two genetic occipital epilepsies are separable because of different genetic abnormalities.

Benign Occipital Epilepsy of Childhood. Genetic transmission is by autosomal dominant inheritance. It may be a phenotypic variation of benign rolandic epilepsy. Both epilepsies are commonly associated with migraine.

Clinical Features. Age at onset is usually between 4 and 8 years. One-third of patients have a family history of epilepsy, frequently benign rolandic epilepsy. The initial seizure manifestation can consist of (1) nonformed visual hallucinations, usually flashing lights or spots;

(2) blindness, hemianopia, or complete amaurosis; (3) visual illusions, such as micropsia, macropsia, or metamorphopsia; or (4) loss of consciousness lasting for up to 12 hours. More than one feature may occur simultaneously. Unilateral clonic seizures, complex partial seizures, or secondary generalized tonic-clonic seizures follow the visual aura. Afterward, the child may have migraine-like headaches and nausea. Attacks occur when the child is awake or asleep, but the greatest frequency is at the transition from wakefulness to sleep. Photic stimulation or playing video games may induce seizures.

Diagnosis. Results of the neurological examination, CT, and MRI are normal. The interictal EEG shows unilateral or bilateral independent high-amplitude, occipital spike-wave discharges with a frequency of 1.5–2.5 cps. Eye opening enhances the discharges, light sleep inhibits them. A similar interictal pattern occurs in some children with absence epilepsy, suggesting a common genetic disorder among different benign genetic epilepsies. During a seizure, rapid firing of spike discharges occurs in one or both occipital lobes.

Epilepsy associated with ictal vomiting is a variant of benign occipital epilepsy (Panayiotopoulos, 1999). Seizures occur during sleep and vomiting, eye deviation, speech arrest, or hemiconvulsions are characteristic.

Management. Standard anticonvulsant drugs usually provide complete seizure control. Typical seizures never persist beyond 12 years of age. However, not all children with occipital discharges have a benign epilepsy syndrome. Persistent or hard-to-control seizures raise the question of a structural abnormality in the occipital lobe, and require MRI examination.

Panayiotopoulos Syndrome

Clinical Features. The age at onset of Panayiotopoulos syndrome is 3 to 6 years, but the range extends from 1 to 14 years. Seizures usually occur in sleep and autonomic and behavioral features predominate. These include vomiting, pallor, sweating, irritability, and tonic eye deviation. The seizures last for hours in one-third of patients. Seizures are infrequent and the overall prognosis is good with remission occurring in 1-2 years. A third of children have only one seizure.

Diagnosis. The interictal EEG shows runs of high amplitude 2–3 Hz sharp and slow wave complexes in the posterior quadrants. Many children may have central-temporal or frontal spikes. The ictal EEG in Panayiotopoulos syndrome is posterior slowing.

Children with idiopathic photosensitive occipital epilepsy, present between 5 and 17 years of age. Television and video games induce seizures. The seizures begin with colorful, moving spots in the peripheral field of vision. With progression of the seizure, tonic head and eye version develops with blurred vision, nausea, vomiting, sharp pain it the head or orbit, and unresponsiveness. Cognitive status, the neurological examination, and brain imaging are normal. The interictal EEG shows bilateral synchronous or asynchronous occipital spikes and spike-wave complexes. Intermittent photic stimulation may induce an occipital photoparyoxysmal response and generalized discharges. The ictal EEG shows occipital epileptiform activity, which may shift from one side to the other. This epilepsy requires distinction from idiopathic generalized epilepsy with photosensitivity.

Management. Standard anticonvulsant drugs usually accomplish seizure control.

Benign Childhood Epilepsy with Centrotemporal Spikes (BECTS)

Benign rolandic epilepsy is an alternate name for BECTS. Genetic transmission is as an autosomal dominant trait. Forty percent of close relatives have a history of febrile seizures or epilepsy.

Clinical Features. The age at onset is between 3 and 13 years, with a peak at 7 to 8 years. Seizures usually stop spontaneously by age 13 to 15 years. This epilepsy is not always benign. In fact, some children have their seizures only partially controlled with polypharmacy. Observations such as "incomplete phenotype penetrance", the incidence of seizures and the response to treatment may be incorrect by the "incomplete observation" in children that may have only mild seizures when everybody is sleeping. Seventy percent of children have seizures only while asleep, 15 % only when awake, and 15 % both awake and asleep.

The typical seizure wakes the child from sleep. Paresthesias occur on one side of the mouth, followed by ipsilateral twitching of the face, mouth, and pharynx, resulting in speech arrest (if dominant hemisphere) or dysarthria (if nondominant hemisphere) and drooling. Consciousness is often preserved. The seizure lasts for 1 or 2 minutes. Daytime seizures do not generalize, but nocturnal seizures in children younger than 5 years old often spread to the arm or evolve into a generalized tonic-clonic seizure. Some children with BECTS have cognitive or behavioral problems, particularly difficulty with sustained attention, reading, and language processing.

Diagnosis. When evaluating a child for a first nocturnal, generalized tonic-clonic seizure, ask the parents if the child's mouth was "twisted." If they answer affirmatively, the child probably has BECTS. They never report this observation spontaneously.

Results of neurological examination and brain imaging studies are normal. Interictal EEG shows unilateral or bilateral spike discharges in the central or centrotemporal region. The spikes are typically of high voltage and activated by drowsiness and sleep. The frequency of spike discharge does not correlate with the subsequent course. Children with both typical clinical seizures and typical EEG abnormalities, especially with a positive family history, do not require neuroimaging. However, those with atypical features or hard-to-control seizures warrant MRI to exclude a low-grade glioma.

Management. Most anticonvulsant drugs are effective. I often prescribe levetiracetam or oxcarbazepine in these children. Most children eventually stop having seizures whether they are treated or not. *However, I am impressed that, in many, the epilepsy is not so benign, and in some continues into adult life.*

Electrical Status Epilepticus During Slow Wave Sleep (ESES)

In ESES, sleep induces paroxysmal EEG activity. The paroxysms may appear continuously or discontinuously during sleep. They are usually bilateral, but sometimes strictly unilateral or with unilateral predominance.

Clinical Features. Age at onset is 3 to 14 years. The seizure types during wakefulness are atypical absence, myoclonic, or akinetic seizures. Children with paroxysmal EEG activity only during sleep tend not to have clinical seizures. Such children are often undiagnosed for months or years. Neuropsychological impairment and behavioral disorders are common. Hyperactivity, learning disabilities and, in some instances, psychotic regressions may persist even after ESES has ceased.

Diagnosis. The most typical paroxysmal discharges of EEG are spike waves of 1.5 and 3.5 Hz, sometimes associated with polyspikes or polyspikes and waves.

Treatment. Standard anticonvulsant drugs are rarely effective. High-dose steroids, ACTH, high-dose benzodiazepines, levetiracetam and intravenous immunoglobulin have all reported some success.

Epilepsia Partialis Continuans

Focal motor seizures that do not stop spontaneously are termed *epilepsia partialis continuans.* This is an ominous symptom and usually indicates an underlying cerebral disorder. Possible causes include infarction, hemorrhage, tumor, hyperglycemia, Rasmussen's encephalitis, and inflammation. Make every effort to stop the seizures with intravenous antiepileptic drugs (see later section on Treatment of Status Epilepticus). The response to anticonvulsant drugs and the outcome depend on the underlying cause.

Hemiconvulsions-Hemiplegia Syndrome (Rasmussen Syndrome)

Rasmussen syndrome is a poorly understood disorder. While originally described as a form of focal, viral encephalitis, an infectious etiology is not established.

Clinical Features. Focal jerking frequently begins in one body part, usually one side of the face or one hand, and then spreads to contiguous parts. Trunk muscles are rarely affected. The rate and intensity of the seizures vary at first, but then become more regular and persist during sleep. By 4 months from first symptom, all have refractory motor seizures (Granata et al, 2003b). The seizures defy treatment and progress to affect first both limbs on one side of the body and then the limbs on the other side. Progressive hemiplegia develops and remains after seizures have stopped.

Diagnosis. EEG and MRI are initially normal and then the EEG shows continuous spike discharges originating in one portion of the cortex, with spread to contiguous areas of the cortex and to a mirror focus on the other side. Secondary generalization may occur. Repeated MRI shows rapidly progressive hemiatrophy with ex vacuo dilation of the ipsilateral ventricle. PET shows widespread hypometabolism of the affected hemisphere at a time when the spike discharges remain localized. The CSF is usually normal, although a few monocytes may be present.

Management. The treatment of Rasmussen syndrome is especially difficult. Standard antiepileptic therapy is not effective for stopping seizures or the progressive hemiplegia. The use of immunosuppressive therapy is recommended by some (Granata et al, 2003a) and antiviral therapy by others. These medical approaches are rarely successful. Early hemispherectomy is the treatment of choice (Kossoff et al, 2003b).

Reading Epilepsy

There was a belief that reading epilepsy and juvenile myoclonic epilepsy were variants because many children with reading epilepsy experience myoclonic jerks of the limbs shortly after arising in the morning. However, recent studies indicate that reading epilepsy is idiopathic epilepsy originating from the left temporal lobe (Archer et al, 2003).

Clinical Features. Age at onset is usually in the second decade. Myoclonic jerks involving orofacial and jaw muscles develop while reading. Reading time before seizure onset is variable. The initial seizure is usually in the jaw and described as "jaws locking or clicking." Other initial features are quivering of the lips, choking in the throat, or difficulty speaking. Myoclonic jerks of the limbs may follow, and some children experience a generalized tonic-clonic seizure if they continue reading. Generalized tonic-clonic seizures may also occur at other times.

Diagnosis. The history of myoclonic jerks during reading and during other processes requiring higher cognitive function is critical to the diagnosis. The interictal EEG usually shows generalized discharges and brief spike-wave complexes can be provoked by reading that are simultaneous with jaw jerks.

Management. Some patients claim to control their seizures without the use of anticonvulsant drugs by quitting reading at the first sign of orofacial or jaw jerks. This seems an impractical approach and an impediment to education. Levetiracetam and lamotrigine are good treatment options.

Temporal Lobe Epilepsy

Temporal lobe epilepsy in children may be primary or secondary. Inheritance of primary temporal lobe epilepsy is often as an autosomal dominant trait. Among children with secondary temporal lobe epilepsy, 30 % give a history of an antecedent illness or event and 40 % show MRI evidence of a structural abnormality.

Clinical Features. Seizure onset in primary temporal lobe epilepsy occurs in adolescence or later. The seizures consist of simple psychic (déjà vu, cognitive disturbances, illusions and hallucinations) or autonomic (nausea, tachycardia, sweating) symptoms. Secondary generalization is unusual. Seizure onset in secondary temporal lobe epilepsy is during the first decade and often occurs during an acute illness. The seizures are usually complex partial in type, and secondary generalization is more common.

Diagnosis. A single EEG in children with primary temporal lobe epilepsy is likely to be normal. The frequency of interictal temporal lobe spikes is low, and diagnosis requires prolonged video-EEG monitoring. The incidence of focal interictal temporal lobe spikes is 78% in children with secondary temporal lobe epilepsy, but detection may require several standard or prolonged EEG studies.

BOX 1-10 Diagnostic Considerations for a First Nonfebrile Tonic-Clonic Seizure after 2 Years of Age

Acute encephalopathy or encephalitis (see Chapter 2)
Isolated unexplained seizure
Partial seizure of any cause with secondary generalization
Primary generalized epilepsy
Progressive disorder of the nervous system (see Chapter 5)

Management. Monotherapy with oxcarbazepine, levetiracetam, lamotrigine or topiramate are usually satisfactory for seizure control in both types. Other anticonvulsants such as phenytoin, carbamazepine and valproate have similar efficacy. I chose medications based on safety, tolerability, potential side effects and cost.

Generalized Seizures

Generalized tonic-clonic seizures are the most common seizures of childhood. They are dramatic and frightening events that invariably demand medical attention. Seizures that are prolonged or repeated without recovery are termed *status epilepticus*. Many children with generalized tonic-clonic seizures have a history of febrile seizures during infancy. Some of these represent a distinct autosomal dominant disorder. Box 1-10 summarizes the diagnostic considerations in a child who has had a generalized tonic-clonic seizure.

Clinical Features. The onset may occur any time after the neonatal period, but the onset of primary generalized epilepsy without absence is usually during the second decade. With absence, the age at onset shifts to the first decade.

Sudden loss of consciousness is the initial feature. The child falls to the floor, and the body stiffens (tonic phase). Repetitive jerking movements of the limbs follow (clonic phase); these movements at first are rapid and rhythmic and then become slower and more irregular as the seizure ends. The eyes roll backward in the orbits; breathing is rapid and deep, causing saliva to froth at the lips; and urinary and fecal incontinence may occur. A postictal sleep follows the seizure from which arousal is difficult. Afterward, the child appears normal but may have sore limb muscles and a painful tongue, bitten during the seizure.

Diagnosis. A first generalized tonic-clonic seizure requires laboratory evaluation. Individualize the evaluation. Important determining factors include neurological findings, family history, and known precipitating factors. An eyewitness report of focal features at the onset of the seizure, or the recollection of an aura, indicates a partial seizure with secondary generalization.

During the seizure, the EEG shows generalized repetitive spikes in the tonic phase and then periodic bursts of spikes in the clonic phase. Movement artifact usually obscures the clonic portion. As the seizure ends, the background rhythms are slow and the amplitude attenuates.

Between seizures, brief generalized spike or spike-wave discharges that are polymorphic in appearance may occur. Discharge frequency sometimes increases with drowsiness and light sleep. The presence of focal discharges indicates secondary generalization of the tonic-clonic seizure.

The CSF is normal following a brief tonic-clonic seizure due to primary epilepsy. However, prolonged or repeated seizures may cause a leukocytosis as many as 80 cells/mm^3 with a polymorphonuclear predominance. The protein concentration can be mildly elevated, but the glucose concentration is normal.

Management. Do not start prophylactic antiepileptic therapy in an otherwise normal child who has had a single unexplained seizure. The recurrence rate is probably less than 50% after 1 year. Several drugs are equally effective in children with recurrent seizures that require treatment.

Epilepsy with Generalized Tonic-Clonic Seizures on Awakening

Epilepsy with generalized tonic-clonic seizures on awakening is a familial syndrome distinct from juvenile myoclonic epilepsy. Onset occurs in the second decade, and 90% of seizures occur on awakening, regardless of the time of day. Seizures also occur with relaxation in the evening. Absence and myoclonic seizures may occur. The mode of inheritance is unknown.

Clinical Features. Onset occurs in the second decade, and 90% of seizures occur on awakening, regardless of the time of day. Seizures also occur with relaxation in the evening. Absence and myoclonic seizures may occur.

Diagnosis. The EEG shows a pattern of idiopathic generalized epilepsies.

Management. Treatment is similar to that of juvenile myoclonic epilepsy with levetiracetam, valproate, lamotrigine, and topiramate (Wheless & Kim, 2002).

Pseudoseizures

Psychogenic symptoms are common. Pseudoseizure is often a psychogenic manifestation in someone with epilepsy or who is familiar with the disease. Children or adolescents with limited coping mechanisms for stress may subconsciously use the complaint of seizure to protect themselves from overwhelming situations. It is important to examine cases of epilepsy "refractory to treatment" for this possibility.

Pseudoseizures occur more often in adolescence than in childhood and more often in females than in males (3:1). Common teenage stressors including school performance, sport performance, social relations, and peer pressure are more frequently the trigger for psychogenic symptoms than sexual abuse, which unfortunately is a common occurrence. People with pseudoseizures may also have true seizures; often, the pseudoseizures begin while epilepsy is controlled when the patient is overwhelmed by stressors and has inadequate coping mechanisms.

Clinical Features. Pseudoseizures are often misdiagnosed as epilepsy. Thirty to forty percent of adults with "refractory seizures" are ultimately diagnosed with pseudoseizures after undergoing inpatient EEG monitoring. Some patients may have both epilepsy and pseudoseizures. The following may raise suspicion for pseudoseizures:

1. Abrupt onset of daily, multiple, "severe" seizures without a preceding neurological insult.
2. Movements with trashing, jerking, asymmetric characteristics including, side to side head motion, asymmetric up and down arm or leg motions, pelvic thrusting, etc.
3. Non-stereotyped events with multiple variable characteristics.
4. Provoked rather than unprovoked events (emotional or other triggers).
5. Periods of unresponsiveness during which attacks may be precipitated and ended by suggestion. Patients usually do not hurt themselves nor experience incontinence. However, incontinence or trauma may occur in pseudoseizures.
6. Epileptic patients bite the side of their tongue or the buccal mucosa. Pseudoseizure patients may bite the tip of their tongue.
7. Epileptics have labored and slow breathing after a convulsion; pseudoseizures typically are followed by tachypnea.

Diagnosis. The diagnosis of most pseudoseizures is by observation alone. A good description or family captured video may be sufficient. When doubt remains, video-EEG monitoring is the best method of diagnosis.

Management. We often use the help of counselors for children with pseudoseizures to identify and address stressors. In addition, SSRIs for children with the comorbidity of anxiety or depression including citalopram 10–20 mg/day, escitalopram 5–10 mg/day or sertraline 50–100 mg/day are often helpful.

Video Game-Induced Seizures

Children who experience seizures while playing video games have a photosensitive seizure disorder demonstrable on EEG during intermittent photic stimulation. Two-thirds have primary generalized epilepsy (generalized tonic-clonic, absence, and juvenile myoclonic epilepsy), and the rest have partial epilepsies, usually benign occipital epilepsy.

MANAGING SEIZURES

Antiepileptic Drug Therapy

The goal when treating epilepsy is to make the child and his or her brain function at the highest level between seizures as often we are unable to provide seizure freedom. In other words, achieve maximum normal function by balancing seizure control against drug toxicity (Hirtz et al, 2003).

Indications for Starting Therapy

Initiate therapy in neurologically abnormal children (symptomatic epilepsy) after the first seizure; more seizures are expected. After a first unexplained and untreated generalized tonic-clonic seizure, less than half of otherwise normal children will have a second seizure. It is reasonable to delay therapy, if the child is not operating a motor vehicle. Always treat juvenile myoclonic epilepsy and absence epilepsy, not only because of expected seizure recurrence, but also because uncontrolled absence impairs education and has higher risks of trauma.

Discontinuing Therapy

Antiepileptic drug therapy is required in children who experience seizures during an acute encephalopathy, e.g., anoxia, head trauma, encephalitis. However, it is reasonable to stop therapy when the acute encephalopathy is over and seizures have stopped if no significant residual deficits.

Pooled data on epilepsy in children suggests that discontinuing antiepileptic therapy is successful after 2 years of complete control. Pooled data is worthless when applied to the individual child. *It is thought that many otherwise normal children started on antiepileptic medication after a first seizure and then remain seizure free for 2 years should not have received medication in the first place.* The decision to stop therapy, like the decision to start therapy, requires an individualized approach to the child and the cause of the epilepsy. Children who are neurologically abnormal (remote symptomatic epilepsy) and those with specific epileptic syndromes that are known to persist into adult life are likely to have recurrences, while some cryptogenic cases have a low incidence of recurrence after the first or second seizure. Three-quarters of relapses occur during the withdrawal phase and in the 2 years thereafter. Contrary to popular belief, the rapid withdrawal of antiepileptic drugs in a person who does not need therapy does not provoke seizures with the probable exception of high-dose benzodiazepines. However, all parents *know* that seizure medication is never abruptly withdrawn and it is foolish to suggest otherwise. Attempt to stop antiepileptic therapy 1 year before driving age in children who are seizure free and neurologically normal without evidence of having a lifelong epileptic tendency.

Principles of Therapy

Start therapy with a single drug. Most children with epilepsy achieve complete seizure control with monotherapy when using the correct drug for the seizure type. Even patients whose seizures are never controlled are likely to do better on the smallest number of drugs. Polypharmacy poses several problems: (1) drugs compete with each other for protein-binding sites; (2) one drug can increase the rate and pathway of metabolism of a second drug; (3) drugs have cumulative toxicity; and (4) compliance is more difficult.

When using more than one drug, change only one drug at a time. When making several changes simultaneously, it is impossible to determine which drug is responsible for a beneficial or an adverse effect.

Administer anticonvulsant drugs no more than twice a day, and urge families to buy pillboxes marked with the 7 days of the week. *It is difficult to remember to take medicine when you are not in pain to prevent something you do not remember from happening. If you ask people if they ever miss their doses the answer is often never, as it is impossible to remember what you forgot.*

Blood Concentrations. The development of techniques to measure blood concentrations of antiepileptic drugs was an important advance in the treatment of epilepsy. However, reference values of drug concentrations are guidelines. Some patients

TABLE 1-2 **Antiepileptic Drugs for Children**

Drug	Initial dose	Target dose	Blood concentration (μg/mL)	Half-life (hours)
Carbamazepine	10 mg/kg/day	20–30 mg/kg/day	4–12	14–27
Clonazepam	0.02 mg/day	0.5–1 mg/day	*	20–40
Ethosuximide	10 mg/kg/day	15–40 mg/kg/day	50–100	30–40
Felbamate	15 mg/kg/day	15–45 mg/kg/day	40–80	20–23
Lamotrigine (non-valproate)	0.5 mg/kg/day	5–10 mg/kg/day	2–20	25 (monotherapy)
Levetiracetam	30 mg/kg/day	60 mg/kg	15–40	5
Oxcarbazepine	10 mg/kg/day	20–40 mg/kg/day	10–40	9
Phenobarbital	3–5 mg/kg/day	5–10 mg/kg/day	15–40	35–73
Phenytoin	5–10 mg/kg/day	5–10 mg/kg/day	10–25	24
Primidone	5 mg/kg/day	10–25 mg/kg/day	8–12	8–22
Topiramate	1-3 mg/kg/day	5–9 mg/kg/day	†	18–30
Valproate	20 mg/kg/day	30–60 mg/kg/day	50–100	6–15
Vigabatrin	40–60 mg/kg/day	60–80 mg/kg/day	†	Days
Zonisamide	1.5 mg/kg/day	6 mg/kg/day	†	24

*Not clinically useful.
†Not established.
Concomitant therapy with other drugs often influences dosages.

are seizure free with concentrations that are below the reference value, and others are unaffected by apparently toxic concentrations. I rely more on patient response than on blood concentration. Fortunately, for children, many of the newer drugs, e.g. lamotrigine, levetiracetam, do not require the measurement of blood concentrations. However, levels may be helpful in some situations.

Measuring total drug concentrations, protein-bound and free fractions, is customary even though the free fraction is responsible for efficacy and toxicity. While the ratio of free to bound fractions is relatively constant, some drugs have a greater affinity for binding protein than other drugs and displace them when used together. The free fraction of the displaced drug increases and causes toxicity even though the measured total drug concentration is "therapeutic."

Most antiepileptic drugs follow first-order kinetics, i.e., blood levels increase proportionately with increases in the oral dose. The main exception is phenytoin, whose metabolism changes from first-order to zero-order kinetics when the enzyme system responsible for its metabolism saturates. Then a small increment in oral dose produces large increments in blood concentration.

The half-lives of the antiepileptic drugs listed in Table 1-2 are at steady state. Half-lives are generally longer when therapy with a new drug begins. Achieving a steady state usually requires five half-lives. Similarly, five half-lives are required to eliminate a drug after discontinuing administration. Drug half-lives vary from individual to individual and may be shortened or increased by the concurrent use of other anticonvulsants or other medications. This is one reason that children with epilepsy may have a toxic response to a drug or increased seizures at the time of a febrile illness.

Some anticonvulsants have active metabolites with anticonvulsant and toxic properties. With the exception of phenobarbital derived from primidone and monohydroxy derived from oxcarbazepine these metabolites are not usually measured. Active metabolites may provide seizure control or have toxic effects when the blood concentration of the parent compound is low.

Adverse Reactions. Some anticonvulsant drugs irritate the gastric mucosa and cause nausea and vomiting. When this occurs, taking smaller doses at shorter intervals, using enteric-coated preparations, and administering the drug after meals may relieve symptoms.

Toxic adverse reactions are dose related. Almost all anticonvulsant drugs cause sedation when blood concentrations are excessive. Subtle cognitive and behavioral disturbances, recognizable only by the patient or family, often occur at low blood concentrations. Never discount the patient's observation of a toxic effect because the blood concentration is within the "therapeutic range." As doses are increased, attention span, memory, and interpersonal relations may become seriously impaired. This is especially common with barbiturates but can occur with any drug.

Idiosyncratic reactions are not dose related. They may occur as hypersensitivity reactions (usually manifest as rash, fever, and lymphadenopathy) or because of toxic metabolites. Idiosyncratic reactions are not always predictable, and respecting the patient's observation is essential. *Notwithstanding package inserts and threats of litigation, routine laboratory studies of blood counts and organ function in a healthy child are neither cost effective nor helpful.* It is preferable to do studies based on clinical features.

Selection of an Antiepileptic Drug

The use of generic drugs is difficult to avoid in managed health care programs. Unfortunately, several different manufacturers provide generic versions of each drug; the bioavailability and half-life of these products vary considerably, and maintaining a predictable blood concentration may be difficult. I usually increase the dose of patients partially controlled when they have a breakthrough seizure and decrease the dose 10 % when they experience side effects. A variation of 10 % up and down from one to the next refill when changing between brands and multiple generics either way is not trivial. These changes may result in loss of seizure control or side effects.

Common reasons for loss of seizure control in children who were previously seizure free are nonadherence and changing from the brand name to a generic drug, or from one generic to another. *Patients should be told when their medication is being changed from brand to generic, generic to brand or generic to different generic.*

For the most part, the basis of drug selection is the neurologist's comfort with using a specific drug, other health conditions and drug use in the patient, the available preparations with respect to the child's age, and the spectrum of antiepileptic activity of the drug. Levetiracetam, lamotrigine, topiramate, valproate, zonisamide, rufinamide and felbamate are drugs with a broad spectrum of efficacy against many different seizure types. The basis of the following comments is personal experience and published reports. Patent extensions granted by the FDA, when research in children is completed, has helped tremendously in the acquisition of knowledge of the use of anticonvulsants in children.

Carbamazepine (Tegretol®, Tegretol-XR®, *Novartis*; Carbatrol®, *Shire Pharmaceuticals*). In my own practice, oxcarbazepine has replaced carbamazepine entirely because of its better side effect profile and tolerability.

Indications. Partial seizures, primary or secondary generalized tonic-clonic seizures. Carbamazepine increases the frequency of absence and myoclonic seizures and is therefore contraindicated.

Administration. Approximately 85 % of the drug is protein bound. Carbamazepine induces its own metabolism, and the initial dose should be 25 % of the maintenance dose to prevent toxicity. The usual maintenance dosage is 15–20 mg/kg/day to provide a blood concentration of 4–12 µg/mL. However, infants often require 30 mg/kg/day. The half-life at steady state is 5–27 hours, and children usually require doses three times a day. Two long-acting preparations are available for twice a day dosing. Concurrent use of cimetidine, erythromycin, grapefruit, fluoxetine, and propoxyphene interferes with carbamazepine metabolism and causes toxicity.

Adverse Effects. A depression of peripheral leukocytes is expected but is rarely sufficient (absolute neutrophil count less than 1000) to warrant discontinuation of therapy. Routine white blood cell counts each time the patient returns for a follow-up visit are not cost effective and do not allow the prediction of life-threatening events. The most informative time to repeat the white blood cell count is concurrently with a febrile illness.

Cognitive disturbances may occur within the therapeutic range. Sedation, ataxia, and nystagmus occur at toxic blood concentrations.

Clobazam (Onfi®, *Lundbeck*)

Indications. Seizures within the spectrum of Lennox-Gastaut, which includes all seizure types other than typical absence seizures.

Administration. For patients with less than 30 Kg of weight, the initial dosage is 5 mg daily titrating up to 20 mg daily (divided into two doses) as tolerated. For patients with more than 30 Kg of weight, the initial dosage is 10 mg daily titrating up to 40 mg daily (divided into two doses) as tolerated.

Adverse Effects. Sedation.

Clonazepam (Klonopin®, *Roche*)

Indications. Clonazepam treats infantile spasms, myoclonic seizures, absence, and partial seizures.

Administration. The initial dosage is 0.025 mg/kg/day in two divided doses. Recommended increments are 0.025 mg/kg every 3 to 5 days as needed and tolerated. The usual maintenance dosage is 0.1 mg/kg/day in three divided doses. Most children cannot tolerate dosages of more than 0.15 mg/kg/day. The therapeutic blood concentration is 0.02–0.07 µg/mL, 47 % of the drug is protein bound, and the half-life is 20–40 hours. Rectal administration is suitable for maintenance if needed.

Adverse Effects. Toxic effects with dosages within the therapeutic range include sedation, cognitive impairment, hyperactivity, and excessive salivation. Idiosyncratic reactions are unusual.

Ethosuximide (Zarontin®, *Pfizer*)

Indications. Ethosuximide is the drug of choice for treating absence epilepsy. It is also useful for myoclonic absence.

Administration. The drug is absorbed rapidly, and peak blood concentrations appear within 4 hours. The half-life is 30 hours in children and up to 60 hours in adults. The initial dosage is 20 mg/kg/day in three divided doses after meals to avoid gastric irritation. Dose increments of 10 mg/kg/day as needed and tolerated to provide seizure control without adverse effects. Levels between 50 and 120 μg/mL are usually therapeutic.

Adverse Effects. The common adverse reactions are nausea and abdominal pain. These symptoms occur from gastric irritation within the therapeutic range and limit the drug's usefulness. The liquid preparation causes more irritation than the capsule. Unfortunately, gel capsules are large and some young children refuse to try this option until older. Always take the medication after eating.

Felbamate (*Meda Pharmaceuticals*)

Indications. Felbamate has a wide spectrum of antiepileptic activity. Its primary use is for refractory partial and generalized seizures, the Lennox-Gastaut syndrome, atypical absence, and atonic seizures.

Administration. Felbamate is rapidly absorbed after oral intake. Maximal plasma concentrations occur in 2–6 hours. The initial dosage is 15 mg/kg/day in three divided doses. Avoid nighttime doses if the drug causes insomnia. To attain seizure control, use weekly dosage increments of 15 mg/kg, as needed, to a total dose of approximately 45 mg/kg/day. Toxicity limits the total dosage. Levels between 50 and 100 μg/mL are usually therapeutic.

Adverse Effects. Initial evidence suggested that adverse effects of felbamate were mild and dose related (nausea, anorexia, insomnia, weight loss) except when in combination with other antiepileptic drugs. The addition of felbamate increases the plasma concentrations of phenytoin and valproate as much as 30 %. The carbamazepine serum concentration falls, but the concentration of its active epoxide metabolite increases almost 50 %.

Post marketing experience showed that felbamate causes fatal liver damage and aplastic anemia in about 1 in 10,000 exposures. Regular monitoring of blood counts and liver function is required and may not help decrease these fatalities. However, this is a valuable drug in refractory epilepsy and has a place when used with caution and informed consent.

Gabapentin (Neurontin®, *Pfizer*)

Indications. Partial seizures with and without secondary generalization and neuropathic pain.

Administration. The usual titration dose is from 10 to 60 mg/kg/day, over two weeks. The mechanism of action is similar to pregabalin, but the efficacy is significantly lower.

Adverse Effects. The adverse effects are sedation, edema, increased weight.

Lacosamide (Vimpat®, *UCB Pharma*)

Indications. Partial seizures with and without secondary generalization.

Administration. The usual titration dose is from 2 to 10 mg/kg/day, over two to four weeks. The mechanism of action is on the sodium channel but different from the traditional sodium channel anticonvulsants.

Adverse Effects. The adverse effects are sedation, ataxia, dizziness.

Lamotrigine (Lamictal®, *GlaxoSmithKline*)

Indications. Lamotrigine is useful in absence epilepsy, atonic seizures, juvenile myoclonic epilepsy, the Lennox-Gastaut syndrome, partial epilepsies, and primary generalized tonic-clonic seizures (Biton et al, 2005). The spectrum of activity is similar to that of valproate.

Administration. The initial dose depends on whether the medication is used as monotherapy (0.3 mg/kg/day), combined with liver enzyme inducing drugs (0.6 mg/kg/day) or with valproate (0.15 mg/kg/day) for the first 2 weeks, then double the dose for 2 weeks and then increase by the same amount weekly until achieving doses of 1–3 mg/kg/day (with valproate), 5–7 mg/kg/day in monotherapy, and 5–15 mg/kg/day when added to liver enzyme inducers.

Plasma concentrations between 2 and 20 μg/mL are usually helpful in reducing or stopping seizures.

Adverse Effects. The main adverse reaction is rash, which is more likely with titrations faster than recommended. Other adverse effects are dizziness, ataxia, diplopia, insomnia and headache.

Levetiracetam (Keppra, *UCB Pharma*)

Indications. Levetiracetam has a broad spectrum of activity and is useful for most seizure types (Berkovic et al, 2007). It is especially effective in the treatment of juvenile myoclonic epilepsy (Sharpe et al, 2007; Noachtar et al, 2008). Its broad spectrum of activity, safety, and lack of drug–drug interactions make it an excellent first-line choice for most epilepsies.

Administration. Levetiracetam is available as a tablet, a suspension, and a solution for intravenous administration. The half-life is short, but the duration of efficacy is longer. Twice daily oral dosing is required. The initial dose in children is 20 mg/kg and the target dose is 20–80 mg/kg.

Adverse Effects. Levetiracetam is minimally liver metabolized. Metabolism occurs in the blood and excretion in the urine. It does not interfere with the metabolism of other drugs and has no life threatening side effects. It makes some children cranky. This was a rare event in the initial studies on the drug, but the incidence approaches 10%. The concomitant use of a small dose of pyridoxine, 50 mg once or twice a day, seems to relieve the irritability. The mechanism of action is probably an effect on GABA as its cofactor.

Oxcarbazepine (Trileptal®, *Novartis*)

Indications. Oxcarbazepine is the active breakdown product of carbamazepine. It has the same therapeutic profile as carbamazepine but much better tolerability and adverse effect profile.

Administration. Oxcarbazepine is available as a tablet and as a suspension. Twice daily dosing is required. The initial dose is 10 mg/kg and then incrementally increased, as needed, to a total dose of 20–60 mg/kg in two divided doses (Glausser et al, 2000; Piña-Garza et al, 2005).

Adverse Effects. The main adverse effect is drowsiness, but this is not as severe as with carbamazepine. Hyponatremia is a potential problem mainly in older populations.

Phenobarbital

Indications. Phenobarbital is effective for partial and generalized tonic-clonic seizures. It is especially useful to treat status epilepticus.

Administration. Oral absorption is slow, and once daily dosing is best when given with the evening meal than at bedtime if seizures are hypnagogic. Since intramuscular absorption requires 1 to 2 hours, the intramuscular route is useless for rapid loading (see Treatment of Status Epilepticus); 50% of the drug is protein bound, and 50% is free.

Initial and maintenance dosages are 3–5 mg/kg/day. The half-life is 50–140 hours in adults, 35–70 hours in children, and 50–200 hours in term newborns. Because of the very long half-life at all ages, once-a-day doses are usually satisfactory, achieving steady state blood concentrations after 2 weeks of therapy. Therapeutic blood concentrations are 15–40 µg/mL.

Adverse Effects. Hyperactivity is the most common and limiting side effect in children. Adverse behavioral changes occur in half of children between ages 2 and 10 years. Cognitive impairment is common. Hyperactivity and behavioral changes are both idiosyncratic and dose-related.

Stevens-Johnson syndrome is more likely when compared with other anticonvulsant agents. Drowsiness and cognitive dysfunction, rather than hyperactivity, are the usual adverse effects after 10 years of age. Allergic rash is the main idiosyncratic reaction.

Phenytoin (Dilantin®, *Pfizer US Pharmaceuticals*)

Indications. Phenytoin treats tonic-clonic and partial seizures.

Administration. Oral absorption is slow and unpredictable in newborns, erratic in infants, and probably not reliable until 3 to 5 years of age. Even in adults, considerable individual variability exists. Once absorbed, phenytoin is 70–95% protein bound. A typical maintenance dosage is 7 mg/kg/day in children. The half-life is up to 60 hours in term newborns, up to 140 hours in premature infants, 5–14 hours in children, and 10–34 hours in adults. Capsules usually require two divided doses, but tablets are more rapidly absorbed and may require three divided doses a day. Administration of three times the maintenance dose achieves rapid oral loading. Fosphenytoin sodium has replaced parenteral phenytoin (see discussion of Status Epilepticus).

Adverse Effects. The major adverse reactions are hypersensitivity, gum hypertrophy, and hirsutism. Hypersensitivity reactions usually occur within 6 weeks of the initiation of therapy. Rash, fever, and lymphadenopathy are characteristic. Once such a reaction has occurred, discontinue the drug. Concurrent use of antihistamines is not appropriate management. Continued use of the drug may produce a Stevens-Johnson syndrome or a lupus-like disorder.

The cause of gum hypertrophy is a combination of phenytoin metabolites and plaque on the teeth. Persons with good oral hygiene are unlikely to have gum hypertrophy. Discuss the importance of good oral hygiene at the onset of therapy. Hirsutism is rarely a problem, and then only for girls. Discontinue the drug when it occurs. Memory impairment, decreased attention span, and personality change may occur at therapeutic concentrations, but they occur less often and are less severe than with phenobarbital.

Pregabalin (Lyrica®, *Pfizer*)

Indications. Partial seizures with and without secondary generalization and neuropathic pain.

Administration. The usual titration dose is from 2 to 10 mg/kg/day, over two weeks. The mechanism of action is similar to gabapentin, but the efficacy is significantly higher.

Adverse Effects. The adverse effects are sedation, edema, increased weight.

Primidone (Mysoline®, *Valeant Pharmaceuticals*)

Indications. Mysoline treats tonic-clonic and partial seizures.

Administration. Primidone metabolizes to at least two active metabolites, phenobarbital and phenyl-ethyl-malonamide (PEMA). The half-life of primidone is 6–12 hours, and that of PEMA is 20 hours. The usual maintenance dosage is 10–25 mg/kg/day, but the initial dosage should be 25 % of the maintenance dosage or intolerable sedation occurs. A therapeutic blood concentration of primidone is 8–12 μg/mL. The blood concentration of phenobarbital derived from primidone is generally four times greater, but this ratio alters with concurrent administration of other antiepileptic drugs.

Adverse Effects. The adverse effects are the same as for phenobarbital, except that the risk of intolerable sedation from the first tablet is greater.

Rufinamide (Banzel®, *Eisai*)

Indications. Seizures within the spectrum of Lennox-Gastaut, which includes all seizure types other than typical absence seizures.

Administration. The initial dosage is 15 mg/Kg/day titrating up to 45 mg/Kg/day (divided into two doses) over two weeks.

Adverse Effects. Sedation, emesis and GI symptoms.

Tiagabine (Gabitril®, *Cephalon Inc.*)

Indications. Adjunctive therapy for partial-onset and generalized seizures.

Administration. The initial single-day dose is 0.2 mg/kg/day. Increase every 2 weeks by 0.2 mg/kg until achieving optimal benefit or adverse reactions occur.

Adverse Effects. The most common adverse effects are somnolence and difficulty concentrating.

Topiramate (Topamax®, *Ortho McNeil*)

Indications. Use for partial-onset and generalized epilepsies, especially the Lennox-Gastaut syndrome. It is also effective for migraine prophylaxis and a reasonable choice in children with both disorders.

Administration. The initial dose is 1–2 mg/kg/day, increased incrementally to up to 10–15 mg/kg/day divided into two doses.

Adverse Effects. Weight loss may occur at therapeutic dosages. When used in overweight children, this is no longer an "adverse" event. Cognitive impairment is common and often detected by relatives rather than the patient. Fatigue and altered mental status occur at toxic dosages. Glaucoma is a rare idiosyncratic reaction. Oligohydrosis is common, and the physician should advise patients to avoid overheating.

Valproate (Depakene®, Depakote®, and Depacon®, *Abbott Pharmaceutical*)

Indications. Use mainly for generalized seizures. It is especially useful for mixed seizure disorders. Included are myoclonic seizures, simple absence, myoclonic absence, myoclonus, and tonic-clonic seizures.

Administration. Oral absorption is rapid, and the half-life is 6–15 hours. Three times a day dosing of the liquid achieves constant blood concentrations. An enteric-coated capsule (Depakote and Depakote sprinkles) slows absorption and allows twice-a-day dosing in children.

The initial dosage is 20 mg/kg/day. Increments of 10 mg/kg/day to a dose of 60 mg/kg/day provide a blood concentration of 50–100 μg/mL. Blood concentrations of 80–120 μg/mL are often required to achieve seizure control. Protein binding is 95 % at blood concentrations of 50 μg/mL and 80 % at 100 μg/mL. Therefore doubling the blood concentration increases the free fraction eightfold. Valproate has a strong affinity for plasma proteins and displaces other antiepileptic drugs.

Valproate is available for intravenous use. A dose of 25 mg/kg leads to a serum level of 100 μg/mL. Maintenance should start 1 to 3 hours after loading at 20 mg/kg/day divided into two doses.

Adverse Effects. Valproate has dose-related and idiosyncratic hepatotoxicity. Dose-related hepatotoxicity is harmless and characterized by increased serum concentrations of transaminases. Important dose-related effects are a reduction in the platelet count, pancreatitis, and hyperammonemia. Thrombocytopenia may result in serious bleeding after trivial injury, while pancreatitis and hepatitis are both associated with nausea and vomiting. Hyperammonemia causes cognitive disturbances and nausea. These adverse reactions are reversible by reducing the daily dose. Reduced plasma carnitine concentrations occur in children taking valproate, and some believe that carnitine supplementation helps relieve cognitive impairment.

The major idiosyncratic reaction is fatal liver necrosis attributed to the production of an aberrant and toxic metabolite. The major risk (1:800) is in children younger than 2 years of age who are receiving polytherapy. Many such cases may result from the combination of valproate on an underlying inborn error of metabolism. Fatal hepatotoxicity is unlikely to occur in children over 10 years of age treated with valproate alone.

The clinical manifestations of idiosyncratic hepatotoxicity are similar to those of Reye syndrome (see Chapter 2). They may begin after 1 day of therapy or may not appear for 6 months. No reliable way exists to monitor patients for idiosyncratic hepatotoxicity or to predict its occurrence.

Vigabatrin (Sabril®, *Lundbeck*)

Indications. Effective treating infantile spasms and partial seizures.

Administration. Vigabatrin is a very-long-acting drug and needs only single day dosing, but twice daily dosing is preferable to reduce adverse effects. The initial dose is 50 mg/kg/day, which increases incrementally, as needed, to 200–250 mg/kg/day.

Adverse Effects. Peripheral loss of vision is the main serious adverse event. The defect is rare and consists of circumferential field constriction with nasal sparing. Behavioral problems, fatigue, confusion, and gastrointestinal upset are usually mild and dose related.

Zonisamide (Zonegran®, *Eisai Inc.*)

Indications. Like levetiracetam, zonisamide has a broad spectrum of activity. It is effective against both primary generalized and partial onset epilepsies and is one of the most effective drugs in myoclonic epilepsies.

Administration. Zonisamide is a long-acting drug and should be given once at bedtime. The initial dose in children is 2 mg/kg/day. The maximum dose is around 15 mg/kg/day.

Adverse Effects. Common adverse effects are drowsiness and anorexia. Of greater concern is the possibility of oligohydrosis and hyperthermia. Monitoring for decreased sweating and hyperthermia is required.

Management of Status Epilepticus

The definition of status epilepticus is a prolonged single seizure (longer than 30 minutes) or repeated seizures without interictal recovery. Generalized tonic-clonic status is life threatening and the most common emergency in pediatric neurology. The prognosis after status epilepticus in newborns is invariably poor (Pisani et al, 2007). The causes of status epilepticus are: (1) a new acute illness such as encephalitis; (2) a progressive neurological disease; (3) loss of seizure control in a known epileptic; or (4) a febrile seizure in an otherwise normal child. The cause is the main determinate of outcome. Recurrence of status epilepticus is most likely in children who are neurologically abnormal and is rare in children with febrile seizures. The assessment of status epilepticus in children is the subject of a Practice Parameter of the Child Neurology Society (Rivello et al, 2006).

Absence status and complex partial status are often difficult to identify as status epilepticus. The child may appear to be in a confusional state.

Immediate Management

Home management of prolonged seizures or clusters of seizures in children with known epilepsy is possible using rectal diazepam to prevent or abort status epilepticus (O'Dell et al, 2005). A rectal diazepam gel is commercially available, or the intravenous preparation can be given rectally. The dose is 0.5 mg/kg for children age 2 to 5 years, 0.3 mg/kg for children age 6 to 12, and 0.2 mg/kg for children >12 years with an upper limit of 20 mg. If the rectal dose fails to stop the seizures, a second dose is recommended 10 minutes after the first dose and hospital emergency services are required. Status epilepticus is a medical emergency requiring prompt attention. Initial assessment should be rapid and includes cardiorespiratory function, a history leading up to the seizure, and a neurological examination. Establish a controlled airway immediately and ventilate. Next, establish venous access. Measures of blood glucose, electrolytes, and anticonvulsant drug concentrations in children with known epilepsy are required. Perform other tests, i.e., a toxic screen, as indicated. Once blood is withdrawn, start an intravenous infusion of saline solution for the administration of anticonvulsant drugs and the administration of an intravenous bolus of a 50% glucose solution, 1 mg/kg.

Drug Treatment

The ideal drug for treating status epilepticus is one that acts rapidly, has a long duration of action, and does not produce sedation. The use of benzodiazepines (diazepam and lorazepam) for this purpose is common. However, they are inadequate by themselves because their duration of action is brief. In addition, children given intravenous benzodiazepines after a prior load of barbiturate often have respiratory depression. The dose of diazepam is 0.2 mg/kg, not to exceed 10 mg at a rate of 1 mg/min. Lorazepam may be preferable to diazepam because of its longer duration of action. The usual dosage in children 12 years of age or younger is 0.1 mg/kg. After age 12 years, it is 0.07 mg/kg.

Intravenous fosphenytoin is an ideal agent because it has a long duration of action, does not produce respiratory depression, and does not impair consciousness. The initial dose is 20 mg/kg (calculated as phenytoin equivalents). Administration can be intravenous or intramuscular, but the intravenous route is greatly preferred. Unlike phenytoin, which requires slow infusions (0.5 mg/kg/min) to avoid cardiac toxicity, fosphenytoin infusions are rapid and often obviate the need for prior benzodiazepine therapy. Infants generally require 30 mg/kg.

Fosphenytoin is usually effective unless a severe, acute encephalopathy is the cause of status. Children who fail to wake up at an expected time after the clinical signs of status have stopped require an EEG to exclude the possibility of electrical status epilepticus.

Intravenous levetiracetam, 20–40 mg/kg, is an excellent alternative to fosphenytoin, because it

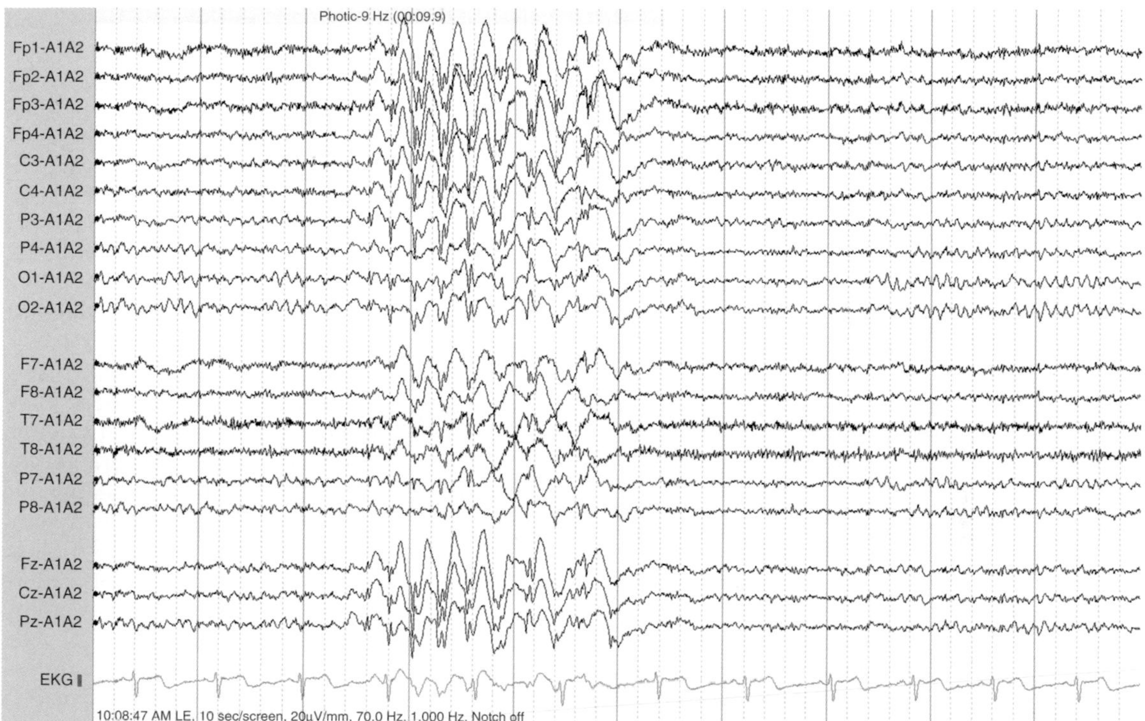

FIGURE 1-4 ■ Juvenile myoclonic epilepsy: 4.7 Hz generalized spike and slow wave discharge lasting 2.5 seconds during photic stimulation.

does not require hepatic metabolism, has minimal interactions, is not cardiotoxic, and can be infused faster; however, it has not undergone the testing to be universally accepted in status protocols. Other attractive options before pentobarbital or midazolam induced coma include lacosamide and Depacon.

When all else fails, several alternatives are available; my preference is pentobarbital coma. Transfer the patient from the emergency department to an intensive care unit. Intubation and mechanically ventilation must be in place. After placing an arterial line, monitor the patient's blood pressure, cardiac rhythm, body temperature, and blood oxygen saturation.

With an EEG monitor recording continuously, infuse 10 mg/kg boluses of pentobarbital until a burst-suppression pattern appears on the EEG (Figure 1-4); a minimum of 30 mg/kg is generally required. Hypotension is the most serious complication and requires treatment with vasopressors. It generally does not occur until after the administration of 40–60 mg/kg. Barbiturates tend to accumulate, and the usual dosage needed to maintain pentobarbital coma is 3 mg/kg/h. Maintaining coma for several days is safe. Continuous EEG recording indicates a burst-suppression pattern. Slow or stop the barbiturate infusion every 24 to 48 hours to see if coma is still required to prevent seizure discharges.

The Ketogenic Diet

The Bible mentions fasting and praying as a treatment for epilepsy. The introduction of diet-induced ketosis to mimic fasting dates to 1921, when barbiturates and bromides were the only available antiepileptic drugs. This method became less popular with the introduction of effective pharmacotherapy. However, it remains an effective method to treat children with seizures refractory to antiepileptic drugs at nontoxic levels. The diet is most effective in infants and young children. A diet that consists of 60% medium-chain triglycerides, 11% long-chain saturated fat, 10% protein, and 19% carbohydrate is commonly used. The main side effects are abdominal pain and diarrhea (Nordli, 2002).

The ketogenic diet causes a prompt elevation in plasma ketone bodies that the brain uses as an energy source. The mechanism of action is not established. The ketogenic diet is most effective for control of myoclonic seizures, infantile spasms, atonic/akinetic seizures, and mixed seizures of the Lennox-Gastaut syndrome. The ketogenic diet is not a "natural" treatment for epilepsy. Side effects are common and alterations in chemistries are more significant than with the use of medications; however, it is a good alternative when epilepsy is not controlled or medications are not tolerated.

Vagal Nerve Stimulation

VNS is a treatment for refractory seizures that uses a programmed stimulus from a chest-implanted generator via coiled electrodes tunneled to the left cervical vagus nerve. Current indications for VNS are for adjunctive treatment of refractory partial seizures. The main adverse effects are voice changes or hoarseness. The ketogenic diet is preferable to VNS in children less than 12 years of age (Wheless & Maggio, 2002). However, VNS is a consideration in children with refractory epilepsy. Many patients seem to have shorter postictal periods and improved mood with this therapy. A 30–40 % reduction in seizures is in general a reasonable expectation.

Surgical Approaches to Childhood Epilepsy

Epilepsy surgery is an excellent option for selected children with intractable epilepsy. Surgery is never a substitute for good medical therapy, and antiepileptic drug therapy often continues after surgery. Lesionectomies, hemispherectomy, interhemispheric commissurotomy, and temporal lobectomy or hippocampectomy are appropriate for different situations. None of these procedures is new, and all have gone through phases of greater or lesser popularity since their introduction. The use of functional MRI, Wada test, single-photon emission computed tomography (SPECT), positron emission tomography (PET), and magnetoencephalography (MEG), when indicated, improves the localization of the epileptogenic foci and the surgical outcomes.

Lesionectomy, Temporal Lobectomy or Hippocampectomy

The resection of an epileptogenic lesion may be needed for diagnosis when neoplasms are suspected. Lesionectomy is often an excellent treatment choice for epilepsies resistant to medical treatment when the MRI shows an underlying structural abnormality in the focus of seizures. Around 80 % of patients with well-circumscribed unifocal epilepsies associated with lesions may remain seizure free after surgical resections. The hippocampus or the temporal lobe are often the target of a potential epilepsy surgery. The success rate decreases in cases where the MRI shows no underlying abnormality or the patient has multiple seizure semiologies and multifocal epilepsies.

Hemispherectomy

The use of hemispherectomy, or more correctly hemidecortication, is exclusively for children with intractable epilepsy and hemiplegia. The original procedure consisted of removing the cortex of one hemisphere along with a variable portion of the underlying basal ganglia. The extent of surgery depended partly upon the underlying disease. The resulting cavity communicated with the third ventricle and developed a subdural membrane lining. The immediate results were good. Seizures were relieved in about 80 % of children, and behavior and spasticity improved without deterioration of intellectual function or motor function in the hemiparetic limbs.

However, late complications of hemorrhage, hydrocephalus, and hemosiderosis occurred in up to 35 % of children and were sometimes fatal. The subdural membrane repeatedly tore, bleeding into the ventricular system and staining the ependymal lining and the pia arachnoid with iron.

Because of these complications, less radical alternatives are generally preferred. These alternatives are the Montreal-type hemispherectomy and interhemispheric commissurotomy. The Montreal-type hemispherectomy is a modified procedure with removal of most of the damaged hemisphere but with portions of the frontal and occipital lobes left in place, but disconnected from the other hemisphere and brainstem. The best results are in children with diseases affecting only one hemisphere, Sturge-Weber syndrome (Kossoff et al, 2002), and Rasmussen encephalitis (Kossoff et al, 2003).

Interhemispheric Commissurotomy

Disconnecting the hemispheres from each other and from the brainstem is an alternative to hemispherectomy in children with intractable epilepsy and hemiplegia. Another use of this procedure is to decrease the occurrence of secondary generalized tonic-clonic seizures from partial or minor generalized seizures. The efficacy of commissurotomy and hemispherectomy in children with infantile hemiplegia is probably comparable, but efficacy of commissurotomy in other forms of epilepsy is unknown.

Complete and partial commissurotomies are in use. Complete commissurotomy entails division of the entire corpus callosum, anterior commissure, one fornix, and the hippocampal commissure. Complete commissurotomies may be one-or two-stage procedures. Partial commissurotomies vary from division of the corpus callosum and hippocampal commissure to division of only the anterior portion of the corpus callosum.

Two immediate, but transitory, postoperative complications may follow interhemispheric commissurotomy: (1) a syndrome of mutism, left arm and leg apraxia, and urinary incontinence;

and (2) hemiparesis. They are both more common after one-stage, complete commissurotomy than after two-stage procedures or partial commissurotomy and probably caused by prolonged retraction of one hemisphere during surgery. Long-term complications may include stuttering and poorly coordinated movements of the hands.

REFERENCES

Archer JS, Briellmann RS, Syngeniotis A, et al. Spike-triggered fMRI in reading epilepsy. Involvement of left frontal cortex working memory area. Neurology 2003;60:415–21.

Berkovic SF, Kowlton RC, Leroy RF, et al. Placebo-controlled study of levetiracetam in idiopathic generalized epilepsy. Neurology 2007;69:1751–60.

Biton V, Sackellares JC, Vuong A, et al. Double-blind, placebo controlled study of lamotrigine in primary generalized tonic-clonic seizures. Neurology 2005;65:1737–43.

Burn J. Closing time for CATCH22. Journal of Medical Genetics 1999;36:737–8.

Camfield P, Camfield C. Epileptic syndromes in childhood: clinical features, outcomes, and treatment. Epilepsia 2002;43:27–32.

Carpio A, Hauser WA. Prognosis for seizure recurrence in patients with newly diagnosed neurocysticercosis. Neurology 2002;59:1730–4.

Connolly MB, Langill L, Wong PKH, et al. Seizures involving the supplementary sensorimotor area in children: A video-EEG analysis. Epilepsia 1995;36:1025–32.

Crest C, Dupont S, Leguern E, et al. Levetiracetam in progressive myoclonic epilepsy. An exploratory study in 9 patients. Neurology 2004;62:640–3.

Dravet C. Les epilepsies graves de l'enfant. Vie Med 1978;8:543–8.

De Koning Tijssen, Rees MI. Hyperekplexia. In: GeneClinics: Medical Genetics Knowledge Base (Database Online). Seattle: University of Washington. Available at http://www.geneclinics.org. PMID: 20301437. Last updated May 19, 2009.

Dulac O. Epileptic encephalopathy. Epilepsia 2001;92 (Suppl 3):23–6.

Freed GE, Martinez F. Atypical seizures as the cause of apnea in a six-month old child. Clinical Pediatrics 2001;40:283–5.

Furwentsches A, Bussmann C, Ramantani G, et al. Levetiracetam in the treatment of neonatal seizures: A pilot study. Seizure 2010;19:185–9.

Glausser TA, Nigro M, Sachdeo R, et al. Adjunctive therapy with oxcarbazepine in children with partial seizures. Neurology 2000;54(12):2237–44.

Gluckman PD, Wyatt JS, Azzopardi D, et al. Selective head cooling with mild systemic hypothermia after neonatal encephalopathy: Multicenter randomized trial. Lancet 2005;365:663–70.

Gospe SM. Pyridoxine-dependent epilepsy. In: GeneClinics: Medical Genetics Knowledge Base [database online]. Seattle: University of Washington. Available at http://www.geneclinics.org. PMID: 20301659. Last updated April 26, 2012.

Granata T, Fusco L, Gobbi G, et al. Experience with immunomodulating treatments in Rasmussen's encephalitis. Neurology 2003a;61:1807–10.

Granata T, Gobbi G, Spreaficio, et al. Rasmussen's encephalitis. Early characteristics allows diagnosis. Neurology 2003b;60:422–5.

Guilleminault C, Palombini L, Pelayo R, et al. Sleepwalking and sleep terrors in prepubertal children: What triggers them? Pediatrics 2003;111:e17–25.

Gümüs H, Kumandas S, Per H. Levetiracetam monotherapy in newly diagnosed cryptogenic West syndrome. Pediatric Neurology 2007;37:350–3.

Hamosh A. Glycine encephalopathy. In: GeneClinics: Medical Genetics Knowledge Base [database online]. Seattle: University of Washington. Available at http://www.geneclinics.org. PMID: 20301531. Last updated November 24, 2009.

Hirtz D, Berg A, Bettis D, et al. Practice parameter: Treatment of the child with a first unprovoked seizure. Report of the Quality Standards Subcommittee of the American Academy of Neurology and the Practice Committee of the Child Neurology Society. Neurology 2003;60:166–75.

Jansen AC, Andermann E. Progressive myoclonus epilepsy, Lafora type. In: GeneClinics: Medical Genetics Knowledge Base [database online]. Seattle: University of Washington. Available at http://www.geneclinics.org. PMID: 20301563. Last updated November 3, 2011.

Jarrar RG, Buchhalter JR, Meyer FB, et al. Long-term follow-up of temporal lobectomy in children. Neurology 2002;59:1635–7.

Korff CM, Nordli DR Jr. Epilepsy syndromes in infancy. Pediatric Neurology 2006;34:253–63.

Kossoff EH, Buck C, Freeman JM. Outcomes of 32 hemispherectomies for Sturge-Weber syndrome worldwide. Neurology 2002;59:1735–8.

Kossoff EH, Boatman D, Freeman JM. Landau-Kleffner syndrome responsive to levetiracetam. Epilepsy and Behavior 2003a;4:571–5.

Kossoff EH, Vining EPG, Pillas DJ, et al. Hemispherectomy for intractable unihemispheric epilepsy. Etiology vs outcome. Neurology 2003b;61:887–90.

Lehesjoki A-E, Koskiniemi M-L. Unverricht-Lundborg Disease. In: GeneClinics: Medical Genetics Knowledge Base [database online]. Seattle: University of Washington. Available at http://www.geneclinics.org. PMID 20301321. Last updated June 18, 2009.

Lotze TE, Wilfong AA. Zonisamide treatment for symptomatic infantile spasms. Neurology 2004;62:296–8.

Mackay MT, Weiss SK, Adams-Webber T, et al. Practice parameter: Medical treatment of infantile spasms. Report of the American Academy of Neurology and the Child Neurology Society. Neurology 2004;62:1668–81.

McDonald-McGinn DM, Emanuel MS, Zackai EH. 22q11.2 deletion syndrome. In: GeneClinics: Medical Genetics Knowledge Base [database online]. Seattle: University of Washington. Available at http://www.geneclinics.org. PMID: 20301696. Last updated December 16, 2005.

Mikati MA, El Bannan D, Sinno D, et al. Response of infantile spasms to levetiracetam. Neurology 2008;70:574–5.

Miller SP, Ramaswamy V, Michelson D, et al. Patterns of brain injury in term neonatal encephalopathy. Journal of Pediatrics 2005;146:453–60.

Minewer M. New evidence for a genetic link between epilepsy and migraine. Neurology 2007;68:1969–70.

Munchau A, Shahidi GA, Eunson LH, et al. A new family with paroxysmal exercise induced dystonia and migraine: a clinical and genetic study. Journal of Neurology, Neurosurgery and Psychiatry 2000;68:609–14.

Nicolai J, Aldenkamp AP, Arends J, et al. Cognitive and behavioral effects of nocturnal epileptiform discharges in children with benign childhood epilepsy with centrotemporal spikes. Epilepsy and Behavior 2006;8:56–70.

Nishino S. Clinical and neurobiological aspects of narcolepsy. Sleep Medicine 2007;8:373–99.

Noachtar S, Andermann E, Meyvisch P, et al. Levetiracetam for the treatment of idiopathic generalized epilepsy with myoclonic seizures. Neurology 2008;70:607–16.

Norcliffe-Kaufman IJ, Kaufman H, Hainsworth R. Enhanced vascular response to hypocapnia in neutrally mediated syncope. Annals of Neurology 2008;63:288–94.

Nordli D. The ketogenic diet, Uses and abuses. Neurology 2002;58(Suppl 7):S21–3.

O'Dell C, Shinnar S, Ballaban-Gil KR, et al. Rectal diazepam gel in the home management of seizures in children. Pediatric Neurology 2005;33:166–72.

Painter MJ. Phenobarbital compared with phenytoin for the treatment of neonatal seizures. New England Journal of Medicine 1999;341:485.

Panayiotopoulos CP. Extraoccipital benign childhood partial seizures with ictal vomiting and excellent prognosis. Journal of Neurology, Neurosurgery and Psychiatry 1999;66:82–5.

Parisi P, Bombardieri R, Curatolo P. Current role of vigabatrin infantile spasms. European Journal of Paediatric Neurology 2007;11:331–6.

Piña-Garza JE, Espinoza R, Nordli D, et al. Oxcarbazepine adjunctive therapy in infants and young children with partial seizures. Neurology 2005;65:1370–5.

Piña-Garza JE, Levinson P, Gucuyener K, et al. Adjunctive lamotrigine for partial seizures in patients ages 1 to 24 months old. Neurology 2008a;70(22, pt 2):2099–108.

Piña-Garza JE, Elterman RD, Ayala R, et al. Long term tolerability and efficacy of lamotrigine in infants 1 to 24 months old. Journal of Child Neurology 2008b;23(8):853–61.

Piña-Garza JE, Nordli D, Rating D, et al. Adjunctive levetiracetam in infants and young children with refractory partial-onset seizures. Epilepsia 2009;50(5):1141–9.

Piña-Garza JE, Schiemann-Delgado J, Yang H, Duncan B. Adjunctive levetiracetam in patients age 1 month to <4 years with partial onset seizures; an open label long term follow-up. Clinical Therapeutics 2010;32:1935–50.

Pisani F, Cerminara C, Fuscio C, et al. Neonatal status epilepticus vs. recurrent neonatal seizures. Clinical findings and outcome. Neurology 2007;69:2177–85.

Porter BE, Judkins AR, Clancy RR, et al. Dysplasia. A common finding in intractable pediatric temporal lobe epilepsy. Neurology 2003;61:365–8.

Rivello JJ, Ashwal S, Hirtz D, et al. Practice parameter: Diagnostic assessment of the child with status epilepticus (an evidence based review). Report of the Quality Standards Subcommittee of the American academy of Neurology and the Child Neurology Society. Neurology 2006;67:1542–50.

Ronen GM, Buckley D, Penney S, et al. Long-term prognosis in children with neonatal seizures. A population study. Neurology 2007;69:1816–22.

Scheuerle AE. Incontinentia pigmenti. In: GeneClinics: Medical Genetics Knowledge Base [database online]. Seattle: University of Washington. Available at http://www.geneclinics.org. PMID: 20301645. Last updated October 28, 2010.

Seashore M. Organic acidemias: An overview. In: GeneClinics: Medical Genetics Knowledge Base [database online]. Seattle: University of Washington. Available at http://www.geneclinics.org. PMID: 20301313. Last updated December 22, 2009.

Scammell TE. The neurobiology, diagnosis, and treatment of narcolepsy. Annals of Neurology 2003;53:154–60.

Sharpe DV, Patel AD, Abou-Khalil B, et al. Levetiracetam monotherapy in juvenile myoclonic epilepsy. Seizure 2008;17:64–8.

Silverstein FS, Jensen FE. Neonatal seizures. Annals of Neurology 2007;62:112–20.

Spacey S, Adams P. Familial nonkinesiogenic dyskinesia. In: GeneClinics: Medical Genetics Knowledge Base [database online]. Seattle: University of Washington. Available at http://www.geneclinics.org. PMID: 20301400. Last updated May 3, 2011.

Striano P, Coppola A, Pezzella M, et al. An open-label trial of levetiracetam in severe myoclonic epilepsy of infancy. Neurology 2007;69:250–4.

Summar ML. Urea cycle disorders overview. In: GeneClinics: Medical Genetics Knowledge Base [database online]. Seattle: University of Washington. Available at http://www.geneclinics.org. PMID: 20301396. Last updated September 1, 2011.

Sutton VR, Van den Veyver IB. Aicardi syndrome. In: GeneClinics: Medical Genetics Knowledge Base [database online]. Seattle: University of Washington. Available at http://www.geneclinics.org. PMID: 20301555. Last updated April 27, 2010.

Strauss KA, Puffenberger EG, Holmes Morton D. Maple syrup urine disease. In: GeneClinics: Medical Genetics Knowledge Base [database online]. Seattle: University of Washington. Available at http://www.geneclinics.org. PMID: 20301495. Last updated December 15, 2009.

Tarkka R, Paakko E, Pyhtinen J, et al. Febrile seizures and mesial temporal sclerosis. No association in a long-term follow-up study. Neurology 2003;60:215–8.

Torres OA, Miller VS, Buist NMR, Hyland K. Folinic acid-responsive neonatal seizures. Journal of Child Neurology 1999;14:529.

Van Hove JLK, Kishnani P, Muenzer J, et al. Benzoate therapy and carnitine deficiency in non-ketotic hyperglycinemia. American Journal of Medical Genetics 1995;59:444–53.

Wheless JW, Kim HL. Adolescent seizures and epilepsy syndromes. Epilepsia 2002;43:33–52.

Wheless JW, Maggio V. Vagus nerve stimulation therapy in patiets younger than 18 years. Neurology 2002;59(Suppl 4):S21–5.

Wolf B. Biotinidase deficiency. In: GeneClinics: Medical Genetics Knowledge Base [database online]. Seattle: University of Washington. Available at http://www.geneclinic.org. PMID: 20301497. Last updated March 15, 2011.

Yang JY, Chan AK, Callen DJ, Paes BA. Neonatal cerebral sinovenous thrombosis: sifting the evidence for a diagnostic plan and treatment strategy. Pediatrics 2010;126:e693–700.

Zimprich F, Ronen GM, Stogmann W, et al. Andreas Rett and benign familial neonatal convulsions revisited. Neurology 2006;67:864–6.

CHAPTER 2

Altered States of Consciousness

The terms used to describe states of decreased consciousness are listed in Table 2-1. With the exception of *coma*, these definitions are not standard. However, they are more precise and therefore more useful than such terms as *semicomatose* and *semistuporous*. The term *encephalopathy* describes a diffuse disorder of the brain in which at least two of the following symptoms are present: (1) altered states of consciousness; (2) altered cognition or personality; and (3) seizures. *Encephalitis* is an encephalopathy accompanied by inflammation and usually cerebrospinal fluid pleocytosis.

Lack of responsiveness is not always lack of consciousness. For example, infants with botulism (see Chapter 6) may have such severe hypotonia and ptosis that they cannot move their limbs or eyelids in response to stimulation. They appear to be in a coma or stupor but are actually alert. The *locked-in syndrome* (a brainstem disorder in which the individual can process information but cannot respond) and catatonia are other examples of diminished responsiveness in the alert state. Lack of responsiveness is also common in psychogenic spells, and transient lack of responsiveness may be seen in children with inattentiveness or obsessive-compulsive traits.

Either increased or decreased neuronal excitability may characterize the progression from consciousness to coma. Patients with increased neuronal excitability (the *high road to coma*) become restless and then confused; next, tremor, hallucinations, and delirium (an agitated confusional state) develop. Myoclonic jerks may occur. Seizures herald the end of delirium and stupor or coma follow. Box 2-1 summarizes the differential diagnosis of the high road to coma. Tumors and other mass lesions are not expected causes. Instead, metabolic, toxic, and inflammatory disorders are likely.

Decreased neuronal excitability (the *low road to coma*) lacks an agitated stage. Instead, awareness progressively deteriorates from lethargy to obtundation, to stupor, and to coma. The differential diagnosis is considerably larger than that with the high road and includes mass lesions and other causes of increased intracranial pressure (Box 2-2). Box 2-3 lists conditions that cause recurrent encephalopathies. A comparison of Box 2-1 and Box 2-2 shows considerable overlap between conditions whose initial features are agitation and confusion and those that begin with lethargy and coma; therefore the disorders responsible for each are described together to prevent repetition.

TABLE 2-1 States of Decreased Consciousness

Term	Definition
Lethargy	Difficult to maintain the aroused state
Obtundation	Responsive to stimulation other than pain*
Stupor	Responsive only to pain*
Coma	Unresponsive to pain

*Responsive indicates cerebral alerting, not just reflex withdrawal.

DIAGNOSTIC APPROACH TO DELIRIUM

Assume that any child with the acute behavioral changes of delirium (agitation, confusion, delusions, or hallucinations) has an organic encephalopathy until proven otherwise. The usual causes of delirium are toxic or metabolic disorders diffusely affecting both cerebral hemispheres. Schizophrenia should not be a consideration in a prepubertal child with acute delirium. Fixed beliefs, unalterable by reason, are *delusions*. The paranoid delusions of schizophrenia are logical to the patient and frequently part of an elaborate system of irrational thinking in which the patient feels menaced. Delusions associated with organic encephalopathy are less logical, not systematized, and tend to be stereotyped.

An *hallucination* is the perception of sensory stimuli that are not present. Organic encephalopathies usually cause visual hallucinations while psychiatric illness usually causes auditory hallucinations, especially if the voices are accusatory. Stereotyped auditory hallucinations that represent a recurring memory are an exception and suggest temporal lobe seizures. Organic encephalopathies usually are associated with less formed and more stereotyped auditory or visual hallucinations.

BOX 2-1 Causes of Agitation and Confusion

EPILEPTIC

- Absence status* (see Chapter 1)
- Complex partial seizure* (see Chapter 1)
- Epileptic encephalopathies*

INFECTIOUS DISORDERS

- Bacterial infections
  - Cat scratch disease*
  - Meningitis* (see Chapter 4)
- Rickettsial infections
  - Lyme disease*
  - Rocky Mountain spotted fever*
- Viral infections
  - Arboviruses
  - Aseptic meningitis
  - Herpes simplex encephalitis*
  - Measles encephalitis
  - Postinfectious encephalomyelitis
  - Reye syndrome

METABOLIC AND SYSTEMIC DISORDERS

- Disorders of osmolality
  - Hypoglycemia*
  - Hyponatremia*
- Endocrine disorders
  - Adrenal insufficiency*
  - Hypoparathyroidism*
  - Thyroid disorders*
- Hepatic encephalopathy
- Inborn errors of metabolism
  - Disorders of pyruvate metabolism (see Chapter 5)
  - Medium-chain acyl-CoA dehydrogenase (MCAD) deficiency
  - Respiratory chain disorders (see Chapters 5, 6, 8, 10)
  - Urea cycle disorder, heterozygote (see Chapter 1)
- Renal disease
  - Hypertensive encephalopathy*
  - Uremic encephalopathy*

MIGRAINE

- Acute confusional*
- Aphasic*
- Transient global amnesia*

PSYCHOLOGICAL

- Panic disorder*
- Schizophrenia

TOXIC

- Immunosuppressive drugs*
- Prescription drugs*
- Substance abuse*
- Toxins*

VASCULAR

- Congestive heart failure*
- Embolism*
- Hypertensive encephalopathy*
- Lupus erythematosus*
- Anti-NMDA antibody encephalitis†
- Subarachnoid hemorrhage*
- Vasculitis*

*Denotes the most common conditions and the ones with disease modifying treatments
†NMDA, **N-methyl-D-aspartate**

BOX 2-2 Causes of Lethargy and Coma

EPILEPSY

- Epileptic encephalopathies
- Postictal state (see Chapter 1)
- Status epilepticus (see Chapter 1)

HYPOXIA-ISCHEMIA

- Cardiac arrest
- Cardiac arrhythmia
- Congestive heart failure
- Hypotension
  - Autonomic dysfunction
  - Dehydration
  - Hemorrhage
  - Pulmonary embolism
- Near-drowning
- Neonatal (see Chapter 1)

INCREASED INTRACRANIAL PRESSURE

- Cerebral abscess (see Chapter 4)
- Cerebral edema (see Chapter 4)
- Cerebral tumor (see Chapters 4 and 10)
- Herniation syndromes (see Chapter 4)
- Hydrocephalus (see Chapters 4 and 18)
- Intracranial hemorrhage
  - Spontaneous (see Chapter 4)
  - Traumatic

INFECTIOUS DISORDERS

- Bacterial infections
  - Cat scratch disease*
  - Gram-negative sepsis*
  - Hemorrhagic shock and encephalopathy syndrome*
  - Meningitis (see Chapter 4)*
  - Toxic shock syndrome
- Postimmunization encephalopathy
- Rickettsial infections
  - Lyme disease*
  - Rocky Mountain spotted fever*
- Viral infections
  - Arboviruses
  - Aseptic meningitis
  - Herpes simplex encephalitis
  - Measles encephalitis

BOX 2-2 Causes of Lethargy and Coma—cont'd

- Postinfectious encephalomyelitis
- Reye syndrome

METABOLIC AND SYSTEMIC DISORDERS

- Disorders of osmolality
  - Diabetic ketoacidosis (hyperglycemia)
  - Hypoglycemia
  - Hypernatremia
  - Hyponatremia
- Endocrine disorders
  - Adrenal insufficiency
  - Hypoparathyroidism
  - Thyroid disorders
- Hepatic encephalopathy
- Inborn errors of metabolism
  - Disorders of pyruvate metabolism (see Chapter 5)
  - Glycogen storage disorders (see Chapter 1)
  - Medium-chain acyl-CoA dehydrogenase (MCAD) deficiency
  - Respiratory chain disorders (see Chapter 5, 6, 8, 10)
  - Urea cycle disorder, heterozygote (see Chapter 1)
- Renal disorders
  - Acute uremic encephalopathy
  - Chronic uremic encephalopathy
  - Dialysis encephalopathy
  - Hypertensive encephalopathy
- Other metabolic disorders
  - Burn encephalopathy
  - Hypomagnesemia
  - Parenteral hyperalimentation
  - Vitamin B complex deficiency

MIGRAINE COMA

- Toxic
  - Immunosuppressive drugs*
  - Prescription drugs*
  - Substance abuse*
  - Toxins*
- Trauma
  - Concussion
  - Contusion
  - Intracranial hemorrhage
    - Epidural hematoma
    - Subdural hematoma
    - Intracerebral hemorrhage
  - Neonatal (see Chapter 1)
- Vascular
  - Hypertensive encephalopathy*
  - Intracranial hemorrhage, nontraumatic* (see Chapter 4)
  - Lupus erythematosus* (see Chapter 11)
  - Neonatal idiopathic cerebral venous thrombosis (see Chapter 1)
  - Vasculitis* (see Chapter 11)

*Denotes the most common conditions and the ones with disease modifying treatments

BOX 2-3 Causes of Recurrent Encephalopathy

- Burn encephalopathy
- Epileptic encephalopathies*
- Hashimoto encephalopathy*
- Hypoglycemia*
- Increased intracranial pressure* (recurrent)
- Medium-chain acyl-CoA dehydrogenase (MCAD) deficiency
- Mental disorders
- Migraine
- Mitochondrial disorders
- Pyruvate metabolism disorders
- Substance abuse
- Urea cycle disorder

*Denotes the most common conditions and the ones with disease modifying treatments

History and Physical Examination

Delirious children, even with stable vital function, require rapid assessment because the potential for deterioration to a state of diminished consciousness is real. Obtain a careful history of the following: (1) the events leading to the behavioral change; (2) drug or toxic exposure (prescription drugs are more often at fault than substances of abuse, and a medicine cabinet inspection should be ordered in every home the child has visited); (3) a personal or family history of migraine or epilepsy; (4) recent or concurrent fever, infectious disease, or systemic illness; and (5) a previous personal or family history of encephalopathy.

Examination of the eyes, in addition to determining the presence or absence of disc edema, provides other etiological clues. Small or large pupils that respond poorly to light, nystagmus, or impaired eye movements suggest a drug or toxic exposure. Fixed deviation of the eyes in one lateral direction may indicate seizure or a significant loss of function in one hemisphere. The general and neurological examinations should specifically include a search for evidence of trauma, needle marks on the limbs, meningismus, lymphadenopathy, and cardiac disease.

Laboratory Investigations

Individualize laboratory evaluation; not every test is essential for each clinical situation. Studies of potential interest include culture; complete blood count; sedimentation rate; urine drug screening; blood concentrations of glucose, electrolytes, calcium and phosphorus, urea nitrogen, ammonia, liver enzymes, thyroid-stimulating hormone, thyroid antibodies, and liver enzymes. If possible, obtain computed tomography (CT) of the head while the results of these tests are pending. If sedation is required to perform the study, a short-acting benzodiazepine is preferred. Nondiagnostic blood studies and normal CT results are an indication for lumbar puncture to look for infection or increased intracranial pressure. A manometer should always be available to measure cerebrospinal fluid pressure.

An electroencephalogram (EEG) is useful in the evaluation of altered mentation. Acute organic encephalopathies will show, at least, a decreased speed in the occipital dominant rhythm during the waking state. The EEG is often normal in psychiatric illnesses. Diffuse theta and delta activity, absence of faster frequencies, and intermittent rhythmic delta activity are characteristic of severe encephalopathies. Specific abnormalities may include epileptiform activity consistent with absence or complex partial status; triphasic waves indicating hepatic, uremic or other toxic encephalopathy; and periodic lateralizing epileptiform discharges in one temporal lobe, suggesting herpes encephalitis.

DIAGNOSTIC APPROACH TO LETHARGY AND COMA

The diagnostic approach to states of diminished consciousness in children is similar to that suggested for delirium, except for greater urgency. The causes of progressive decline in the state of consciousness are diffuse or multifocal disturbances of the cerebral hemispheres or focal injury to the brainstem. Physical examination reveals the anatomic site of abnormality in the brain.

History and Physical Examination

Obtain the same historical data as for delirium, except that mass lesions are an important consideration. Inquire further concerning trauma or preceding symptoms of increasing intracranial pressure. Direct the physical examination at determining both the anatomical site of disturbed cerebral function and its cause. The important variables in locating the site of abnormality are state of consciousness, pattern of breathing, pupillary size and reactivity, eye movements, and motor responses. The cause of lethargy and obtundation is usually mild depression of hemispheric function. Stupor and coma are characteristic of much more extensive disturbance of hemispheric function or involvement of the diencephalon and upper brainstem. Derangements of the dominant hemisphere may have a greater effect on consciousness than derangements of the nondominant hemisphere.

Cheyne-Stokes respiration, in which periods of hyperpnea alternate with periods of apnea, is usually caused by bilateral hemispheric or diencephalic injuries, but can result from bilateral damage anywhere along the descending pathway between the forebrain and upper pons. Alertness, pupillary size, and heart rhythm may vary during Cheyne-Stokes respiration. Alertness is greater during the waxing portion of breathing. Lesions just ventral to the aqueduct or fourth ventricle cause a sustained, rapid, deep hyperventilation (central neurogenic hyperventilation). Abnormalities within the medulla and pons affect the respiratory centers and cause three different patterns of respiratory control: (1) *apneustic breathing*, a pause at full inspiration; (2) *ataxic breathing*, haphazard breaths and pauses without a predictable pattern; and (3) *Ondine's curse*, failure of automatic breathing when asleep.

In metabolic encephalopathies, retention of the pupillary light reflex is usual. Absence of the pupillary reflex in a comatose patient indicates a structural abnormality. The major exception is drugs: the cause of fixed dilation of pupils in an alert patient is topical administration of mydriatics. In comatose patients, hypothalamic damage causes unilateral pupillary constriction and a Horner's syndrome; midbrain lesions cause midposition fixed pupils; pontine lesions cause small but reactive pupils; and lateral medullary lesions cause a Horner's syndrome.

Tonic lateral deviation of both eyes indicates a seizure originating in the frontal lobe opposite to the direction of gaze (saccade center); the parietal lobe ipsilateral to the direction of gaze (pursuit center); or a destructive lesion in the ipsilateral frontal lobe in the direction of gaze. The assessment of ocular motility in comatose patients is the instillation of ice water sequentially 15 minutes apart in each ear to chill the tympanic membrane. Ice water in the right ear causes both eyes to deviate rapidly to the right and then slowly return to the midline. The rapid movement to the right is a brainstem reflex, and its presence indicates that much of the brainstem is intact. Abduction of the right eye with failure of left eye adduction indicates a lesion in the medial longitudinal fasciculus (see Chapter 15). The slow movement that returns the eyes to the left requires a corticopontine pathway originating in the right hemisphere and terminating in the left pontine lateral gaze center. Its presence indicates unilateral hemispheric function. Skew deviation, the deviation of one eye above the other (hypertropia), usually indicates a lesion of the brainstem or cerebellum.

Carefully observe trunk and limb position at rest, spontaneous movements, and response to noxious stimuli. Spontaneous movement of all limbs generally indicates a mild depression of hemispheric function without structural disturbance. Monoplegia or hemiplegia, except when in the postictal state, suggests a structural disturbance of the contralateral hemisphere. An extensor response of the trunk and limbs to a noxious stimulus is termed *decerebrate rigidity*. The most severe form is *opisthotonos*: the neck is hyperextended and the teeth clenched; the arms adducted, hyperextended, and hyperpronated; and the legs extended with the feet plantar flexed. Decerebrate rigidity indicates brainstem compression and considered an ominous sign whether present at rest or in response to noxious stimuli. Flexion of the arms and extension of the legs is termed *decorticate rigidity*. It is uncommon in children except following head injury and indicates hemispheric dysfunction with brainstem integrity.

Laboratory Investigations

Laboratory investigations are similar to those described for the evaluation of delirium. Perform head CT with contrast enhancement promptly in order to exclude the possibility of a mass lesion and herniation. It is a great error to send a child whose condition is uncertain for CT without someone in attendance who knows how to monitor deterioration and intervene appropriately.

HYPOXIA AND ISCHEMIA

Hypoxia and ischemia usually occur together. Prolonged hypoxia causes personality change first and then loss of consciousness; acute anoxia results in immediate loss of consciousness.

Prolonged Hypoxia

Clinical Features. Prolonged hypoxia can result from severe anemia (oxygen-carrying capacity reduced by at least half), congestive heart failure, chronic lung disease, and neuromuscular disorders.

The best-studied model of prolonged, mild hypoxia involves ascent to high altitudes. Mild hypoxia causes impaired memory and judgment, confusion, and decreased motor performance. Greater degrees of hypoxia result in obtundation, multifocal myoclonus, and sometimes focal neurological signs such as monoplegia and hemiplegia. Children with chronic cardiopulmonary disease may have an insidious alteration in behavioral state as the arterial oxygen concentration slowly declines.

The neurological complications of cystic fibrosis result from chronic hypoxia and hypercapnia leading to lethargy, somnolence, and sometimes coma. Neuromuscular disorders that weaken respiratory muscles, such as muscular dystrophy, often produce nocturnal hypoventilation as a first symptom of respiratory insufficiency. Frequent awakenings and fear of sleeping are characteristic (see Chapter 7).

Diagnosis. Consider chronic hypoxia in children with chronic cardiopulmonary disorders who become depressed or undergo personality change. Arterial oxygen pressure (P_aO_2) values below 40 mmHg are regularly associated with obvious neurological disturbances, but minor mental disturbances may occur at P_aO_2 concentrations of 60 mmHg, especially when hypoxia is chronic.

Management. Encephalopathy usually reverses when P_aO_2 is increased, but persistent cerebral dysfunction may occur in mountain climbers after returning to sea level, and permanent cerebral dysfunction may develop in children with chronic hypoxia. As a group, children with chronic hypoxia from congenital heart disease have a lower IQ than nonhypoxic children. The severity of mental decline relates to the duration of hypoxia. Treat children with neuromuscular disorders who develop symptoms during sleep with overnight, intermittent positive-pressure ventilation (see Chapter 7).

Acute Anoxia and Ischemia

The usual circumstance in which acute anoxia and ischemia occur is cardiac arrest or sudden hypotension. Anoxia without ischemia occurs with suffocation (near drowning, choking). Prolonged anoxia leads to bradycardia and cardiac arrest. In adults, hippocampal and Purkinje cells begin to die after 4 minutes of total anoxia and ischemia. Exact timing may be difficult in clinical situations when ill-defined intervals of anoxia and hypoxia occur. Remarkable survivals are sometimes associated with near drowning in water cold enough to lower cerebral temperature and metabolism. The pattern of hypoxic-ischemic brain injury in newborns is different and depends largely on brain maturity (see Chapter 1).

Clinical Features. Consciousness is lost within 8 seconds of cerebral circulatory failure, but the loss may take longer when anoxia occurs without ischemia. Presyncopal symptoms of lightheadedness and visual disturbances sometimes precede loss of consciousness. Initially, myoclonic movements due to lack of cortical spinal inhibition may occur. Seizures may follow.

Prediction of outcome after hypoxic-ischemic events depends on age and circumstances. Only 13% of adults who have had a cardiac arrest regain independent function in the first year after arrest. The outcome in children is somewhat better because the incidence of preexisting cardiopulmonary disease is lower. Absence of pupillary responses on initial examination is an ominous sign; such patients do not recover independent function. Twenty-four hours after arrest, lack of motor responses in the limbs and eyes identifies patients with a poor prognosis. Persistent early-onset myoclonus is a negative prognostic sign (Krumholz & Berg, 2002). In contrast, a favorable outcome is predictable for patients who rapidly recover roving or conjugate eye movements and limb withdrawal from pain. Children who are unconscious for longer than 60 days will not regain language skills or the ability to walk.

Two delayed syndromes of neurological deterioration follow anoxia. The first is *delayed postanoxic encephalopathy*, the appearance of apathy or confusion 1 to 2 weeks after apparent recovery. Motor symptoms follow, usually rigidity or spasticity, and may progress to coma or death. Demyelination is the suggested mechanism. The other syndrome is *postanoxic action myoclonus*. This usually follows a severe episode of anoxia and ischemia caused by cardiac arrest. All voluntary activity initiates disabling myoclonus (see Chapter 14). Symptoms of cerebellar dysfunction are also present.

Diagnosis. Cerebral edema is prominent during the first 72 hours after severe hypoxia. CT during that time shows decreased density with loss of the differentiation between gray and white matter. Severe, generalized loss of density on the CT correlates with a poor outcome. An EEG that shows a burst-suppression pattern or absence of activity is associated with a poor neurological outcome or death; lesser abnormalities typically are not useful in predicting the prognosis. Magnetic resonance imaging (MRI) is a more sensitive imaging modality that shows the extent of hypoxia very well in diffusion weighted T_2 and FLAIR images; however, some of the changes noted with this technique may be reversible.

Management. The principles of treating patients who have sustained hypoxic-ischemic encephalopathy do not differ substantially from the principles of caring for other comatose patients. Maintaining oxygenation, circulation, and blood glucose concentration is essential. Regulate intracranial pressure to levels that allow satisfactory cerebral perfusion (see Chapter 4). Anticonvulsant drugs manage seizures (see Chapter 1). Anoxia is invariably associated with lactic acidosis. Restoration of acid-base balance is essential.

The use of barbiturate coma to slow cerebral metabolism is common practice, but neither clinical nor experimental evidence indicates a beneficial effect following cardiac arrest or near drowning. Hypothermia prevents brain damage during the time of hypoxia and ischemia and has some value after the event. Corticosteroids do not improve neurological recovery in patients with global ischemia following cardiac arrest. Postanoxic action myoclonus sometimes responds to levetiracetam, zonisamide or valproate.

Persistent Vegetative State

The term *persistent vegetative state* (PVS) describes patients who, after recovery from coma, return to a state of wakefulness without cognition. PVS is a form of eyes-open permanent unconsciousness with loss of cognitive function and awareness of the environment but preservation of sleep-wake cycles and vegetative function. Survival is indefinite with good nursing care. The usual causes, in order of frequency, are anoxia and ischemia, metabolic or encephalitic coma, and head trauma. Anoxia-ischemia has the worst prognosis. Children who remain in a PVS for 3 months do not regain functional skills.

The American Academy of Neurology has adopted the policy that discontinuing medical treatment, including the provision of nutrition and hydration, is ethical in a patient whose diagnosed condition is PVS, when it is clear that the patient would not want maintenance in this state, and the family agrees to discontinue therapy.

BRAIN DEATH

The guidelines for brain death suggested by the American Academy of Neurology (1995) are generally accepted. Box 2-4 summarizes the important features of the report. The Academy urged caution in applying the criteria to children younger than 5 years, but subsequent experience supports the validity of the standards in the newborn and through childhood. Absence of cerebral blood flow is the earliest and most definitive proof of brain death.

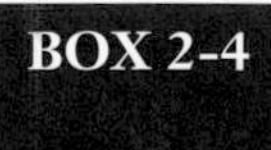

BOX 2-4 Diagnostic Criteria for the Clinical Diagnosis of Brain Death

PREREQUISITES

Cessation of all brain function
Proximate cause of brain death is known
Condition is irreversible

CARDINAL FEATURES

Coma
- Absent brainstem reflexes
- Pupillary light reflex
- Corneal reflex
- Oculocephalic reflex
- Oculovestibular reflex
- Oropharyngeal reflex

Apnea (established by formal apnea test)

CONFIRMATORY TESTS (OPTIONAL)

Cerebral angiography
Electroencephalography
Radioisotope cerebral blood flow study
Transcranial Doppler ultrasonography

INFECTIOUS DISORDERS

Bacterial Infections

Cat-Scratch Disease

The causative agent of cat-scratch disease is *Bartonella (Rochalimaea) henselae*, a Gram-negative bacillus transmitted by a cat scratch and perhaps by cat fleas. It is the most common cause of chronic benign lymphadenopathy in children and young adults. The estimated incidence in the United States is 22 000 per year, and 80 % of cases occur in children less than 12 years of age.

Clinical Features. The major feature is lymphadenopathy proximal to the site of the scratch. Fever is present in only 60 % of cases. The disease is usually benign and self-limited. Unusual systemic manifestations are oculoglandular disease, erythema nodosum, osteolytic lesions, and thrombocytopenic purpura. The most common neurological manifestation is encephalopathy. Transverse myelitis, radiculitis, cerebellar ataxia, and neuroretinitis are rare manifestations. Neurological manifestations when present occur 2 or 3 weeks after the onset of lymphadenopathy.

Neurological symptoms occur in 2 % of cases of cat-scratch disease, and 90 % of them manifest as encephalopathy. The mechanism is unknown, but the cause may be either a direct infection or vasculitis. The male-to-female ratio is 2:1. Only 17 % of cases occur in children less than 12 years old and 15 % in children 12 to 18 years old. The frequency of fever and the site of the scratch are the same in patients with encephalitis compared to those without encephalitis. The initial and most prominent feature is a decreased state of consciousness ranging from lethargy to coma. Seizures occur in 46–80 % of cases and combative behavior in 40 %. Focal findings are rare (Florin et al, 2008), but neuroretinitis, Guillain-Barré syndrome, and transverse myelitis can be seen.

Diagnosis. The diagnosis requires local lymphadenopathy, contact with a cat, and an identifiable site of inoculation. Enzyme-linked immunosorbent assay (ELISA) tests and polymerase chain reaction (PCR) amplification from infected tissues are available for diagnosis. The cerebrospinal fluid is normal in 70 % of cases. Lymphocytosis in the cerebrospinal fluid, when present, does not exceed 30 cells/mm^3. The EEG is diffusely slow. Only 19 % of patients have abnormal findings on CT scan or MRI of the brain, and these include lesions of the cerebral white matter, basal ganglia, thalamus, and gray matter (Florin et al., 2008).

Management. All affected children recover completely, 50 % within 4 weeks. For neuroretinitis, doxycycline is preferred because of its excellent intraocular and central nervous system (CNS) penetration. For children younger than 8 years of age in whom tooth discoloration is a concern, erythromycin is a good substitute. When coupled with rifampin, these antibiotics seem to promote disease resolution, improve visual acuity, decrease optic disk edema, and decrease the duration of encephalopathy. We use the combination of doxycycline and rifampin for 2 to 4 weeks in immunocompetent patients and 4 months for immunocompromised patients in cases of encephalopathy or neuroretinitis (Florin et al., 2008)

Gram-Negative Sepsis

Clinical Features. The onset of symptoms in Gram-negative sepsis may be explosive and characterized by fever or hypothermia, chills, hyperventilation, hemodynamic instability, and mental changes (irritability, delirium, or coma). Neurological features may include asterixis, tremor, and multifocal myoclonus. Multiple organ failure follows (1) renal shutdown caused by hypotension; (2) hypoprothrombinemia caused by vitamin K deficiency; (3) thrombocytopenia caused by nonspecific binding of immunoglobulin; (4) disseminated intravascular coagulation with infarction or hemorrhage in several organs; and (5) progressive respiratory failure.

Diagnosis. Always consider sepsis in the differential diagnosis of shock, and obtain blood cultures. When shock is the initial feature, Gram-negative sepsis is the likely diagnosis. In *Staphylococcus aureus* infections, shock is more likely to occur during the course of the infection and not as an initial feature. The cerebrospinal fluid is usually normal or may have an elevated concentration of protein. MRI or CT of the brain is normal early in the course and shows edema later on.

Management. Septic shock is a medical emergency. Promptly initiate antibiotic therapy at maximal doses (see Chapter 4). Treat hypotension by restoration of intravascular volume, and address each factor contributing to coagulopathy. Mortality is high even with optimal treatment.

Hemorrhagic Shock and Encephalopathy Syndrome

Bacterial sepsis is the presumed cause of the hemorrhagic shock and encephalopathy syndrome.

Clinical Features. Most affected children are younger than 1 year of age, but cases occur in children up to 26 months. Half of children have mild prodromal symptoms of a viral gastroenteritis or respiratory illness. In the rest, the onset is explosive; a previously well child is found unresponsive and having seizures. Fever of 38°C or higher is a constant feature. Marked hypotension with poor peripheral perfusion is the initial event. Profuse watery or bloody diarrhea with metabolic acidosis and compensatory respiratory alkalosis follows. Disseminated intravascular coagulopathy develops, and bleeding occurs from every venipuncture site. The mortality rate is 50 %; the survivors have mental and motor impairment.

Diagnosis. The syndrome resembles toxic shock syndrome, Gram-negative sepsis, heat stroke, and Reye syndrome. Abnormal renal function occurs in every case, but serum ammonia concentrations remain normal, hypoglycemia is unusual, and blood cultures yield no growth.

Cerebrospinal fluid is normal except for increased pressure. CT shows small ventricles and loss of sulcal marking caused by cerebral edema. The initial EEG background is diffusely slow or may be isoelectric. A striking pattern called *electric storm* evolves over the first hours or days. Runs of spikes, sharp waves, or rhythmic slow waves that fluctuate in frequency, amplitude, and location characterize the pattern.

Management. Affected children require intensive care with ventilatory support, volume replacement, correction of acid–base and coagulation disturbances, anticonvulsant therapy, and control of cerebral edema.

Rickettsial Infections

Lyme Disease. A spirochete (*Borrelia burgdorferi*) causes Lyme disease. The vector is hard-shelled deer ticks: *Ixodes dammini* in the eastern United States, *I. pacificus* in the western United States, and *I. ricinus* in Europe. Lyme disease is now the most common vector-borne infection in the United States. Six northeastern states account for 80 % of cases.

Clinical Features. The neurological consequences of disease are variable and some are uncertain. Those associated with the early stages of disease enjoy the greatest acceptance. The first symptom (stage 1) in 60–80 % of patients is a skin lesion of the thigh, groin, or axillae (erythema chronicum migrans), which may be associated with fever, regional lymphadenopathy, and arthralgia. The rash begins as a red macule at the site of the tick bite and then spreads to form a red annular lesion with partial clearing, sometimes appearing as alternating rings of rash and clearing.

Neurological involvement (neuroborreliosis) develops weeks or months later when the infection disseminates (stage 2) (Halperin, 2005). Most children have only headache, which clears completely within 6 weeks; the cause may be mild aseptic meningitis or encephalitis. Fever may not occur. Facial palsy, sleep disturbances, and papilledema are rare. Polyneuropathies are uncommon in children. Transitory cardiac involvement (myopericarditis and atrioventricular block) may occur in stage 2.

A year or more of continual migratory arthritis begins weeks to years after the onset of neurological features (stage 3). Only one joint, often the knee, or a few large joints are affected. During stage 3, the patient feels ill. Encephalopathy with memory or cognitive abnormalities and confusional states, with normal cerebrospinal fluid results, may occur. Other psychiatric or fatigue syndromes appear less likely to be causally related (Halperin, 2005).

Diagnosis. The spirochete grows on cultures from the skin rash during stage 1 of the disease. At the time of meningitis, the cerebrospinal fluid may be normal at first but then shows a lymphocytic pleocytosis (about 100 cells/mm^3), an elevated protein concentration, and a normal glucose concentration. *B. burgdorferi* grows on culture from the cerebrospinal fluid during the meningitis. A two-test approach establishes the diagnosis of neuroborreliosis. The first step is to show the production of specific IgG and IgM antibodies in cerebrospinal fluid. Antibody production begins 2 weeks after infection, and IgG is always detectable at 6 weeks. The second step, used when the first is inconclusive, is PCR (polymerase chain reaction) to detect the organism.

Management. Either ceftriaxone (2 g once daily intravenously) or penicillin (3–4 mU intravenously every 3–4 hours) for 2–4 weeks treats encephalitis. Examine the cerebrospinal fluid toward the end of the 2- to 4-week treatment course to assess the need for continuing treatment and again 6 months after the conclusion of therapy. Intrathecal antibody production may persist for years following successful treatment, and in isolation it does not indicate active disease. Patients in whom cerebrospinal fluid pleocytosis fails to resolve within 6 months, however, should be retreated.

The treatment of peripheral or cranial nerve involvement without cerebrospinal fluid abnormalities is with oral agents, either doxycycline, 100 mg twice daily for 14–21 days, or amoxicillin, 500 mg every 8 hours for 10–21 days. An effective vaccine against Lyme disease is available and may be used for children who live in endemic areas.

A subcommittee from the American Academy of Neurology concluded in 2007 that some evidence supports the use of penicillin, ceftriaxone, cefotaxime, and doxycycline in both adults and children with neuroborreliosis (Halperin et al, 2007).

Rocky Mountain Spotted Fever. Rocky Mountain spotted fever is an acute tick-borne disorder caused by *Rickettsia rickettsii.* Its geographic name is a misnomer; the disease is present in the northwestern and eastern United States, Canada, Mexico, Colombia, and Brazil.

Clinical Features. Fever, myalgia, and rash are constant symptoms and begin 2–14 days after tick bite. The rash first appears around the wrist and ankles 3–5 days after onset of illness and spreads to the soles of the feet and forearms. It may be maculopapular, petechial, or both. Headache is present in 66 % of affected individuals, meningitis or meningoencephalitis in 33 %, focal neurological signs in 14 %, and seizures in 6 %. The focal abnormalities result from microinfarcts.

Diagnosis. *R. rickettsii* are demonstrable by direct immunofluorescence or immunoperoxidase staining of a skin biopsy specimen of the rash. Other laboratory tests may indicate anemia, thrombocytopenia, coagulopathy, hyponatremia, and muscle tissue breakdown. Serology retrospectively confirms the diagnosis. The cerebrospinal fluid shows a mild pleocytosis.

Management. Initiate treatment when the diagnosis is first suspected. Delayed treatment results in 20 % mortality. Oral or intravenous tetracycline (25–50 mg/kg/day), chloramphenicol (50–75 mg/kg/day) in four divided doses, or oral doxycycline (100 mg twice a day for 7 days) is effective. Continue treatment for 2 days after the patient is afebrile.

Toxic Shock Syndrome

Toxic shock syndrome is a potentially lethal illness caused by infection or colonization with some strains of *Staphylococcus aureus.*

Clinical Features. The onset is abrupt. High fever, hypotension, vomiting, diarrhea, myalgia, headache, and a desquamating rash characterize the onset. Multiple organ failure may occur during desquamation. Serious complications include cardiac arrhythmia, pulmonary edema, and oliguric renal failure. Initial encephalopathic features are agitation and confusion. These may be followed by lethargy, obtundation, and generalized tonic-clonic seizures.

Many pediatric cases have occurred in menstruating girls who use tampons, but they may also occur in children with occlusive dressings after burns or surgery, and as a complication of influenza and influenza-like illness in children with staphylococcal colonization of the respiratory tract.

Diagnosis. No diagnostic laboratory test is available. The basis for diagnosis is the typical clinical and laboratory findings. Over half of the patients have sterile pyuria, immature granulocytic leukocytes, coagulation abnormalities, hypocalcemia, low serum albumin and total protein concentrations, and elevated concentrations of blood urea nitrogen, transaminase, bilirubin, and creatine kinase. Cultures of specimens from infected areas yield *S. aureus.*

Management. Hypotension usually responds to volume restoration with physiological saline solutions. Some patients require vasopressors or fresh-frozen plasma. Initiate antibiotic therapy promptly with an agent effective against *S. aureus.*

Viral Infections

Because encephalitis usually affects the meninges as well as the brain, the term *meningoencephalitis* is more accurate. However, distinguishing encephalitis from aseptic meningitis is useful for viral diagnosis because most viruses cause primarily one or the other, but not both. In the United States, the most common viruses that cause meningitis are enteroviruses, herpes simplex virus (HSV), and arboviruses. However, despite the best diagnostic effort, the cause of 70% of cases of suspected viral encephalitis is unknown (Glaser et al, 2003).

Routine childhood immunization has reduced the number of pathogenic viruses circulating in the community. Enteroviruses and HSV are now the most common viral causes of meningitis and encephalitis in children. However, specific viral identification is possible in only 15–20% of cases.

The classification of viruses undergoes frequent change, but a constant first step is the separation of viruses with a DNA nucleic acid core from those with an RNA core. The only DNA viruses that cause acute postnatal encephalitis in immunocompetent hosts are herpes viruses. RNA viruses causing encephalitis are myxoviruses (influenza and measles encephalitis), arboviruses (St Louis encephalitis, eastern equine encephalitis, western equine encephalitis, La Crosse-California encephalitis), retroviruses (acquired immune deficiency syndrome encephalitis), and rhabdoviruses (rabies). RNA viruses (especially enteroviruses and mumps) are responsible for aseptic meningitis.

Some viruses, such as HSV, are highly neurotropic (usually infect the nervous system) but rarely neurovirulent (rarely cause encephalitis), whereas others, such as measles, are rarely neurotropic but are highly neurovirulent. In addition to viruses that directly infect the brain and meninges, encephalopathies may also follow systemic viral infections. These probably result from demyelination caused by immune-mediated responses of the brain to infection.

Aseptic Meningitis

The term *aseptic meningitis* defines a syndrome of meningismus and cerebrospinal fluid leukocytosis without bacterial or fungal infection. Drugs or viral infections are the usual cause. Viral meningitis is a benign, self-limited disease from which 95% of children recover completely.

Clinical Features. The onset of symptoms is abrupt and characterized by fever, headache, and stiff neck, except in infants who do not have meningismus. Irritability, lethargy, and vomiting are common. "Encephalitic" symptoms are not part of the syndrome. Systemic illness is uncommon, but its presence may suggest specific viral disorders. The acute illness usually lasts less than 1 week, but malaise and headache may continue for several weeks.

Diagnosis. In most cases of aseptic meningitis, the cerebrospinal fluid contains 10–200 leukocytes/mm^3, but cell counts of 1000 cells/mm^3 or greater may occur with lymphocytic choriomeningitis. The response is primarily lymphocytic, but polymorphonuclear leukocytes may predominate early in the course. The protein concentration is generally between 50 and 100 mg/dL (0.5 and 1 g/L) and the glucose concentration is normal, although it may be slightly reduced in children with mumps and lymphocytic choriomeningitis.

Aseptic meningitis usually occurs in the spring or summer, and enteroviruses are responsible for most cases in children. Nonviral causes of aseptic meningitis are rare but considerations include Lyme disease, Kawasaki disease, leukemia, systemic lupus erythematosus, and migraine.

Individuals with a personal or family history of migraine may have attacks of severe headache associated with stiff neck and focal neurological disturbances, such as hemiparesis and aphasia. Cerebrospinal fluid examination shows a pleocytosis of 5–300 cells/mm^3 that is mainly lymphocytes, and a protein concentration of 50–100 mg/dL (0.5–1 g/L). Unresolved is whether the attacks are migraine provoked by intercurrent aseptic meningitis or represent a "meningitic" form of migraine. The recurrence of attacks in some people suggests that the mechanism is wholly migrainous. Nonsteroidal anti-inflammatory drugs may also contribute to pleocytosis.

Bacterial meningitis is the major concern when a child has meningismus. Although cerebrospinal fluid examination provides several clues that differentiate bacterial from viral meningitis, initiate antibiotic therapy for every child with a clinical syndrome of aseptic meningitis until cerebrospinal fluid culture is negative for bacteria (see Chapter 4). This is especially true for children who received antibiotic therapy before examination of the cerebrospinal fluid.

Management. Treatment for herpes encephalitis with acyclovir is routine in children with viral meningitis or encephalitis until excluding that diagnosis. Treatment of viral aseptic meningitis is symptomatic. Bed rest in a quiet environment and mild analgesics provide satisfactory relief of symptoms in most children.

Arboviral (Arthropod-Borne) Encephalitis

The basis of arbovirus classification is ecology rather than structure. Ticks and mosquitoes are the usual vectors, and epidemics occur in the spring and summer. Each type of encephalitis has a defined geographic area. Arboviruses account for 10% of encephalitis cases reported in the United States.

La Crosse-Californa Encephalitis. The California serogroup viruses, principally La Crosse encephalitis, are the most common cause of arboviral encephalitis in the United States (McJunkin et al, 2001). The endemic areas are the midwest and western New York State. Most cases occur between July and September. Small woodland mammals serve as a reservoir and mosquitoes as the vector.

Clinical Features. Most cases of encephalitis occur in children, and asymptomatic infection is common in adults. The initial feature is a flu-like syndrome that lasts for 2 or 3 days. Headache heralds the encephalitis. Seizures and rapid progression to coma follows. Focal neurological disturbances are present in 20 % of cases. Symptoms begin to resolve 3–5 days after onset, and most children recover without neurological sequelae. Death is uncommon and occurs mainly in infants.

Diagnosis. Examination of cerebrospinal fluid shows a mixed pleocytosis with lymphocytes predominating. The count is usually 50–200 cells/mm^3, but it may range from 0 to 600 cells/mm^3. The virus is difficult to culture, and diagnosis depends on showing a 4-fold or greater increase in hemagglutination inhibition and neutralizing antibody titers between acute and convalescent sera.

Management. Treatment is supportive. No effective antiviral agent is available.

Eastern Equine Encephalitis. Eastern equine encephalitis is the most severe type of arboviral encephalitis, with a mortality rate of 50–70%. Fewer than 10 cases occur per year in the United States.

Clinical Features. Eastern equine encephalitis is a perennial infection of horses from New York State to Florida. Human cases do not exceed five each year, and they follow epidemics in horses. The mortality rate is high. Wild birds serve as a reservoir and mosquitoes as a vector. Consequently, almost all cases occur during the summer months.

Onset is usually abrupt and characterized by high fever, headache, and vomiting, followed by drowsiness, coma, and seizures. A long duration of non-neurological prodromal symptoms predicts a better outcome. In infants, seizures and coma are often the first clinical features. Signs of meningismus are often present in older children. Children usually survive the acute encephalitis, but expected sequelae include mental impairment, epilepsy, and disturbed motor function.

Diagnosis. The cerebrospinal fluid pressure is usually elevated, and examination reveals 200–2000 leukocytes/mm^3, of which half are polymorphonuclear leukocytes. MRI shows focal lesions in the basal ganglia and thalamus. Diagnosis relies on showing a 4-fold or greater rise in complement fixation and neutralizing antibody titers between acute and convalescent sera.

Management. Treatment is supportive. No effective antiviral agent is available.

Japanese B Encephalitis. Japanese B encephalitis is a major form of encephalitis in Asia and is an important health hazard to nonimmunized travelers during summer months. The virus cycle is among mosquitoes, pigs, and birds.

Clinical Features. The initial features are malaise, fever, and headache or irritability lasting for 2–3 days. Meningismus, confusion, and delirium follow. During the second or third week, photophobia and generalized hypotonia develop. Seizures may occur at any time. Finally, rigidity, a mask-like facies, and brainstem dysfunction ensue. Mortality rates are very high among indigenous populations and lower among Western travelers, probably because of a difference in the age of the exposed populations.

Diagnosis. Examination of the cerebrospinal fluid shows pleocytosis (20–500 cells/mm^3). The cells are initially mixed, but later lymphocytes predominate. The protein concentration is usually between 50 and 100 mg/dL (0.5 and 1 mg/L), and the glucose concentration is normal. Diagnosis depends on demonstrating a 4-fold or greater elevation in the level of complement-fixing antibodies between acute and convalescent sera.

Management. Treatment is supportive. No effective antiviral agent is available, but immunization with an inactivated vaccine protects against encephalitis in more than 90 % of individuals.

St Louis Encephalitis. St Louis encephalitis is endemic in the western United States and epidemic in the Mississippi valley and the Atlantic states. It is the most common cause of epidemic viral encephalitis in the United States. The vector is a mosquito, and birds are the major reservoir.

Clinical Features. Most infections are asymptomatic. The spectrum of neurological illness varies from aseptic meningitis to severe encephalitis leading to death. The mortality rate is low. Headache, vomiting, and states of decreased consciousness are the typical features. A slow evolution of neurological symptoms, the presence of generalized weakness and tremor, and the absence of focal findings and seizures favor a diagnosis of St Louis encephalitis over HSV encephalitis. The usual duration of illness is 1–2 weeks. Children usually recover completely, but adults may have residual mental or motor impairment.

Diagnosis. Cerebrospinal fluid examination reveals a lymphocytic pleocytosis (50 to 500 cells/mm^3) and a protein concentration between 50 and 100 mg/dL (0.5 and 1 g/L). The glucose concentration is normal.

The virus is difficult to grow on culture, and diagnosis requires a 4-fold or greater increase in complement fixation and hemagglutination inhibition antibody titers between acute and convalescent sera.

Management. Treatment is supportive. No effective antiviral agent is available.

West Nile Virus Encephalitis. West Nile virus is one of the world's most widely distributed viruses. It emerged in eastern North America in 1999 and subsequently become the most important cause of arboviral meningitis, encephalitis, and acute flaccid paralysis in the continental United States. Most transmission occurs by the bite of an infected mosquito. However, person-to-person transmission through organ transplantation, blood and blood product transfusion, and intrauterine spread can occur. Mosquitoes of the genus Culex are the principal maintenance vectors; wild birds serve as the principal amplifying hosts (Bode et al, 2006).

Clinical Features. Most infections are asymptomatic. A nonspecific febrile illness characterizes the onset. Encephalitis occurs in less than 1 % of infected individuals, mainly the elderly. Clinical features suggestive of infection include movement disorders, e.g., tremor, myoclonus, parkinsonism, and severe weakness of the lower motor neuron (DeBiasi & Tyler, 2006). The weakness results from spinal cord motor neuron injury resulting in flaccid weakness and areflexia. Approximately 1 in 150 infected persons will develop encephalitis or meningitis (DeBiasi & Tyler, 2006). Case fatality is 12–14 %.

Diagnosis. In patients with weakness, electromyographic and nerve conduction velocity studies are consistent with motor neuron injury. Detection of IgM antibodies in cerebrospinal fluid or IgM and IgG antibodies in serum are diagnostic.

Management. Treatment is supportive. No effective antiviral agent is available.

Herpes Simplex Encephalitis

Two similar strains of HSV are pathogenic to humans. HSV-1 is associated with orofacial infections and HSV-2 with genital infections. Both are worldwide in distribution. Forty percent of children have antibodies to HSV-1, but routine detection of antibodies to HSV-2 occurs at puberty. HSV-1 is the causative agent of acute herpes simplex encephalitis after the newborn period and HSV-2 of encephalitis in the newborn (see Chapter 1).

Initial orofacial infection with HSV-1 may be asymptomatic. The virus replicates in the skin, infecting nerve fiber endings and then the trigeminal ganglia. Further replication occurs within the ganglia before the virus enters a latent stage during which it is not recoverable from the ganglia. Reactivation occurs during times of stress, especially intercurrent febrile illness. The reactivated virus ordinarily retraces its neural migration to the facial skin but occasionally spreads proximally to the brain, causing encephalitis. The host's immunocompetence maintains the virus in a latent state. An immunocompromised state results in frequent reactivation and severe, widespread infection.

HSV is the single most common cause of nonepidemic encephalitis and accounts for 10–20% of cases (Whitley, 2006). The estimated annual incidence is 2.3 cases per million population. Thirty-one percent of cases occur in children.

Clinical Features. Primary infection is often the cause of encephalitis in children. Only 22 % of those with encephalitis have a history of recurrent labial herpes infection. Typically, the onset is acute and characterized by fever, headache, lethargy, nausea, and vomiting. Eighty percent of children show focal neurological disturbances (hemiparesis, cranial nerve deficits, visual field loss, aphasia, and focal seizures), and the remainder show behavioral changes or generalized seizures without clinical evidence of focal neurological deficits. However, both groups have focal abnormalities on neuroimaging studies or EEG. Once a seizure occurs, the child is comatose. The acute stage of encephalitis lasts for approximately a week. Recovery takes several weeks and is often incomplete.

Herpes meningitis is usually associated with genital lesions. The causative agent is HSV-2. The clinical features are similar to those of aseptic meningitis caused by other viruses.

Diagnosis. Prompt consideration of herpes simplex encephalitis is important because treatment is available. Cerebrospinal fluid pleocytosis is present in 97 % of cases. The median count is 130 leukocytes/mm^3 (range, 0–1000). Up to 500 red blood cells/mm^3 may be present as well. The median protein concentration is 80 mg/dL (0.8 g/L), but 20 % of those affected have normal protein concentrations and 40 % have concentrations exceeding 100 mg/dL (1 g/L). The glucose concentration in the cerebrospinal fluid is

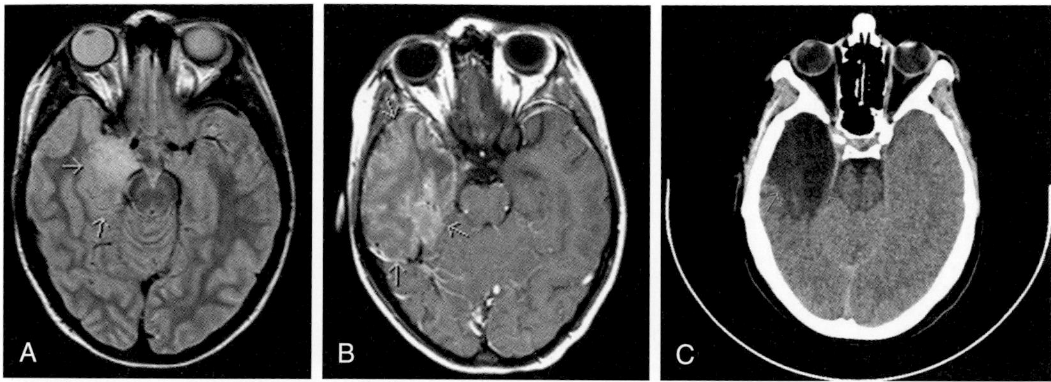

FIGURE 2-1 ■ Herpes encephalitis (same patient over time). (A) Axial T_2 MRI shows high signal in mesial temporal region in early encephalitis. (B) Axial T_2 MRI shows involvement of the whole temporal lobe. (C) CT scan shows residual encephalomalacia of the temporal lobe.

usually normal, but in 7 % of cases it is less than half of the blood glucose concentration.

In the past, the demonstration of periodic lateralizing epileptiform discharges on EEG was presumptive evidence of herpes encephalitis. However, MRI has proved to be a more sensitive early indicator of herpes encephalitis. T_2-weighted studies show increased signal intensity involving the cortex and white matter in the temporal and inferior frontal lobes (Figure 2-1). The areas of involvement then enlarge and coalesce. The identification of the organism in the cerebrospinal fluid by PCR has obviated the need for brain biopsy to establish the diagnosis.

Management. Most physicians begin intravenous acyclovir treatment in every child with a compatible clinical history. The standard course of treatment is 10 mg/kg every 8 hours in adolescents and 20 mg/kg every 8 hours in neonates and children for 14 to 21 days. Such treatment reduces mortality from 70 % in untreated patients to 25–30 %. The highest mortality rate is in patients already in coma at treatment onset. Function returns to normal in 38 %. New neurological disturbances may occur in some children after cessation of therapy (De Tiege et al, 2003). These syndromes are more likely when the original treatment course is short. The role of corticosteroids remains uncertain. Retrospective studies suggest no obvious harm and perhaps some benefit by adding corticosteroids to acyclovir treatment (Kamei et al, 2006).

A syndrome of choreoathetosis occurs within 1 month of the original encephalitis. Brain MRI does not show new necrotic areas and the mechanism may be immune mediated. A second syndrome, which may occur early or years later, lacks choreoathetosis but more resembles the initial infection. The cause is probably renewed viral replication.

Measles (Rubeola) Encephalitis

Compulsory immunization had almost eliminated natural measles infection in the United States, but the incidence began climbing again in 1990 because of reduced immunization rates. The risk of encephalitis from natural disease is 1:1000. The mechanism of measles encephalitis may be either direct viral infection, an allergic demyelination, or both. Chapter 5 contains a description of a chronic form of measles encephalitis (see subacute sclerosing panencephalitis).

Clinical Features. Measles is a neurotropic virus, and EEG abnormalities are often present even without clinical symptoms of encephalopathy. Symptoms of encephalitis usually begin 1 to 8 days after the appearance of rash or delayed for 3 weeks. The onset is usually abrupt and characterized by lethargy or obtundation that rapidly progress to coma. Generalized seizures occur in half of children. The spectrum of neurological disturbances includes hemiplegia, ataxia, and involuntary movement disorders. Acute transverse myelitis may occur as well (see Chapter 12). The incidence of neurological morbidity (cognitive impairment, epilepsy, and paralysis) is high but does not correlate with the severity of acute encephalitis.

Measles immunization does not cause an acute encephalopathy or any chronic brain damage syndrome. Generalized seizures may occur following immunization. These are mainly febrile seizures, and recovery is complete.

Diagnosis. Examination of cerebrospinal fluid shows a lymphocytic pleocytosis. The number of lymphocytes is usually highest in the first few days but rarely exceeds 100 cells/mm^3. Protein concentrations are generally between 50 and 100 mg/dL (0.5 and 1 g/L), and the glucose concentration is normal.

Management. Treatment is supportive. Anticonvulsant drugs usually provide satisfactory seizure control.

ACUTE DISSEMINATED ENCEPHALOMYELITIS

Acute disseminated encephalomyelitis (ADEM) is a central demyelinating disorder of childhood. The belief was that ADEM was a monophasic immunological reaction to a viral illness because fever is an initial feature. *This belief is incorrect on two counts. First, consider the fever as part of the ADEM and not evidence of prior infection; second, ADEM often is not monophasic, but the first attack of a recurring disorder similar to multiple sclerosis.* An immune-mediated mechanism is the presumed pathophysiology (Tenembaum et al, 2007).

Examples of postinfectious disorders appear in several chapters of this book and include the Guillain-Barré syndrome (see Chapter 7), acute cerebellar ataxia (see Chapter 10), transverse myelitis (see Chapter 12), brachial neuritis (see Chapter 13), optic neuritis (see Chapter 16), and Bell's palsy (see Chapter 17). The cause-and-effect relationship between viral infection and many of these syndromes is impossible to establish, especially when 30 days is the accepted latency period between viral infection and onset of neurological dysfunction. *The average school-age child has at least four to six "viral illnesses" each year, so that as many as half of children report a viral illness 30 days before the onset of any life event.* This average is probably higher for preschool-age children in day care.

Clinical Features. MRI has expanded the spectrum of clinical features associated with ADEM by allowing the demonstration of small demyelinating lesions. Often, the encephalopathy is preceded by lethargy, headache, and vomiting. Whether these "systemic features" are symptoms of a viral illness or of early encephalopathy is not clear. The onset of neurological symptoms is abrupt and characterized by focal motor signs, altered states of consciousness, or both. Optic neuritis, transverse myelitis, or both may precede the encephalopathy (see Chapter 12). Some children never have focal neurological signs, whereas in others the initial feature suggests a focal mass lesion. Mortality is highest in the first week. A favorable outcome is not the rule. Many children experience repeated episodes and follow a course similar to multiple sclerosis (Banwell et al, 2007). The burden of involvement noted in MRI correlates with the amount of symptoms more than in multiple sclerosis.

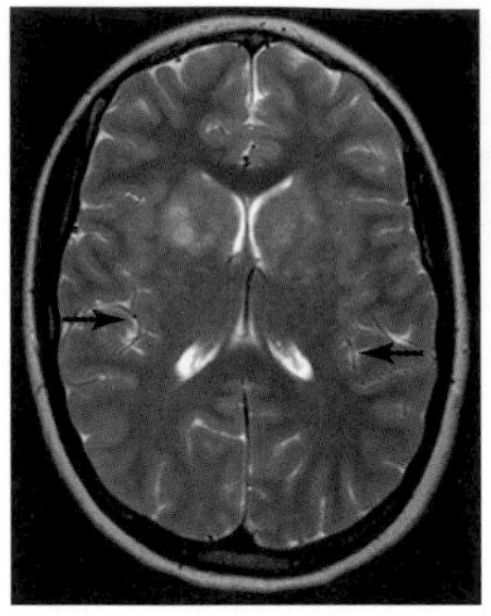

FIGURE 2-2 ■ Acute disseminated encephalomyelitis. T_2 axial MRI shows high signal in basal ganglia and surrounding white matter.

Diagnosis. T_2-weighted MRI reveals a marked increase in signal intensity throughout the white matter (Figure 2-2), but also involves the gray matter. The corpus callosum and periventricular region are commonly affected (Hynson et al, 2001). The lesions may resolve in the weeks that follow. In boys, consider the diagnosis of adrenoleukodystrophy (see Chapter 5). The cerebrospinal fluid is frequently normal. Occasional abnormalities are a mild lymphocytic pleocytosis and elevation of the protein concentration.

Management. Treatment with intravenous high-dose methylprednisolone helps in about 50% of cases. Intravenous immunoglobulin and plasma exchange may benefit children who fail to respond to corticosteroids (Khurana et al, 2005). All treatment protocols are empirical.

Reye Syndrome

Reye syndrome is a systemic disorder of mitochondrial function that occurs during or following viral infection. The occurrence is higher with salicylate use for symptomatic relief during viral illness. Recognition of this relationship has led to decreased use of salicylates in children and a marked decline in the incidence of Reye syndrome.

Clinical Features. In the United States, sporadic cases are generally associated with varicella (chickenpox) or nonspecific respiratory infections; small epidemics are associated with influenza B infection. When varicella is the precipitating infection, the initial stage of Reye syndrome occurs 3 to 6 days after the appearance of rash.

The clinical course is relatively predictable and divisible into five stages:

Stage 0: Vomiting, but no symptoms of brain dysfunction.

Stage I: Vomiting, confusion, and lethargy.

Stage II: Agitation, delirium, decorticate posturing, and hyperventilation.

Stage III: Coma, and decerebrate posturing.

Stage IV: Flaccidity, apnea, and dilated, fixed pupils.

The progression from stage I to stage IV may be explosive, evolving in less than 24 hours. More commonly, the period of recurrent vomiting and lethargy lasts for a day or longer. In most children with vomiting and laboratory evidence of hepatic dysfunction following varicella or respiratory infection, liver biopsy shows the features of Reye syndrome, despite normal cerebral function. The designation of this stage is Reye stage 0. Stages I and II represent metabolic dysfunction and cerebral edema. Stages III and IV indicate generalized increased intracranial pressure and herniation.

Focal neurological disturbances and meningismus are not part of the syndrome. Fever is not a prominent feature, and hepatomegaly occurs in one half of patients late in the course. The outcome is variable, but, as a rule, infants do worse than do older children. Progression to stages III and IV at all ages is associated with a high death rate and with impaired neurological function in survivors.

Diagnosis. Typical blood abnormalities are hypoglycemia, hyperammonemia, and increased concentrations of hepatic enzymes. Serum bilirubin concentrations remain normal, and jaundice does not occur. Acute pancreatitis sometimes develops and is identified by increased concentrations of serum amylase. The cerebrospinal fluid is normal except for increased pressure. The EEG shows abnormalities consistent with a diffuse encephalopathy.

Liver biopsy is definitive. Light microscopy shows panlobular accumulation of small intracellular lipid droplets and depletion of succinic acid dehydrogenase in the absence of other abnormalities. Electron microscopic changes include characteristic mitochondrial abnormalities, peroxisomal proliferation and swelling, proliferation of smooth endoplasmic reticulum, and glycogen depletion.

Conditions that mimic Reye syndrome are disorders of fatty acid oxidation, ornithine transcarbamylase deficiency, and valproate hepatotoxicity. Assume an inborn error of metabolism in any child with recurrent Reye syndrome (Box 2-3) or a family history of similar illness. Metabolic products of valproate are mitochondrial poisons that produce an experimental model of Reye syndrome.

Management. Admit all children to a pediatric intensive care unit. Treatment of children with stage I or II disease is intravenous hypertonic (10–15 %) glucose solution at normal maintenance volumes. Stages III and IV require treatment of increased intracranial pressure (see Chapter 4) by elevation of the head, controlled mechanical ventilation, and mannitol. Corticosteroids are of limited benefit and not used routinely. Some authorities continue to advocate intracranial pressure monitors and pentobarbital coma, despite failure to affect outcome. Fortunately, this once common and deadly disease has nearly disappeared in the United States with discontinuation of salicylate therapy for children.

POSTIMMUNIZATION ENCEPHALOPATHY

Three types of vaccine are in general use in the United States: live-attenuated viruses, whole or fractionated-killed organisms, and toxoids.

Live-attenuated virus vaccines (measles, mumps, rubella, varicella, and oral poliomyelitis) produce a mild and usually harmless infection with subsequent immunity. However, even under ideal circumstances of vaccine preparation and host resistance, symptoms of the natural disease and its known neurological complications may develop in vaccine recipients.

Whole-killed organisms (pertussis, influenza, rabies, and inactivated poliomyelitis) do not reproduce their natural disease, but alleged injury to the nervous system is by a toxic or allergic mechanism. Whole-cell pertussis vaccine may cause seizures, and while causation of chronic brain damage was never established, this was a concern. Fortunately, a safe acellular vaccine replaced whole-cell vaccine. Semple rabies vaccine had been an important cause of encephalitis, but the newer vaccine, prepared from virus grown on human diploid cells, is safe and only rarely implicated as a cause of polyneuropathy. Semple vaccine, still in use in some parts of the world, contains myelin-basic protein and is known to cause encephalomyelitis. None of the other whole-killed organism vaccines cause encephalopathy.

Toxoid production is by the inactivation of toxins produced by bacteria. Diphtheria and tetanus toxoids are the only such vaccines now in use. Tetanus toxoid is associated with the Guillain-Barré syndrome and brachial plexitis; neither is associated with encephalopathy.

METABOLIC AND SYSTEMIC DISORDERS

Disorders of Osmolality

The number of particles in a solution determines the osmolality of a solution. Sodium salts, glucose, and urea are the primary osmoles of the extracellular space, potassium salts of the intracellular space, and plasma proteins of the intravascular space. Because cell membranes are permeable to water and osmotic equilibrium is constant, the osmolality of the extracellular space determines the volume of intracellular fluid. Hypernatremia and hyperglycemia are the major causes of serum hyperosmolality, and hyponatremia is the main cause of serum hypo-osmolality.

Diabetic Ketoacidosis

The major cause of symptomatic hyperglycemia in children is diabetic ketoacidosis. Nonketotic hyperglycemic coma, associated with mild or non-insulin-requiring diabetes, is unusual in children.

Clinical Features. Diabetic ketoacidosis develops rapidly in children who have neglected to take prescribed doses of insulin or who have a superimposed infection. Initial features are polydipsia, polyuria, and fatigue. The child hyperventilates to compensate for metabolic acidosis. Lethargy rapidly progresses to coma. Ketoacidosis is the leading cause of death in children with diabetes, and mortality rates are still as high as 10%.

Cerebral edema develops in 1% of cases of diabetic ketoacidosis. The attributed mechanism is retention of intracellular osmolytes in the brain during hydration, causing a shift of water into the intracellular space. Signs of cerebral edema include agitation, confusion, lethargy, headache, emesis, and incontinence. The severity of cerebral edema correlates with changes in level of consciousness. Other, less common, neurological complications of diabetic ketoacidosis are venous sinus thrombosis and intracerebral hemorrhage. Both are associated with focal or generalized seizures.

Diagnosis. The basis for diagnosis is the combination of a blood glucose level greater than 400 mg/dL (22 mmol/L), the presence of serum and urinary ketones, an arterial pH less than 7.25, and a serum bicarbonate concentration less than 15 mmol/L.

Management. In children with moderate to severe diabetic ketoacidosis, avoid the rapid administration of hypotonic fluids at a time of high serum osmolality. Replace fluid deficits evenly over 48 hours. Reduce the sodium deficit by half in the first 12 hours and the remainder eliminated over the next 36 hours. Provide bicarbonate ion in physiological proportions.

Hypoglycemia

Symptomatic hypoglycemia after the neonatal period is usually associated with insulin use in the treatment of diabetes mellitus. Only a minority of cases are caused by sepsis and inborn errors of metabolism.

Clinical Features. Clinical features are not precisely predictable from the blood glucose concentration. Hypoglycemia does not usually become symptomatic until blood concentrations are less than 50 mg/dL (2.8 mmol/L). The rate of fall may be important in determining the clinical features. Dizziness and tremor may occur at blood concentrations below 60 mg/dL (3.1 mmol/L) and serve as a warning of insulin overdose. Greater declines in blood glucose concentration result in confusion, delirium, and loss of consciousness. Sudden hemiplegia, usually transitory and sometimes shifting between the two sides, is a rare feature of hypoglycemia. The mechanism is unknown, and CT shows no evidence of infarction.

Diagnosis. Always suspect hypoglycemia in diabetic children with altered mental status or decreased consciousness. Measure the blood glucose concentration promptly.

Management. Diabetic children should be encouraged to carry a source of sugar for use at the first symptom of hypoglycemia. Children who are comatose from hypoglycemia should receive immediate intravenous glucose replacement. Complete recovery is the rule.

Hypernatremia

The usual causes of hypernatremia are: (1) dehydration in which water loss exceeds sodium loss; (2) over-hydration with hypertonic saline solutions. Hypernatremia is a medical emergency and, if not corrected promptly, may lead to permanent brain damage and death.

Clinical Features. Hypernatremic dehydration may be a consequence of vomiting or diarrhea, especially if water intake is restricted. Overzealous correction of hyponatremia causes iatrogenic hypernatremia. Rapid alterations in sodium concentration are much more likely to cause encephalopathy than are equivalent concentrations attained slowly. The symptoms of hypernatremia are referable to the nervous system and include irritability, lethargy progressing to coma, and seizures. The presence of focal neurological deficits suggests cerebral venous sinus thrombosis.

Diagnosis. Symptomatic hypernatremia develops at sodium concentrations greater than 160mEq/L (160mmol/L). EEG shows the nonspecific slowing associated with metabolic encephalopathies. Focal slowing on the EEG or focal abnormalities on examination warrants neuroimaging to look for venous sinus thrombosis.

Chronic or recurrent episodes of hypernatremia may result from hypodipsia (lack of thirst), a rare condition encountered in children with congenital or acquired brain disorders. The syndrome is usually associated with a defect in secretion of antidiuretic hormone.

Management. Rapid water replacement can lead to cerebral edema. The recommended approach is to correct abnormalities of intravascular volume before correcting the water deficit.

Hyponatremia

Hyponatremia may result from water retention, sodium loss, or both. The syndrome of inappropriate antidiuretic hormone secretion (SIADH) is an important cause of water retention. Sodium loss results from renal disease, vomiting, and diarrhea. Permanent brain damage from hyponatremia is uncommon, but may occur in otherwise healthy children if the serum sodium concentration remains less than 115mEq/L for several hours.

Syndrome of Inappropriate Antidiuretic Hormone Secretion

SIADH occurs in association with several neurological disorders, including head trauma, infections, and intracranial hemorrhage.

Clinical Features. Most patients with SIADH have a preexisting loss of consciousness from their underlying neurological disorder. In such patients, hyponatremia is the only feature of SIADH. In those who are alert, lethargy develops from the hyponatremia but rarely progresses to coma or seizures.

Diagnosis. The care of children with acute intracranial disorders requires vigilance for SIADH. Repeated determinations of the serum sodium concentration are required. Measure the urinary sodium concentration once documenting hyponatremia and low serum osmolality. The urine osmolality in SIADH does not always exceed the serum osmolality, but the urine is less than maximally dilute, which excludes the dilutional hyponatremia of water intoxication.

Management. All signs of SIADH respond to fluid restriction. An intake of 50–75 % of daily water maintenance is generally satisfactory.

Sodium Loss

Clinical Features. Movement of water into the brain causes *hyponatremic encephalopathy*. Serum sodium concentrations below 125mEq/L (125mmol/L) are associated with nausea, vomiting, muscular twitching, and lethargy. Seizures and coma are associated with a further decline to less than 115mEq/L (115mmol/L).

Diagnosis. Hyponatremia is a potential problem in children with vomiting or diarrhea or with renal disease. Both serum and urinary sodium concentrations are low.

Management. Infuse hypertonic sodium chloride (514mEq/L) with the goal of increasing the serum sodium concentration to 125–130mEq/L (125–130mmol/L) but by no more than 25mEq/L (25mmol/L) in the first 48 hours. More rapid corrections are associated with seizures, hypernatremic encephalopathy, and the possibility of central pontine myelinolysis.

Endocrine Disorders

Adrenal Disorders

Adrenal hypersecretion causes agitation or depression but does not produce coma. Adrenal failure may result from sepsis, abrupt withdrawal of corticosteroid therapy, or adrenal hemorrhage. Initial symptoms are nausea, vomiting, abdominal pain, and fever. Lethargy progresses to coma and is associated with hypovolemic shock. Prompt intravenous infusion of fluids, glucose, and corticosteroids is lifesaving.

Parathyroid Disorders

All of the neurological features of hyperparathyroidism relate to hypercalcemia. Weakness and myopathy are relatively common. Alterations in mental status occur in 50 % of patients and include apathy, delirium, paranoia, and dementia. Apathy and delirium occur at serum calcium concentrations greater than 11mg/dL (2.75mmol/L), and psychosis and dementia develop at concentrations of 16mg/dL (4.0mmol/L) or greater.

Seizures are the main feature of hypoparathyroidism and hypocalcemia. They may be generalized or focal and often preceded by tetany. Hypocalcemic seizures do not respond to anticonvulsant drugs; calcium replacement is the only treatment.

Thyroid Disorders

Hyperthyroidism causes exhilaration bordering on mania and may be associated with seizures, tremor, and chorea (see Chapter 14). Thyroid storm (crisis) is a life-threatening event characterized by restlessness, cardiac arrhythmia, vomiting, and diarrhea. Delirium is an early feature and may progress to coma.

Acquired hypothyroidism affects both the central and peripheral nervous systems. Peripheral effects include neuropathy and myopathy. Central effects are cranial nerve abnormalities, ataxia, psychoses, dementia, seizures, and coma. Delusions and hallucinations occur in more than half of patients with long-standing disease. Myxedema coma, a rare manifestation of long-standing hypothyroidism in adults, is even less common in children. A characteristic feature is profound hypothermia without shivering.

Hashimoto's Encephalopathy. Hashimoto's encephalopathy is a steroid-responsive encephalopathy associated with high titers of antithyroid antibodies (Castillo et al, 2006). It often occurs in association with other immune-mediated disorders.

Clinical Features. The progression of symptoms is variable. In some, it begins with headache and/or confusion that progress to stupor. In others, a progressive encephalopathy characterized by dementia occurs. Focal or generalized seizures and transitory neurological deficits (stroke-like episodes) may be an initial or a late feature. Tremulousness and/or myoclonus occur during some stage in the illness. Other symptoms including cognitive decline may occur (Vasconcellos et al, 1999). The encephalopathy lasts for days to months and often gradually disappears. Recurrent episodes are the rule and may coincide with the menstrual cycle (Sellal et al, 2002).

Diagnosis. Suspect Hashimoto's encephalopathy in every case of recurrent or progressive encephalopathy. The cerebrospinal fluid protein concentration is usually elevated, sometimes above 100mg/dL (1g/L), but the pressure and cell count are normal. Affected individuals are usually euthyroid. The diagnosis depends on the presence of antithyroid antibodies. Antibodies against thyroglobulin and the microsomal fraction are most common, but antibodies against other thyroid elements and other organs may be present as well. Antithyroid antibodies and circulating immune complexes are detectable in the cerebrospinal fluid but do not correlate with clinical symptoms (Ferracci et al, 2003). MRI may show diffuse signal abnormalities in the white matter.

Management. Corticosteroids are beneficial in ending an attack and preventing further episodes. The long-term prognosis is good.

Hepatic Encephalopathy

Children with acute hepatic failure often develop severe cerebral edema. Viral hepatitis, drugs, toxins, and Reye syndrome are the main causes of acute hepatic failure. The cause of encephalopathy is hepatic cellular failure and the diversion of toxins from the hepatic portal vein into the systemic circulation. Severe viral hepatitis with marked elevation of the unconjugated bilirubin concentration may even lead to kernicterus in older children.

In children with chronic cholestatic liver disease, demyelination of the posterior columns and peripheral nerves may result from vitamin E deficiency. The major features are ataxia, areflexia, and gaze paresis, without evidence of encephalopathy (see Chapter 10).

Clinical Features. The onset of encephalopathy can be acute or slowly evolving (Tessier et al, 2002). Malaise and fatigue are early symptoms that accompany the features of hepatic failure: jaundice, dark urine, and abnormal results of liver function tests. Nausea and vomiting occur with fulminating hepatic failure. The onset of coma may be spontaneous or induced by gastrointestinal bleeding, infection, high protein intake, and excessive use of tranquilizers or diuretics. The first features are disturbed sleep and a change in affect. Drowsiness, hyperventilation, and asterixis, a flapping tremor at the wrist with arms extended and wrists flexed, follow. Hallucinations sometimes occur during early stages, but a continuous progression to coma is more common. Seizures and decerebrate rigidity develop as the patient becomes comatose.

Diagnosis. In hepatic coma, the EEG pattern is not specific but is always abnormal and suggests a metabolic encephalopathy: loss of posterior rhythm, generalized slowing of background, and frontal triphasic waves. Biochemical markers of liver failure include a sharp rise in serum transaminase, increased prothrombin time, mixed hyperbilirubinemia, hyperammonemia, and a decline in serum albumin concentration.

Management. The goal of treatment is to maintain cerebral, renal, and cardiopulmonary function until liver regeneration or transplantation can occur. Cerebral function is impaired, not only by abnormal concentrations of metabolites but also by cerebral edema.

Inborn Errors of Metabolism

The inborn errors of metabolism that cause states of decreased consciousness are usually associated with hyperammonemia, hypoglycemia, or organic aciduria. Neonatal seizures are

BOX 2-5 Differential Diagnosis of Carnitine Deficiency

INBORN ERRORS OF METABOLISM

- Aminoacidurias
  - Glutaric aciduria
  - Isovaleric acidemia
  - Methylmalonic acidemia
  - Propionic acidemia
- Disorders of pyruvate metabolism
  - Multiple carboxylase deficiency
  - Pyruvate carboxylase deficiency
  - Pyruvate dehydrogenase deficiency
- Disorders of the respiratory chain
- Medium-chain acyl-CoA dehydrogenase (MCAD) deficiency
- Phosphoglucomutase deficiency

ACQUIRED CONDITIONS

- Hemodialysis
- Malnutrition
- Pregnancy
- Reye syndrome
- Total parenteral nutrition
- Valproate hepatotoxicity

an early feature in most of these conditions (see Chapter 1), but some may not cause symptoms until infancy or childhood. Inborn errors with a delayed onset of encephalopathy include disorders of pyruvate metabolism and respiratory chain disorders (see Chapters 5, 6, 8, and 10); hemizygotes for ornithine carbamylase deficiency and heterozygotes for carbamyl phosphate synthetase deficiency (see Chapter 1); glycogen storage diseases (see Chapter 1); and primary carnitine deficiency.

Medium-Chain Acyl-CoA Dehydrogenase Deficiency

Medium-chain acyl-coenzyme A dehydrogenase (MCAD) is one of the enzymes involved in mitochondrial fatty acid oxidation. Mitochondrial fatty acid oxidation fuels hepatic ketogenesis, a major source of energy when hepatic glycogen stores deplete during prolonged fasting and periods of higher energy demands (Matern & Rinaldo, 2012). Transmission of the trait is by autosomal recessive inheritance. MCAD deficiency is the main cause of the syndrome of *primary carnitine deficiency* (Box 2-5). Carnitine has two main functions: (1) the transfer of long-chain fatty acids into the inner mitochondrial membrane to undergo β-oxidation and generate energy; and (2) the modulation of the acyl-CoA/CoA ratio and the esterification of potentially toxic acyl-CoA metabolites. The transfer of fatty acids across the mitochondrial membrane requires the conversion of acyl-CoA to acylcarnitine and the enzyme carnitine palmitoyl transferase. If the carnitine concentration is deficient, toxic levels of acyl-CoA accumulate and impair the citric acid cycle, gluconeogenesis, the urea cycle, and fatty acid oxidation.

Clinical Features. The characteristic features of the disorder are intolerance to prolonged fasting, recurrent episodes of hypoglycemia, and coma. Affected children are normal at birth. Recurrent attacks of nonketotic hypoglycemia, vomiting, confusion, lethargy, and coma are provoked by intercurrent illness or fasting during infancy and early childhood. Cardiorespiratory arrest and sudden infant death may occur, but MCAD is not an important cause of the sudden infant death syndrome. Between attacks, the child may appear normal. In some families the deficiency causes cardiomyopathy, whereas in others it causes only mild to moderate proximal weakness (see Chapters 6 and 7). Deficiencies of long-chain and short-chain acyl-CoA dehydrogenase cause a similar clinical phenotype.

Diagnosis. All affected children have low or absent urinary ketones during episodes of hypoglycemia and elevated serum concentrations of aspartate aminotransferase and lactate dehydrogenase. Blood carnitine concentrations are less than 20 μmol/mg noncollagen protein. Showing the enzyme deficiency or the genetic mutation establishes the diagnosis. Abnormal acylcarnitine profile in plasma or urine organic acids is suspicious, and the diagnosis can be confirmed with measurement of MCAD enzyme activity in fibroblasts or other tissues.

Management. The prognosis is excellent once the diagnosis is established and institution of frequent feedings avoids prolonged period of fasting. L-Carnitine supplementation, initially 50 mg/kg/day, and increased as tolerated (up to 800 mg/kg/day), further reduces the possibility of attacks. Adverse effects of carnitine include nausea, vomiting, diarrhea, and abdominal cramps.

During an acute attack, provide a diet rich in medium-chain triglycerides and low in long-chain triglycerides in addition to carnitine. General supportive care is required for hypoglycemia and hypoprothrombinemia.

Renal Disorders

Children with chronic renal failure are at risk for acute or chronic uremic encephalopathy, dialysis encephalopathy, hypertensive encephalopathy, and neurological complications of the immunocompromised state.

Acute Uremic Encephalopathy

Clinical Features. In children with acute renal failure, symptoms of cerebral dysfunction develop over several days. Asterixis is often the initial feature. Periods of confusion and headache, sometimes progressing to delirium and then to lethargy, follow. Weakness, tremulousness, and muscle cramps develop. Myoclonic jerks and tetany may be present. If uremia continues, decreasing consciousness and seizures follow.

The *hemolytic-uremic syndrome* is a leading cause of acute renal failure in children younger than 5 years old. The combination of thrombocytopenia, uremia, and Coombs-negative hemolytic anemia are characteristic features. Encephalopathy is the usual initial feature, but hemiparesis and aphasia caused by thrombotic stroke can occur in the absence of seizures or altered states of consciousness. Most children recover, but may have chronic hypertension. Survivors usually have normal cognitive function, but may have hyperactivity and inattentiveness.

Diagnosis. The mechanism of uremic encephalopathy is multifactorial and does not correlate with concentrations of blood urea nitrogen alone. Hyperammonemia and disturbed equilibrium of ions between the intracellular and extracellular spaces are probably important factors. Late in the course, acute uremic encephalopathy may be confused with hypertensive encephalopathy. A distinguishing feature is that increased intracranial pressure is an early feature of hypertensive encephalopathy but not of acute uremic encephalopathy. Early in the course, the EEG shows slowing of the background rhythms and periodic triphasic waves (Palmer, 2002).

Management. Hemodialysis reverses the encephalopathy and should be accomplished as quickly as possible after diagnosis.

Chronic Uremic Encephalopathy

Clinical Features. Congenital renal hypoplasia is the usual cause of chronic uremic encephalopathy. Renal failure begins during the first year, and encephalopathy occurs between 1 and 9 years of age. Growth failure precedes the onset of encephalopathy. Three stages of disease occur sequentially.

Stage 1 consists of delayed motor development, dysmetria and tremor, or ataxia. Examination during this stage shows hyperreflexia, mild hypotonia, and extensor plantar responses. Within 6 to 12 months, the disease progresses to stage 2.

Stage 2 includes myoclonus of the face and limbs, partial motor seizures, dementia, and then generalized seizures. Facial myoclonus and lingual apraxia make speech and feeding difficult, and limb myoclonus interferes with ambulation. The duration of stage 2 is variable and may be months to years.

Stage 3 consists of progressive bulbar failure, a vegetative state, and death.

Diagnosis. The basis for diagnosis is the clinical findings. Serial EEG shows progressive slowing and then superimposed epileptiform activity; serial CT shows progressive cerebral atrophy. Hyperparathyroidism with hypercalcemia occurs in some children with chronic uremic encephalopathy, but parathyroidectomy does not reverse the process.

Management. Hemodialysis and renal transplantation.

Dialysis Encephalopathy

Long-term dialysis may be associated with acute, transitory neurological disturbances attributed to the rapid shift of fluids and electrolytes between intracellular and extracellular spaces (*dialysis disequilibrium syndrome*). Most common are headaches, irritability, muscle cramps, and seizures. Seizures usually occur toward the end of dialysis or up to 24 hours later. Lethargy or delirium may precede the seizures.

Progressive encephalopathies associated with dialysis are often fatal. Two important causes exist: (1) opportunistic infections in the immunodeficient host usually caused by cytomegalovirus and mycoses in children; and (2) the dialysis dementia syndrome.

Dialysis Dementia Syndrome

Clinical Features. The mean interval between commencement of dialysis and onset of symptoms is 4 years (range, 1–7 years), and subsequent progression of symptoms varies from weeks to years. A characteristic speech disturbance develops either as an initial feature or later in the course. It begins as intermittent hesitancy of speech (stuttering and slurring) and may progress to aphasia. Agraphia and apraxia may be present as well. Subtle personality changes suggestive of depression occur early in the course. A phase of hallucinations and agitation may occur, and progressive dementia develops.

Myoclonic jerking of the limbs is often present before the onset of dementia. First noted during dialysis, it soon becomes continuous and interferes with normal activity. Generalized tonic-clonic seizures often develop and become more frequent and severe as the encephalopathy progresses. Complex partial seizures may occur, but focal motor seizures are unusual.

Neurological examination reveals the triad of speech arrest, myoclonus, and dementia. In addition, symmetric proximal weakness (myopathy) or distal weakness and sensory loss (neuropathy) with loss of tendon reflexes may occur.

Diagnosis. EEG changes correlate with disease progress. A characteristic early feature is the appearance of paroxysmal high-amplitude delta activity in the frontal areas, despite a normal posterior rhythm. Eventually the background becomes generally slow, and frontal triphasic waves are noted. Epileptiform activity develops in all patients with dialysis dementia and is the EEG feature that differentiates dialysis dementia from uremic encephalopathy. The activity consists of sharp, spike, or polyspike discharges that may have a periodic quality.

Management. Aluminum toxicity derived from the dialysate fluid is the probable cause of most cases. Removal of aluminum from dialysate prevents the appearance of new cases and progression in some established cases.

Hypertensive Encephalopathy

Hypertensive encephalopathy occurs when increases in systemic blood pressure exceed the limits of cerebral autoregulation. The result is damage to small arterioles, which leads to patchy areas of ischemia and edema. Therefore, focal neurological deficits are relatively common.

Clinical Features. The initial features are transitory attacks of cerebral ischemia and headache. Misinterpretation of such symptoms as part of uremic encephalopathy is common, despite the warning signs of focal neurological deficits. Headache persists and is accompanied by visual disturbances and vomiting. Seizures and diminished consciousness follow. The seizures are frequently focal at onset and then generalized. Examination reveals papilledema and retinal hemorrhages.

Diagnosis. Because the syndrome occurs in children receiving long-term renal dialysis while awaiting transplantation, the differential diagnosis includes disorders of osmolality, uremic encephalopathy, and dialysis encephalopathy. A posterior cerebral edema syndrome associated with hypertensive encephalopathy is evident on MRI (Figure 2-3). This syndrome, otherwise known as posterior reversible encephalopathy syndrome, or PRES, has been described with hypertension, immunosuppressants, renal failure and eclampsia (Yusuhara et al, 2011). Hypertensive encephalopathy is distinguishable from other encephalopathies associated with renal disease by the greater elevation of blood pressure and the presence of focal neurological disturbances.

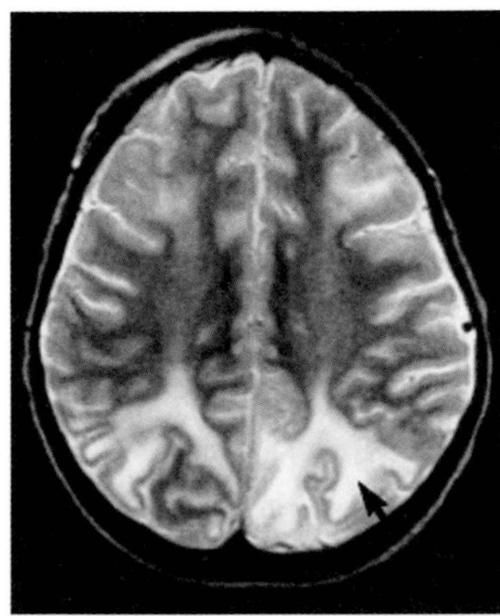

FIGURE 2-3 ■ MRI in hypertensive encephalopathy. The arrow points to increased signal intensity in both occipital lobes.

Management. Hypertensive encephalopathy is a medical emergency. Treatment consists of anticonvulsant therapy and aggressive efforts to reduce hypertension. Measures to reduce cerebral edema are required in some patients.

Other Metabolic Encephalopathies

Box 2-2 lists several less common causes of metabolic encephalopathy. Some are attributable to derangements of a single substance, but most are multifactorial.

In 5% of children with burns covering 30% of the body surface, an encephalopathy that may have an intermittent course develops (burn encephalopathy). The onset is days to weeks after the burn. Altered mental states (delirium or coma) and seizures (generalized or focal) are the major features. The encephalopathy is not attributable to a single factor.

Encephalopathies that occur during total parenteral hyperalimentation are generally due to hyperammonemia caused by excessive loads of amino acids. The causes of hypomagnesemia in infancy include prematurity, maternal deficiency, maternal or infant hypoparathyroidism, a high phosphorus diet, exchange transfusion, intestinal disorders, and specific defects in magnesium absorption. These conditions are often associated with hypocalcemia. Excessive use of diuretics causes hypomagnesemia in older children. Symptoms develop when plasma magnesium concentrations are less than 1.2 mg/dL (0.5 mmol/L), and include jitteriness, hyperirritability, and seizures. Further decline in serum magnesium concentrations leads to obtundation and coma.

Deficiency of one or more B vitamins may be associated with lethargy or delirium, but only thiamine deficiency causes coma. Thiamine deficiency is relatively common in alcoholic adults and produces Wernicke encephalopathy but is uncommon in children. Subacute necrotizing encephalopathy (Leigh disease) is a thiamine deficiency-like state in children (see Chapters 5 and 10).

Systemic Lupus Erythematosus

Systemic lupus erythromatosus (SLE) is a multisystem autoimmune disease, characterized by the presence of antinuclear antibodies, especially antibodies to double-standard DNA. It accounts for 5 % of patients seen in pediatric rheumatology clinics. The onset of SLE is uncommon before adolescence. In childhood, the ratio of girls affected to boys is 5:1.

The pathophysiology of the neurological dysfunction is immune complex deposition in the brain rather than vasculitis. The clinical and imaging features are consistent with diffuse encephalopathy rather than stroke.

Clinical Features. The female to male gender bias is 8:1. CNS manifestations are the initial feature of SLE in 20 % of cases and occur in half of children with SLE during the course of their illness. Neuropsychiatric abnormalities occur in up to 95 % of patients. Patients with CNS involvement have usually a more severe course. Other common features are recurrent headache, cognitive disorders, and seizures. Some degree of cognitive dysfunction is measurable in most patients, but dementia is uncommon. Depression and anxiety are relatively common. It is uncertain whether depression is symptomatic of the disease or a reaction to chronic illness. Corticosteroids, which are a mainstay of treatment, may also contribute to the anxiety. Frank psychosis, as defined by impaired reality testing and hallucinations, occurs in less than 15 % of patients.

Diagnosis. Other criteria establish the diagnosis of SLE before the development of encephalopathy. Patients with encephalopathy usually have high serum titers of anti-DNA and lymphocytotoxic antibodies and high cerebrospinal fluid titers of antineural antibodies. This further supports the concept that the encephalopathy is immune mediated.

Management. The usual treatment of the CNS manifestations of SLE is high-dose oral or intravenous corticosteroids after ruling out an infectious process. Several studies support the use of both steroids and cyclophosphamide in treating CNS lupus.

Anti-N-Methyl-D-Aspartate (NMDA) Receptor Antibody Encephalopathy

This condition was recently recognized and is an important treatable condition seen in children as young as 2 years old.

Clinical Features. Most children and adolescents present with behavioral personality changes (including symptoms of depression, anxiety or psychosis), seizures or sleep disorders, with a lesser percentage presenting with dyskinesias or dystonias (9.5 %), and speech reduction (3 %). Malignant catatonia with autonomic instability is possible. Ultimately, 77 % of children develop seizures, 84 % stereotyped movements, and 86 % autonomic instability. Ovarian teratomas are an important potential cause of the syndrome in girls (31 %), but less so than in adult women (56 %). Tumors are rare in males.

Diagnosis. Confirmation by ELISA of antibodies against the NR1 subunit of the NMDA receptors is diagnostic.

Management. When possible, tumor removal offers the best prognosis, in addition to immunosuppressant therapy. Most patients have significant or full recovery after tumor removal or immunotherapy, but up to one-quarter experience relapses. Intravenous immunoglobulin, steroids and plasmapheresis have all been associated with improvement or resolution of symptoms (Florance et al, 2009).

MIGRAINE

Migraine causes several neurological syndromes and is discussed in many chapters. Among its less common syndromes are a confusional state, an amnestic state, and coma.

Acute Confusional Migraine

Clinical Features. A confused and agitated state resembling toxic-metabolic psychosis occurs as a migraine variant in children between the ages of 5 and 16. Most affected children are 10 years of age or older. The symptoms develop rapidly. The child becomes delirious and appears to be in pain but does not complain of headache. Impaired awareness of the environment, retarded responses to painful stimuli, hyperactivity, restlessness, and combative behavior are evident. The duration of an attack is usually 3–5 hours but may be as long as 20 hours. The child eventually falls into a deep sleep, appears normal on awakening, and has no memory of the episode. Confusional attacks tend to recur over days or months and then evolve into typical migraine episodes.

Diagnosis. Migraine is always a clinical diagnosis and other possibilities require exclusion. The diagnosis relies heavily on a family history of migraine, but not necessarily of confusional migraine. During or shortly after a confusional attack the EEG shows unilateral temporal or occipital slowing.

Management. Most individuals experiencing a first attack come for emergency services. Intramuscular chlorpromazine, 1 mg/kg, treats the acute attack. After the end of the attack, suggest a prophylactic agent to prevent further episodes (see Chapter 3).

Migraine Coma

Migraine coma is a rare, extreme form of migraine.

Clinical Features. The major features of migraine coma are: (1) recurrent episodes of coma precipitated by trivial head injury; and (2) apparent meningitis associated with life-threatening cerebral edema. Migraine coma occurs in kindred with familial hemiplegic migraine (see Chapter 11), but a similar syndrome may also occur in sporadic cases. Coma develops following trivial head injury and is associated with fever. Cerebral edema causes increased intracranial pressure. States of decreased consciousness may last for several days. Recovery is then complete.

Diagnosis. Coma following even trivial head injury causes concern for intracranial hemorrhage. The initial CT scan may be normal, especially if obtained early in the course. Scans obtained between 24 and 72 hours show either generalized or focal edema. Examination of the cerebrospinal fluid reveals increased pressure and pleocytosis (up to 100 cells/mm^3). The combination of fever, coma, and cerebrospinal fluid pleocytosis suggests viral encephalitis, and herpes is a possibility if edema localizes to one temporal lobe.

Management. Treat children who have experienced migraine coma with a prophylactic agent to prevent further attacks (see Chapter 3). The major treatment goal during the acute attack is to decrease intracranial pressure by reducing cerebral edema (see Chapter 4).

Transient Global Amnesia

Sudden inability to form new memories and repetitive questioning about events, without other neurological symptoms or signs, characterizes transient global amnesia. It usually occurs in adults and is not a migraine symptom. However, migraine is the probable cause when such attacks occur in children or in more than one family member.

Clinical Features. Attacks last for periods ranging from 20 minutes to several hours, and retrograde amnesia is present on recovery. Many adults with transient global amnesia have a history of migraine, and a similar syndrome occurs in children with migraine following trivial head injury. The attacks are similar to acute confusional migraine except that the patient has less delirium and greater isolated memory deficiency.

Diagnosis. A personal or family history of migraine is essential for diagnosis. The CT scan shows no abnormalities, but the EEG may show slowing of the background rhythm in one temporal lobe.

Management. Management is the same as for migraine with aura (see Chapter 3).

PSYCHOLOGICAL DISORDERS

Panic disorders and schizophrenia may have an acute onset of symptoms suggesting delirium or confusion and must be distinguished from acute organic encephalopathies.

Panic Disorder

Clinical Features. Recognition of panic attacks as a disorder of adolescents and school-age children is relatively recent. A panic attack is an agitated state caused by anxiety. Principal features are paroxysmal dizziness, headache, and dyspnea. Hyperventilation often occurs and results in further dizziness, paresthesias, and light-headedness. The attacks are usually unprovoked, but some factors, such as phobias or situational anxieties, may provoke them. They can last for minutes to hours and recur daily. The person may feel drained afterwards, different from the confusion and psychomotor slowing noted after a generalized seizure.

Diagnosis. Panic attacks simulate cardiac, pulmonary or neurological disease, and many children undergo extensive and unnecessary medical evaluation or treatments before a correct diagnosis is reached. Suspect panic disorder in children with recurrent attacks of hyperventilation, dizziness, or dyspnea. The attacks are self-limited. Cessation after any intervention such as a breathing treatment often leads to the wrong diagnosis.

Management. Selective serotonin reuptake inhibitors are very helpful in decreasing anxiety and the occurrence of panic attacks. Citalopram at doses between 5 and 20 mg/day and escitalopram at doses of 2.5–10 mg/day are our first line of treatment.

Schizophrenia

Clinical Features. Schizophrenia is a disorder of adolescence or early adult life and almost never seen in prepubertal children. Schizophrenic individuals do not have an antecedent history of an affective disorder. An initial feature is often declining work performance simulating dementia. Intermittent depersonalization (not knowing where or who one is) may occur early in the course and suggests complex partial seizures.

Thoughts move with loose association from one idea to another until they become incoherent. Delusions and hallucinations are common and usually have paranoid features. Motor activity is either lacking or excessive and purposeless. This combination of symptoms in an adolescent may be difficult to distinguish clinically from drug encephalopathy.

Diagnosis. Establishing the diagnosis is by careful evaluation of mental status. The family may have a history of schizophrenia. Neurological and laboratory findings are normal. A normal EEG in an alert child with the clinical symptoms of an acute encephalopathy points to a psychiatric disturbance, including schizophrenia.

Management. Antipsychotic drugs may alleviate many of the symptoms.

TOXIC ENCEPHALOPATHIES

Accidental poisoning with drugs and chemicals left carelessly within reach is relatively common in children from ages 1 to 4 years. Between ages 4 and 10, a trough occurs in the frequency of poisoning, followed by increasing frequency of intentional and accidental poisoning with substances of abuse and prescription drugs in adolescents.

Immunosuppressive Drugs

Immunosuppressive drugs are in extensive use for children undergoing organ transplantation. The drugs themselves, secondary metabolic disturbances, and cerebral infection may cause encephalopathy at times of immunosuppression. Children treated with amphotericin B used to treat aspergillosis after bone marrow transplantation for leukemia have been repored to develop a severe encephalopathy with parkinsonian features.

Corticosteroid Psychosis

Daily use of corticosteroids at doses lower than 1 mg/kg may cause hyperactivity, insomnia, and anxiety. The higher dosages used for immunosuppression, generally >2 mg/kg/day, may precipitate a psychosis similar to schizophrenia or delirium. Stopping the drug reverses the symptoms.

Cyclosporine Encephalopathy

Cyclosporine, the drug most commonly used to prevent organ rejection, causes encephalopathy in 5 % of recipients. The blood concentration of the drug does not correlate simply with any neurological complication. The more common syndrome consists of lethargy, confusion, cortical blindness, and visual hallucinations without any motor disturbances. A similar syndrome also occurs in children with hypertension from other causes who are not taking cyclosporine (posterior reversible encephalopathy syndrome). A second syndrome is a combination of motor symptoms (ataxia, tremor, paralysis) and altered states of consciousness and cognition.

MRI shows widespread edema and leukoencephalopathy more prominent in the posterior regions (PRES). In children with the syndrome of visual disturbances and encephalopathy, the most intense disturbances are in the occipital lobes (see Figure 2-3) (Yasuhara et al, 2011). The encephalopathy clears completely after stopping the drug. Sometimes restarting the drug at a lower dose does not cause encephalopathy.

OKT3 Meningoencephalitis

OKT3 is an anti-T-cell monoclonal antibody used to initiate immunosuppression and to treat rejection. Up to 14 % of patients develop fever and sterile meningitis 24 to 72 hours after the first injection, and up to 10 % develop encephalopathy within 4 days. The encephalopathy slowly resolves over the next 2 weeks, even when the drug is continued. This toxicity is also associated with the posterior reversible encephalopathy syndrome (Yasuhara et al, 2011)

Prescription Drugs Overdoses

Most intentional overdoses are with prescription drugs, because they are readily available. The drugs usually found in homes are benzodiazepines, salicylates, acetaminophen, barbiturates, and tricyclic antidepressants. Delirium or coma may be due to toxic effects of psychoactive drugs (anticonvulsants, antidepressants, antipsychotics, and tranquilizers).

Clinical Features. As a rule, toxic doses of psychoactive drugs produce lethargy, nystagmus, or ophthalmoplegia and loss of coordination. Higher concentrations cause coma and seizures. Involuntary movements may occur as an idiosyncratic or dose-related effect. Diazepam is remarkably safe, and an overdose typically does not cause coma or death when taken alone. Other benzodiazepines are also reasonably safe.

Tricyclic antidepressants are among the most widely prescribed drugs in the United States and account for 25% of serious overdoses. The major features of overdose are coma, hypotension, and anticholinergic effects (flushing, dry skin, dilated pupils, tachycardia, decreased gastrointestinal motility, and urinary retention). Seizures and myocardial depression may be present as well.

Following phenothiazine or haloperidol ingestion, symptom onset may be delayed for 6 to 24 hours, and then occur intermittently. Extrapyramidal disturbances (see Chapter 14) and symptoms of anticholinergic poisoning are prominent features. Fatalities are uncommon and probably caused by cardiac arrhythmia.

Diagnosis. Most drugs are laboratory identified within 2 hours. Perform a urine drug screen in all cases of unidentified coma or delirium. If an unidentifiable product is in the urine, identification may be possible in the plasma. The blood drug concentration should be determined.

Management. The specificities and degree of supportive care needed depend on the drug and the severity of the poisoning. Most children need an intravenous line and careful monitoring of cardiorespiratory status. A continuous electrocardiogram is often required because of concern for arrhythmia. Remove unabsorbed drug from the stomach by lavage and repeated doses of activated charcoal (30 mg every 6 hours) administered to prevent absorption and increase drug clearance. Treat extrapyramidal symptoms with intravenous diphenhydramine, 2 mg/kg.

Poisoning

Most accidental poisonings occur in small children ingesting common household products. Usually, the ingestion quickly comes to attention because the child is sick and vomits. Insecticides, herbicides, and products containing hydrocarbons or alcohol are commonly at fault. Clinical features vary depending on the agent ingested. Optimal management requires identification of constituent poisons, estimation of the amount ingested, interval since exposure, cleansing of the gastrointestinal tract, specific antidotes when available, and supportive measures.

Substance Abuse

Alcohol remains the most common substance of abuse in the United States. More than 90% of high school seniors have used alcohol one or more times, and 6% are daily drinkers. Approximately 6% of high school seniors use marijuana daily, but less than 0.1% use hallucinogens or opiates regularly. The use of cocaine, stimulants, and sedatives has been increasing in recent years. Daily use of stimulants is up to 1% of high school seniors.

Clinical Features. The American Psychiatric Association defines the diagnostic criteria for substance abuse as: (1) a pattern of pathological use with inability to stop or reduce use; (2) impairment of social or occupational functioning, which includes school performance in children; and (3) persistence of the problem for 1 month or longer.

The clinical features of acute intoxication vary with the substance used. Almost all disturb judgment, intellectual function, and coordination. Alcohol and sedatives lead to drowsiness, sleep, and obtundation. In contrast, hallucinogens cause bizarre behavior, which includes hallucinations, delusions, and muscle rigidity. Such drugs as phencyclidine (angel dust) and lysergic acid diethylamide (LSD) produce a clinical picture that simulates schizophrenia.

The usual symptoms of marijuana intoxication are euphoria and a sense of relaxation at low doses and a dream-like state with slow response time at higher doses. Very high blood concentrations produce depersonalization, disorientation, and sensory disturbances. Hallucinations and delusions are unusual with marijuana and suggest mixed-drug use.

Consider amphetamine abuse when an agitated state couples with peripheral evidence of adrenergic toxicity: mydriasis, flushing, diaphoresis, and reflex bradycardia caused by peripheral vasoconstriction. Cocaine affects the brain and heart. Early symptoms include euphoria, mydriasis, headache, and tachycardia. Higher doses produce emotional lability, nausea and vomiting, flushing, and a syndrome that simulates paranoid schizophrenia. Life-threatening complications are hyperthermia, seizures, cardiac arrhythmia, and stroke. Associated stroke syndromes include transient ischemic attacks in the distribution of the middle cerebral artery, lateral medullary infarction, and anterior spinal artery infarction.

Diagnosis. The major challenge is to differentiate acute substance intoxication from schizophrenia or psychosis. Important clues are a history of substance abuse obtained from family or friends, associated autonomic and cardiac disturbances, and alterations in vital signs. Urinary and plasma screening generally detects the substance or its metabolites.

Management. Management of acute substance abuse depends on the substance used and the amount ingested. Physicians must be alert to the possibility of multiple drug or substance exposure. An attempt should be made to empty the gastrointestinal tract of substances taken orally. Support of cardiorespiratory function and correction of metabolic disturbances are generally required. Intravenous diazepam reduces the hallucinations and seizures produced by stimulants and hallucinogens. Standard cardiac drugs are useful to combat arrhythmias.

Toxicity correlates poorly with drug blood concentrations with regard to the following substances: amphetamines, benzodiazepines, cocaine, hallucinogens, and phencyclidine. The basis for management decisions is the patient's condition.

The most vexing problem with substance abuse is generally not the acute management of intoxication, but rather breaking the habit. This requires the patient's motivation and long-term inpatient and outpatient treatment.

TRAUMA

Pediatric neurologists are rarely involved in the acute care of severe head trauma. More often, request for consultation comes later when some symptoms persist. Trivial head injuries, without loss of consciousness, are commonplace in children and an almost constant occurrence in toddlers. Suspect migraine whenever transitory neurological disturbances: for example, amnesia, ataxia, blindness, coma, confusion, and hemiplegia follow trivial head injuries. Important causes of significant head injuries are child abuse in infants, sports and play injuries in children, and motor vehicle accidents in adolescents. *Suspect juvenile myoclonic epilepsy in an adolescent driver involved in a single motor vehicle accident, when the driver has no memory of the event but never sustained a head injury.* It is likely that an absence seizure caused loss of control of the vehicle.

Concussion

Concussion is an alteration in mental status following a blow to the head. Loss of consciousness may or may not occur. Guidelines are available from the American Academy of Neurology (1997) and The American Academy of Pediatrics pertaining to the management of concussions in sports.

Clinical Features. Confusion and amnesia are the main features. The confusion and amnesia may occur immediately after the blow to the head or several minutes later. Frequently observed features of concussion include a befuddled facial expression, slowness in answering questions or following instructions, easy distractibility, disorientation, slurred or incoherent speech, incoordination, emotionality, and memory deficits.

In the following days to weeks, the child may have any of these symptoms: low-grade headache, light-headedness, poor attention and concentration, memory dysfunction, easy fatigability, irritability, difficulty with focusing vision, noise intolerance, anxiety, and sleep disturbances

Among children who have lost consciousness, the child is invariably tired and sleeps long and soundly if left undisturbed after regaining consciousness. Many children complain of headache and dizziness for several days or weeks following concussion (see Post-Traumatic Headache in Chapter 3). They may be irritable and have memory disturbances. The severity and duration of these symptoms usually correlate with the severity of injury but sometimes seem disproportionate.

Focal or generalized seizures, and sometimes status epilepticus, may occur 1 or 2 hours following head injury. Seizures may even occur in children who did not lose consciousness. Such seizures rarely portend later epilepsy.

Diagnosis. Obtain a cranial CT, without contrast and with windows adjusted for bone and soft tissue, whenever loss of consciousness, no matter how brief, follows a head injury. This is probably cost-effective because it reduces the number of hospital admissions. MRI in children with moderate head injury may show foci of hypointensity in the white matter, which indicates axonal injury as the mechanism of lost consciousness. Order an EEG for any suspicion that the head injury occurred during a seizure or if neurological disturbances are disproportionate to the severity of injury.

Management. Mild head injuries do not require immediate treatment, and a child whose neurological examination and CT scan findings are normal does not require hospitalization. Tell the parents to allow the child to sleep.

Severe Head Injuries

The outcome following severe head injuries is usually better for children than for adults, but children less than 1 year of age have double the mortality of those between 1 and 6 years, and three times the mortality of those between 6 and 12 years. CT evidence of diffuse brain swelling on the day of injury is associated with a 53% mortality rate.

Shaking Injuries

Clinical Features. Shaking is a common method of child abuse in infants (Duhaime et al, 1998). An unconscious infant arrives at the emergency department with bulging fontanelles. Seizures may have precipitated the hospital visit. The history is fragmentary and inconsistent among informants, and there may be a history of prior social services involvement with the family.

The child shows no external evidence of head injury, but ophthalmoscopic examination shows retinal and optic nerve sheath hemorrhages. Retinal hemorrhages are more common after inflicted injuries than after accidental injuries and may be due to rotational forces. Many of the hemorrhages may be old, suggesting repeated shaking injuries. On the thorax or back, the examiner notes bruises that conform to the shape of a hand that held the child during the shaking. Healing fractures of the posterior rib cage indicate prior child abuse. Death may result from uncontrollable increased intracranial pressure or contusion of the cervicomedullary junction.

Diagnosis. The CT shows a swollen brain but may not show subdural collections of blood if bleeding is recent. MRI reveals subdural collections of blood.

Management. The first step should always be protecting other children in the home or around the possible perpetrator. Neurosurgery consultation for intracranial monitoring, blood evacuation, ventriculoperitoneal shunting or decompressive procedures is indicated. Seek protective service to prevent further injuries. Overall, the neurological and visual outcomes among victims of shaking are poor. Most have considerable residual deficits.

Closed Head Injuries

Supratentorial subdural hematomas are venous in origin, are frequently bilateral, and usually occur without associated skull fracture. Supratentorial epidural hematomas are usually associated with skull fracture. Epidural and subdural hematomas are almost impossible to distinguish on clinical grounds alone. Progressive loss of consciousness is a feature of both types, and both may be associated with a lucid interval between the time of injury and neurological deterioration. Posterior fossa epidural and subdural hemorrhages occur most often in newborns (see Chapter 1) and older children with posterior skull fractures.

TABLE 2-2 **Glasgow Coma Scale***

Eye Opening (E)	
Spontaneously	4
To speech	3
To pain	2
None	1
Best Motor Response (M)	
Obeys	6
Localizes	5
Withdraws	4
Abnormal flexion	3
Abnormal extension	2
None	1
Verbal Response (V)	
Oriented	5
Confused conversation	4
Inappropriate words	3
Incomprehensible sounds	2
None	1

*Coma score = E + M + V.

Clinical Features. Loss of consciousness is not always immediate; a lucid period of several minutes may intervene between injury and onset of neurological deterioration. The Glasgow Coma Scale quantifies the degree of responsiveness following head injuries (Table 2-2). Scores of 8 or less correlate well with severe injury.

Acute brain swelling and intracranial hemorrhage cause the clinical features. Increased intracranial pressure is always present and may lead to herniation if uncontrolled. Focal neurological deficits suggest intracerebral hemorrhage.

Mortality rates in children with severe head injury are usually between 10% and 15% and have not changed substantially in the past decade. Low mortality rates are sometimes associated with higher percentages of survivors in chronic vegetative states. Duration of coma is the best guide to long-term morbidity. Permanent neurological impairment is an expected outcome when coma persists for 1 month or longer.

Diagnosis. Perform cranial CT as rapidly as possible after closed head injuries. Typical findings are brain swelling and subarachnoid hemorrhage with blood collecting along the falx. Intracranial hemorrhage may be detectable as well. Immediately after injury, some subdural hematomas are briefly isodense and not observed. Later the hematoma appears as a region of increased density, convex toward the skull and concave toward the brain. With time, the density decreases.

Intracerebral hemorrhage is usually superficial but may extend deep into the brain. Frontal or temporal lobe contusion is common. Discrete deep hemorrhages without a superficial extension are not usually the result of trauma. Keep the neck immobilized in children with head injuries until radiographic examination excludes fracture-dislocation of the cervical spine. The force of a blow to the skull frequently propagates to the neck. Examine the child for limb and organ injury when head injury occurs in a motor vehicle accident.

Management. Manage all severe head injuries in an intensive care unit. Essential support includes controlled ventilation, prevention of hypotension, and sufficient reduction in brain swelling to maintain cerebral perfusion. Chapter 4 contains a review of methods to reduce cerebral edema. Barbiturate coma does not affect the outcome.

Acute expanding intracranial hematomas warrant immediate surgery. Small subdural collections, not producing a mass effect, can remain in place until the patient's condition stabilizes and options considered. Consult neurosurgery as early as possible for possible intracranial pressure monitoring, shunting, hematoma evacuation or decompressive procedures.

Open Head Injuries

The clinical features, diagnosis, and management of open head injuries are much the same as described for closed injuries. The major differences are the greater risk of epidural hematoma and infection and the possibility of damage to the brain surface from depression of the bone.

Supratentorial epidural hematomas are usually temporal or temporoparietal in location. The origin of the blood may be arterial (tearing of the middle meningeal artery), venous, or both. Skull fracture is present in 80% of cases. Increased intracranial pressure accounts for the clinical features of vomiting and decreased states of consciousness. Epidural hematoma has a characteristic lens-shaped appearance (Figure 2-4).

Infratentorial epidural hematoma is venous in origin and associated with occipital fracture. The clinical features are headache, vomiting, and ataxia. Skull fractures, other than linear fractures, are associated with an increased risk of infection. A depressed fracture is one in which the inner table fragment is displaced by at least the thickness of the skull. A *penetrating* fracture is one in which the dura is torn. Most skull fractures heal spontaneously. Skull fractures that do not heal are usually associated with a dural tear and feel pulsatile. In infants, serial radiographs of the skull may suggest that the fracture is enlarging because the rapid growth of the brain causes the fracture line to spread further in order to accommodate the increasing intracranial volume.

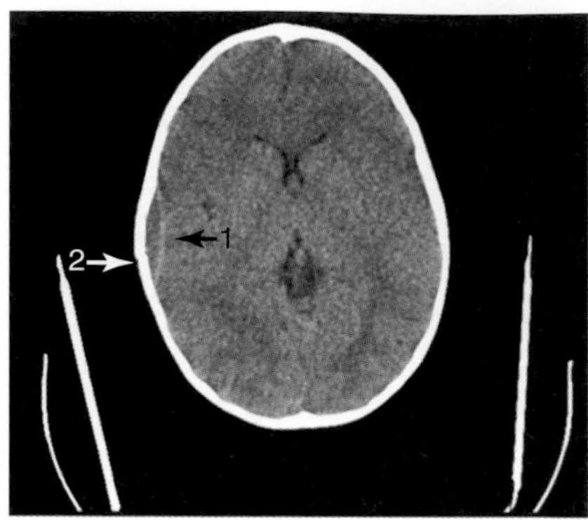

FIGURE 2-4 ■ Chronic epidural hematoma. CT scan shows a lens shaped chronic epidural hematoma (1) under a skull fracture (2).

Depressed fractures of the skull vault may injure the underlying brain and tear venous sinuses. The result is hemorrhage into the brain and subdural space. Management includes elevation of depressed fragments, debridement and closure of the scalp laceration, and systemic penicillin.

Basilar skull fractures with dural tear may result in leakage of cerebrospinal fluid from the nose or ear and meningitis. Such leaks usually develop within 3 days of injury. The timing and need for dural repair are somewhat controversial, but the need for intravenous antibiotic coverage is established.

Post-Traumatic Epilepsy

The rates of late post-traumatic epilepsy from the military (28–53%), which include missile injuries, are higher than the civilian rates (3–14%). Post-traumatic epilepsy follows 34% of missile injuries but only 7.5% of nonmissile injuries. Late seizures after closed head injury are more likely to occur in association with intracranial hematoma or depressed skull fracture. The prophylactic use of anticonvulsant therapy after a head injury to prevent post-traumatic seizures had been customary. Phenytoin prophylaxis decreases the risk of early post-traumatic seizures but not late post-traumatic epilepsy.

REFERENCES

American Academy of Neurology. Practice parameters for determining brain death in adults (summary statement). Neurology 1995;45:1012–4.

American Academy of Neurology. Practice parameters for concussion in sports. Neurology 1997;48:581–5.

Banwell B, Ghezzi A, Bar-Or A, et al. Multiple sclerosis in children: clinical diagnosis therapeutic strategies, and future directions. Lancet Neurology 2007;6:887–902.

Bode AV, Sejvar JJ, Pape WJ, et al. West Nile virus disease: a descriptive study of 228 patients hospitalized in a 4-county region of Colorado in 2003. Clinical Infectious Diseases 2006;42:1234–40.

Castillo P, Woodruff B, Caselli R, et al. Steroid-responsive encephalopathy associated with autoimmune thyroiditis. Archives of Neurology 2006;63:197–202.

De Tiege X, Rozenberg F, Des Portes V, et al. Herpes encephalitis relapses in children. Differentiation of two neurologic entities. Neurology 2003;61:241–3.

DeBiasi RL, Tyler KL. West Nile virus meningoencephalitis. Nature Clinical Practice Neurology 2006;2:264–75.

Duhaime A-C, Christian CW, Rorke LB, et al. Nonaccidental head injury in infants–the "shaken baby syndrome." New England Journal of Medicine 1998;338:1822–9.

Ferracci F, Moretto G, Candeago RM, et al. Antithyroid antibodies in the CSF. Their role in the pathogenesis of Hashimoto's encephalopathy. Neurology 2003;60:712–4.

Florance NR, Davis RL, Lam C, et al. Anti-N-methyl-D-aspartate receptor (NMDAR) encephalitis in children and adolescents. Annals of Neurology 2009;66:11–8.

Florin TA, Zaoutis TE, Zaoutis LB. Beyond cat scratch disease: Widening spectrum of Bartonella henselae infection. Pediatrics 2008;121:e1413–25.

Glaser CA, Gilliam S, Schnurr D, et al. California Encephalitis Project, 1998-2000. In search of encephalitis etiologies: diagnostic challenges in the California Encephalitis Project, 1998-2000. Clinical Infectious Diseases 2003;36:731–42.

Halperin JJ. Central nervous system Lyme disease. Current Neurology and Neuroscience Reports 2005;5:446–52.

Halperin JJ, Shapiro ED, Logigian E, et al. Practice parameter: Treatment of nervous system Lyme disease (an evidence-based review): Report of the Quality Standards Subcommittee of the American Academy of Neurology. Neurology 2007;69(1):91–102.

Hynson JL, Kornberg AJ, Coleman LT, et al. Clinical and radiological features of acute disseminated encephalomyelitis in children. Neurology 2001;56:1308–12.

Kamei S, Sekizawa T, Shiota H, et al. Evaluation of combination therapy using acyclovir and corticosteroid in adult patients with herpes simplex virus encephalitis. Journal of Neurology, Neurosurgery and Psychiatry 2006;76:1544–9.

Khurana DR, Melvin JM, Kothare SV, et al. Acute disseminated encephalomyelitis in children: Discordant neurologic and neuroimaging abnormalities and response to plasmapheresis. Pediatrics 2005;116:431–6.

Krumholz A, Berg AT. Further evidence that for status epilepticus "one size fits all" does not fit. Neurology 2002;58:515–6.

Matern D, Rinaldo P. Medium chain acyl-coenzyme A dehydrogenase deficiency. In: GeneClinics: Medical Genetics Knowledge Base [database online]. Seattle: University of Washington. Available at http://www.geneclinics.org. PMID: 20301597. Last updated January 19, 2012.

McJunkin JE, de los Reyes EC, Irazuzta JE, et al. La Crosse encephalitis in children. New England Journal of Medicine 2001;344:801–7.

Palmer CA. Neurological manifestations of renal disease. Neurology Clinics 2002;20:23–40.

Sellal F, Berton C, Andriantseheno M, et al. Hashimoto's encephalopathy: exacerbation associated with menstrual cycle. Neurology 2002;59:1633–5.

Tenembaum S, Chitnis T, Ness J, et al. Acute disseminated encephalomyelitis. Neurology 2007;68(Suppl 2):1–7.

Tessier G, Villeneuve E, Villeneuve JP. Etiology and outcome of acute liver failure: Experience from a liver transplantation centre in Montreal. Canadian Journal of Gastroenterology 2002;16:672–6.

Vasconcellos E, Piña-Garza JE, Fakhoury T, et al. Pediatric manifestations of Hashimoto's encephalopathy. Pediatric Neurology 1999;20:394–8.

Whitley RJ. Herpes simplex encephalitis: Adolescents and adults. Antiviral Research 2006;71:141–8.

Yasuhara T, Tokunaga K, Hishikawa T, et al. Posterior reversible encephalopathy syndrome. Journal of Clinical Neuroscience 2011;18:406–9.

CHAPTER 3

HEADACHE

APPROACH TO HEADACHE

Headache is one of the most common neurological symptoms and the source of frequent referrals to neurology. Proper diagnosis and management of headache has a positive impact on the lives of many children and their parents, and may significantly reduce the direct and indirect cost associated with this symptom. The World Health Organization ranks migraines as one of the top 20 disabilities in the world. Magnetic resonance imaging (MRI) and computed tomography (CT) scan are not always necessary or justified, and exposing the patient to radiation or anesthesia when not needed is not a good practice. A thorough history and neurological examination serves the child better than imaging studies in most cases. Migraine is the most common headache diagnosis in children. Some of these children develop more frequent and less disabling headaches due to additional contributing factors (analgesics, caffeine, stress, depression, etc.). The prevalence of migraines increases from 3 % in children age 3 to 7 years to 4–11 % in children age 7 to 11 years and 8–23 % in adolescents. The mean age of onset for boys is 7 years and for girls 11 years (Lewis et al, 2004). Children with migraine average twice as many days lost from school as those without migraine.

Sources of Pain

Box 3-1 summarizes pain-sensitive structures of the head and neck. The main pain-sensitive structures inside the skull are blood vessels. Mechanisms that stimulate pain from blood vessels are vasodilatation, inflammation, and traction-displacement. Increased intracranial pressure causes pain mainly by the traction and displacement of intracranial arteries (see Chapter 4). The brain parenchyma, its ependymal lining, and the meninges, other than the basal dura, are insensitive to pain.

BOX 3-1 Sources of Headache Pain

INTRACRANIAL

- Cerebral and dural arteries
- Dura mater at base of brain
- Large veins and venous sinuses

EXTRACRANIAL

- Cervical roots
- Cranial nerves
- Extracranial arteries
- Muscles attached to skull
- Periosteum/sinuses

Pain transmission from supratentorial intracranial vessels is by the trigeminal nerve, whereas pain transmission from infratentorial vessels is by the first three cervical nerves. The ophthalmic division of the trigeminal nerve innervates the arteries in the superficial portion of the dura and refers pain to the eye and forehead. The second and third divisions of the trigeminal nerve innervate the middle meningeal artery and refer pain to the temple. All three divisions of the trigeminal nerve innervate the cerebral arteries and refer pain to the eye, forehead, and temple. In contrast, referred pain from all structures in the posterior fossa is to the occiput and neck.

Several extracranial structures are pain sensitive. Major scalp arteries are present around the eye, forehead, and temple and produce pain when dilated or stretched. Cranial bones are insensitive, but periosteum, especially in the sinuses and near the teeth, is painful when inflamed. The inflamed periosteum is usually tender to palpation or other forms of physical stimulation. Muscles attached to the skull such as the neck extensors, the masseter muscles, the temporalis, and the frontalis are a possible source of pain. Understanding of the mechanism of muscle pain is incomplete, but probably involves prolonged contraction (literally *uptight*). The extraocular muscles are a source of muscle contraction pain in patients with heterophoria. When an imbalance exists, especially in convergence, long periods of close work cause difficulty in maintaining conjugate gaze and pain localizes to the orbit and forehead. Decreased visual acuity causes blurred vision, not headaches. Impaired vision is a common delay in the diagnosis and management of migraines.

Pain from the cervical roots and cranial nerves is generally due to mechanical traction from injury or malformation. Pain follows this nerve distribution: the neck and back of the head up to the vertex for the cervical roots and the face for the cranial nerves.

Taking the History

History is the most important tool in diagnosing headaches. The first step is to identify the headache temporal pattern:

Acute generalized headaches: This pattern is common with systemic or central nervous system (CNS) infections, exertional, cerebrospinal fluid (CSF) leak, postseizure, CNS hemorrhage, hypertension or metabolic causes (hypoglycemia, hypercapnea, and hypoxia).

Acute localized headaches: Sinusitis, otitis, temporomandibular joint (TMJ), ocular disease, neuralgia (trigeminal, glossopharyngeal, occipital), trauma or dental disease.

Acute recurrent headaches: Migraine, cluster, paroxysmal hemicranias, episodic tension headache, ice-pick, exertional, cough and intercourse headaches.

Chronic progressive headaches: CNS neoplasm, pseudotumor cerebri, brain abscess, subdural hematoma, hydrocephalus.

Chronic nonprogressive headaches: Depression, chronic tension, post-concussion, analgesic and caffeine induced, psychogenic and malingering headaches.

The following four questions are useful in determining the headache pattern:

1. "*Is the headache chronic but not disabling, or does it occur occasionally and prevent normal activity?*" The number of school days missed because of headache is a good indication of frequency, severity, and disability.
2. "*What is the longest period of time that you have been headache free?*" This identifies a common headache pattern in which the child has a flurry of headaches over a period of a week or two and then, after a prolonged headache-free interval, experiences another flurry of daily headaches.
3. "*How many different kinds of headache do you have?*" A common response is that child has two kinds of headache: one headache is severe and causes the child to look sick (migraine), and the other is a mild headache that is almost constant but not disabling (analgesic rebound headache).
4. "*What analgesics have you used and how often?*" This helps establish what has worked and what has failed, and may establish the diagnosis of analgesic rebound headache as a contributing factor.

Helpful responses to traditional questions concerning the history of headache can be obtained from children 10 years of age or older. Several typical headache patterns, when present, allow recognition of either the source or the mechanism of pain:

1. A continuous, low-intensity, chronic headache, in the absence of associated symptoms or signs, is unlikely to indicate a serious intracranial disease.
2. Intermittent headaches, especially those that make the child look and feel sick, from which the child recovers completely and is normal between attacks, are likely to be migraine.
3. A severe headache of recent onset, unlike anything previously experienced, from which the child never returns to a normal baseline, is probably due to significant intracranial disease.
4. Brief, intense pain lasting for seconds, in an otherwise normal child, is unusual and suggests *ice-pick headache.*
5. Periosteal pain, especially inflammation of the sinuses, localizes to the affected sinus and the area is tender to palpation. Sinusitis and allergies as a cause of headache are grossly overstated. Evidence of "sinusitis" is a common feature of CT studies on children evaluated for other reasons.
6. Cervical root and cranial nerve pain has a radiating or shooting quality.

Evaluation

A routine brain imaging study on every child with chronic headache is not cost effective and is not a substitute for an adequate history and physical examination. A joint committee of the American Academy of Neurology and The Child Neurology Society published a practice parameter for the evaluation of children and adolescents with recurrent headaches. Those with normal neurological examinations require neither electroencephalography (EEG) nor neuroimaging (Lewis et al, 2002). A CT scan of the head is helpful in most cases of suspected intracranial pathology as cause of headache. Lumbar puncture, magnetic resonance angiography and/or CT angiogram are useful when suspecting aneurysm leaks. MRI with magnetic resonance venogram may be useful when suspecting venous thrombosis in cases of increased intracranial pressure (see Chapter 4).

MIGRAINE

Ten percent of children aged 5 to 15 years old have migraine, and migraine accounts for 75 % of headaches in young children referred for neurological consultation. Children with migraine average twice as many days lost from school as those without migraine. Migraine is an hereditary disorder with a multifactorial inheritance pattern. When interviewing both parents, at least one parent gives a history of migraine in 90 % of cases. The figure drops to 80 % if only the mother is present. The prevalence of migraine is 2.5 % under the age of 7 (both genders equally affected), 5 % from age 7 to puberty (female-to-male ratio of 3:2), 5 % in postpubertal boys, and 10 % in postpubertal girls. The higher incidence of migraine in pubertal girls than in boys probably relates to the triggering effect of the menstrual cycle on migraine attacks. Approximately one-quarter of children will be migraine free by age 25 years, boys significantly more often than girls, and more than half will still have headaches at age 50 years. Of those who become parents, 50 % will have at least one child who suffers from migraine (Bille, 1997). When evaluating for family history of migraine, it is useful to expand your questioning if the parent initially reports a negative family history. Often the family labels their headaches as "normal headaches," "sinus headaches," or "allergy headache," and when asked about the qualities of these headaches they describe typical migraines.

Genetics of Migraine

Familial hemiplegic migraine is the only well-established monogenic migraine syndrome (Gardner, 2009). This condition is mapped to chromosome 19 and seems to affect calcium and sodium channels, resulting in enhanced neurotransmission and probable facilitation of the cortical spreading depression that occurs in migraines (Pietrobon, 2010). Other migraine types are more complex, appearing to result from the interaction of genetic susceptibility and environmental factors. Genetic factors are more evident in migraine with aura than in migraine without aura. Migraine and migraine-like headaches are part of several known genetic disorders.

Triggering Factors

Among persons with a predisposition to migraine, the provocation of individual attacks is usually an idiosyncratic triggering factor. Common triggering factors are stress, exercise, head trauma, the premenstrual decline in circulating estrogen, and barometric pressure changes. An allergic basis for migraine is not established. I accept without comment parental statements implicating specific foods and food additives, but discourage extensive evaluation of food as a trigger.

Stress and Exercise

Migraine symptoms may first occur during stress or exercise or, more often, during a time of relaxation following a period of stress. When stress is the triggering factor, attacks are most likely to occur in school or just after returning home. Attacks rarely occur upon awakening. Children with migraine do not have a specific personality type. Migraine is just as likely in a "slug" as in an overachiever. However, the overachiever is more likely to reach the threshold for a migraine, and sometimes the management of anxiety or obsessive-compulsiveness results in decreased migraine frequency in these patients.

Head Trauma

The mechanism by which blows to the head and whiplash head movements provoke migraine attacks is unknown. Trivial blows to the head during competitive sports are significant triggering factors because they occur against a background of vigorous exercise and stress. A severe migraine attack – headache, vomiting, and transitory neurological deficits, following a head injury – suggests the possibility of intracranial hemorrhage. Appreciating the cause-and-effect relationship between head trauma and migraine reduces the number of diagnostic tests requested.

Transitory cerebral blindness, as well as other transitory neurological deficits, sometimes occurs after head trauma in children with migraine (see Chapter 16).

Menstrual Cycle

The higher rate of migraine among postpubertal girls as compared with prepubertal children of both genders or with postpubertal boys supports the observation that hormonal changes in the normal female cycle trigger attacks of migraine. The widespread use of oral contraceptives has provided some insight into the relationship between the female hormonal cycle and migraine. Some oral contraceptives increase the frequency and intensity of migraine attacks in many women with a history of migraine and may precipitate the initial attack in genetically predisposed women who have previously been migraine free. Among women taking oral contraceptives, the greatest increase in frequency of migraine occurs at midcycle.

The decline in the concentration of circulating estrogens is probably the critical factor in precipitating an attack.

Clinical Syndromes

Migraine in children is divisible into three groups: (1) migraine with aura (classic migraine); (2) migraine without aura (common migraine); and (3) migraine equivalent syndromes. Migraine without aura is more than twice as common as migraine with aura in school-age children. Migraine with and without aura are variable expressions of the same genetic defect, and both kinds of attacks may occur in the same individual at different times. The main feature of migraine equivalent syndromes is a transitory disturbance in neurological function. Headache is a minor feature or is not present. One percent of migraineurs do not experience headache. Discussion of these syndromes occurs in several other chapters (Box 3-2).

Ice-pick headache, called *primary stabbing headache* by the International Headache Society (2004), is a peculiar migraine equivalent that occurs mainly during adolescence or later. A severe pain on top of the head drives the patient to the floor. It ends as quickly as it comes. Bouts may repeat over days or months and then remit spontaneously. Ice-pick headaches end so quickly that treatment is not required, only reassurance.

Migraine with Aura

Migraine with aura is a biphasic event. In the initial phase, a wave of excitation followed by depression of cortical function spreads (cortical spreading depression) over both hemispheres from back to front associated with decreased regional cerebral blood flow and transient neurological dysfunction. The cause of dysfunction is primarily neuronal depression rather than ischemia. The second phase is usually, but not necessarily, associated with increased blood flow in both the internal and external carotid circulations. Headache, nausea, and sometimes vomiting occur in the second phase.

BOX 3-2 Migraine Equivalents

- Acute confusional migraine* (see Chapter 2)
- Basilar migraine (see Chapter 10)
- Benign paroxysmal vertigo* (see Chapter 10)
- Cyclic vomiting
- Hemiplegic migraine* (see Chapter 11)
- Ophthalmoplegic migraine (see Chapter 15)
- Paroxysmal torticollis (see Chapter 14)
- Transient global amnesia (see Chapter 2)

*Denotes the most common conditions and the ones with disease modifying treatments

During an attack, the main clinical features (aura) may reflect only the first phase, only the second phase, or both phases. The usual features of the aura are visual aberrations: the perception of sparkling lights or colored lines, blind spots, blurred vision, hemianopia, transient blindness, micropsia, or visual hallucinations. Only a third of children describe visual symptoms. The visual aura tends to be stereotyped and unique to the child. The perception of the imagery may be limited to one eye, one visual field, or without localization.

Visual hallucinations and other visual distortions may disturb time sense and body image. This symptom complex in migraine is called *the Alice-in-Wonderland syndrome*. More extreme disturbances in mental state – amnesia, confusion, and psychosis – are discussed in the sections on confusional migraine and transient global amnesia (see Chapter 2).

Dysesthesias of the limbs and perioral region are the next most common sensory features. Other possible features of the aura are focal motor deficits, usually hemiplegia (see Hemiplegic Migraine) or ophthalmoplegia (see Ophthalmoplegic Migraine), and aphasia. Such deficits, although alarming, are transient; normal function usually returns within 24 hours and always within 72 hours.

A migraine attack may terminate at the end of the initial phase without headache. Alternatively, the initial phase may be brief or asymptomatic and headache is the major symptom (see Migraine without Aura). The pain is usually dull at first and then becomes throbbing, pulsating, or pounding. A severe headache that is maximal at onset is not suggestive of migraine. Pain is unilateral in approximately two-thirds of patients and bilateral in the rest. It is most intense in the region of the eye, forehead, and temple. Eventually the pain becomes constant and diffuse. Most headaches last for 2 to 6 hours, and are associated with nausea and sometimes vomiting. Anorexia and photophobia are concomitant symptoms. The child looks sick and wants to lie down; always ask the parent, "Does the child look sick?" With migraine, the answer is always "Yes." Vomiting frequently heralds the end of the attack, and the fatigued child falls into a deep sleep. Normal function resumes when the child awakens. Most children average one attack per month but may have long intervals without attacks and other intervals when attacks occur weekly.

The intervals with frequent headaches are probably times of stress.

Migraine without Aura

The attacks of migraine without aura are monophasic. The typical initial symptoms are personality change, malaise, and nausea. Recurrent vomiting may be the only feature of the attack in preschool children.

The headache may be unilateral and pounding, but more often the child has difficulty localizing the pain and describing its quality. When the headache is prolonged, the pain is not of uniform intensity; instead, intermittent severe headaches superimpose on a background of chronic discomfort in the neck and other pericranial muscles. Physical activity aggravates the pain. Migraine without aura may be difficult to separate from other headache syndromes or from intercurrent illness. The important clues are that the child appears sick, wants to lie down, and is sensitive to light and sound. Nausea and vomiting may occur repeatedly, need not herald the termination of the attack, and can be more prominent than the headache.

Diagnosis

The clinical features are the basis for migraine diagnosis; migraine is one of the few remaining neurological disorders in which the physician cannot stumble on the diagnosis by imaging the brain. Salient features are a family history of migraine and some combination of recurrent headache, nausea, or neurological disturbances, especially if aggravated by activity and relieved by rest and sleep. Many children will also have an increased perception of all sensory modalities including photophobia (lights), sonophobia (sounds), and osmophobia (smells). The physician should be reluctant to make the diagnosis if questioning of both biological parents does not elicit a family history of migraine. When obtaining the history, be certain that you are speaking with the biological parents and you ask for a family history of headaches and not only migraines as they usually classify their headaches as "normal headaches," "sinus headaches" or "allergy headaches." Almost half of children with migraine also have a history of motion sickness.

Diagnostic tests are unnecessary when the family history and clinical features clearly establishe a migraine diagnosis. Brain imaging is indicated only when uncertainty exists. The main reason is new abnormalities on examination. Lesser reasons are a negative family history or atypical features of the attack. The only reason to request an EEG in children with migraine-like headaches is to exclude the possibility of benign occipital epilepsy (see Chapter 1).

Management

Some improvement is common after the initial diagnosis of migraine. This is probably due to a reassurance given to the child and the family of not having a tumor or other more serious problem. Once the child's parents are convinced that the headache is due to migraine and not brain tumor, they are less anxious, the child is more relaxed, and headaches either decrease in frequency or become less a topic of discussion and concern.

The two approaches to migraine therapy are treatment of the acute attack and prophylaxis. Many children need both. Most boys do not have migraine attacks during adult life, but girls often continue having attacks until menopause.

Good advice for all migraineurs includes: (1) healthy eating and sleep habits: (2) avoid use of caffeine; (3) avoid overuse of analgesics; (4) avoid triggers when identified and possible; and (5) avoid narcotics as this may compound the problem.

Treating the Acute Attack

Acute treatment of migraines is always more effective when given early during the attack. Medication should be available at home, when traveling and at school if possible. The first line of medications includes ibuprofen or naproxen 10 mg/kg or acetaminophen 15 mg/kg. Nonprescription analgesics and nonsteroidal anti-inflammatory drugs, especially ibuprofen, are more effective than placebo in controlling pain (Mather, 2003). Nasal sumatriptan 5 or 20 mg and oral triptans such as sumitriptan (50–100 mg), rizatriptan (5–10 mg), eletriptan (20–40 mg) or zolmitriptan (2.5–5 mg) may be useful. Sumatriptan nasal spray is well tolerated, more effective that placebo, and recommended (Lewis et al, 2004). Adverse effects include fatigue, tingling of the head and arms, and a sensation of pressure or stiffness in the neck, throat, and chest.

The orally dissolved formulations of zolmitriptan and rizatriptan may be useful for children unable to swallow pills. The time of absorption is the same as other tablets as the absorption is not sublingual. For patients requiring faster onset, or when vomiting precludes oral medications, the nasal (5–20 mg) or injectable (3–6 mg) sumatriptan and the nasal or injectable (0.5–1 mg) dihydroergotamine (DHE) is a better option. The triptans and DHE are not FDA approved for children, but off-label use is common among headache specialists.

Rectal promethazine (12.5–25 mg) or prochloperazine injectable (5–10 mg) are also used when vomit interferes with oral administrations. Both promethazine and prochlorperazine can be given orally but sedation from this medication occurs in about 90 % of patients and may be as disabling as the illness. These options are helpful and less expensive when the treatment is needed at bedtime.

The following is one possible protocol for the management of severe migraine in the emergency room and hospital (Kabbouche & Linder, 2005). Prochlorperazine maleate 0.15 mg/kg with a maximum of 10 mg injected intravenously. If headache is not completely relieved, then use intravenous DHE. Pregnancy testing is required for girls over 12 years of age. Use 0.5 mg for children younger than 9 years and 1 mg for children 9 years or older. Doses may be repeated every 6 to 8 hours. If DHE fails, load with intravenous valproate sodium, 15 mg/kg followed by 5 mg/kg every 8 hours.

Migraine Prophylaxis

An extraordinarily large number of agents with diverse pharmacological properties are available for daily use to prevent migraine attacks. The use of prophylaxis agents should be considered in the following situations:

1. Migraines once a week (frequent abortive therapy may lead to medication induced headaches).
2. Failure to respond to abortive therapy.
3. Only responsive to abortive medications that also cause sedation (sedation may be as disabling in terms of loss of productivity).
4. Disability (loss of school or social activities).

The drugs with proven efficacy in older populations include amitriptyline, propranolol, valproate, topiramate. Cyproheptadine, commonly used by pediatricians, is only slightly better than placebo in controlled clinical trials.

Amitriptyline. Amitriptyline is inexpensive and has an acceptable side effect profile at low dosages, 0.5–1 mg/kg up to 50 mg at bedtime. Amitriptyline is our first choice. The mechanism of action is unknown. Nortriptyline has less sedation and may be used in patients sensitive to this side effect the morning after their dose.

Propranolol. Propranolol is a β-adrenergic blocking agent. It decreases headache frequency by at least half in 80 % of patients. The mechanism of action is probably central and not by β-adrenergic blockade. Propranolol must have central action because depression is a common side effect. This and exercise intolerance are the main reason it is often not used in children and adolescents.

The dosage in children is 2 mg/kg in three divided doses. Because depression is a dose-related adverse reaction and because lower doses may be effective, start treatment at 1 mg/kg/day. Asthma and diabetes are contraindications to usage. The maintenance dose of the sustained-release tablet is one-third greater than that of the short-acting preparation. Plasma levels of propranolol are not useful in determining the effective dose for migraine.

People who respond to propranolol do not develop tolerance. However, if abruptly stopping the drug after 6 to 12 months of therapy, some individuals will have rebound headaches of increased frequency. Others will continue to show the benefits achieved during therapy.

Topiramate and Valproate. Topiramate and valproate are widely used for epilepsy prophylaxis. In children, a dose of topiramate 50–100 mg daily or divided twice a day, or valproate 250–500 mg twice a day is effective for migraine prophylaxis. Side effects at low dosages are minimal. Be cautious with the use of valproate in adolescent females because of the significant potential for birth defects. I suggest topiramate for children who are overweight and valproate in those who are underweight or have bipolar traits. These are also good options for children with epilepsy and migraine as comorbidity.

CLUSTER HEADACHE

Cluster headache is rare in children, but may have adolescent onset. It occurs mainly in males and rarely affects other family members (Russell et al, 1995). Cluster headache is distinct from chronic paroxysmal hemicrania and hemicrania continua (see following section on Indomethacin-Responsive Headache).

Clinical Features. The onset is almost exclusively after age 10. Clusters of headaches recur over periods of weeks or months separated by intervals of months to years. A cluster of daily attacks lasting for 4 to 8 weeks may occur once or twice a year, often in the autumn or spring. Headaches do not occur in the interim.

Headache is the initial feature, often beginning during sleep. The pain occurs in bursts lasting for 30 to 90 minutes and repeats two to six times each day. It is always unilateral and affects the same side of the head in each attack. Pain begins behind and around one eye before spreading to the entire hemicrania. During an attack, the affected individual cannot lie still but typically walks the floor in anguish. This feature distinguishes cluster headache from migraine, in which the child wants to avoid motion and rest or sleep. Pain is intense and described either as throbbing, sharp or constant. The scalp may seem edematous and tender. One-third of individuals with cluster headache experience sudden intense jabs of pain suggesting trigeminal neuralgia/tic douloureux. Nausea and vomiting do not occur, but symptoms of hemicranial autonomic dysfunction – injection of the conjunctiva, tearing of the eye, Horner syndrome, sweating, flushing of the face, and stuffiness of the nose – develop ipsilateral to the headache.

Diagnosis. The clinical features alone establish the diagnosis of cluster headache. Laboratory or imaging studies have no value.

Management. The management of cluster headache consists of suppressing recurrences of a bout in progress and relieving acute pain. Prednisone suppresses bouts of cluster headache. An initial dose is 1 mg/kg/day for the first 5 days, followed by a tapering dose over 2 weeks. If headaches reappear during the tapering process, the dose is increased and maintained at a level sufficient to keep the patient headache free. If the bout of cluster headache is prolonged, alternative therapies should be considered to prevent adverse effects from long-term steroid administration.

Sumatriptan or oxygen inhalation or both treat the acute attack. The dose of sumatriptan in adults is a 6 mg injection. Most adolescents would require the same. Inhalation of 100 % oxygen at a rate of 8–10 L/min relieves an acute attack in most patients. Lithium is useful for patients with a chronic form of cluster headache in which the headache never ceases. Provide increasing doses to achieve a blood concentration of 1.2 mEq/L (1.2 mmol/L). Most patients have at least a partial response to lithium, but only 50 % are relieved completely. The addition of daily oral ergotamine enhances the beneficial effect of lithium. Verapamil, a calcium channel blocker, may be used at doses of 2–6 mg/kg/day. Topiramate may also work as prophylaxis for cluster headaches at 50–100 mg nightly. Indomethacin is another treatment option (0.5–1 mg/kg/day).

INDOMETHACIN-RESPONSIVE HEADACHE

Indomethacin-responsive headache syndromes are a group of seemingly unrelated headache disorders that respond to indomethacin and to nothing else. The syndromes include chronic paroxysmal hemicrania, hemicrania continua, and benign exertional headache.

Chronic Paroxysmal Hemicrania

Clinical Features. As with cluster headache, the main features of chronic paroxysmal hemicrania are unilateral throbbing pain associated with ipsilateral autonomic features. However, the attack duration is briefer but more frequent than in cluster headache (Goadsby & Lipton, 1997). Attacks last for weeks to months followed by remissions that last for months to years. The pain is located in the frontal and retro-orbital regions and is accompanied by conjunctival injection and tearing.

Diagnosis. The clinical features are the basis for diagnosis and laboratory or imaging studies are normal.

Management. Chronic paroxysmal hemicrania responds to indomethacin. The typical adult dosage is 75 mg/day. Successive attacks often require larger dosages. Acetazolamide may prove successful when indomethacin fails.

Hemicrania Continua

Clinical Features. Hemicrania continua is a continuous unilateral headache of moderate severity. Autonomic symptoms may be associated but are not prominent. Some patients have continuous headaches lasting for weeks to months separated by pain-free intervals; others never experience remissions. The episodic form may later become continuous.

Diagnosis. The clinical features establish the diagnosis after excluding other causes of chronic headache, such as increased intracranial pressure and chronic use of analgesics.

Management. The headaches usually respond to indomethacin at dosages of 25–250 mg/day.

Benign Exertional Headache

Exertion, especially during competitive sports, is a known trigger for migraine in predisposed individuals (see Migraine earlier in this chapter). Persons who do not have migraine may also experience headaches during exercise. Headache during sexual intercourse may be a form of exertional headache or is at least a comorbid condition (Frese et al, 2003). Some adolescents experience this headache type with weight lifting.

Clinical Features. Exertional headaches tend to be acute and severe, starting early in the course of exercise, while headaches with sexual activity increase with sexual excitement and may have a dull or throbbing quality. Headache may occur during prolonged sexual arousal, as well as during sexual intercourse.

Diagnosis. The association between exertion and headache is easily recognized. Requests for medical consultation are unusual unless the patient is a competitive athlete whose performance is impaired.

Management. Indomethacin use prior to exertion may prevent headache. The prophylactic use of indomethacin, 25 mg three times a day, or propranolol, 1–2 mg/kg/day, also reduces the incidence of attacks.

CHRONIC LOW-GRADE NON-PROGRESSIVE HEADACHES

These are almost constant or intermittent daily headaches. Most of the time, the headaches start in a child with a history of migraines and gradually increase in frequency until they occur daily. When presenting to the clinic at this stage, the headaches tend to be multifactorial in origin. The child or adolescent does not appear sick except when having a superimposed migraine attack, but is constantly complaining of headache.

In some cases, the daily headaches precede migraines. Many adolescents with chronic daily headache later convert to migraine (Wang et al, 2007). In our experience, most patients with daily headaches have a previous history suggestive of migraines.

The most common contributing factors to these multifactorial headaches are: (1) frequent analgesic use; (2) frequent caffeine use; (3) stressors, with school being the most frequent; (4) depressed mood; and (5) psychogenic etiology. The best way to treat these patients is to address all possible factors from onset to avoid delays in recovery.

Analgesic Rebound Headache

Clinical Features. Analgesic rebound is one of the more common causes of chronic headache in people of all ages. Individuals with migraine are especially predisposed to analgesic rebound headaches (*extended migraine*). The term refers to a vicious cycle of headache–analgesic use–headache when the analgesic effect wears off–more analgesic use. The pain is generalized, of low intensity, and dull. It interferes with but does not prevent routine activities and activity is not an aggravating factor (Zwart et al, 2003). This phenomenon has been described in children and adolescents, and in infants as young as 17 months (Piña-Garza & Warner, 2000; Vasconcellos et al, 1998; Warner et al, 2002).

Diagnosis. Any child using nonprescription analgesics every day, or even most days, is likely to suffer from analgesic rebound headache. The risk of chronic daily headache is high if taking analgesics, triptans or narcotics two or more doses per week.

Management. Stop all analgesic use and avoid caffeine as well. Bedtime amitriptyline (0.– 1 mg/kg) often helps the transition to the analgesic-free state. Gabapentin 2400 mg/day has proven efficacy in the treatment of chronic daily headache and may be useful for analgesic rebound headache as well (Spira et al, 2003). The first few days may be difficult, but a positive effect within weeks reinforces the recommended management. During the first months, the patient should keep a headache calendar to document the decline in headache frequency. Most of the time the migraines or rebound pain may be worse after the initial discontinuation of the offender and abortive medications for pain such as promethazine, prochloperazine and DHE are the only options. Most other medications may have a medication-induced headache effect.

Caffeine Headache

Clinical Features. Many children, especially adolescents, drink large volumes of carbonated beverages containing caffeine each day. The amount of caffeine in many popular beverages is equivalent to that in a cup of brewed coffee. The exact mechanism of the caffeine headache is not established; it could be a withdrawal effect or a direct effect of caffeine. Individuals who regularly drink large amounts of caffeine-containing beverages often notice a dull frontotemporal headache an hour or more after the last use. More caffeine relieves the headache, initiating a caffeine addiction. Withdrawal symptoms may become severe and include throbbing headache, anxiety, and malaise. In our experience, the daily use of caffeine alone is rarely the offender leading to daily headaches in a migraineur, but if the caffeine is not stopped completely, recovery is almost impossible.

Diagnosis. Most people associate caffeine with coffee and are unaware of the caffeine content of soft drinks. In addition to coffee, tea, and colas, other popular drinks with high caffeine content are deceptive because they do not have a cola color. Caffeine is also found in chocolate milk, chocolates, and other chocolate products. Adolescent girls frequently use diet colas as a substitute for food and become caffeine dependent.

Management. Caffeine addiction, like other addictions, is often hard to break. Most patients require abrupt cessation. As in analgesic rebound headache, amitriptyline at bedtime may be useful in breaking the cycle.

Stress, Depression and Psychogenic Headaches

Most migraine sufferers have an increase in headaches with stress. For children and adolescents, school is a common source of stress. The disability imposed by their migraines and the interference of this with their learning and absences from school further increases the level of stress. Not acknowledging and correcting this cycle may interfere with recovery. Temporary home schooling or abbreviated days are sometime necessary to relieve the pressure experienced by the patient.

We also have to acknowledge that chronic pain and disability may lead to depression, and that mild to moderate depression may present as headaches, body aches, gastrointestinal complaints, decreased stamina or change in sleeping or eating habits. Some children require management of their depressed mood to regain headache control.

In addition, psychogenic symptoms are common in all ages and headache is likely the most common. Children or adolescents with limited coping mechanisms for stress may subconsciously use the complaint of headache to protect themselves from overwhelming situations. It is important to examine cases of chronic daily headaches for all these factors.

Clinical Features. Chronic headaches without autonomic changes, tachycardia or hypertension during acute episodes of severe pain. Normal neurological examination, and history of depressed mood or psychosocial stressors.

Diagnosis. There is no confirmatory testing. The diagnosis should be suspected in children or adolescents with chronic headaches unresponsive to medical treatment, with a normal neurological examination, and normal vital signs during a "severe headache."

Management. We often use the help of counselors for children with daily headaches and stressors. In addition, selective serotonin reuptake inhibitors (SSRIs) for children with the comorbidity of anxiety or depression, including citalopram 10–20 mg/day, escitalopram 5–10 mg qd or sertraline 50–100 mg qd, are often helpful.

Post-Traumatic Headache

Several different kinds of headache are associated with head trauma. Forty percent of people experience a vascular headache the first day or two after head injury. It is a diffuse, pounding headache made worse by movement of the head or by coughing and straining. Dizziness may be associated. *Post-traumatic vascular headaches always subside spontaneously. Chronic post-traumatic headache is not a clinical entity; prolonged post-traumatic headaches are analgesic rebound headaches.*

Clinical Features. The individual sustains a head injury, with or without loss of consciousness, or a whiplash injury. CT scans of the head or neck do not reveal intracranial or vertebral injury. Shortly afterward, the child experiences head and/or neck pain requiring analgesic treatment – first a narcotic and then a nonprescription analgesic. A dull daily headache develops, for which a variety of analgesic medications provide no permanent relief.

Diagnosis. In the absence of imaging evidence of intracranial or vertebral injury, consider all chronic low-grade head or neck pain following trauma an analgesic rebound headache.

Management. See previous discussion of Analgesic Rebound Headache.

Tension Headache

The term tension headache is time honored (Lewis et al, 2005). The name suggests that the cause of headache is stress. This etiology is usually true with regard to episodic tension headaches (see section on Pain from Other Cranial Structures that follows), but the mechanism of chronic tension headache is less well established and is probably multifactorial. One often obtains a family history of chronic tension headache, and about half of adults with chronic tension headache date the onset to childhood. One study found tension headache the most common subtype of chronic daily headache in adolescence (Wang et al, 2006). Indeed, adolescence may cause tension headache in all family members. In our opinion, chronic tension headache is a diagnosis that has been overused or incorrectly used without fully evaluating for other contributing factors for headaches. Many of these patients suffer from depression and caffeine- and medication-induced headaches. Tension headache seems to be the most appropriate diagnosis for patients who have underlying obsessive-compulsiveness and anxiety traits, which makes them prone to respond in this way to stressors.

Clinical Features. Individuals with chronic headache of any cause may be depressed and anxious. Pain is usually bilateral and diffuse, and the site of most intense pain may shift during the course of the day. Much of the time, the headache is dull and aching; sometimes it is more intense. Headache is generally present upon awakening and may continue all day but not aggravated by routine physical activity. Most children describe an undulating course characterized by long periods in which headache occurs almost every day and shorter intervals when they are headache free.

Nausea, vomiting, photophobia, phonophobia, and transitory neurological disturbances are not associated with chronic tension headache. When these features are present, they usually occur only a few times a month and suggest intermittent migraine against a background of chronic tension headache. The neurological examination is normal.

Diagnosis. The diagnosis of chronic tension headache is to some extent a diagnosis of exclusion. Common causes of chronic headache in children that require distinction are migraine and analgesic rebound headache. Both may coexist with chronic tension headache. Brain imaging is sometimes required to exclude the specter of brain tumor. The management of chronic tension headache is often easier after a normal head CT.

Management. Chronic tension headache is by definition difficult to treat or it would not be a chronic headache. Most children have tried and received no benefit from several nonprescription analgesics before coming to a physician, and analgesic rebound headache often complicates management. The use of more powerful analgesics or analgesic–muscle relaxant combinations has limited value and generally adds upset stomach to the child's distress.

It is not always clear that a child with chronic tension headache is experiencing stress. When a stressful situation is identified, e.g., divorce of the parents, custody battle, unsuitable school placement, physical or sexual abuse, the headache cannot be managed without resolution of the stress. If the child has comorbid anxiety or obsessive-compulsiveness, SSRIs may be helpful.

HEADACHES ASSOCIATED WITH DRUGS AND FOODS

Many psychotropic drugs, analgesics, and cardiovascular agents cause headache. Cocaine use produces a migraine-like headache in individuals who do not have migraine at other times. Drug-induced headache is suspect in a child who has headache following the administration of any drug. These headaches tend to be intermittent rather than daily.

Food Additives

Clinical Features. The addition of chemicals to foods preserves shelf life and enhances appearance. Ordinarily concentrations are low, and adverse effects occur only in genetically sensitive individuals. Nitrites are powerful vasodilators used to enhance the appearance of cured meats such as hot dogs, salami, bacon, and ham. Diffuse, throbbing headaches may occur just after ingestion.

Monosodium glutamate (MSG), primarily used in Chinese cooking, may cause generalized vasodilatation. Sensitive individuals develop a throbbing bi-temporal headache and a band headache, sometimes associated with pressure and tightness of the face and a burning sensation over the body. Symptom onset is 20 minutes after MSG ingestion.

Diagnosis. The association between ingestion of a specific food and headache is quickly evident to the patient.

Management. Avoiding the offending chemical prevents headache. This avoidance is not easy, as prepared foods often do not contain a list of all additives.

Marijuana

Marijuana is a peripheral vasodilator and causes a sensation of warmth, injection of the conjunctivae, and, sometimes, frontal headache. The headache is mild and ordinarily is experienced only during marijuana use. However, marijuana metabolites remain in the blood for several days, and chronic headaches occur in children who are regular users.

HEADACHE AND SYSTEMIC DISEASE

Vasculitis

Headaches caused by vasculitis, especially temporal arteritis, are important in the differential diagnosis of vascular headaches in adults. Cerebral vasculitis is uncommon in children and usually occurs as part of a collagen vascular disease, as a result of hypersensitivity, or as part of an infection of the nervous system.

Connective Tissue Disorders

Headache is a feature of systemic lupus erythematosus (SLE) and mixed connective tissue disease. In patients with connective tissue disease, it is not clear that the cause of neurological symptoms, including headache, is vasculitis of the cerebral arteries.

Clinical Features. Severe headache occurs in up to 10 % of children with SLE. It may occur in the absence of other neurological manifestation and can be the initial feature of SLE.

Mixed connective tissue disease is a syndrome with features of SLE, scleroderma, and polymyositis. Its course is usually less severe than that of lupus. Thirty-five percent of people with mixed connective tissue disease report vascular headaches. The headaches are moderate and generally do not interfere with activities of daily living. They may be unilateral or bilateral but are generally throbbing. More than half of patients report a visual aura, and some have nausea and vomiting. Some of these children may be experiencing migraine aggravated by the underlying vasculitis; in others, the cause of headache is the vasculitis itself.

Diagnosis. The diagnosis of connective tissue disease depends on the combination of a compatible clinical syndrome and the demonstration of antinuclear antibodies in the blood. The presence of antinuclear antibodies in a child with headache who has no systemic symptoms of connective tissue disease should suggest the possibility of a hypersensitivity reaction.

Management. The ordinary treatment of children with connective tissue disease is corticosteroids. In many cases, headaches develop while the child is already taking corticosteroids; this occurrence is not an indication to increase the dose. Symptomatic treatment may be adequate.

Hypersensitivity Vasculitis

The important causes of hypersensitivity vasculitis in children are serum sickness, Henoch-Schönlein purpura (see Chapter 11), amphetamine abuse, and cocaine abuse. Children with serum sickness or Henoch-Schönlein purpura have systemic symptoms that precede the headache. Persistent headache and behavioral changes are often the only neurological consequences of Henoch-Schönlein purpura. In contrast, substance abuse can cause a cerebral vasculitis in the absence of systemic symptoms. The features are headache, encephalopathy, focal neurological deficits, and subarachnoid hemorrhage.

Hypertension

A sudden rise in systemic blood pressure causes the explosive, throbbing headache associated with pheochromocytoma. Children with chronic hypertension may have low-grade occipital headache on awakening that diminishes as they get up and begin activity or frontal throbbing headache during the day. However, most children with chronic hypertension are asymptomatic. When a child with renal disease develops headache, hypertension is probably not the cause (see Chapter 2). Instead, pursue alternative causes. Headaches are common in patients undergoing dialysis and may be due to psychological tension, the precipitation of migraine attacks, and dialysis itself. Dialysis headache begins a few hours after terminating the procedure and is characterized by a mild bifrontal throbbing headache, sometimes associated with nausea and vomiting.

PAIN FROM OTHER CRANIAL STRUCTURES

Eyestrain

Clinical Features. Prolonged ocular near-fixation in a child with a latent disturbance in convergence may cause dull, aching pain behind the eyes that is quickly relieved when the eyes are closed. The pain is of muscular origin and caused by the continuous effort to maintain conjugate gaze. If work continues despite ocular pain, episodic tension headache may develop.

Diagnosis. Refractive errors are often a first consideration in children with eyestrain. Eyeglasses do not correct the headache. Refractive errors do not cause eyestrain in children, as presbyopia does in adults. Refractive errors cause poor vision and not headaches; when present they delay the diagnosis and management of migraines. These children are often referred with excellent corrected vision and persistent migraines.

Management. Resting the eyes relieves eyestrain.

Episodic Tension Headache

Clinical Features. Episodic tension headache is common in people of all ages and both genders. Fatigue, exertion, and temporary life stress cause the headache. The mechanism is probably prolonged contraction of muscles attached to the skull. The pain is constant, aching, and tight. Localization is mainly to the back of the head and neck, sometimes becomes diffuse, and then described as a constricting band around the head. Nausea, vomiting, photophobia, and phonophobia are not present. Headaches usually last for periods ranging from 30 minutes to all day. One episode may last for several days, with some waxing and waning, but not for a week.

Diagnosis. Episodic tension headache differs from chronic tension, which has similar clinical features but persists for weeks, months, or years. Most episodic tension headaches are self-diagnosed, and the individual rarely seeks medical attention.

Management. Rest, relaxation, warm compresses to the neck, massage and nonprescription analgesics relieve pain.

Sinusitis

When questioned about migraine symptoms, most parents identify their own episodic headache, preceded by scintillating scotomata, and followed by nausea and vomiting, as sinusitis. This diagnosis, favored by physicians and patients to describe chronic or episodic headaches, is usually wrong. The vasodilation that occurs in the trigeminal vasculature of a migraine patient during an attack may confuse them and make them feel their symptoms are respiratory in origin. The turbinates during an acute attack of migraine get "puffy" and "shrink" with the use of triptans.

Clinical Features. Children with sinusitis are usually sick. They are febrile, feel stuffy, and have difficulty maintaining a clear airway. Localized tenderness is present over the infected frontal or maxillary sinuses, and inflammation of the ethmoidal or sphenoidal sinuses causes deep midline pain behind the nose. Blowing the nose or quick movements of the head, especially bending forward, exaggerate the pain. Concurrent vascular headache caused by fever is common.

Diagnosis. Radiographs reveal clouding of the sinuses and sometimes a fluid level. CT of the skull is exceptionally accurate in identifying sinusitis but usually an unnecessary expense. It is impressive how often CT of the head, performed for reasons other than headache, shows radiographic evidence of asymptomatic sinus disease. Clearly, radiographic evidence of sinus disease does not necessarily explain many patients' headache.

Management. The primary objective of treatment is to allow the sinus to drain. Decongestants usually accomplish drainage, but sometimes surgery is required. Antibiotics have limited usefulness if drainage is not established.

Temporomandibular Joint Syndrome

The TMJ syndrome does not cause chronic generalized daily headache. The pain is unilateral and centered over and below the TMJ (Rothner, 1995).

Clinical Features. TMJ syndrome is a rare disease in children, occurring as young as 8 years of age. The duration of symptoms before diagnosis may be as long as 5 years and averages 2 years. The primary disturbance is arthritis of the TMJ causing localized pain in the lower face and crepitus in the joint. Because of pain on one side, chewing occurs on the other, with unwanted overuse of the affected side. The overused masseter muscle becomes tender; a muscle contraction headache ensues. Localization of pain is on the side of the face and the vertex. Bruxism or dental malocclusion is the usual cause of arthritis, but a prior injury of the jaw accounts for one-third of TMJ syndromes in children.

Diagnosis. Radiographs of the TMJ usually show some internal derangement of the joint and may show degenerative arthritis. MRI using surface coils is the most effective technique to show the disturbed joint architecture.

Management. TMJ syndrome treatment based on controlled experiments is not established. Placebos provide considerable benefit, and TMJ syndrome is not an indication for extensive oral surgery. Nonsteroidal anti-inflammatory agents, application of heat to the tense muscles, and dental splints may prove useful.

Whiplash and Other Neck Injuries

Whiplash and other neck injuries cause pain by rupturing cervical disks, damaging soft tissue, injuring occipital nerves, and causing excessive muscle contraction. The muscles contract in an effort to splint the area of injury and thereby reduce further tissue damage.

Clinical Features. Constant contraction of the neck extensors causes a dull, aching pain not only in the neck but also in the shoulders and upper arms. This pain may persist for up to 3 months after the injury. Holding the head in a fixed position is common. Nausea and vomiting are not associated symptoms.

Diagnosis. Cervical spine radiographs are required after any neck or head injury to determine the presence of fracture or dislocation. Shooting pains, radiating either to the occiput or down the arm and into the fingers, suggest the possibility of disk herniation and require further study with MRI.

Management. Warn the patient and family at the onset that prolonged head and neck pain is an expected outcome after injury and does not indicate a serious condition. Several different interventions achieve pain relief. Lying or sitting with the head supported, superficial application of heat to the painful muscles, muscle relaxants, and non-narcotic analgesics are potentially effective. When pain persists after 3 months and affects the head as well, the possibility of analgesic rebound headache is more likely.

SEIZURE HEADACHE

Diffuse headache caused by vasodilatation of cerebral arteries is a frequent occurrence following a generalized tonic-clonic convulsion. In patients who have both epilepsy and migraine, one can trigger the other; frequently, headache and seizure occur concurrently. Approximately 1 % of epileptic patients report headache as a seizure manifestation (seizure headache). Most patients with seizure headaches have epilepsy prior to the development of headache. In rare children, headache is the only feature of their seizure disorder.

Clinical Features. Headache is part of several epilepsy syndromes. The most common syndrome in children is *benign occipital epilepsy* (see Chapter 1). The sequence of events suggests migraine. One of the authors evaluated one eloquent adolescent who complained of paroxysmal "head pain unlike other headaches" that was associated with EEG evidence of generalized epileptiform activity. Anticonvulsants relieved head pain.

Headache may also occur as a seizure manifestation in patients known to have epilepsy. Such individuals usually have a long history of partial or generalized seizures before headache becomes part of the syndrome. Associated ictal events depend on the site of the cortical focus and may include auditory hallucinations, visual disturbances, vertigo, déjà vu, and focal motor seizures. Headache may be the initial feature of the seizure or can follow other partial seizure manifestations, such as déjà vu and vertigo. Headache description may be throbbing, sharp, or without an identified quality. Complex partial seizures, simple partial seizures, or generalized tonic-clonic seizures follow the headache phase. Spike foci in patients with seizure headaches are usually temporal in location.

Diagnosis. Chronic headache in children is not an indication for EEG. Interictal discharges, especially rolandic spikes, do not indicate that the headaches are a seizure manifestation, only that the child has a genetic marker for epilepsy. Children with paroxysmal headaches, clearly not migraine, may require an EEG study. If interictal spike discharges are seen, an effort should be made to record a seizure headache with an EEG monitor. The observation of continuous epileptiform activity during a headache provides reassurance that headache is a seizure manifestation and anticonvulsant drugs will prove effective.

Management. The response to anticonvulsant therapy is both diagnostic and therapeutic. Because the seizure focus is usually cortical and most often in the temporal lobe, use antiepileptic drugs useful for partial epilepsies (see Chapter 1).

REFERENCES

Bille B. A 40-year follow-up of school children with migraine. Cephalalgia 1997;17:488–91.

Frese A, Eikermann A, Frese K. Headache associated with sexual activity: demography, clinical features, and comorbidity. Neurology 2003;61:796–800.

Gardner KL. Familial hemiplegic migraine. In: GeneClinics: Medical Genetics Knowledge Base [database online]. Seattle: University of Washington. Available at http://www.geneclinics.org. PMID: 20301562. Last updated September 8, 2009.

Goadsby PJ, Lipton RB. A review of paroxysmal hemicranias, SUNCT syndrome and other short lasting headaches with autonomic features, including new cases. Brain 1997;120:193–209.

International Headache Society. The International Classification of Headache Disorders, 2nd ed. Cephalalgia 2004;24(Suppl 1):9–160.

Kabbouche M, Linder SL. Management of migraine in children and adolescents in the emergency department and inpatient setting. Pediatric Annals 2005;34:466–71.

Lewis DW, Ashwal S, Dahl G, et al. Practice parameter: Evaluation of children and adolescents with recurrent headaches. Report of the Quality Standards Committee of the American Academy of Neurology and the Practice Committee of the Child Neurology Society. Neurology 2002;59:490–8.

Lewis DW, Gozzo YF, Avner MT. The "other" primary headaches in children and adolescents. Pediatric Neurology 2005;33:303–13.

Lewis D, Ashwal S, Hershey A, et al. Practice parameter: Pharmacological treatment of migraine headache in children and adolescents. Report of the American Academy of Neurology Quality Standards Subcommittee and the Practice Committee of the Child Neurology Society. Neurology 2004;63:2215–24.

Mathew NT, Loder EW. Evaluating the triptans. American Journal of Medicine 2005;118(Suppl 1):29S–35S.

Mather DB. Acute management of migraine. Highlights of the US Headache Consortium. Neurology 2003;60(Suppl 2):S21–3.

Pietrobon D. Insight into migraine mechanisms and Cav2.1 calcium channel function from mouse models of familial hemiplegic migraine. Journal of Physiology 2010;588(11):1871–8.

Piña-Garza JE, Warner JS. Analgesic rebound headaches in a 17 month old infant. Journal of Child Neurology 2000;15:261.

Rothner AD. Miscellaneous headache syndromes in children and adolescents. Seminars in Pediatric Neurology 1995;21:59–164.

Russell MB, Andersson PG, Thomsen LL. Familial occurrence of cluster headache. Journal of Neurology, Neurosurgery and Psychiatry 1995;58:341–3.

Silberstein SD, McCory DC. Ergotamine and dihydroergotamine: History, pharmacology, and efficacy. Headache 2003;43:144–66.

Spira PJ, Beran RG. The Australian Gabapentin Chronic Daily Headache Group. Gabapentin in the prophylaxis of chronic daily headache. A randomized placebo-controlled study. Neurology 2003;61:1753–9.

Vasconcellos E, Piña-Garza JE, Millan EJ, Warner JS. Analgesic rebound headaches in children and adolescents. Journal of Child Neurology 1998;13:443–7.

Wang S-J, Fuh J-L, Lu S-R, et al. Chronic daily headache in adolescents. Prevalence, impact, and medication overuse. Neurology 2006;66:193–7.

Wang S-J, Fuh J-L, Lu S-R, et al. Outcomes and predictors or chronic daily headache in adolescents. A two-year longitudinal study. Neurology 2007;68:591–6.

Warner JS, Lavin PJ. Piña-Garza JE. Rebound headaches: Keys to effective therapy. Consultant February 2002:139–42.

Zwart JA, Dyb G, Hagen K, et al. Analgesic use: A predictor of chronic pain and medication overuse headache. The Head-HUNT study. Neurology 2003;61:160–4.

CHAPTER 4

INCREASED INTRACRANIAL PRESSURE

The presenting complaint when dealing with increased intracranial pressure (Box 4-1) varies with age. Infants may present with bulging fontanelle, macrocephaly or failure to thrive. Older children often present with headache, emesis, diplopia or change in mentation. The basis of referral for some children is the detection of disc edema during an eye examination. Some conditions causing increased intracranial pressure are discussed elsewhere in this book (see Chapters 2, 3, 10, and 15). This chapter is restricted to conditions in which symptoms of increased intracranial pressure are initial and prominent features. The timely management of increased intracranial pressure prevents secondary brain insult, regardless of the original cause, which is often a primary central nervous sytem (CNS) process (infection, abscess, tumor, infarct, others). When treating increased intracranial pressure the goal is to reduce the pressure while maintaining adequate cerebral perfusion.

PATHOPHYSIOLOGY

Normal intracranial pressure in the resting state is approximately 10 mmHg (136 mmH_2O). Pressures greater than 20 mmHg are abnormal. When the cranial bones fuse during childhood, the skull is a rigid box enveloping its content. Intracranial pressure is then the sum of the individual pressures exerted by the brain, blood, and cerebrospinal fluid (CSF). An increase in the volume of any one component requires an equivalent decrease in the size of one or both of the other compartments if intracranial pressure is to remain constant. Because the provision of oxygen and nutrients to the brain requires relatively constant cerebral blood flow, the major adaptive mechanisms available to relieve pressure are the compressibility of the brain and the rapid reabsorption of cerebrospinal fluid (CSF) by arachnoid villi. Infants and young children, in whom the cranial bones are still unfused, have the additional adaptive mechanism of spreading the cranial bones apart and bulging of the anterior fontanelle to increase cranial volume.

BOX 4-1 Features of Increased Intracranial Pressure

IN INFANTS

- Bulging fontanelle
- Failure to thrive
- Impaired upward gaze (setting sun sign)
- Large head (see Chapter 18)
- Shrill cry
- Split sutures

IN CHILDREN

- Diplopia (see Chapter 15)
- Headache (see Chapter 3)
- Mental changes
- Papilledema
- Projectile vomiting

Cerebrospinal Fluid

The choroid plexus accounts for at least 70% of CSF production, and the transependymal movement of fluid from the brain to the ventricular system accounts for the remainder. The average volumes of CSF are 90 mL in children 4 to 13 years old and 150 mL in adults. The rate of formation is approximately 0.35 mL/min or 500 mL/day. Approximately 14% of total volume turns over every hour. The rate at which CSF forms remains relatively constant and declines only slightly as CSF pressure increases. In contrast, the rate of absorption increases linearly as CSF pressure exceeds 7 mmHg. At a pressure of 20 mmHg, the rate of absorption is three times the rate of formation.

Impaired absorption, not increased formation, is the usual mechanism of progressive hydrocephalus. Choroid plexus papilloma is the only pathological process in which formation sometimes can overwhelm absorption. However, even in cases of choroid plexus papillomas, obstruction of the CSF flow rather than overproduction may be the cause of hydrocephalus. When absorption is impaired, efforts to decrease the formation of CSF are not likely to have a significant effect on volume and intracranial pressure.

Cerebral Blood Flow

Systemic arterial pressure is the primary determinant of cerebral blood flow. Normal cerebral blood flow remains remarkably constant from birth to adult life and is generally 50–60 mL/min/100 g brain weight. The autonomic innervation of blood vessels on the surface and at the base of the brain is richer than vessels of any other organ. These nerve fibers allow the autoregulation of cerebral blood flow. Autoregulation refers to a buffering effect by which cerebral blood flow remains constant despite changes in systemic arterial perfusion pressure. Alterations in the arterial blood concentration of carbon dioxide have an important effect on total cerebral blood flow. Hypercarbia dilates cerebral blood vessels and increases blood flow, whereas hypocarbia constricts cerebral blood vessels and decreases flow. Alterations in blood oxygen content have the reverse effect, but are less potent stimuli for vasoconstriction or vasodilation than are alterations in the blood carbon dioxide concentration.

Cerebral perfusion pressure is the difference between mean systemic arterial pressure and intracranial pressure. Reducing systemic arterial pressure or increasing intracranial pressure reduces perfusion pressure to dangerous levels. The autoregulation of the cerebral vessels is lost when cerebral perfusion pressure decreases to less than 50 cmH_2O or in the presence of severe acidosis. Arterial vasodilation or obstruction of cerebral veins and venous sinuses increases intracranial blood volume. Increased intracranial blood volume, similar to increased CSF volume, results in increased intracranial pressure.

Cerebral Edema

Cerebral edema is an increase in the brain's volume caused by an increase in its water and sodium content. Increased intracranial pressure results from either localized or generalized cerebral edema. The categories of cerebral edema are vasogenic, cytotoxic, or interstitial.

Increased capillary permeability causes vasogenic edema; this occurs with brain tumor, abscess, and infection, and to a lesser degree with trauma and hemorrhage. The fluid is located primarily in the white matter and responds to treatment with corticosteroids. Osmotic agents have no effect on vasogenic edema, but they reduce total intracranial pressure by decreasing normal brain volume. Cytotoxic edema, characterized by swelling of neurons, glia, and endothelial cells, constricts the extracellular space. The usual causes are hypoxia and ischemia. Corticosteroids do not decrease this type of edema, but osmotic agents may relieve intracranial pressure by reducing brain volume.

Transependymal movement of fluid causes interstitial edema from the ventricular system to the brain; this occurs when CSF absorption is blocked and the ventricles enlarge. The fluid collects chiefly in the periventricular white matter. Agents intended to reduce CSF production, such as acetazolamide, topiramate (Stevenson, 2008), and furosemide, may be useful. Corticosteroids and osmotic agents are not effective.

Mass Lesions

Mass lesions, e.g., tumor, abscess, hematoma, arteriovenous malformation, increase intracranial pressure by occupying space at the expense of other intracranial compartments, provoking cerebral edema, blocking the circulation and absorption of CSF, increasing blood flow, and obstructing venous return.

SYMPTOMS AND SIGNS

The clinical features of increased intracranial pressure depend on the child's age and the rate at which pressure increases. Newborns and infants present a special case because expansion of skull volume allows partial venting of increased pressure. The rate of intracranial pressure increase is important at all ages. Intracranial structures accommodate slowly increasing pressure remarkably well, but sudden changes are intolerable and result in some combination of headache, personality change, and states of decreasing consciousness.

Increased Intracranial Pressure in Infancy

Measurement of head circumference and palpation of the anterior fontanelle are readily available methods of assessing intracranial volume and pressure rapidly. The measure of head circumference is the greatest anteroposterior circumference. Normal standards are different for premature and full-term newborns. Normal head growth in a term newborn is 2 cm/month for the first 3 months, 1 cm/month for the second 3 months, and 0.5 cm/month for the next 6 months. Excessive head growth is a major feature of increased intracranial pressure throughout the first year up to 3 years of age. Normal head growth does not preclude the presence of increased intracranial pressure; for example, in posthemorrhagic hydrocephalus, considerable ventricular dilation precedes any measurable change in head circumference by compressing the brain parenchyma.

The palpable tension of the anterior fontanelle is an excellent measure of intracranial pressure. In a quiet infant, a fontanelle that bulges above the level of the bone edges and is sufficiently tense to cause difficulty in determining where bone ends and fontanelle begins is abnormal and indicates increased intracranial pressure. A full fontanelle, which is clearly distinguishable from the surrounding bone edges, may indicate increased intracranial pressure, but alternate causes are crying, edema of the scalp, subgaleal hemorrhage, and extravasation of intravenous fluids. The normal fontanelle clearly demarcates from bone edges, falls below the surface, and pulsates under the examining finger. Although the size of the anterior fontanelle and its rate of closure are variable, increased intracranial pressure should be suspected when separation of the metopic and coronal sutures is sufficient to accomodate a fingertip.

The infant experiences lethargy, vomiting, and failure to thrive when cranial suture separation becomes insufficient to decompress increased intracranial pressure. Sixth cranial nerve palsies, impaired upward gaze (setting sun sign), and disturbances of blood pressure and pulse may ensue. Optic disc edema is uncommon.

Increased Intracranial Pressure in Children

Headache

Headache is a common symptom of increased intracranial pressure at all ages. Traction and displacement of intracranial arteries are the major causes of headache from increased intracranial pressure (see Chapter 3). As a rule, the trigeminal nerve innervates pain from supratentorial intracranial vessels, and referral of pain is to the eye, forehead, and temple. In contrast, cervical nerves innervate infratentorial intracranial vessels, and referral of pain is to the occiput and neck.

With generalized increased intracranial pressure, as occurs from cerebral edema or obstruction of the ventricular system, headache is generalized and more prominent on awakening and when rising to a standing position. Pain is constant but may vary in intensity. Coughing, sneezing, straining, and other maneuvers, such as Valsalva, that transiently increase intracranial pressure exaggerate headache. The quality of the pain is often difficult to describe. Vomiting in the absence of nausea, especially on arising in the morning, is often a concurrent feature. In the absence of generalized increased intracranial pressure, localized, or at least unilateral, headache can occur if a mass causes traction on contiguous vessels.

In children younger than 10 years old, separation of sutures may relieve symptoms of increased intracranial pressure temporarily. Such children may have a symptom-free interval of several weeks after weeks or months of chronic headache and vomiting. The relief of pressure is temporary, and symptoms eventually return with their prior intensity. An intermittent course of symptoms should not direct attention away from the possibility of increased intracranial pressure.

An individual who was previously well and then experienced abrupt onset, intense headache probably has suffered a subarachnoid hemorrhage. A small hemorrhage may not cause loss of consciousness but still produces sufficient meningeal irritation to cause intense headache and some stiffness of the neck. Fever may be present.

BOX 4-2 Differential Diagnosis of a Swollen Disk

Congenital disk elevation
Increased intracranial pressure
Ischemic neuropathy
Optic glioma
Optic nerve drusen
Papillitis
Retrobulbar mass

Diplopia and Strabismus

Paralysis or paresis of one or both abducens nerves is a common feature of generalized increased intracranial pressure and may be a more prominent feature than headache in children with idiopathic intracranial hypertension (pseudotumor cerebri).

Optic Disc Edema

Optic disc edema ("papilledema") is passive swelling of the optic disc caused by increased intracranial pressure (Box 4-2). Extension of the arachnoid sheath of the optic nerve to the retina is essential for the of optic disc edema. This extension does not occur in a small percentage of people, and they can have severe increased intracranial pressure without disc edema. The edema is usually bilateral and when unilateral suggests a mass lesion behind the affected eye. Early disc edema is asymptomatic. Only with advanced papilledema does transitory obscuration of vision occur. Preservation of visual acuity differentiates papilledema from primary optic nerve disturbances, such as optic neuritis, in which visual acuity is always profoundly impaired early in the course (see Chapter 16).

The observation of papilledema in a child with headache or diplopia confirms the diagnosis of increased intracranial pressure. The diagnosis of papilledema is not always easy, however, and congenital variations of disc appearance may confuse the issue. The earliest sign of papilledema is loss of spontaneous venous pulsations in the vessels around the disc margin. Spontaneous venous pulsations occur in approximately 80 % of normal adults, but the rate is closer to 100 % in children. Spontaneous venous pulsations cease when intracranial pressure exceeds 200 mmH_2O. Papilledema is not present if spontaneous venous pulsations are present, no matter how obscure the disc margin may appear to be. Conversely, when spontaneous venous pulsations are lacking in children, one should suspect papilledema even though the disc margin is flat and well visualized.

As edema progresses, the disc swells and is raised above the plane of the retina, causing obscuration of the disc margin and tortuosity of the veins (Figure 4-1). Associated features include small flame-shaped hemorrhages and nerve fiber infarcts known as cotton wool. If the process continues, the retina surrounding the disc becomes edematous so that the disk appears greatly enlarged (Figure 4-2), and retinal exudates radiate from the fovea. Eventually the hemorrhages and exudates clear, but optic atrophy ensues, and blindness may be permanent. Even if increased intracranial pressure is relieved during the early stages of disc edema, 4 to 6 weeks is required before the retina appears normal again.

Congenitally elevated discs, usually caused by hyaline bodies (drusen) within the nerve head, give the false impression of papilledema. The actual drusen are not observable before age 10, and only the elevated nerve head is apparent. Drusen continue to grow and can be seen in older children and in their parents (Figure 4-3). Drusen are an autosomal dominant trait and occur more often in Europeans than other ethnic groups. Spontaneous venous pulsations differentiate papilledema from anomalous nerve head elevations. Their presence excludes papilledema.

Herniation Syndromes

Increased intracranial pressure may cause portions of the brain to shift from their normal

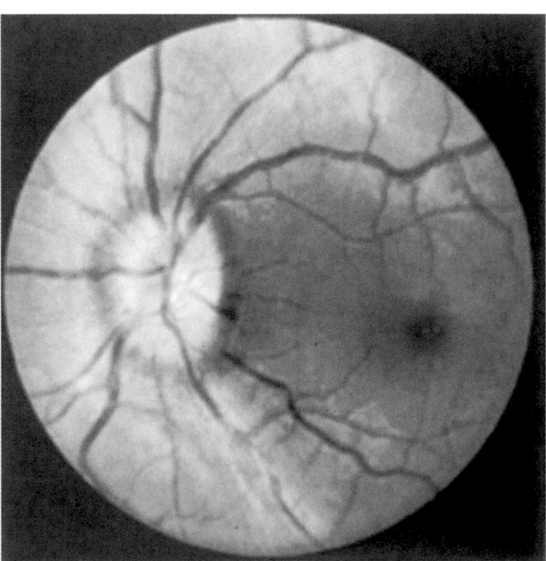

FIGURE 4-2 ■ Established papilledema. The optic disk is elevated, and opacification of the nerve fiber layer shows around the disk margin and retinal folds (Paton lines) temporally.

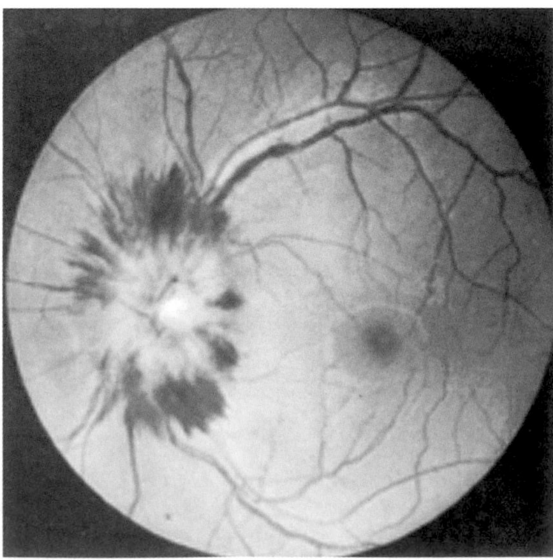

FIGURE 4-1 ■ Acute papilledema. The optic disk is swollen, and peripapillary nerve fiber layer hemorrhages are evident.

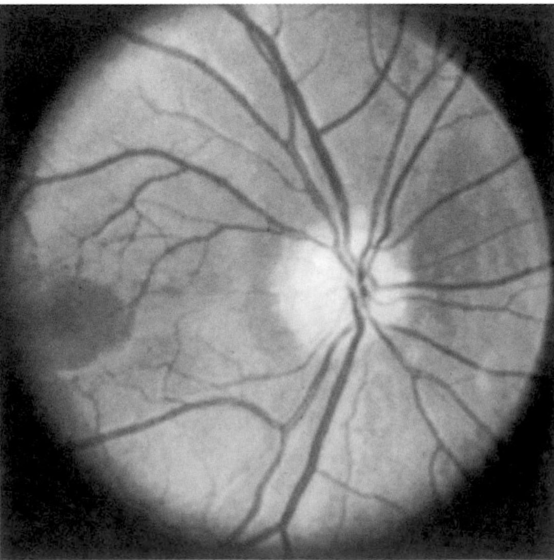

FIGURE 4-3 ■ Drusen. The disk margin is indistinct, the physiological cup is absent, and yellowish globular bodies are present on the surface.

location into other compartments, compressing structures already occupying that space. These shifts may occur under the falx cerebri, through the tentorial notch, and through the foramen magnum (Box 4-3).

Increased intracranial pressure is a relative contraindication for lumbar puncture. The change in fluid dynamics causes herniation in certain circumstances. The hazard is greatest when pressure between cranial compartments is unequal. This prohibition is relative, and early lumbar puncture is the rule in infants and children with suspected infections of the nervous system despite the presence of increased intracranial pressure. In other situations, lumbar puncture is rarely essential for diagnosis, but usually accomplished safely in the absence of papilledema. The following computed tomography (CT) criteria define people at increased risk of herniation after lumbar puncture:

- Lateral shift of midline structures
- Loss of the suprachiasmatic and basilar cisterns
- Obliteration of the fourth ventricle
- Obliteration of the superior cerebellar and quadrigeminal plate cisterns.

Falx Herniation

Herniation of one cingulate gyrus under the falx cerebri is more common in the presence of one enlarged hemisphere. The major feature is compression of the internal cerebral vein and the anterior cerebral artery, resulting in still greater increased intracranial pressure because of reduced venous outflow and arterial infarction.

> **BOX 4-3 Herniation Syndromes**
>
> **UNILATERAL (UNCAL) TRANSTENTORIAL HERNIATION**
>
> Declining consciousness
> Increased blood pressure, slow pulse
> Dilated and fixed pupil
> Homonymous hemianopia
> Respiratory irregularity
> Decerebrate rigidity
>
> **BILATERAL (CENTRAL) TRANSTENTORIAL HERNIATION**
>
> Decerebrate or decorticate rigidity
> Declining consciousness
> Impaired upward gaze
> Irregular respiration
> Pupillary constriction or dilation
>
> **CEREBELLAR (DOWNWARD) HERNIATION**
>
> Declining consciousness
> Impaired upward gaze
> Irregular respirations
> Lower cranial nerve palsies
> Neck stiffness or head tilt

Unilateral (Uncal) Transtentorial Herniation

The tentorial notch allows structures to pass from the posterior to the middle fossa. The brainstem, the posterior cerebral artery, and the third cranial nerve are its normal components. Unilateral transtentorial herniation characteristically occurs when enlargement of one temporal lobe causes the uncus or hippocampus to bulge into the tentorial notch. Falx herniation is usually an associated feature. Because considerable intracranial pressure is required to cause such a shift, consciousness decreases even before the actual herniation. It declines continuously as the brainstem com. Direct pressure on the oculomotor nerve causes ipsilateral dilation of the pupil; sometimes dilation of the contralateral pupil occurs because the displaced brainstem compresses the opposite oculomotor nerve against the incisura of the tentorium. Contralateral homonymous hemianopia occurs (but is impossible to test in an unconscious patient) because of compression of the ipsilateral posterior cerebral artery. With further pressure on the midbrain, both pupils dilate and fix, respirations become irregular, decerebrate posturing is noted, and death results from cardiorespiratory collapse.

Bilateral (Central) Transtentorial Herniation

Central herniation usually is associated with generalized cerebral edema. Both hemispheres displace downward, pushing the diencephalon and midbrain caudad through the tentorial notch. The diencephalon becomes edematous, and the pituitary stalk is avulsed. The clinical features are states of decreasing consciousness, pupillary constriction followed by dilation, impaired upward gaze, irregular respiration, disturbed control of body temperature, decerebrate or decorticate posturing, and death.

Cerebellar Herniation

Increased pressure in the posterior fossa may cause upward herniation of the cerebellum through the tentorial notch or downward displacement of one or both cerebellar tonsils through the foramen magnum. Upward displacement causes compression of the midbrain, resulting in impairment of upward gaze, dilated or fixed pupils, and respiratory irregularity. Downward cerebellar herniation

BOX 4-4 Medical Measures to Decrease Intracranial Pressure

- Corticosteroids
- Elevation of head
- Hyperosmolality
  - Glycerol
  - Hypertonic saline
  - Mannitol
- Hyperventilation
- Hypothermia
- Pentobarbital coma

causes compression of the medulla, resulting in states of decreasing consciousness, impaired upward gaze, and lower cranial nerve palsies. One of the earliest features of cerebellar herniation into the foramen magnum is neck stiffness or head tilt in an effort to relieve the pressure by enlarging the surface area of the foramen magnum.

MEDICAL TREATMENT

Several measures to lower increased intracranial pressure are available, even in circumstances in which surgical intervention is required (Box 4-4).

Monitoring Intracranial Pressure

Severe head trauma is the usual reason for continuous monitoring of intracranial pressure in children. Despite advances in technology, the effect of pressure monitoring on the outcome in medical diseases associated with increased intracranial pressure is questionable. It has no value in children with hypoxic-ischemic encephalopathies and has marginal value in children with other kinds of encephalopathies.

Head Elevation

Elevating the head of the bed 30–45° above horizontal improves jugular venous drainage and decreases intracranial pressure. Systemic blood pressure remains unchanged, resulting in increased cerebral perfusion.

Homeostasis

Maintain normal glucose. Both hypo- and hyperglycemia may cause further insult. Hyperglycemia may increase oxidative stress. Maintain adequate oxygenation (95 %) and CO_2 (35–45 mmHg). Avoid hypotension, and maintain systolic pressure at least above the 5th percentile for age; permissive hypertension is often preferred. Prevent hyponatremia and maintain osmolalities between 300 and 320 mOsml/L to decrease possible edema with hyponatremia or decreased osmolality. Maintain normal body temperature, as every 1 °C increases brain metabolism by 5 %. Prevent seizures as they may further increase intracranial pressure and brain metabolism. Pain and agitation management are important to prevent further elevations in intracranial pressure; however, sedation should not compromise blood pressure as decrements may result in decreased cerebral perfusion (Pitfield et al, 2012).

Hyperventilation

Children with Glasgow Scale scores of less than 8 should have intubation to maintain oxygen saturations above 95 % and end tidal carbon dioxide between 35 and 40 mmHg. Intracranial pressure decreases within seconds of the initiation of hyperventilation. The mechanism is vasoconstriction resulting from hypocarbia. The goal is to lower the arterial pressure of carbon dioxide to 25–30 mmHg. Ischemia may result from further or prolonged reductions. Avoid hyperventilation in patients with head trauma. The use of hyperventilation is only a transient benefit and should always be followed by immediate neurosurgical consultation (Pitfield et al, 2012).

Osmotic Diuretics

Mannitol is the osmotic diuretic most widely used in the United States. A 20 % solution of mannitol, 0.25 g to 1 g/kg infused intravenously over 15 minutes, exerts its beneficial effects as a plasma expander and as an osmotic diuretic. Hypertonic saline causes similar vascular changes to mannitol. The typical dosage is 5–10 mL/kg of 3 % hypertonic saline solution given over 5 to 10 minutes (Pitfield et al, 2012). Excretion is by the kidneys, and large doses may cause renal failure, especially when using nephrotoxic drugs concurrently. Maintain serum osmolarity at less than 320 mOsm and adequate intravascular volume.

Corticosteroids

Corticosteroids, such as dexamethasone, are effective in the treatment of vasogenic edema. The intravenous dosage is 0.1–0.2 mg/kg every 6 hours. Onset of action is 12 to 24 hours; peak action may be longer. The mechanism is uncertain. Cerebral blood flow is not affected. Corticosteroids are most useful for reducing edema surrounding mass lesions and are not useful in the treatment of edema secondary to head injury.

Hypothermia

Hypothermia decreases cerebral blood flow and frequently is used concurrently with pentobarbital coma. Body temperature maintained between 27°C and 31°C is ideal. The gain of using hypothermia in addition to other measures that decrease cerebral blood flow is uncertain.

Pentobarbital Coma

Barbiturates reduce cerebral blood flow, decrease edema formation, and lower the brain's metabolic rate. These effects do not occur at anticonvulsant plasma concentrations but require brain concentrations sufficient to produce a burst-suppression pattern on the electroencephalogram. Barbiturate coma is particularly useful in patients with increased intracranial pressure resulting from disorders of mitochondrial function, such as Reye syndrome. Pentobarbital is preferred to phenobarbital (see Chapter 1).

HYDROCEPHALUS

Hydrocephalus is a condition marked by an excessive volume of intracranial CSF. It is termed communicating or noncommunicating, depending on whether or not the CSF communicates between the ventricular system and the subarachnoid space. Congenital hydrocephalus occurs in approximately 1:1000 births. It is generally associated with other congenital malformations, and the causes are genetic disturbances or intrauterine disorders, such as infection and hemorrhage. Often, no cause is determined. Congenital hydrocephalus is discussed in Chapter 18 because its initial feature is usually macrocephaly.

The causes of acquired hydrocephalus are brain tumor, intracranial hemorrhage, or infection. Solid brain tumors generally produce hydrocephalus by obstructing the ventricular system, whereas nonsolid tumors, such as leukemia, impair the reabsorptive mechanism in the subarachnoid space.

Intracranial hemorrhage and infection may produce communicating and noncommunicating hydrocephalus and may increase intracranial pressure through the mechanisms of cerebral edema and impaired venous return. Because several factors contribute to increased intracranial pressure, acquired hydrocephalus is discussed by cause in the sections that follow.

BOX 4-5 Brain Tumors in Children

Hemispheric Tumors

- Choroid plexus papilloma
- Glial tumors
  - Astrocytoma
  - Ependymoma
  - Oligodendroglioma
  - Primitive neuroectodermal tumors
- Pineal region tumors
  - Pineal parenchymal tumors
    - Pineoblastoma
    - Pineocytoma
  - Germ cell tumors
    - Embryonal cell carcinoma
    - Germinoma
    - Teratoma
  - Glial tumors
    - Astrocytoma
    - Ganglioglioma
- Other tumors
  - Angiomas
  - Dysplasia
  - Meningioma
  - Metastatic tumors

Middle Fossa Tumors

- Optic glioma (see Chapter 16)
- Sellar and parasellar tumors (see Chapter 16)

Posterior Fossa Tumors

- Astrocytoma (see Chapter 10)
- Brainstem glioma (see Chapter 15)
- Ependymoma (see Chapter 10)
- Hemangioblastoma (see Chapter 10)
- Medulloblastoma (see Chapter 10)

BRAIN TUMORS

Primary tumors of the posterior fossa and middle fossa are discussed in Chapters 10, 15, and 16 (Box 4-5). This section discusses tumors of the cerebral hemispheres. Supratentorial tumors comprise approximately half of brain tumors in children. They occur more commonly in children younger than 2 years old and adolescents.

Choroid Plexus Tumors

Choroid plexus tumors arise from the epithelium of the choroid plexus of the cerebral ventricles. They represent only 2–4 % of all pediatric brain tumors, but 10–20 % of tumors that develop in infancy. Three histological variants exist: choroid plexus papillomas, atypical papillomas, and choroid plexus carcinomas. Choroid plexus papillomas are five times more common than choroid plexus carcinoma. Choroid plexus tumors usually are located in one lateral ventricle, but also may arise in the third ventricle.

Clinical Features. Onset is usually during infancy, and the tumor may be present at birth. The main features are those of increased intracranial pressure from hydrocephalus. Communicating hydrocephalus may result from excessive production of CSF by the tumor, but noncommunicating hydrocephalus caused by obstruction of the ventricular foramen is the rule. If the tumor is pedunculated, its movement may cause intermittent ventricular obstruction by a ball-valve mechanism. The usual course is one of rapid progression, with only a few weeks from first symptoms to diagnosis.

Infants with choroid plexus tumors usually have macrocephaly and are thought to have congenital hydrocephalus. Older children have nausea, vomiting, diplopia, headaches, and weakness. Papilledema is the rule.

Diagnosis. Multilobular, calcified, contrast-enhancing intraventricular masses are characteristic of choroid plexus tumors. Because affected children show clear evidence of increased intracranial pressure, CT is usually the first test performed. The tumor is located within one ventricle as a mass of increased density with marked contrast enhancement. Hydrocephalus of one or both lateral ventricles is present. Choroid plexus papillomas are vascular and many tumors bleed spontaneously. The spinal fluid may be xanthochromic or grossly bloody. The protein concentration in the CSF is usually elevated.

Management. The choroid plexus receives its blood supply from the anterior and posterior choroidal arteries, branches of the internal carotid artery, and the posterior cerebral artery. The rich vascular network within the tumors is a major obstacle to complete surgical removal. Yet the extent of surgical resection is the single most important factor that determines the prognosis of a choroid plexus papilloma.

Preliminary evidence suggests that choroid plexus carcinomas are chemosensitive tumors. The role of adjuvant radiation is controversial. The indications for radiation are age younger than age 3 years, subtotal resection, malignant features within the tumor, or dissemination of the tumor along the neuraxis.

The 5-year survival rate is 50 %, with most deaths occurring within 7 months of surgery. Complete tumor removal completely relieves hydrocephalus without the need of a shunt.

Glial Tumors

Tumors of glial origin constitute approximately 40 % of supratentorial tumors in infants and children. The common glial tumors of childhood in order of frequency are astrocytoma, ependymoma, and oligodendroglioma. A mixture of two or more cell types is the rule. *Oligodendroglioma* occurs exclusively in the cerebral hemispheres, whereas astrocytoma and ependymoma have either a supratentorial or an infratentorial location. Oligodendroglioma is mainly a tumor of adolescence. These tumors grow slowly and tend to calcify. The initial symptom is usually a seizure rather than increased intracranial pressure.

Astrocytoma

The grading of hemispheric astrocytomas is by histological appearance: low-grade, anaplastic, and glioblastoma multiforme. Low-grade astrocytomas confined to the posterior fossa constitute 12–18 % of all pediatric intracranial tumors and 20–40 % of all brainstem tumors. No gender predilection exists; the peak age at diagnosis is 6 to 10 years. Low-grade astrocytomas are more common than high-grade astrocytomas in children. The incidence of low-grade astrocytomas has increased in recent years because of the widespread availability and use of MRI in the diagnosis of presymptomatic lesions (Wrensch et al, 2002).

Anaplastic tumors and glioblastoma multiforme are high-grade tumors. Glioblastoma multiforme accounts for fewer than 10 % of childhood supratentorial astrocytomas and is more likely to occur in adolescence than in infancy. High-grade tumors may evolve from low-grade tumors.

Clinical Features. The initial features of glial tumors in children depend on location and may include seizures, hemiparesis, and movement disorders affecting one side of the body. Seizures are the most common initial feature of low-grade gliomas. Tumors infiltrating the basal ganglia and internal capsule are less likely to cause seizures than tumors closer to cortical structures. A slow-growing tumor may not cause a mass effect because surrounding neural structures accommodate infiltrating tumors. Such tumors may cause only seizures for several years before causing weakness of the contralateral limbs.

Headache is a relatively common complaint. Pain localizes if the tumor produces focal displacement of vessels without increasing intracranial pressure. A persistent focal headache usually correlates well with tumor location.

The initial features in children with medullary tumors may be progressive dysphagia, hoarseness, ataxia, and hemiparesis. Cervicomedullary tumors cause neck discomfort, weakness or numbness of the hands, and an asymmetric quadriparesis. Midbrain tumors cause features of increased intracranial pressure, diplopia, and hemiparesis.

Symptoms of increased intracranial pressure, generalized headache, nausea, and vomiting are initial features of hemispheric astrocytoma in only one-third of children but are common at the time of diagnosis. Intracranial pressure is likely to increase when rapidly growing tumors provoke edema of the hemisphere. A mass effect collapses one ventricle, shifts midline structures, and puts pressure on the aqueduct. When herniation occurs or when the lateral ventricles are dilated because of pressure on the aqueduct, the early features of headache, nausea, vomiting, and diplopia are followed by generalized weakness or fatigability, lethargy, and declining consciousness.

Papilledema occurs in children with generalized increased intracranial pressure, but macrocephaly occurs in infants. When papilledema is present, abducens palsy is usually an associated symptom. Other neurological findings depend on the site of the tumor and may include hemiparesis, hemisensory loss, or homonymous hemianopia.

Diagnosis. MRI is always preferable to CT when suspecting a tumor. In a CT scan, a low-grade glioma appears as low-density or cystic areas that enhance with contrast material (Figure 4-4). A low-density area surrounding the tumor that does not show contrast enhancement indicates edema.

High-grade gliomas have patchy areas of low and high density, sometimes evidence of hemorrhage, and cystic degeneration. Marked contrast enhancement, often in a ring pattern, is noted. When a mass effect is present, imaging studies show a shift of midline structures, deformity of the ipsilateral ventricle, and swelling of the affected hemisphere with obliteration of sulcal markings (Figure 4-5). A mass effect occurs in half of low-grade astrocytomas and almost all high-grade tumors.

Management. Treat all children with increased intracranial pressure caused by hemispheric astrocytoma with dexamethasone to reduce vasogenic cerebral edema and with ventriculoperitoneal shunting when hydrocephalus coexists. Headache and nausea frequently are relieved within 24 hours; neurological deficits improve as well.

Surgical resection of the tumor is the next step in treatment. Long-term survival for children with completely resected supratentorial low-grade astrocytoma is good, with the notable exception of those with diffuse pontine gliomas, in whom the prognosis is poor (Jallo et al, 2004; Mauffrey, 2006). Gemistocytic astrocytoma, a variant of astrocytoma characterized by the presence of gemistocytic neoplastic astrocytes with eosinophilic cytoplasm, has a less predictable clinical course, because these tumors tend to rapidly progress to higher-grade lesions such as anaplastic astrocytoma and glioblastoma. The prognosis for focal midbrain tumors is also favorable in spite of the fact that complete resection is not possible (Stark et al, 2005).

Children with low-grade astrocytomas of the cerebral hemisphere have a 20-year survival rate of 85% after surgical resection alone (Pollack et al, 1995). Postoperative radiotherapy impairs cognition without increasing survival. Postoperative radiation should be recommended for anaplastic astrocytomas. Children with anaplastic

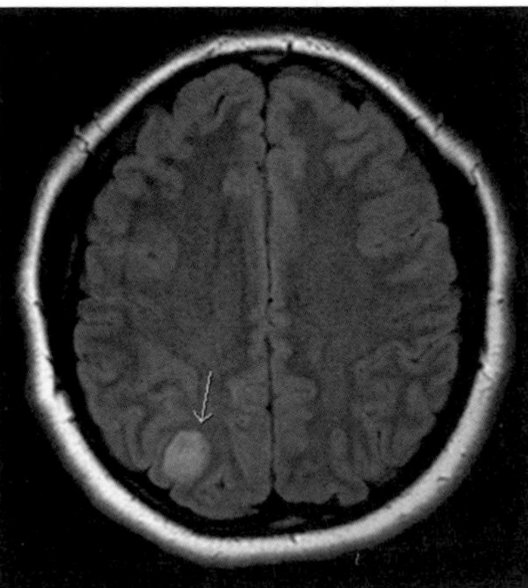

FIGURE 4-4 ■ Low grade glioma. Axial T_2 flair MRI shows a well circumscribed and homogeneous neoplasm (arrow).

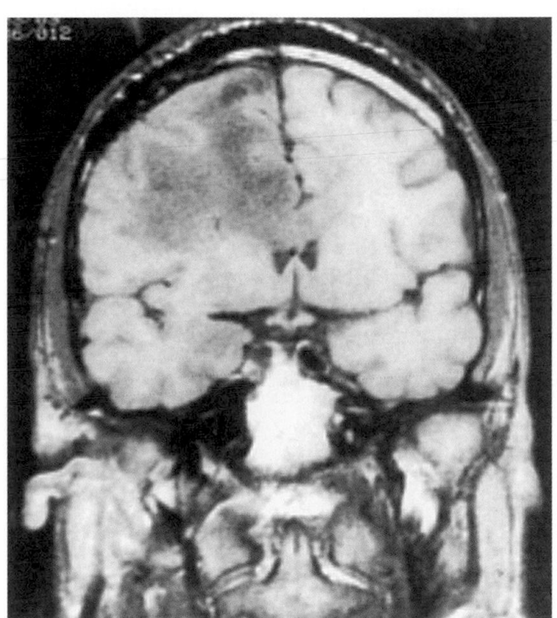

FIGURE 4-5 ■ Malignant glioma. MRI shows a malignant astrocytoma invading the corpus callosum.

astrocytomas have less than a 30 % 5-year survival rate even with radiotherapy, and children with glioblastoma multiforme have less than a 3 % 5-year survival. Because the 5-year survival rate of children with high-grade astrocytomas is poor, several chemotherapy protocols are being tried.

Ependymoma

Ependymomas are tumors derived from cells that line the ventricular system and may be either supratentorial or infratentorial in location. Infratentorial ependymoma is discussed in Chapter 10 because the initial symptom is often ataxia. Symptoms of increased intracranial pressure are the first feature in 90 % of children with posterior fossa ependymoma, and papilledema is present in 75 % at the time of initial examination.

Approximately 60 % of children with ependymoma are younger than 5 years old at the time of diagnosis, and only 4 % are older than 15 years. As a rule, infratentorial ependymoma occurs at a younger age than supratentorial ependymoma.

The expected location of supratentorial ependymoma is in relation to the third and lateral ventricles. Ependymal tumors may arise within the hemispheres, however, at a site distant from the ventricular system. Such tumors probably derive from ependymal cell rests.

Clinical Features. Symptoms of increased intracranial pressure are less prominent with supratentorial tumors than with infratentorial tumors. Common manifestations are focal weakness, seizures, and visual disturbances. Papilledema is a common feature in all patients with ependymoma. Hemiparesis, hyperreflexia, and hemianopia are typical features, but some children show only ataxia. The duration of symptoms before diagnosis averages only 7 months but can be 1 month for malignant tumors and several years for low-grade tumors.

Diagnosis. A typical MRI appearance of a fourth ventricular ependymoma is that of a homogeneously enhancing solid mass extending out of the foramina of Luschka or the foramen of Magendie with associated obstructive hydrocephalus. Tumor density on CT is usually greater than brain density, and contrast enhancement is present. Small cysts within the tumor are relatively common. Approximately one-third of supratentorial ependymomas contain calcium.

Tumors within the third ventricle cause marked dilation of the lateral ventricles, with edema of the hemispheres and obliteration of sulcal markings. High-grade tumors are likely to seed the subarachnoid space, producing metastases in the spinal cord and throughout the ventricular system. In such cases, tumor cells may line the lateral ventricles and produce a "cast" of contrast enhancement around the ventricles.

Management. Complete surgical resection is possible in only 30 % of cases. Even after complete resection, the 5-year rate of progression-free survival is 60–80 %. Survival relates directly to the effectiveness of surgical removal followed by either radiation therapy or chemotherapy. The use of radiation in young children with ependymomas was avoided in the past because the risks of cognitive, endocrine, and developmental side effects. However, the advent of more selective radiation delivery techniques has made postoperative radiation therapy an attractive option for pediatric patients (Mansur et al, 2004). Several studies suggest that radiation therapy prolongs progression-free survival after subtotal resection of an ependymoma. As such, there is now growing evidence supporting the use of adjuvant radiation for spinal cord and supratentorial ependymomas (Merchant et al, 2004).

Primitive Neuroectodermal Tumors

Medulloblastoma represents approximately 85 % of intracranial primitive neuroectodermal tumors (PNETs) and 15 % of all pediatric brain tumors.

Clinical Features. Age at onset may be anytime during childhood but is usually before age 10 (McNeil et al, 2002). The incidence in males is twice that of females, and the median age at diagnosis is 5 to 7 years. Because PNETs are highly malignant, the progression of symptoms is rapid, and the time to diagnosis is usually less than 3 months.

Many clinical features of medulloblastoma relate to its location in the fourth ventricle. Obstructive hydrocephalus and increased intracranial pressure are prominent. Headache occurs early and usually precedes diagnosis by 4 to 8 weeks. Morning nausea, vomiting, and irritability are early features. Lethargy, diplopia, head tilt, and truncal ataxia lead to evaluation. The common signs on examination are papilledema, ataxia, dysmetria, and cranial nerve involvement. Abducens nerve palsy is the cause of diplopia and head tilt. Torticollis can be a sign of cerebellar tonsil herniation.

Diagnosis. On CT, PNETs are high-density lesions that enhance and produce hydrocephalus. The tumor mass is surrounded by cerebral edema, and midline structures frequently are shifted under the falx. MRI shows homogeneous to mixed signal intensity in the

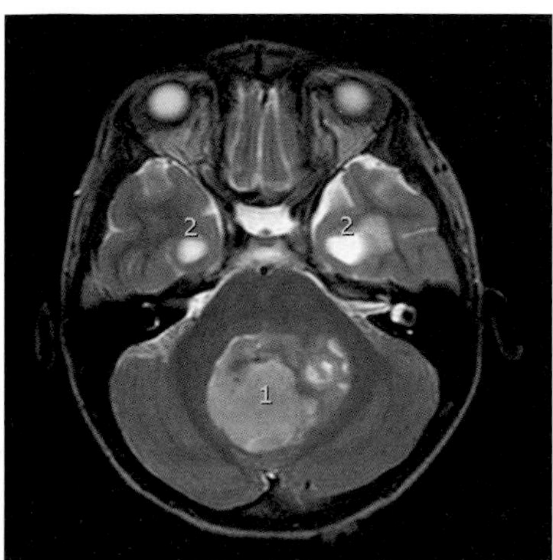

FIGURE 4-6 ■ Primitive neuroectodermal tumor. T_2 axial MRI shows (1) a 6.5 cm × 3 cm heterogeneous mass with cysts and (2) secondary dilation of temporal horns/hydrocephalus.

tumor. On T_2-weighted images, the lesions are nearly isointense to brain parenchyma, but they enhance intensely after contrast administration (Figure 4-6).

Management. Dexamethasone often relieves cerebral edema. Complete tumor resection is rarely accomplished. PNETs are radiosensitive and radiation of the entire craniospinal axis is required. Survival is usually less than 1 year. Several chemotherapeutic trials are ongoing.

Pineal Region Tumors

The derivation of tumors in the pineal region is from several histological types. Germ cell tumors are the most common, followed by tumors of the pineal parenchyma. The incidence of pineal region tumors is 10 times higher in Japan than in the United States or western Europe. Pineal region tumors are more common in boys than in girls and generally become symptomatic during adolescence.

Clinical Features. Because pineal region tumors are in a midline location, where they can invade or compress the third ventricle or aqueduct, symptoms of increased intracranial pressure are common. The first symptoms may be acute and accompanied by midbrain dysfunction. Midbrain dysfunction resulting from pressure by pineal region tumors on the periaqueductal gray is *Parinaud syndrome*: loss of pupillary light reflex, supranuclear palsy of upward gaze with preservation of downward gaze, and retraction-convergence nystagmus when upward gaze is attempted. Eventually, paralysis of upward and downward gaze and loss of accommodation may occur.

Tumors growing into or compressing the anterior hypothalamus produce loss of vision, diabetes insipidus, precocious puberty, and emaciation. Precocious puberty occurs almost exclusively in boys. Extension of tumor into the posterior fossa produces multiple cranial neuropathies and ataxia, and lateral extension causes hemiparesis.

Diagnosis. Pineal germinomas are well circumscribed and relatively homogeneous. The MRI appearance is low signal intensity on T_2-weighted images and marked enhancement with intravenous contrast. Teratomas appear lobulated and have hyperdense and multicystic areas. Calcification may be present, and contrast enhancement is not uniform. Tumors that spread into the ventricular system and have intense contrast enhancement are likely to be malignant. Tumors that contain abundant amounts of calcium are likely to be benign.

CT or MRI sometimes identifies asymptomatic non-neoplastic pineal cysts in children undergoing imaging for other reasons. These are developmental variants of the pineal gland, which may contain calcium. They only rarely grow to sufficient size to obstruct the aqueduct or cause Parinaud syndrome.

Management. Stereotactic biopsy is essential to establish the histological type and to plan therapy. Ventricular drainage relieves hydrocephalus when needed. Resection of pure germinomas is never appropriate, because of their sensitivity to radiation and chemotherapy. Resection is the procedure of choice for nongerminomatous pineal region tumors once the diagnosis is established. It may be curative for benign lesions such as a pure teratoma and may improve prognosis for patients with malignant tumors. The common complications of pineal region surgery are ocular dysmotility, ataxia, and altered mental status.

Other Tumors

Cerebral metastatic disease is unusual in childhood. Tumors that produce cerebral metastases most frequently are osteogenic sarcoma and rhabdomyosarcoma in patients younger than 15 years old and testicular germ cell tumors after age 15. The cerebral hemispheres, more often than posterior fossa structures, are affected. Pulmonary involvement always precedes cerebral metastasis. Brain metastasis is rarely present at the time of initial cancer diagnosis.

Meningioma is uncommon in children. The initial features may be focal neurological signs, seizures, or increased intracranial pressure.

INTRACRANIAL ARACHNOID CYSTS

Primary arachnoid cysts are CSF-filled cavities within the arachnoid. The cause of cyst formation is uncertain. They represent a minor disturbance in arachnoid formation and not a pathological process. Arachnoid cysts are found in 0.5 % of postmortem examinations; two-thirds are supratentorial and one-third are infratentorial.

Clinical Features. Most cysts are asymptomatic structures identified by CT or MRI. The detection of an arachnoid cyst is often easily perceived as an incidental finding; however, deciding whether the cyst caused the symptom for which the imaging study was required is sometimes problematic. Subarachnoid cysts are usually present from infancy, but may develop, or at least enlarge enough to detect, during adolescence.

Large cysts can produce symptoms by compressing adjacent structures or by increasing intracranial pressure. Focal neurological disturbances vary with the location but are most often hemiparesis or seizures when the cyst is supratentorial and ataxia when the cyst is infratentorial. Compression of the frontal lobe from early infancy may result in undergrowth of contralateral limbs.

Increased intracranial pressure can result from mass effect or from hydrocephalus and is associated with cysts in all locations. Clinical features include macrocephaly, headache, and behavioral change.

Diagnosis. It has become common for children with headache, learning or behavioral disorders, and suspected seizure disorders to undergo imaging studies of the brain. Many of these studies show incidental arachnoid cysts. A cause-and-effect relationship is a consideration only if the cyst is large and clearly explains the symptoms. Positron emission tomography may be useful in deciding whether an arachnoid cyst is having a pressure effect on the brain. Hypometabolism in the surrounding brain indicates brain compression.

Management. Simple drainage of the cyst often results in reaccumulation of fluid and recurrence of symptoms. Superficial cysts require excision, and deeply located cysts require a shunt into the peritoneal space.

INTRACRANIAL HEMORRHAGE

Head Trauma

Head trauma is a major cause of intracranial hemorrhage from the newborn period through childhood and adolescence. It is associated with intracerebral hemorrhage, subarachnoid hemorrhage, subdural hematoma, and epidural hematoma. Increased intracranial pressure is a constant feature of intracranial hemorrhage and may occur from cerebral edema after concussion without hemorrhage. Intracranial hemorrhage from head trauma is discussed in Chapter 2.

Intraventricular Hemorrhage in the Newborn

Intraventricular hemorrhage is primarily a disorder of live-born premature neonates with respiratory distress syndrome. The autoregulation of cerebral blood flow, which meets local tissue needs by altering cerebrovascular resistance, is impaired in premature newborns with respiratory distress syndrome. During episodes of systemic hypotension, decreased cerebral blood flow increases the potential for cerebral infarction. Such infarctions usually occur symmetrically in the white matter adjacent to the lateral ventricles. The late finding of these infarcts is termed *periventricular leukomalacia*.

During episodes of systemic hypertension, cerebral blood flow increases. Hemorrhage occurs first in the subependymal germinal matrix, then bursts through the ependymal lining into the lateral ventricle. Such hemorrhages are termed *periventricular-intraventricular hemorrhages* (PIVHs). The predilection of the germinal matrix for hemorrhage during episodes of increased cerebral blood flow is unknown. The likely explanation is prior ischemic injury that weakens the capillary walls and their supporting structures, making them vulnerable to rupture during episodes of increased cerebral blood flow. Intraventricular hemorrhage also occurs in full-term newborns, but the mechanism of hemorrhage at term is different from that before term.

Periventricular-Intraventricular Hemorrhage in Premature Newborns

The incidence of PIVH in premature newborns with birth weight less than 2000 g has been declining. The reason for the decline is probably attributable to advances in ventilatory care. PIVH occurs in approximately 20 % of premature newborns of birth weight less than 1500 g (Roland & Hill, 1997). It occurs on the first day in 50 % and before the fourth day in 90 % of affected newborns. PIVH originates from rupture of small vessels in the subependymal germinal matrix. Approximately 80 % of germinal matrix hemorrhages extend into the ventricular system. Hemorrhagic lesions into the cerebral parenchyma accompany severe hemorrhages. Parenchymal hemorrhages are usually unilateral and result from hemorrhagic venous infarction in the periventricular region (Volpe, 2000).

The following is a grading system for PIVH:

Grade I: isolated subependymal hemorrhage.

Grade II: intraventricular hemorrhage without ventricular dilation.

Grade III: intraventricular hemorrhage with ventricular dilation.

Grade IV: intraventricular hemorrhage with ventricular dilation and hemorrhage into the parenchyma of the brain.

Hemorrhage into the parenchyma of the brain (grade IV) is a coexistent process caused by hemorrhagic infarction (periventricular hemorrhagic infarction) and is not an extension of the first three grades of intraventricular hemorrhage.

Clinical Features. Routine ultrasound examinations are standard in the care for all newborns whose birth weight is 1800 g or less and often reveal PIVH in newborns in which no clinical suspicion existed. Among this group, some have blood in the CSF, and others have clear CSF. Only newborns with grade III or IV hemorrhage have predictable clinical features.

In some premature newborns, PIVH produces rapid neurological deterioration characterized by decreasing states of consciousness, severe hypotonia, and respiratory insufficiency. Within minutes to hours, the infant shows obvious evidence of increased intracranial pressure: bulging fontanelle, decerebrate posturing, loss of pupillary reflexes, and respiratory arrest. Hypothermia, bradycardia, hypotension, and hematocrit may decrease by 10%.

Often the hemorrhage manifests by stepwise progression of symptoms over hours or days. The initial symptoms are subtle and include change in behavior, diminished spontaneous movement, and either an increase or a decrease in appendicular tone. The fontanelles remain soft, and vital signs are normal. These first symptoms may correspond to grade I hemorrhage. Some newborns become stable and have no further difficulty. Others undergo clinical deterioration characterized by hypotonia and declining consciousness. This deterioration probably corresponds to the presence of blood in the ventricles. The child becomes lethargic or obtunded, then may stabilize. If continued bleeding causes acute ventricular dilation, apnea and coma follow. Seizures occur when blood dissects into the cerebral parenchyma.

Newborns with PIVH are at risk for progressive hydrocephalus. The likelihood is much greater among children with grade III or IV hemorrhage. Initial ventricular dilation is probably due to plugging of the arachnoid villi and impaired reabsorption of CSF. The ventricles can enlarge by compressing the brain without causing a measurable change in head circumference. Weekly ultrasound studies are imperative to follow the progression of hydrocephalus.

BOX 4-6 Prevention of Intra- and Periventricular Hemorrhage

ANTENATAL

- Delivery in specialized center
- Prevention of prematurity

POSTNATAL

- Avoidance of rapid volume expansion
- Correction of coagulation abnormalities
- Maintenance of stable systemic blood pressure
- Muscle paralysis of ventilated premature newborns
- Potential pharmacological agents
  - Indomethacin
  - Phenobarbital
- Vitamin K

Diagnosis. Ultrasound is the standard for the diagnosis of intraventricular hemorrhage in the newborn. Ultrasound is preferred over other brain imaging techniques because it is accurate and easily performed in the intensive care nursery. MRI during infancy or childhood is useful to show the extent of brain damage from the combination of periventricular strokes (leading later to leukomalacia) and PIVH.

Prevention. Box 4-6 lists some methods to prevent PIVH. A premature newborn has a significant risk of PIVH and this increases with the amount of intensive care required. Unnecessary manipulation of a premature infant should be avoided, and a quiet environment maintained. Muscle paralysis with pancuronium bromide in ventilated premature newborns reduces the incidence and severity of PIVH by stabilizing fluctuations of cerebral blood flow velocity. Phenobarbital may dampen fluctuations of systemic blood pressure and cerebral blood flow, and indomethacin inhibits prostaglandin synthesis, regulating cerebral blood flow; however, the efficacy of both agents is inconclusive and some concerns about the use of phenobarbital must be considered.

Extension of hemorrhage occurs in 20–40% of cases. Serial ultrasound scans provide early diagnosis of posthemorrhagic hydrocephalus, which develops in 10–15% of premature newborns with PIVH. Factors that influence the management of posthemorrhagic hydrocephalus are the rate of progression, ventricular size, and intracranial pressure. The hydrocephalus ultimately arrests or regresses in 50 % of children and progresses to severe hydrocephalus in the remainder. Rapid ventricular enlargement requires intervention in less than 4 weeks.

Management. When intraventricular hemorrhage has occurred, the direction of treatment is towards the prevention or stabilization of progressive posthemorrhagic hydrocephalus. The efficacy of treatment for posthemorrhagic hydrocephalus is difficult to assess because the role of ventricular dilation in causing chronic neurological impairment is not established. Newborns with progressive posthemorrhagic hydrocephalus also have experienced asphyxial encephalopathy, germinal matrix hemorrhage, and periventricular insult. Neurological morbidity correlates better with the degree of parenchymal damage than with ventricular size.

The definitive treatment is placement of a ventriculoperitoneal shunt. Early shunt placement, while the ventricles still contain blood, has a high incidence of shunt failure and infection, so temporizing measures are required. These measures include CSF drainage by serial lumbar punctures, external ventriculostomy, and drugs that reduce CSF production with carbonic anhydrase inhibitors such as topiramate and zonisamide and diuretics such as acetazolamide and furosemide.

Intraventricular Hemorrhage at Term

In contrast to intraventricular hemorrhage in a premature newborn, which originates almost exclusively from the germinal matrix, intraventricular hemorrhage at term may originate from the veins of the choroid plexus, from the germinal matrix, or both.

Clinical Features. Full-term newborns with intraventricular hemorrhage form two groups. In more than half, delivery was difficult, frequently from breech position, and some degree of intrauterine asphyxia sustained. Usually, these newborns show bruising and require resuscitation. At first, they appear to be improving, then, multifocal seizures occur on the second day postpartum. The fontanelle is tense, and the CSF is bloody.

The other half of affected infants have experienced neither trauma nor asphyxia and appear normal at birth. During the first hours postpartum, apnea, cyanosis, and a tense fontanelle develop. The mechanism of hemorrhage is unknown. Posthemorrhagic hydrocephalus is common in both groups, and 35 % require shunt placement.

Diagnosis. Ultrasound is as useful for diagnosis of intraventricular hemorrhage in full-term newborns as in premature newborns.

Management. The treatment of full-term newborns with intraventricular hemorrhage is the same as for premature newborns with intraventricular hemorrhage.

Arterial Aneurysms

Arterial aneurysms are vestiges of the embryonic circulation and are present in a rudimentary form before birth. Only rarely do they rupture during childhood. Symptomatic arterial aneurysms in childhood may be associated with coarctation of the aorta or polycystic kidney disease. Aneurysms tend to be located at the bifurcation of major arteries at the base of the brain.

Clinical Features. Subarachnoid hemorrhage is usually the first feature of a ruptured aneurysm. The initial symptoms may be catastrophic: sudden loss of consciousness, tachycardia, hypotension, and evidence of increased intracranial pressure, but in most patients the first bleeding is a "warning leak" that may go unrecognized. Severe headache, stiff neck, and low-grade fever characterize the warning leak. Occasionally, aneurysms produce neurological signs by exerting pressure on adjacent cranial nerves. Oculomotor nerve dysfunction is common, resulting in disturbances of gaze and pupillary function.

Physical activity does not relate to the time of rupture. Aneurysmal size is the main predictor of rupture; aneurysms smaller than 1 cm in diameter have a low probability of rupture.

The patient's state of consciousness is the most important predictor of survival. Approximately 50 % of patients die during the first hospitalization, some from the initial hemorrhage during the first 14 days. Untreated, another 30 % die from recurrent hemorrhage in the next 10 years. Unruptured aneurysms may cause acute severe headache without nuchal rigidity. The mechanism of headache may be aneurysmal thrombosis or localized meningeal inflammation.

Diagnosis. On the day of aneurysmal rupture, CT shows intracranial hemorrhage in all patients, but the blood rapidly reabsorbs, and only two-thirds have visible hemorrhage on the fifth day using standard MRI or magnetic resonance angiography (MRA). Lumbar puncture is common because the stiff neck, headache, and fever suggest bacterial meningitis. The fluid is grossly bloody and thought traumatic, unless centrifugation reveals xanthochromic fluid. When a diagnosis of subarachnoid hemorrhage is established, all vessels need to be visualized to determine the aneurysmal site and the presence of multiple aneurysms. Four-vessel cerebral arteriography had been the standard imaging study, but improved MRA technology and CT angiography are often diagnostic and less invasive.

Management. The definitive treatment is surgical clipping and excision of the aneurysm. Early surgery prevents rebleeding in conscious patients (Olafsson et al, 1997). Cerebral vasospasm and ischemia are the leading causes of death and disability among survivors of an initial aneurysm rupture. Pharmacological means to prevent rebleeding are becoming less important with the increasing frequency of early operative intervention. Medical therapy for the prevention and treatment of vasospasm includes a regimen of volume expansion and induced systemic hypertension. Nimodipine is effective for the prevention of delayed ischemia due to vasospasm.

The 6-month survival rate in patients who are conscious at the time of admission is approximately 86%. In contrast, only 20% of patients comatose on admission live 6 months.

Arteriovenous Malformations

Approximately 0.1 % of children have an arteriovenous malformation, of which 12–18% become symptomatic in childhood (Menovsky & van Overbeeke, 1997). These are not on a genetic basis. Two types of malformations occur. One type arises early in gestation from an abnormal communication between primitive choroidal arteries and veins. Such malformations are in the midline and give rise to the vein of Galen malformation, malformations involving the choroid plexus, and shunts between cerebellar arteries and the straight sinus. The other type arises later in gestation or even after birth between superficial arteries and veins. The result is an arteriovenous malformation within the parenchyma of the cerebral hemisphere. Interconnections exist between the vessels of the scalp, skull, and dura, causing anastomotic channels between the extracranial and intracranial circulations to remain patent. Approximately 90% of arteriovenous malformations are supratentorial, and 10% are infratentorial.

Deep Midline Malformations

Hydrocephalus and cardiac failure during infancy are the presenting features of large deep midline malformations, especially malformations involving the great vein of Galen. They rarely bleed (Meyers et al, 2000). These malformations are discussed in Chapter 18.

Clinical Features. Small, deep midline malformations are rarely symptomatic in childhood. Bleeding into the parenchyma of the brain or into the subarachnoid space brings the problem to attention. Secondary venous changes reroute the drainage to the pial veins, which then bleed. Because the bleeding is from the venous rather than the arterial side of the malformation, the initial symptoms are not as catastrophic as with arterial aneurysms. Symptoms may evolve over several hours, and no characteristic clinical syndrome is associated. Most patients describe sudden severe headache, neck stiffness, and vomiting. Fever is frequently an associated symptom. The presence of focal neurological deficits depends on the location of the malformation and may include hemiparesis, sensory disturbances, and oculomotor palsies. Many patients recover completely from the first hemorrhage; the risk of recurrent hemorrhage is small.

Diagnosis. Contrast-enhanced MRI or CT easily reveals most arteriovenous malformations and shows the degree of ventricular enlargement. Four-vessel arteriography, CT angiogram or MRA defines all arterial and venous channels.

Management. Microsurgical excision, when feasible, is the treatment modality of choice. Management of deep midline malformations is by venous embolization. The results vary with the size and location of the malformation.

Supratentorial Malformations

Clinical Features. Among children with arteriovenous malformations in and around the cerebral hemispheres, the initial feature is intracranial hemorrhage in half and seizures in half. Recurrent vascular headache may precede the onset of hemorrhage and seizures or may develop concurrently. Headaches are usually unilateral but may not occur consistently on the same side. In some patients, the headaches have a migraine quality: scintillating scotomata and unilateral throbbing pain. The incidence of these migraine-like headaches in patients with arteriovenous malformations does not seem to be greater than in the general population. The malformation probably provokes a migraine attack in people who are genetically predisposed. Most patients who have seizures have at least one focal seizure, but, among the seizures associated with arteriovenous malformations, half are focal seizures and half are secondary generalized seizures. No specific location of the malformation is associated with a higher incidence of seizures. Small superficial malformations, especially in the centroparietal region, are associated with the highest incidence of hemorrhage. Hemorrhage may be subarachnoid only or may dissect into the brain parenchyma.

Diagnosis. Contrast-enhanced MRI and CT provide excellent visualization of the malformation in most children. Four-vessel arteriography is typically required to define all arterial and venous channels prior to surgical intervention.

Management. The photon knife is becoming the standard of treatment for small malformations. Other options for management include microsurgical excision and embolization. Superficial malformations are more accessible for direct surgical excision than malformations deep in the midline. In considering treatment modes, the physician must balance the decision to do something against the decision to do nothing based on the likelihood of further bleeding and the morbidity due to intervention.

Cocaine Abuse

Intracranial hemorrhage is associated with cocaine abuse, especially crack, in young adults. The hemorrhages may be subarachnoid or intracerebral in location. Sudden transitory increases in systemic blood pressure are the cause.

INFECTIOUS DISORDERS

Infections of the brain and meninges produce increased intracranial pressure by causing cerebral edema, by obstructing the flow and reabsorption of CSF, and by impairing venous outflow. Symptoms of increased intracranial pressure are frequently the initial features of bacterial and fungal infections and, occasionally, viral encephalitis. Viral infections are more likely to cause seizures, personality change, or decreased consciousness and are discussed in Chapter 2.

Bacterial Meningitis

The offending organism and the clinical features of bacterial meningitis vary with age. It is useful to discuss the syndromes of bacterial meningitis by age group: newborn, infants and young children (28 days to 5 years), and school-age children.

Meningitis in the Newborn

Meningitis occurs in approximately 1:2000 term newborns and 3:1000 premature newborns and accounts for 4% of all neonatal deaths. It is a consequence of septicemia, and organs other than the brain are infected. Maternal infection is the main risk factor for sepsis and meningitis.

An early-onset (first 5 days) and a late-onset (after 5 days) pattern of meningitis have been identified in newborns. In early-onset meningitis, acquisition of infection is at the time of delivery, and the responsible organisms are usually *Escherichia coli* or group B *Streptococcus*. The newborn becomes symptomatic during the first week, and the mortality rate is 20–50%. In late-onset meningitis, acquisition of infection is postnatal, and symptoms may begin the fourth day postpartum but usually begin after the first week. Newborns requiring intensive care are specifically at risk for late-onset meningitis because of excessive instrumentation. The responsible organisms are *E. coli*, group B *Streptococcus*, enterococci, Gram-negative enteric bacilli (*Pseudomonas* and *Klebsiella*), and *Listeria monocytogenes*. The mortality rate is 10–20%.

Clinical Features. Newborns infected in utero or during delivery may experience respiratory distress and shock within 24 hours of birth. Other features that may be associated with septicemia include hyperthermia, hypothermia, jaundice, hepatomegaly, lethargy, anorexia, and vomiting.

In late-onset meningitis, the clinical manifestations are variable. Initial symptoms are usually nonspecific and include lethargy, disturbed feeding, and irritability. As the meningitis worsens, hyperthermia, respiratory distress or apnea, and seizures are present in about half of newborns, but bulging of the fontanelle occurs in only a quarter, and nuchal rigidity does not occur. Shock is the usual cause of death.

Diagnosis. The diagnosis of septicemia and meningitis in the newborn is often difficult to establish based on symptoms. The first suspicion of septicemia should prompt lumbar puncture. Even in the absence of infection, the CSF of febrile newborns averages 11 leukocytes/mm^3 (range 0–20 leukocytes/mm^3). Less than 6% are polymorphonuclear leukocytes. The protein concentration has a mean value of 84 mg/dL (0.84 g/L), with a range of 40–130 mg/dL (0.4–1.3 g/L), and the glucose concentration has a mean value of 46 mg/dL (0.46 g/L), with a range of 36–56 mg/dL (0.36–0.56 g/L).

In newborns with meningitis, the leukocyte count is usually in the thousands, and the protein concentration may vary from less than 30 mg/dL (<0.3 g/L) to greater than 1000 mg/dL (>10 g/L). A Gram-stained smear of CSF permits identification of an organism in less than half of cases. Even when the smear is positive, identification may be inaccurate. Rapid detection of bacterial antigens by immunoelectrophoresis, latex agglutination, and radioimmunoassays is helpful in the diagnosis of several bacterial species.

Management. Start treatment with the first suspicion of sepsis. Laboratory confirmation is not required. The choice of initial antibiotic coverage varies, but usually includes ampicillin and gentamicin. An alternative regimen is ampicillin and cefotaxime, but cefotaxime-resistant strains are emerging rapidly. Identification of an organism leads to specific therapy.

Ampicillin and cefotaxime is used to treat *E. coli*, penicillin or ampicillin treats group B *Streptococcus*, and cefotaxime and an aminoglycoside treat *Klebsiella pneumoniae*. *Pseudomonas* is difficult to eradicate, and combined intravenous and intrathecal therapy may be required.

The duration of treatment for neonatal meningitis is at least 2 weeks beyond the time the CSF becomes sterile. Two days after discontinuing antibiotic therapy, reculture the CSF. A positive culture indicates the need for a second course of therapy. *Citrobacter diversus* infections often cause a hemorrhagic necrosis of the brain, with liquefaction of the cerebral white matter and abscess formation. CT readily identifies the abscesses.

Mortality is 20–30% and is highest for Gram-negative infections. The type of infecting organism and the gestational age of the infant are the main variables that determine mortality. Permanent neurological sequelae occur in 30–50% of survivors, including hydrocephalus, cerebral palsy, epilepsy, cognitive impairment, and deafness. Even when the head circumference is normal, exclusion of hydrocephalus requires CT evaluation.

Meningitis in Infants and Young Children

For children 6 weeks to 3 months old, group B *Streptococcus* remains a leading cause of meningitis, and *E. coli* is less common. The other important organism is *Neisseria meningitidis*. *Haemophilus influenzae*, which had been an important pathogen after 3 months of age, has almost disappeared because of routine immunization. *S. pneumoniae* and *N. meningitidis* are now the principal causes of meningitis in children older than 1 month.

Clinical Features. The onset of meningitis may be insidious or fulminating. The typical clinical findings include fever, irritability, and neck stiffness. A bulging fontanelle is a feature in young infants. After the fontanelle closes, headache, vomiting, and lethargy are initial features. Seizures occur in about one-third of children with meningitis. They usually occur during the first 24 hours of illness and often bring the child to medical attention. When seizures occur, state of consciousness declines. Seizures can be focal or secondary generalized and often difficult to control.

Examination reveals a sick and irritable child who resists being touched or moved. Ophthalmoscopic findings are usually normal or show only minimal papilledema. Focal neurological signs are unusual except in tuberculous meningitis or in cases in which abscess formation has occurred.

The rapidity with which neurological function declines depends on the severity of cerebral edema and cerebral vasculitis. Death may ensue from brainstem compression caused by transtentorial herniation. Peripheral vascular collapse can result from brainstem herniation, endotoxic shock, or adrenal failure. Of children with meningococcemia, 60% have a characteristic petechial or hemorrhagic rash. The rash, although generalized, is most prominent below the waist.

Meningeal irritation causes neck stiffness, characterized by limited mobility and pain on attempted flexion of the head. With the child supine, meningeal irritation is tested. Pain and resistance to extending the knee with the leg flexed at the hip is the Kernig sign. Spontaneous flexion at the hips when passively flexing the neck is the Brudzinski sign. These signs of meningeal irritation also occur with subarachnoid hemorrhage and infectious meningitis. The signs of meningeal irritation are rare below the age of 6 months.

Diagnosis. Lumbar puncture and examination of the CSF are essential for the diagnosis of bacterial meningitis. Because bacterial meningitis is often associated with septicemia, however, the blood, urine, and nasopharynx are cultured. The peripheral white blood cell count, especially immature granulocytes, is usually increased. Peripheral leukocytosis is much more common in bacterial than in viral infections but does not rule out viral meningitis. The platelet count is important because some infections are associated with thrombocytopenia. Proper evaluation of the CSF concentration of glucose requires a concurrent measure of the blood glucose concentration. The diagnosis of syndrome of inappropriate antidiuretic hormone secretion (SIADH) requires measurement of serum electrolytes, especially sodium. SIADH occurs in most patients with acute bacterial meningitis. Every child at risk for tuberculous meningitis requires a tuberculin skin test.

Perform lumbar puncture as quickly as possible when bacterial meningitis is suspected. Cranial CT before lumbar puncture has become routine, but has questionable value and adds considerably to the cost of care. When the need for CT scanning significantly delays lumbar puncture, obtain blood cultures and initiate antimicrobial therapy. Generalized increased intracranial pressure is always part of acute bacterial meningitis and is not a contraindication to lumbar puncture.

Information derived from lumbar puncture includes opening and closing pressures, appearance, white blood cell count with differential count, red blood cell count, concentrations of glucose and protein, and identification of microorganisms as shown by Gram stain and culture. The characteristic findings are increased pressure, a cloudy appearance, a cellular response of several thousand polymorphonuclear leukocytes, a reduction in the concentration of glucose to less than half of that in the plasma, and an elevated protein concentration. The expected findings of bacterial meningitis may vary, however, with the organism, the timing of the lumbar puncture, the prior use of antibiotics, and the immunocompetence of the host.

Management. Administer antimicrobials immediately. Do not delay treatment until after obtaining the results of lumbar puncture. Vancomycin and a third-generation cephalosporin are the initial treatment of meningitis. The final choice awaits the results of culture and antibiotic sensitivity.

The outcome for infants and children with bacterial meningitis depends on the infecting organism and the speed of initiating appropriate antibiotic therapy. Ten percent of children have persistent bilateral or unilateral hearing loss after bacterial meningitis, and 4 % have neurological deficits. The incidence of hearing loss is 31 % after infection with *S. pneumoniae* and 6 % after infection with *H. influenzae*. Hearing loss occurs early and probably is not related to the choice of antibiotic. Children with neurological deficits are at risk for epilepsy.

Meningitis in School-Age Children

S. pneumoniae and *N. meningitidis* account for most cases of bacterial meningitis in previously healthy school-age children in the United States, whereas *Mycobacterium tuberculosis* is a leading cause of meningitis in economically deprived populations. The symptoms of bacterial meningitis in school-age children do not differ substantially from the symptoms encountered in preschool children (see previous section on clinical features and treatment). In one retrospective study of children treated for bacterial meningitis in the 1980s, 8.5 % had major neurological deficits (cognitive impairment, seizures, hydrocephalus, cerebral palsy, blindness, or hearing loss), and 18.5 % had learning disabilities (Grimwood et al, 1995). Vancomycin and a third-generation cephalosporin are recommended.

Special Circumstances

Pneumococcus. Conditions associated with pneumococcal meningitis are otitis media, skull fractures, and sickle cell disease. Children with asplenia and chronic illnesses require immunization with Pneumovax. Penicillin G and ampicillin are equally effective in treating meningitis caused by penicillin-sensitive strains of *S. pneumoniae*. Vancomycin is part of the treatment because of the frequent occurrence of bacteria resistant to penicillin and ceftriaxone.

Meningococcus. Children with complement deficiency or asplenia require immunization for meningococcus. All household members who may have had saliva-exchange contact also require prophylaxis for meningococcal meningitis. A 2-day course of oral rifampin is prescribed, 10 mg/kg every 12 hours for children 1 month to 12 years old and 5 mg/kg every 12 hours for infants younger than 1 month old.

Tuberculous Meningitis. Worldwide, tuberculosis remains a leading cause of morbidity and death in children. In the United States, tuberculosis accounts for less than 5 % of bacterial meningitis cases in children, but it occurs with higher frequency where sanitation is poor. Infection of children follows inhalation of the organism from adults. Tuberculosis occurs first in the lungs, then disseminates to other organs within 6 months.

Clinical Features. The peak incidence of tuberculous meningitis is between 6 months and 2 years of age. The first symptoms tend to be more insidious than with other bacterial meningitides, but they sometimes progress in a fulminating fashion. Tuberculous meningitis, in contrast to fungal meningitis, is not a cause of chronic meningitis. If not treated, a child with tuberculous meningitis dies within 3 to 5 weeks.

Most often, fever develops first, and the child becomes listless and irritable. Headache may cause the irritability. Vomiting and abdominal pain are sometimes associated symptoms. Headache and vomiting become increasingly frequent and severe. Signs of meningismus develop during the second week after onset of fever. Cerebral infarction occurs in 30–40 % of affected children. Seizures may occur early, but more often they occur after meningismus is established. Consciousness declines progressively, and focal neurological deficits are noted. Most common are cranial neuropathies and hemipareses. Papilledema occurs relatively early in the course.

Diagnosis. Consider the diagnosis of tuberculosis in any child with a household contact. General use of tuberculin skin testing in children is crucial to early detection. In the early stages, children with tuberculous meningitis may have only fever. The peripheral white blood cell count generally is elevated (10 000–20 000 cells/mm^3). Hyponatremia and hypochloremia are frequently present because of ISADH. The CSF is usually cloudy and increased in pressure. The leukocyte count in the CSF may range from 10 to 250 cells/mm^3 and rarely exceeds 500 cells/mm^3.

Lymphocytes predominate. The glucose concentration declines throughout the course of the illness and is generally less than 35 mg/dL (<1.8 mmol/L). Conversely, the protein concentration increases steadily and is usually greater than 100 mg/dL (>1 g/L).

Smears of CSF stained by the acid-fast technique generally show the bacillus, if obtained from large CSF samples prepared by centrifuge. Recovery of the organism from the CSF is not always successful even when guinea pig inoculation is used. Newer diagnostic tests include a polymerase chain reaction technique with reported sensitivities of 70–75% and enzyme-linked immunosorbent assay and radioimmunoassay tests for anti-mycobacterial antigens in the CSF.

Management. Early treatment enhances the prognosis for survival and for neurological recovery. A positive skin test is reason to initiate isoniazid therapy in an asymptomatic child. However, immigrants from endemic areas may skin test positive as they often have been immunized against tuberculosis. Complete neurological recovery is unlikely when the child becomes comatose. Mortality rates of 20% are recorded even when treatment is initiated early.

The recommended initial drug regimen for treatment of tuberculous meningitis in the first 2 months is isoniazid, 20 mg/kg/day orally up to 500 mg/day; streptomycin, 20 mg/kg/day intramuscularly up to 1 g/day until establishing drug susceptibility; rifampin, 15 mg/kg/day orally up to 600 mg/day; and pyrazinamide, 30 mg/kg/day. Continue isoniazid and rifampin therapy for an additional 10 months. The use of corticosteroids is appropriate to reduce inflammation and cerebral edema.

Communicating hydrocephalus is a common complication of tuberculous meningitis because of impaired reabsorption of CSF. Periodic CT assessment of ventricular size is routine and specifically indicated when mental function deteriorates. Before the infection is controlled, treatment of communicating hydrocephalus is by repeated lumbar punctures and acetazolamide. In many cases, obstructive hydrocephalus develops later; in these cases, a surgical shunt is required.

Brain Abscess

The factors commonly predisposing to pyogenic brain abscess in children are meningitis, chronic otitis media, sinusitis, and congenital heart disease. Brain abscesses in the newborn are usually the result of meningitis caused by *C. diversus* and other species of Enterobacteriaceae. Pyogenic abscesses in children younger than 5 months but older than the neonatal period are uncommon and usually occur in children with hydrocephalus and shunt infection. The organisms most often responsible are *Staphylococcus* species. After 5 months of age, the infecting organisms are diverse, and many abscesses contain a mixed flora. Coagulase-positive *S. aureus* and anaerobic *Streptococcus* are the organisms most frequently recovered.

Clinical Features. The clinical features of brain abscess, similar to those of any other space-occupying lesion, depend on the age of the child and the location of the mass. A period of cerebritis, characterized by fever, headache, and lethargy, precedes encapsulation of the abscess. Seizures also may occur, but, in the absence of seizures, the initial symptoms may not be severe enough to arouse suspicion of cerebral infection. If the period of cerebritis is not recognized, the initial clinical manifestations are the same as those of other mass lesions. Infants have abnormal head growth, a bulging fontanelle, failure to thrive, and sometimes seizures. Older children show signs of increased intracranial pressure and focal neurological dysfunction. Fever is present in only 60 % of cases, and meningeal irritation is relatively uncommon. Based on clinical features alone, pyogenic brain abscess is difficult to separate from other mass lesions, such as brain tumor. About 80 % of abscesses are in the cerebral hemispheres. Hemiparesis, hemianopia, and seizures are the usual clinical features. Cerebellar abscess most often results from chronic otitis and is manifest as nystagmus and ataxia.

Diagnosis. The combination of headache and papilledema, with or without focal neurological dysfunction, suggests the possibility of a mass lesion and calls for neuroimaging. Most abscesses appear on CT as an area of decreased density surrounded by a rim of intense enhancement referred to as a ring lesion. This lesion, although characteristic, is not diagnostic. Malignant brain tumors may have a similar appearance. Ring enhancement occurs during the late stages of cerebritis, just before capsule formation. After the capsule forms, the diameter of the ring decreases and the center becomes more hypodense. Multiple abscesses may be present.

Management. The development of neuroimaging has altered the management of cerebral abscess. Previously, surgical drainage was immediate on diagnosis of abscess formation. Antimicrobials are the initial therapy now even for encapsulated abscesses, with progress followed with serial scans.

The initial step in treatment is to reduce brain swelling by the use of corticosteroids. Follow the steroids with an intravenous antimicrobial regimen that generally includes a penicillinase-resistant penicillin, such as methicillin, 300 mg/kg/day, and chloramphenicol, 100 mg/kg/day. This combination is effective against *Staphylococcus* and mixed Gram-negative organisms. Identification of a specific organism by culture of CSF or blood allows specific antimicrobial therapy. In general, penicillin G is preferable to ampicillin for penicillin-sensitive organisms. If medical therapy does not resolve the abscess, surgical drainage is necessary. Even in such cases, prolonged medical therapy before surgery increases the success of total excision.

Subdural and Epidural Empyema

Meningitis in infants and sinusitis in older children are the most common factors causing infection in the subdural space. The subdural space is sterile in children with bacterial meningitis, but contamination may occur when a subdural tap occurs before sterilizing the subarachnoid space with antibiotics. In older children, the usual cause of subdural and epidural abscesses is by penetrating head injuries or chronic mastoiditis. Infections of the subdural space are difficult to contain and may extend over an entire hemisphere.

Clinical Features. Subdural empyema produces increased intracranial pressure because of mass effect, cerebral edema, and vasculitis. Vasculitis leads to thrombosis of cortical veins, resulting in focal neurological dysfunction and increased intracranial pressure. Children with subdural infections have headache, fever, vomiting, seizures, and states of decreasing consciousness. Unilateral and alternating hemipareses are common.

Diagnosis. Suspect subdural empyema in children with meningitis whose condition declines after an initial period of recovery or in children who continue to have increased intracranial pressure of uncertain cause. Examination of the CSF may not be helpful, but the usual abnormality is a mixed cellular response, generally less than 100 cells/mm^3 and with a lymphocytic predominance. The glucose concentration is normal, and the protein concentration is only mildly elevated.

CT is particularly helpful in showing a subdural or epidural abscess. The infected collection appears as a lens-shaped mass of increased lucency just beneath the skull. A shift of midline structures is generally present. In infants, subdural puncture provides an abscess specimen for identification of the organism. Subdural puncture also drains much of the abscess.

BOX 4-7 Common Fungal Pathogens

Yeast Forms

- *Candida*
- *Cryptococcus neoformans*

Dimorphic Forms

- *Blastomyces dermatitidis*
- *Coccidioides immitis*
- *Histoplasma capsulatum*

Mold Forms

- *Aspergillus*

Management. The treatment of subdural or epidural empyema requires corticosteroids to decrease intracranial pressure, antimicrobials to eradicate the organisms, and anticonvulsants for seizures. Medical therapy and CT to monitor progress may replace surgical drainage of subdural empyema in some situations.

Fungal Infections

Fungi exist in two forms: molds and yeasts. Molds are filamentous and divided into segments by hyphae. Yeasts are unicellular organisms surrounded by a thick cell wall and sometimes a capsule. Several fungi exist as yeast in tissue but are filamentous when grown in culture. Such fungi are dimorphic. Box 4-7 lists common fungal pathogens. Fungal infections of the CNS system may cause an acute, subacute, or chronic meningitis; solitary or multiple abscesses; and granulomas. Fungal infections of the nervous system are most common in children who are immunosuppressed, especially children with leukemia or acidosis. Fungal infections also occur in immunocompetent children.

Cryptococcus neoformans and *Coccidioides immitis* are the leading causes of fungal meningitis in immunocompetent children. Among clinically recognized fungal CNS disease, *Cryptococcus* and *Candida* infections are the most common, followed by *Coccidioides*, *Aspergillus*, and zygomycetes. Other fungi rarely involve the CNS.

Candidal Meningoencephalitis

Candida is a common inhabitant of the mouth, vagina, and intestinal tract. Ordinarily it causes no symptoms; however, *Candida* can multiply and become an important pathogen in immunosuppressed children taking multiple antibiotics, children with debilitating diseases, transplant recipients, and critically ill neonates undergoing treatment with long-term vascular catheters. The most common sites of infection are the mouth (thrush), skin, and vagina. Candidal meningitis is almost unheard of in healthy, nonhospitalized children.

Clinical Features. *Candida* reaches the brain and other organs by vascular dissemination. The brain is involved less often than other organs, and fever, lethargy, and vomiting are the prominent features. Hepatosplenomegaly and arthritis may be present.

Cerebral involvement can be in the form of meningitis, abscess formation, or both. The clinical features of meningoencephalitis are fever, vomiting, meningismus, papilledema, and seizures leading to states of decreased consciousness. In some individuals, a single large cerebral abscess forms that causes focal neurological dysfunction and papilledema.

Diagnosis. Suspect cerebral *Candida* infection when unexplained fever develops in children with risk factors for disseminated disease. The organism can be isolated from blood, joint effusion fluid, or CSF. When meningitis is present, a predominantly neutrophilic response is present in the CSF associated with a protein concentration that is generally 100 mg/dL (1 g/L). Reduction of the glucose concentration is small. Children who have a candidal abscess rather than meningitis are likely to have normal or near-normal CSF. CT reveals a mass lesion resembling a pyogenic abscess or tumor.

Management. When candidal infection develops in a child because of an indwelling vascular catheter, remove the catheter. Treat with amphotericin B and flucytosine, which have a synergistic effect. Dosages are the same as for other fungal infections; administer the drugs for 6 to 12 weeks, depending on the efficacy of therapy and the presence of adverse reactions.

Coccidioidomycosis

C. immitis is endemic in the San Joaquin Valley of California and all southwestern states. Inhalation is the route of infection, and almost 90 % of individuals become infected within 10 years of moving into an endemic area. Only 40 % of patients become symptomatic; the other 60 % are positive only by skin test.

Clinical Features. Malaise, fever, cough, myalgia, and chest pain follow respiratory infection. The pulmonary infection is self-limiting. The incidence of fungal dissemination from the lung to other organs is 1:400. The dissemination rate is considerably higher in infants than in older children and adults.

The usual cause of coccidioidal meningitis is hematogenous spread from lung to meninges, but sometimes meningitis occurs by direct extension after infection of the skull. Symptoms of meningitis develop 2 to 4 weeks after respiratory symptoms begin. The main features are headache, apathy, and confusion. These symptoms may persist for weeks or months without concurrent seizures, meningismus, or focal neurological disturbances. If the meningitis becomes chronic, hydrocephalus eventually develops because the basilar meningitis prevents reabsorption of CSF.

Diagnosis. Suspect coccidioidal meningitis in patients living in endemic areas when headache develops after an acute respiratory infection. Skin hypersensitivity among individuals living in an endemic area is not helpful because a large percentage of the population is exposed and has a skin test positive for the organism. The CSF generally shows increased pressure, and the lymphocytic cellular response is 50–500 cells/mm^3. Often, eosinophils also are present. The protein concentration ranges from 100 to 500 mg/dL (1–5 g/L), and the glucose concentration is less than 35 mg/dL (<1.8 mmol/L).

In *C. immitis* meningitis, CSF culture is often negative and serological tests may be more useful. Complement-fixing antibody titers above 1:32 or 1:64 are significant. In early infection, serology is positive in 70 % of patients and increases to 100 % in later stages of untreated coccidioidal meningitis.

Management. Amphotericin B is the drug of choice for coccidioidal meningitis. It must be administered intravenously (Box 4-8) and intrathecally. The initial intrathecal dose is 0.1 mg for the first three injections. An increased dose of 0.25–0.5 mg three or four times each week completes the course. Prolonged treatment is required, and some clinicians recommend weekly intrathecal injections indefinitely.

BOX 4-8 Dosage Schedule for Amphotericin B

- Administer amphotericin B first intravenously in a single test dose of 0.1 mg/kg (not to exceed 1 mg) over at least 20 minutes to assess the child's temperature and blood pressure responses
- If the response is acceptable, administer the first therapeutic dose of 0.25 mg/kg over 2 hours the same day as the test dose
- Increase the dose in daily increments of 0.1–0.25 mg/kg, depending on the severity of infection, until achieving the daily maintenance dose of 1 mg/kg
- In life-threatening situations, use daily dosages of 1.25–1.5 mg/kg

Adverse reactions to intrathecal administration include aseptic meningitis and pain in the back and legs. Miconazole may be administered intravenously and intrathecally to patients unable to tolerate high doses of amphotericin B.

Cryptococcal Meningitis

Birds, especially pigeons, carry *C. neoformans* and disseminate it widely in soil. Acquisition of human infection is by inhalation. Dissemination is bloodborne, but the CNS is a favorite target, causing subacute and chronic meningoencephalitis.

Clinical Features. Cryptococcal meningitis is uncommon before age 10, and perhaps only 10 % of cases occur before age 20. Male infection rates are greater than female rates. Most children with cryptococcal meningitis are immunocompetent.

The first symptoms are usually insidious; chronic headache is the major feature. The headache waxes and wanes, but eventually becomes continuous and associated with nausea, vomiting, and lethargy. Body temperature may remain normal, especially in older children and adults, but younger children often have low-grade fever. Personality and behavioral changes are relatively common. The child becomes moody, listless, and sometimes frankly psychotic. Characteristic features of increased intracranial pressure are blurred vision, diplopia, and papilledema. Seizures and focal neurological dysfunction are not early features but are signs of vasculitis, hydrocephalus, and granuloma formation.

Diagnosis. Even when suspected, the diagnosis of cryptococcal meningitis fails to be established. The CSF may be normal but more often shows an increased opening pressure and less than 100 cells/mm^3 lymphocytes. The protein concentration is elevated, generally greater than 100 mg/dL (>1 g/L), and the glucose concentration is less than 40 mg/dL (<2 mmol/L).

The diagnosis of cryptococcal meningitis relies on detection of cryptococcal polysaccharide antigen by latex agglutination, demonstration of the organism in India ink preparations of CSF, or CSF culture. Approximately 50 % of India ink preparations and 75 % of culture results are positive. The latex agglutination test for cryptococcal polysaccharide antigen is sensitive and specific for cryptococcal infection.

Management. The treatment of choice is intravenous amphotericin B (0.3–0.5 mg/kg/day) combined with oral flucytosine (150 mg/kg/day) in four divided doses (Sanchez & Noskin, 1996). Amphotericin B, diluted with 5 % dextrose and water in a drug concentration no greater than 1 mg/10 mL of fluid, constitutes the intravenous solution. Nephrotoxicity is the limiting factor in achieving desirable blood levels. Box 4-8 summarizes the intravenous regimen, which is generally the same for all fungal infections of the nervous system. The total dose varies with the response and the side effects, but is usually 1500–2000 mg/1.7 m^2 of body surface. Continuous therapy for 4 to 6 weeks is required.

The toxic effects include chills, fever, nausea, and vomiting. Frequent blood counts and urinalyses monitor for anemia and nephrotoxicity. Manifestations of renal impairment are the appearance of cells or casts in the urine, an elevated blood concentration of urea nitrogen, and decreased creatinine clearance. When renal impairment occurs, discontinue the drug and restart at a lower dose.

Cytopenia limits the use of flucytosine. Seriously ill patients, treated late in the course of the disease, also should be given intrathecally administered amphotericin B and miconazole. A decline of the agglutination titer in the CSF indicates therapeutic efficacy. Periodic cranial CT monitors for the development of hydrocephalus.

Other Fungal Infections

Histoplasmosis is endemic in the central United States and causes pulmonary infection. Miliary spread is unusual. Neurological histoplasmosis may take the form of leptomeningitis, focal abscess, or multiple granulomas. Blastomycosis is primarily a disease of North America. Hematogenous spread from the lungs infects the brain. Multiple abscesses form, which give the CT appearance of metastatic disease. The cellular response in the CSF is markedly increased when fungi produce meningitis and may be normal or only mildly increased with abscess formation. Amphotericin B is the mainstay of therapy for fungal infections; the combination of itraconazole and amphotericin B treats *Histoplasma capsulatum*.

IDIOPATHIC INTRACRANIAL HYPERTENSION (PSEUDOTUMOR CEREBRI)

The term idiopathic intracranial hypertension (IIH) characterizes a syndrome of increased intracranial pressure, normal CSF content, and a normal brain with normal or small ventricles on brain imaging studies. IIH may have an identifiable underlying cause or may be idiopathic. Identification of a specific cause is usual in children younger than 6 years old, whereas most idiopathic cases occur after age 11 years. Box 4-9 lists some causes

BOX 4-9 Causes of Intracranial Hypertension

DRUGS

- Corticosteroid withdrawal
- Doxicycline
- Nalidixic acid
- Oral contraceptives
- Tetracycline
- Thyroid replacement
- Vitamin A

SYSTEMIC DISORDERS

- Guillain-Barré syndrome
- Iron deficiency anemia
- Leukemia
- Polycythemia vera
- Protein malnutrition
- Systemic lupus erythematosus
- Vitamin A deficiency
- Vitamin D deficiency

HEAD TRAUMA

INFECTIONS

- Otitis media (sinus thrombosis)
- Sinusitis (simus thrombosis)

METABOLIC DISORDERS

- Adrenal insufficiency
- Diabetic ketoacidosis (treatment)
- Galactosemia
- Hyperadrenalism
- Hyperthyroidism
- Hypoparathyroidism
- Pregnancy

of IIH. An established cause-and-effect relationship is uncertain in many of these conditions. The most frequent causes are obesity, otitis media, head trauma, the use of certain drugs and vitamins, and feeding after malnutrition.

Clinical Features. Patients with IIH have headaches that are diffuse, are worse at night, and often wake them from sleep in the early hours of the morning. Sudden movements, such as coughing, aggravate headache. Headaches may be present for several months before establishing a diagnosis. Some patients complain of dizziness. Transitory loss of vision may occur with change of position. Prolonged papilledema may lead to visual loss (Friedman & Jacobson, 2002).

Young children may have only irritability, somnolence, or apathy. Less common symptoms are transitory visual obscurations, neck stiffness, tinnitus, paresthesias, and ataxia. Most children are not acutely ill, and mental ability is normal.

Neurological examination is normal except for papilledema and abducens nerve palsy. Features of focal neurological dysfunction are lacking. Loss of vision is the main concern. Untreated IIH may lead to progressive papilledema and optic atrophy. Loss of vision may be rapid and severe. Early diagnosis and treatment are essential to preserve vision.

Diagnosis. IIH is a diagnosis of exclusion. Brain imaging including magnetic resonance venograpy is required in every child with headache and papilledema to exclude a mass lesion or hydrocephalus. The results of imaging studies are usually normal in children with IIH. In some, the ventricles are small, and normal sulcal markings are absent. Assess visual fields, with special attention to the size of the blind spot, at baseline and after treatment is initiated. Exclude known underlying causes of IIH by careful history and physical examination. Ordinarily, identification of an underlying cause is easily established.

Management. The goals of therapy are to relieve headache and preserve vision. A single lumbar puncture, with the closing pressure reduced to half of the opening pressure, is sufficient to reverse the process in many cases. The mechanism by which lumbar puncture is effective is unknown, but a transitory change in CSF dynamics seems sufficient to readjust the pressure. Remove any possible triggers such as vitamin A, doxycycline, and tetracycline, and address weight reduction when applicable.

The usual treatment of children with IIH is acetazolamide, 10 mg/kg/day, after the initial lumbar puncture. Whether the acetazolamide is an important addition to lumbar puncture is not clear. If symptoms return, the lumbar puncture is repeated on subsequent days. Some children require serial lumbar punctures.

Occasionally, children continue to have increased intracranial pressure and evidence of progressive optic neuropathy despite the use of lumbar puncture and acetazolamide. In such patients, studies should be repeated to look for a cause other than idiopathic pseudotumor cerebri. If studies are negative, lumboperitoneal shunt is the usual option to reduce pressure. Optic nerve fenestration relieves papilledema but does not relieve increased intracranial pressure. A newly proposed technique is stenting the venous sinus to reduce pressure (Higgins et al, 2003). Usefulness of this technique is not yet established.

REFERENCES

Friedman DI, Jacobson DM. Diagnostic criteria for idiopathic intracranial hypertension. Neurology 2002;59:1492–5.

Grimwood K, Anderson VA, Bond L, et al. Adverse outcome of bacterial meningitis in school-age survivors. Pediatrics 1995;95:646–56.

Higgins JN, Cousins C, Owler BK, et al. Idiopathic intracranial hypertension. 12 cases treated by venous sinus stenting. Journal of Neurology, Neurosurgery and Psychiatry 2003;12:1662–6.

Jallo GI, Biser-Rohrbaugh A, Freed D. Brainstem gliomas. Childs Nervous System 2004;20:143–53.

Mansur DB, Drzymala RE, Rich KM, et al. The efficacy of stereotactic radiosurgery in the management of intracranial ependymoma. Journal of Neuro-oncology 2004;66:187–90.

Mauffrey C. Pediatric brainstem gliomas: prognostic factors and management. Journal of Clinical Neuroscience 2006;13:431–7.

McNeil DE, Cote TR, Clegg L, et al. Incidence and trends in pediatric malignancies medulloblastoma/primitive neuroectodermal tumor: A SEER update. Medical and Pediatric Oncology 2002;39:190–4.

Menovsky T, van Overbeeke JJ. Cerebral arteriovenous malformations in childhood. State of the art with special reference to treatment. European Journal of Pediatrics 1997;56:741–6.

Merchant TE, Mulhern RK, Krasin MJ, et al. Preliminary results from a phase II trial of conformation radiation therapy and evaluation of radiation-related CNS effects for pediatric patients with localized ependymoma. Journal of Clinical Oncology 2004;22:3156–62.

Meyers PM, Halbach VV, Phatouros CP, et al. Hemorrhagic complications in vein of Galen malformations. Annals of Neurology 2000;47:748–55.

Olafsson E, Hauser A, Gudmundsson G. A population-based study of prognosis of ruptured cerebral aneurysm. Mortality and recurrence of subarachnoid hemorrhage. Neurology 1997;48:1191–5.

Pitfield AF, Carroll AB, Kissoon N. Emergency management of increased intracranial pressure. Pediatric Emergency Care 2012;28:200–4.

Pollack IF, Gerszten PC, Martinez AJ, et al. Intracranial ependymomas of childhood. Long-term outcome and prognostic factors. Neurosurgery 1995;37:655–67.

Roland EH, Hill A. Intraventricular hemorrhage and posthemorrhagic hydrocephalus. Clinical Perinatology 1997;24:589–605.

Sanchez JL, Noskin GA. Recent advances in the management of opportunistic fungal infections. Comprehensive Therapy 1996;22:703–12.

Stark A, Fritsch M, Claviez A, et al. Management of tectal glioma in childhood. Pediatric Neurology 2005;33:33–8.

Stevenson SB. Pseudotumor cerebri: Yet another reason to fight obesity. Journal of Pediatric Health Care 2008;22:40–3.

Volpe JJ. Neurology of the Newborn, 4th ed. Philadelphia: WB Saunders; 2000.

Wrensch M, Minn Y, Chew T, et al. Epidemiology of primary brain tumors: current concepts and review of the literature. Neuro-oncology 2002;4:278–99.

CHAPTER 5

PSYCHOMOTOR RETARDATION AND REGRESSION

Psychomotor retardation or developmental delay refers to the slow progress in the attainment of developmental milestones. This may be caused by either static (Box 5-1) or progressive (Box 5-2) encephalopathies. In contrast, psychomotor regression refers to the loss of developmental milestones previously attained. This is usually due to a progressive disease of the nervous system. In some cases, reports of regression may also result from parental misperception of attained milestones or by the development of new clinical features from an established static disorder as the brain matures (Box 5-3).

DEVELOPMENTAL DELAY

Delayed achievement of developmental milestones is one of the more common problems evaluated by child neurologists. Two important questions require answers. Is developmental delay restricted to specific areas or is it global? Is development delayed or regressing?

BOX 5-1 Diagnosis of Developmental Delay: No Regression

PREDOMINANT SPEECH DELAY

- Bilateral hippocampal sclerosis
- Congenital bilateral perisylvian syndrome (see Chapter 17)
- Hearing impairment* (see Chapter 17)
- Infantile autism

PREDOMINANT MOTOR DELAY

- Ataxia (see Chapter 10)
- Hemiplegia (see Chapter 11)
- Hypotonia (see Chapter 6)
- Neuromuscular disorders* (see Chapter 7)
- Paraplegia (see Chapter 12)

GLOBAL DEVELOPMENTAL DELAY

- Cerebral malformations
- Chromosomal disturbances
- Intrauterine infection
- Perinatal disorders
- Progressive encephalopathies (see Box 5-2)

*Denotes the most common conditions and the ones with disease modifying treatments

In infants, the second question is often difficult to answer. Even in static encephalopathies, new symptoms such as involuntary movements and seizures may occur as the child gets older, and delayed acquisition of milestones without other neurological deficits is sometimes the initial feature of progressive disorders. However, once it is clear that milestones previously achieved are lost or that focal neurological deficits are evolving, a progressive disease of the nervous system is a consideration.

The *Denver Developmental Screening Test* (DDST) is an efficient and reliable method for assessing development in the physician's office. It rapidly assesses four different components of development: personal–social, fine motor adaptive, language, and gross motor. Several psychometric tests amplify the results, but the DDST in combination with neurological assessment provides sufficient information to initiate further diagnostic studies.

Language Delay

Normal infants and children have a remarkable facility for acquiring language during the first decade. Those exposed to two languages concurrently learn both. Vocalization of vowels occurs in the first month, and, by 5 months, laughing and squealing are established. At 6 months, infants begin articulating consonants, usually M, D, and B. Parents translate these to mean "mama," "dada," and "bottle" or "baby," although this is not the infant's intention. These first attempts at vowels and consonants are automatic and sometimes occur even in deaf children. In the months that follow, the infant imitates many speech sounds, babbles and coos, and finally learns the specific use of "mama" and "dada" by 1 year of age. Receptive skills are always more highly developed than expressive skills, because language must be decoded before it is encoded. By 2 years of age, children have learned to combine at least two words, understand more than 250 words, and follow many simple verbal directions.

Developmental disturbances in the language cortex of the dominant hemisphere that occur before 5 years of age, and possibly later, displace

BOX 5-2 Progressive Encephalopathy: Onset Before Age 2

ACQUIRED IMMUNE DEFICIENCY SYNDROME ENCEPHALOPATHY*

DISORDERS OF AMINO ACID METABOLISM
- Guanidinoacetate methyltransferase deficiency*
- Homocystinuria (21q22)*
- Maple syrup urine disease (intermediate and thiamine response forms)*
- Phenylketonuria
- Guanidinoacetate methyltransferase deficiency*

DISORDERS OF LYSOSOMAL ENZYMES
- Ganglioside storage disorders
  - GM_1 gangliosidosis
  - GM_2 gangliosidosis (Tay-Sachs disease, Sandhoff disease)
- Gaucher disease type II (glucosylceramide lipidosis)*
- Globoid cell leukodystrophy (Krabbe disease)
- Glycoprotein degradation disorders
- I-cell disease
  - Mucopolysaccharidoses*
  - Type I (Hurler Syndrome)*
  - Type III (Sanfilippo disease)
- Niemann-Pick disease type A (sphingomyelin lipidosis)
- Sulfatase deficiency disorders
  - Metachromatic leukodystrophy (sulfatide lipidoses)
  - Multiple sulfatase deficiency

CARBOHYDRATE-DEFICIENT GLYCOPROTEIN SYNDROMES

HYPOTHYROIDISM*

MITOCHONDRIAL DISORDERS
- Alexander disease
- Mitochondrial myopathy, encephalopathy, lactic acidosis, stroke (see Chapter 11)
- Progressive infantile poliodystrophy (Alpers disease)
- Subacute necrotizing encephalomyelopathy (Leigh disease)
- Trichopoliodystrophy (Menkes disease)

NEUROCUTANEOUS SYNDROMES
- Chediak-Higashi syndrome
- Neurofibromatosis*
- Tuberous sclerosis*

OTHER DISORDERS OF GRAY MATTER
- Infantile ceroid lipofuscinosis (Santavuori-Haltia disease)
- Infantile neuroaxonal dystrophy
- Lesch-Nyhan disease*
- Progressive neuronal degeneration with liver disease
- Rett syndrome

OTHER DISORDERS OF WHITE MATTER
- Aspartoacylase deficiency (Canavan disease)
- Galactosemia: Transferase deficiency*
- Neonatal adrenoleukodystrophy (see Chapter 6)*
- Pelizaeus-Merzbacher disease
- Progressive cavitating leukoencephalopathy

PROGRESSIVE HYDROCEPHALUS*

*Denotes the most common conditions and the ones with disease modifying treatments

BOX 5-3 Causes of Apparent Regression in Static Encephalopathy

- Increasing spasticity (usually during the first year)
- New onset movement disorders (usually during the second year)
- New onset seizures
- Parental misperception of attained milestones
- Progressive hydrocephalus

language to the contralateral hemisphere. This does not occur in older children.

Autistic Spectrum Disorders

Infantile autism is not a single disorder, but rather many different disorders described by a broad behavioral phenotype that has a final common pathway of atypical development (Volkmar et al, 2005). The terms autistic spectrum disorders (ASD) and pervasive developmental disorders are used to classify the spectrum of behavioral symptoms. Asperger disorder represents the high-functioning end of the autistic disorder spectrum. Many different gene loci are identifiable, some or all of which contribute to the phenotype (Schellenberg et al, 2006). The "broad autism phenotype" includes individuals with some symptoms of autism who do not meet the full criteria for autism or other disorders.

Autism has become an increasingly popular diagnosis. An apparent increasing incidence of diagnosis suggests to some an environmental factor. However, data does not confirm the notion of an autism epidemic nor causation by any environmental factor. The definition of ASD has become so wide that it is likely contributing to the apparent increase in prevalence. Most biological studies indicate genetic or other prenatal factors. Anxiety and obsessive-compulsive traits are highly represented in parents of children with ASD. It is possible that these children will have an overload of these genetic traits contributing to some of their symptoms.

Clinical Features. The major diagnostic criteria are impaired sociability, impaired verbal and nonverbal communication skills, and restricted activities and interests (Rapin, 2002). Failure of language development is the feature most likely to bring autistic infants to medical attention and correlates best with the outcome; children who fail to develop language before the age 5 years have the worst outcome. The IQ is less than 70 in most children with autism. However, IQ may be significantly underestimated due to their impaired interactive skills, which make testing difficult and less reliable. Some autistic children show no affection to their parents or other care providers, while others are affectionate on their own terms. Autistic children do not show normal play activity; some have a morbid preoccupation with spinning objects, stereotyped behaviors such as rocking and spinning, and relative insensitivity to pain. An increased incidence of epilepsy in autistic children is probable.

Diagnosis. Infantile autism is a clinical diagnosis and not confirmable by laboratory tests. Infants with profound hearing impairment may display autistic behavior, and tests of hearing are diagnostic. Electroencephalography (EEG) is indicated when seizures are suspected and to evaluate the less likely possibility of Landau-Kleffner syndrome. The study should be obtained with sedation in most cases, since sleep recording is needed and autistic children often become distressed by the procedure and do not cooperate with electrode placement.

Management. Autism is not curable, but several drugs may be useful to control specific behavioral disturbances. Behavior modification techniques improve some aspects of the severely aberrant behavior. However, despite the best program of treatment, these children function in a moderately to severely retarded range despite their level of intelligence. In our experience most children benefit from the use of selective serotonin reuptake inhibitors. csf Citalopram (10–20 mg/day) and escitalopram (5–10 mg/day) are commonly used. Children with ASD often suffer from anxiety and obsessive-compulsive behaviors that may interfere with their development and social skills. Obsessive-compulsive traits are often difficult to discern in patients with autism. Autistic children are typically unable to express themselves, and their obsessive thinking only becomes visible when associated with compulsions. Therefore a trial with the above medications should be offered in most cases. Many children also benefit from a management of hyperactive behaviors when present. Clonidine 0.05–0.1 mg bid or guanfacine 0.5–1 mg bid are good options.

Bilateral Hippocampal Sclerosis

Both bilateral hippocampal sclerosis and *the congenital bilateral perisylvian syndrome* cause a profound impairment of language development. The former also causes failure of cognitive capacity that mimics infantile autism, while the latter causes a pseudobulbar palsy (see Chapter 17). Infants with medial bilateral hippocampal sclerosis generally come to medical attention for refractory seizures. However, the syndrome emphasizes that the integrity of one medial hippocampal gyrus is imperative for language development.

Hearing Impairment

The major cause of isolated delay in speech development is a hearing impairment (see Chapter 17). Hearing loss may occur concomitantly with global developmental retardation, as in rubella embryopathy, cytomegalic inclusion disease, neonatal meningitis, kernicterus, and several genetic disorders. Hearing loss need not be profound; it can be insidious, yet delay speech development. The loss of high-frequency tones, inherent in telephone conversation, prevents the clear distinction of many consonants that we learn to fill in through experience; infants do not have experience in supplying missing sounds.

The hearing of any infant with isolated delay in speech development requires audiometric testing. Crude testing in the office by slamming objects and ringing bells is inadequate. Hearing loss is suspected in children with global retardation caused by disorders ordinarily associated with hearing loss or in retarded children who fail to imitate sounds. Other clues to hearing loss in children are excessive gesturing and staring at the lips of people who are talking. Brain auditory evoked potentials offer good screening for neonatal hearing deficits and are standard practice in many institutions.

Delayed Motor Development

Infants with delayed gross motor development but normal language and social skills are often hypotonic and may have a neuromuscular disease (see Chapter 6). Isolated delay in motor function is also caused by ataxia (see Chapter 10), mild hemiplegia (see Chapter 11), and mild paraplegia (see Chapter 12). Many such children have a mild form of cerebral palsy, sufficient to delay the achievement of motor milestones but not severe enough to cause a recognizable disturbance in cognitive function during infancy. The detection of mild disturbances in cognitive function more often occur when the child enters school. Children with benign macrocephaly may have isolated motor delay in the first 18 months, due to the difficulty achieving adequate head control with their larger head size.

Global Developmental Delay

Most infants with global developmental delay have a static encephalopathy caused by an antenatal or perinatal disturbance. However, 1 % of infants with developmental delay and no evidence of regression have an inborn error of metabolism and 3.5–10 % have a chromosomal disorder (Shevell et al, 2003). An exhaustive search for an underlying cause in every infant whose development is slow but not regressing is not cost effective. Factors that increase the likelihood of finding a progressive disease are an affected family member, parental consanguinity, organomegaly, and absent tendon reflexes. Unenhanced cranial magnetic resonance imaging (MRI) and chromosome analysis/microarray is a reasonable screening test in all infants with global developmental delay. MRI often detects a malformation or other evidence of prenatal disease and provides a diagnosis that ends the uncertainty.

Chromosomal Disturbances

Abnormalities in chromosome structure or number are the single most common cause of severe mental retardation, but they still comprise only one-third of the total. Abnormalities of autosomal chromosomes are always associated with infantile hypotonia (see Chapter 6). In addition, multiple minor face and limb abnormalities are usually associated features. These abnormalities in themselves are common, but they assume diagnostic significance in combination. Box 5-4 summarizes the clinical features that suggest chromosomal aberrations and Table 5-1 lists some of the more common chromosome syndromes.

Fragile X Syndrome. The fragile X syndrome is the most common chromosomal cause of cognitive impairment. Its prevalence in males is approximately 20:100 000. The name derives from a fragile site (constriction) detectable in folate-free culture medium at the Xq 27 location. The unstable fragment contains a trinucleotide repeat in the *FMR1* gene that becomes larger

BOX 5-4 Clinical Indications for Chromosome Analysis

GENITOURINARY
- Ambiguous genitalia
- Polycystic kidney

HEAD AND NECK
- High nasal bridge
- Hypertelorism or hypotelorism
- Microphthalmia
- Mongoloid slant (in non-Asians)
- Occipital scalp defect
- Small mandible
- Small or fish mouth (hard to open)
- Small or low-set ears
- Upward slant of eyes
- Webbed neck

LIMBS
- Abnormal dermatoglyphics
- Low-set thumb
- Overlapping fingers
- Polydactyly
- Radial hypoplasia
- Rocker-bottom feet

TABLE 5-1 Selected Autosomal Syndromes*

Defect	Features
5p monosomy	Characteristic "cri du chat" cry Moonlike face Hypertelorism Microcephaly
10p trisomy	Dolichocephaly "Turtle's beak" Osteoarticular anomalies
Partial 12p monosomy	Microcephaly Narrow forehead Pointed nose Micrognathia
18 trisomy	Pointed ears Micrognathia Occipital protuberance Narrow pelvis Rocker-bottom feet
21 trisomy	Hypotonia Round flat (mongoloid) facies Brushfield spots Flat nape of neck

*Growth retardation and cognitive impairment are features of all autosomal chromosome disorders.

in successive generations (*DNA amplification*), causing more severe phenotypic expression. A decrease in the repeat size to normal may also occur. Because *FMR1* mutations are complex and may involve several gene-disrupting alterations, abnormal individuals may show atypical presentations with an IQ above 70 (Saul & Tarleton, 2012).

Clinical Features. Males with a complete phenotype have a characteristic appearance (large head, long face, prominent forehead and chin, protruding ears), connective tissue findings (joint laxity), and large testes after puberty. Behavioral abnormalities, sometimes including ASD, are common. The phenotypic features of males with full mutations vary in relation to puberty. Prepubertal males grow normally but have an occipitofrontal head circumference larger than the 50th percentile. Achievement of motor and speech milestones is late and temperament is abnormal, sometimes suggesting autism. Other physical features that become more obvious after puberty include a long face, prominent forehead, large ears, prominent jaw, and large genitalia.

The phenotype of females depends on both the nature of the *FMR1* mutation and random X-chromosome inactivation. About 50 % of females who inherit a full fragile X mutation are cognitively impaired; however, they are usually less severely affected than males with a full mutation. Approximately 20 % of males with a fragile X chromosome are normal, while 30 % of carrier females are mildly affected. An asymptomatic male can pass the abnormal chromosome to his daughters, who are usually asymptomatic as well. The daughters' children, both male and female, may be symptomatic.

Diagnosis. DNA-based testing has replaced the use of chromosome analysis using modified culture techniques to induce fragile sites (Saul & Tarleton, 2012). Molecular genetic testing is now the standard of diagnosis.

Management. Treatment consists of pharmacological management of behavior problems and educational intervention.

Cerebral Malformations

Approximately 3 % of all children have at least one major malformation, but the responsible etiological factors are identifiable in only 20 % of these cases. Many intrauterine diseases cause destructive changes that cause malformation of the developing brain. The exposure of an embryo to infectious or toxic agents during the first weeks after conception can disorganize the delicate sequencing of neural development at a time when the brain is incapable of generating a cellular response. Alcohol, lead, prescription drugs, and substances of abuse are factors in the production of cerebral malformations. Although a cause-and-effect relationship is difficult to establish in any individual, maternal cocaine use is probably responsible for vascular insufficiency and infarction of many organs, including the brain.

Suspect a cerebral malformation in any cognitively impaired child who is dysmorphic, has malformations of other organs, or has an abnormality of head size and shape (see Chapter 18). Noncontrast-enhanced computed tomography (CT) is satisfactory to show major malformations, but MRI is the better method to show migrational defects and is more cost-effective for diagnosis of malformations.

Intrauterine Infections

The most common intrauterine infections are human immunodeficiency virus (HIV) and cytomegalovirus (CMV). HIV infection can occur in utero, but acquisition of most infections occurs perinatally. Infected infants are asymptomatic in the newborn period and later develop progressive disease of the brain (see the section below: Progressive Encephalopathies with Onset Before Age 2). Rubella embryopathy has almost disappeared because of mass immunization but reappears when immunization rates decline.

Congenital Syphilis. Reported cases of congenital syphilis have increased since 1988, partly because of an actual increase in case number but also because the case definition has broadened. By the current definition, all stillborn infants and live infants born to a woman with a history of untreated or inadequately treated syphilis have congenital syphilis.

Clinical Features. Infection of the fetus is transplacental. Two-thirds of infected newborns are asymptomatic and are identified only on screening tests. The more common features in symptomatic newborns and infants are hepatosplenomegaly, periostitis or osteochondritis, pneumonia (pneumonia alba), persistent rhinorrhea (snuffles), and a maculopapular rash that can involve the palms and soles. If left untreated, the classic stigmata of Hutchinson's teeth, saddle nose, interstitial keratitis, saber shins, cognitive impairment, hearing loss, and hydrocephalus develop.

The onset of neurological disturbances is usually after age 2 years and includes eighth nerve deafness and cognitive impairment. The combination of nerve deafness, interstitial keratitis, and peg-shaped upper incisors is the *Hutchinson triad.*

Diagnosis. Every newborn infant's mother should have serologic testing to exclude syphilis infection prior to discharge from the nursery. Nontreponemal antibody tests (Venereal Disease Research Laboratory [VDRL] and rapid plasma reagin card tests) are screening tests and the fluorescent treponemal antibody test absorbed with nonpallidum treponemas is confirmatory. Suspect concomitant HIV infection in every child with congenital syphilis.

Management. Consultation with an infectious disease specialist is beneficial in all children suspected of having congenital syphilis. Treatment typically consists of intravenous aqueous penicillin G at a dose of 50 000 units/kg/dose q12 hours for the first 7 days of life, then q8h thereafter, for a total of 10 days. Alternatively, administer procaine penicillin G intramuscularly at a dose of 50 000 units/kg/day for 10 days.

Cytomegalic Inclusion Disease. Cytomegalovirus (CMV) is a member of the herpes virus group and produces a chronic infection characterized by long periods of latency punctuated by intervals of reactivation. CMV is the most common congenital viral infection (1–2 % of all live births) and results either from primary maternal infection or from reactivation of the virus in the mother. Pregnancy may cause reactivation of maternal infection. Risks to the fetus are greatest during the first half of gestation. Fortunately, less than 0.05 % of newborns with viruria have symptoms of cytomegalic inclusion disease.

Clinical Features. Less than 10 % of infected newborns are symptomatic. Clinical manifestations include intrauterine growth retardation, jaundice, petechiae/purpura, hepatosplenomegaly, microcephaly, hydrocephaly, intracerebral calcifications, glaucoma, and chorioretinitis. Except for the brain, most organ involvement is self-limited.

Migrational defects (lissencephaly, polymicrogyria, and cerebellar agenesis) are the main consequence of fetal infection during the first trimester. Some infants have microcephaly secondary to intrauterine infection without evidence of systemic infection at birth.

Diagnosis. Virus must be isolated within the first 2 to 3 weeks of life to confirm congenital infection. Afterwards, virus shedding no longer differentiates congenital from postnatal infection. While CMV can be isolated from many sites, urine and saliva are preferred samples for congenital CMV infection, because of their viral content. For these samples, a shell vial technique using monoclonal antibodies to detect CMV early antigens in inoculated fibroblasts grown on cover slips after centrifugation is diagnostic. Detection of CMV DNA by polymerase chain reaction (PCR) or in situ hybridization of tissues and fluids is available in specialized laboratories. Infected newborns should be isolated from women of childbearing age.

In infants with developmental delay and microcephaly, establishing the diagnosis of cytomegalic inclusion disease is by serological demonstration of prior infection and a consistent pattern of intracranial calcification.

Management. Much of the brain damage from congenital CMV occurs in utero and is not influenced by postnatal treatment. The antiviral agents currently approved for CMV treatment are ganciclovir (and its prodrug, valganciclovir), foscarnet, and cidofovir. The risk–benefit ratio of these agents in treating congenital CMV infection is uncertain.

Congenital Lymphocytic Choriomeningitis

Clinical Features. The lymphocytic choriomeningitis virus (LCMV) causes minor respiratory symptoms when inhaled postnatally, but prenatal infection causes severe brain malformation (Bonthius et al, 2007). Because the virus targets the developing brain all infected children have retinal injury and brain malformations.

The most commonly described congenital anomalies are chorioretinopathy, macrocephaly, and microcephaly. LCMV is a common cause of hydrocephalus. Up to one-third of newborns with hydrocephalus have positive serology to LCMV, and conversely almost 90 % of children with serologically confirmed perinatal infection with LCMV have hydrocephalus. Almost 40 % have hydrocephalus at birth; the remainder develop it over the first 3 months of age. Blindness and psychomotor retardation are potential long-term complications. Outcome severity depends on the timing of infection; early infection produces the worse outcomes.

Diagnosis. Imaging of the brain reveals major malformations. Viral culture of blood, cerebrospinal fluid (CSF), and urine are diagnostic. Immunofluorescent antibody tests or enzyme-linked immunosorbent assays are currently available for serum and CSF. PCR for detection of LCMV RNA may be available in the near future.

Management. Much of the brain damage from congenital LCMV occurs in utero and is not influenced by postnatal treatment.

Rubella Embryopathy. The rubella virus is a small, enveloped RNA virus with worldwide distribution and is responsible for an endemic mild exanthematous disease of childhood (German measles). Major epidemics, in which significant numbers of adults are exposed and infected, occurred every 9 to 10 years in both the United States and the United Kingdom. However, the incidence of rubella embryopathy in the United States has steadily declined with introduction of the rubella vaccine.

Clinical Features. Rubella embryopathy is a multisystem disease characterized by intrauterine growth retardation, cataracts, chorioretinitis, congenital heart disease, sensorineural deafness, hepatosplenomegaly, jaundice, anemia, thrombocytopenia, and rash. Eighty percent of children with a congenital rubella syndrome have nervous system involvement. The neurological features are bulging fontanelle, lethargy, hypotonia, and seizures. Seizure onset is from birth to 3 months of age.

Diagnosis. In order to provide accurate counseling, make every effort to confirm rubella infection in the exposed pregnant woman. Virus isolation is complicated and the diagnosis is established best by documenting rubella-specific IgM antibody in addition to a 4-fold or greater rise in rubella-specific IgG.

Management. Prevention is by immunization and avoiding possible exposure during pregnancy. No treatment is available for active infection in the newborn.

Toxoplasmosis. *Toxoplasma gondii* is a protozoan estimated to infect 1 per 1000 live births in the United States each year. The symptoms of toxoplasmosis infection in the mother usually go unnoticed. Transplacental transmission of toxoplasmosis is possible in situations of primary maternal infection during pregnancy or in immunocompromised mothers who have chronic or recurrent infection. The rate of placental transmission is highest during the last trimester, but fetuses infected at that time are least likely to have symptoms later on. The transmission rate is lowest during the first trimester, but fetuses infected at that time have the most serious sequelae.

Clinical Features. One-quarter of infected newborns have multisystem involvement (fever, rash, hepatosplenomegaly, jaundice, and thrombocytopenia) at birth. Neurological dysfunction is manifest as seizures, altered states of consciousness, and increased intracranial pressure. The triad of hydrocephalus, chorioretinitis, and intracranial calcification is the hallmark of congenital toxoplasmosis in older children. About 8% of infected newborns, who are asymptomatic at birth, later show neurological sequelae, especially psychomotor retardation.

Diagnosis. Detection of the organism is diagnostic, as are commercially available serological techniques. Presume any patient with positive IgG and IgM titers to be recently infected. In the United States the Toxoplasma Serology Laboratory of the Palo Alto Medical Foundation Research Institute offers confirmatory serological and PCR testing and methods for isolation of the organism. In addition, medical consultants are available for interpretation of test results and advice on management

The presence of positive or rising IgM and IgG titers confirms acute *T. gondii* infection in a pregnant woman. Detection of *T. gondii* DNA in amniotic fluid by PCR is less invasive and more sensitive than isolating parasites from fetal blood or amniotic fluid. Serial fetal ultrasonographic examinations monitor for ventricular enlargement and other signs of fetal infection.

In older children, the diagnosis requires not only serological evidence of prior infection but also compatible clinical features.

Management. A combined prenatal and postnatal treatment program for congenital toxoplasmosis can reduce the neurological morbidity. When seroconversion indicates acute maternal infection, fetal blood and amniotic fluid are cultured and fetal blood tested for *Toxoplasma*-specific IgM. The mother requires only spiramycin treatment unless proven fetal infection exists, when pyrimethamine and sulfadoxine are required. In newborns with clinical evidence of toxoplasmosis, administer pyrimethamine (Daraprim®) and sulfadiazine for 1 year. Because pyrimethamine is a folic acid antagonist, administer folinic acid (leucovorin) during therapy and for 1 week after termination of treatment. Routine monitoring of the peripheral platelet count is required. Newborns with a high protein concentration in the CSF or chorioretinitis also require prednisone, 1–2 mg/kg/day. The optimal duration of therapy for congenital toxoplasmosis is unknown but 1 year is the rule. Because of the high likelihood of fetal damage, termination of pregnancy is frequently recommended if *T. gondii* infection is confirmed and infection is thought to have occurred at less than 16 weeks of gestation or if the fetus shows evidence of hydrocephalus.

Perinatal Disorders

Perinatal infection, asphyxia, maternal drug use, and trauma are the main perinatal events that cause psychomotor retardation (see Chapter 1). The important infectious diseases are bacterial meningitis (see Chapter 4) and herpes encephalitis (see Chapter 1). Although the overall mortality rate for bacterial meningitis is now less than 50%, half of survivors show significant neurological disturbances almost immediately. Mental and motor disabilities, hydrocephalus, epilepsy, deafness, and visual loss are the most common sequelae. Psychomotor retardation may be the only or the most prominent sequelae. Progressive mental deterioration can occur if meningitis causes a secondary hydrocephalus.

Telling Parents Bad News

It is not possible to make bad news sound good or even half-bad. The goal of telling parents that their child will have neurologic or cognitive impairment is that they hear and understand what you are saying. The mind must be prepared to hear bad news. It is a mistake to tell people more than they are ready to accept. Too often, parents bring their child for a second opinion because previous doctors "didn't tell us anything." In fact, they may have said too much too fast and the parents tuned out.

My goal for the first visit is to establish that the child's development is not normal (not a normal variation), that something is wrong with the brain, and that I share the parents' concern. I order imaging of the brain, usually MRI, in every developmentally delayed child. When abnormal, review the MRI with the parents to help their understanding of the problem. Unfortunately, many mothers come alone for this critical visit and must later restate your comments to doubting fathers and grandparents. Most parents cannot handle more information than "the child is not normal" at the first consultation and further discussion awaits a later visit. However, always answer probing questions fully. Parents must never lose confidence in your willingness to be forthright. The timing of the next visit depends on the age of the child and the severity of the cognitive impairment. The more the child falls behind in reaching developmental milestones, the more ready parents will be to accept the diagnosis of cognitive impairment.

When the time comes to tell a mother that her child has cognitive impairment, it is not helpful to describe the deficit as mild, moderate, or severe. Parents want to know what the child will do. Will he walk, need special schools, and live alone? The next question is "What can I do to help my child?" Direct them to programs that provide developmental specialists and other parents who can help them learn how to live with a chronic handicapping disorder and gain access to community resources.

Providing a prognosis after a brain insult in a neonate or young infant is often difficult. Fortunately, the plasticity of the young brain may offer improved outcomes in some cases, making it difficult to provide a definite prognosis. Prognosis is often better in cases that affect only one hemisphere. In fact, complete encephalomalacia of one hemisphere may be associated with better development than having a very injured but still "functional" hemisphere. In all cases we have to make families aware of the spectrum of possibilities and high probability of deficits.

PROGRESSIVE ENCEPHALOPATHIES WITH ONSET BEFORE AGE 2

The differential diagnosis of progressive diseases of the nervous system that start before age 2 years is somewhat different from those that begin during childhood (see Box 5-5). The history and physical examination must answer three questions before initiating laboratory diagnosis:

1. Is this multi-organ or only central nervous system (CNS) disease? Other organ involvement suggests lysosomal, peroxisomal, and mitochondrial disorders.
2. Is this a (CNS) or both central and peripheral nervous systems process? Nerve or muscle involvement suggests mainly lysosomal and mitochondrial disorders.
3. Does the disease affect primarily the gray matter or the white matter? Early features of gray matter disease are personality change, seizures, and dementia. Characteristic of white matter disease is focal neurological deficits, spasticity, and blindness. Whether the process begins in the gray matter or the white matter, eventually clinical features of dysfunction develop in both. The EEG is usually abnormal early in the course of gray matter disease and late in the course of white matter disease. MRI shows cortical atrophy in gray matter disease and cerebral demyelination in white mater disease (Figure 5-1). Visual evoked responses and motor conduction velocities are useful in documenting demyelination, even subclinical, in the optic and peripheral nerves, respectively.

Acquired Immune Deficiency Syndrome Encephalopathy

Acquired immune deficiency syndrome (AIDS) is a human retroviral disease caused by the lentivirus subfamily now designated as human immunodeficiency virus (HIV). Adults spread HIV by sexual contact, intravenous drug abuse, and blood transfusion. Pediatric AIDS cases result from transplacental or perinatal transmission. Transmission may occur by breastfeeding. The mother may be asymptomatic when the child becomes infected.

BOX 5-5 Progressive Encephalopathy: Onset after Age 2 years

DISORDERS OF LYSOSOMAL ENZYMES
- Gaucher disease type III (glucosylceramide lipidosis)
- Globoid cell leukodystrophy (late-onset Krabbe disease)
- Glycoprotein degradation disorders
- Aspartylglycosaminuria
- Mannosidosis type II
- GM_2 gangliosidosis (juvenile Tay-Sachs disease)
- Metachromatic leukodystrophy (late-onset sulfatide lipidoses)
- Mucopolysaccharidoses types II and VII
- Niemann-Pick type C (sphingomyelin lipidosis)

INFECTIOUS DISEASE
- Acquired immune deficiency syndrome encephalopathy*
- Congenital syphilis*
- Subacute sclerosing panencephalitis

OTHER DISORDERS OF GRAY MATTER
- Ceroid lipofuscinosis
  - Juvenile
  - Late infantile (Bielschowsky-Jansky disease)
- Huntington disease
- Mitochondrial disorders
  - Late-onset poliodystrophy
  - Myoclonic epilepsy and ragged-red fibers
- Progressive neuronal degeneration with liver disease
- Xeroderma pigmentosum

OTHER DISORDERS OF WHITE MATTER
- Adrenoleukodystrophy
- Alexander disease
- Cerebrotendinous xanthomatosis
- Progressive cavitating leukoencephalopathy

*Denotes the most common conditions and the ones with disease modifying treatments

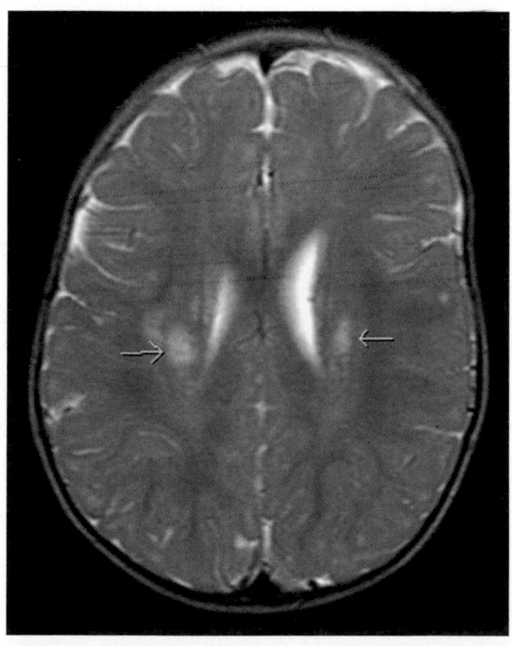

FIGURE 5-1 ■ Krabbe's disease. T_2 axial MRI shows an early stage of symmetric demyelination (arrows).

Clinical Features. Evidence of infection is apparent during the first year in 30% of children born to AIDS-infected mothers. As a rule, the outcome is worse when the onset of symptoms is early, and the rate of progression in the child relates directly to the severity of disease in the mother.

Twenty percent of children with HIV present with severe symptoms or die in infancy (Galli et al, 2000). The cause of their poor prognosis is unknown. The spectrum of neurological and non-neurological manifestations in HIV-infected children is somewhat different from adults. Hepatosplenomegaly and bone marrow failure, lymphocytic interstitial pneumonia, chronic diarrhea and failure to thrive, acquired microcephaly, cerebral vasculopathy, and basal ganglia calcification occur more frequently in children. Opportunistic infections that represent recrudescence of previously acquired infections in adults, e.g., cerebral toxoplasmosis, progressive multifocal leukoencephalopathy, are rare in infants.

AIDS encephalopathy may be subacute or indolent and is not necessarily associated with failure to thrive or opportunistic infections. The onset of encephalopathy may occur from 2 months to 5 years after exposure to the virus. Ninety percent of affected infants show symptoms by 18 months of age. Progressive loss of developmental milestones, microcephaly, dementia, and spasticity characterize the encephalopathy. Other features in less than 50% of children are ataxia, pseudobulbar palsy, involuntary movement disorders, myoclonus, and seizures. Death usually occurs a few months after the onset of AIDS encephalopathy.

Diagnosis. HIV DNA PCR is the preferred method for the diagnosis of HIV infection in infants and children younger than 18 months of age. It is performed on peripheral blood mononuclear cells and is highly sensitive and specific by 2 weeks of age. Approximately 30% of infants with HIV infection will have a positive DNA PCR assay result by 48 hours, 93% by 2 weeks, and almost all infants by 1 month of age.

Management. The introduction of routine maternal treatment with highly active antiretroviral therapy (HAART) in 1996 has greatly decreased the incidence of pediatric AIDS. Combined treatment with zidovudine (azidothymidine, AZT), didanosine, and nevirapine is well tolerated and may have sustained efficacy against HIV-1. Bone marrow suppression is the only important evidence of toxicity.

Disorders of Amino Acid Metabolism

Disorders of amino acid metabolism impair neuronal function by causing excessive production of toxic intermediary metabolites and reducing the production of neurotransmitters. The clinical syndromes are either an acute neonatal encephalopathy with seizures and cerebral edema (see Chapter 1) or cognitive impairment and dementia. Some disorders of amino acid metabolism cause cerebral malformations, such as agenesis of the corpus callosum. Although the main clinical features of aminoaciduria are referable to gray matter dysfunction (cognitive impairment and seizures), myelination is often profoundly delayed or defective.

Guanidinoacetate Methyl transferase (GAMT) Deficiency

Amidinotransferase converts glycine to guanidoacetate and GAMT converts guanidoacetate to creatine. GAMT deficiency causes cognitive impairment, hypotonia, and a movement disorder (Caldeira et al, 2005). Transmission is by autosomal recessive inheritance. Gene map locus is 19p13.3. This disorder is rare but treatable.

Clinical Features. Affected children appear normal at birth and may develop normally during infancy. By the end of the first year, development fails to progress and hypotonia is noted. Regression of development follows and is associated with dyskinesias, dystonia, and myoclonic jerks.

Diagnosis. MRI reveals marked demyelination and magnetic resonance spectroscopy shows creatine depletion and guanidinoacetate phosphate accumulation.

Management. Early oral administration of creatine monohydrate significantly prevents and reverses all symptoms and late treatment provides some reduction in abnormal movements.

Homocystinuria

The main defect responsible for the syndrome is almost complete deficiency of the enzyme cystathionine-β-synthase (Picker & Levy, 2011). Two variants are recognized: *B6-responsive homocystinuria* and *B6-nonresponsive homocystinuria.* B6-responsive homocystinuria is usually milder than the nonresponsive variant. Transmission of all forms is by autosomal recessive inheritance. Heterozygotes have partial deficiencies. Cystathionine synthase catalyzes the condensation of serine and homocysteine to form cystathionine (Figure 5-2). When the enzyme is deficient, the blood and urine concentrations of homocysteine, homocystine, and methionine are increased. Newborn screening programs detect hypermethioninemia.

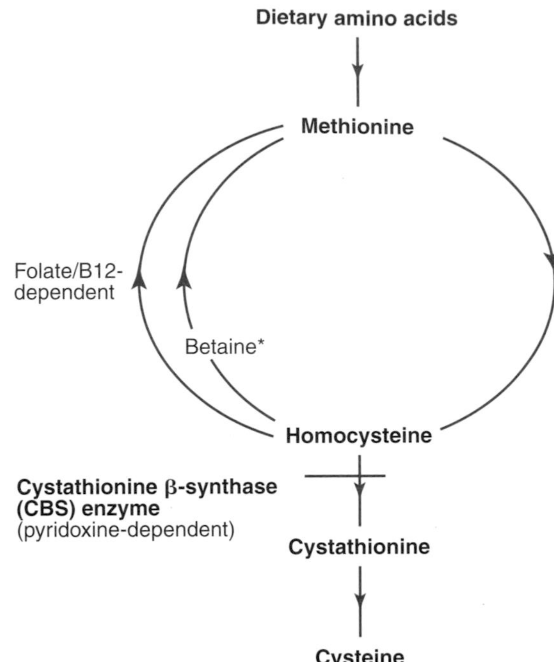

FIGURE 5-2 ■ Metabolic disturbance in homocystinuria. Absence of cystathionine β-synthase (cystathionine synthetase) blocks the metabolism of homocysteine, causing the accumulation of homocystine and methionine.

*Alternate pathway with betaine treatment.

(Modified and redrawn from Picker JD, Levy HL. Homocystinuria caused by cystathionine beta-synthase deficiency. In: Pagon RA, Bird TD, Dolan CR, et al., eds. Seattle University of Washington. Available at http://www.geneclinics.org. PMID: 20301697. Last updated April 26, 2011.)

Clinical Features. Affected individuals appear normal at birth. Neurological features include mild to moderate cognitive impairment, ectopia lentis, and cerebral thromboembolism. Developmental delay occurs in half of cases, and intelligence declines progressively with age in untreated children. Most will eventually function in the mildly cognitive impaired range. Intelligence is generally higher in B6-responsive than B6-nonresponsive homocystinuria.

High plasma homocysteine concentrations adversely affect collagen metabolism and are responsible for intimal thickening of blood vessel walls, leading to arterial and venous thromboembolic disease. Cerebral thromboembolism is a life-threatening complication. Emboli may occur in infancy, but is usually in adult life. Young adult heterozygotes are also at risk. Occlusion of the coronary or carotid arteries can lead to sudden death or severe neurological handicap. Thromboembolism is the first clue to the diagnosis in 15 % of cases.

Dislocation of the lens, an almost constant feature of homocystinuria, typically occurs between 2 and 10 years of age. Almost all patients have lens dislocation by age 40 years. Older children have osteoporosis, often first affecting the spine resulting in scoliosis. Many children are tall and thin, with blond, sparse, brittle hair and a Marfan syndrome habitus. This habitus does not develop until middle or late childhood and serves as a clue to the diagnosis in fewer than 40 % of cases.

The diagnosis is suspect in any infant with isolated and unexplained developmental delay, since disease-specific features may not appear until later childhood. The presence of either thromboembolism or lens dislocation strongly suggests homocystinuria.

Diagnosis. The biochemical features of homocystinuria are increased concentrations of plasma homocystine, total homocysteine, and methionine; increased concentration of urine homocystine; and reduced cystathionine β-synthase enzyme activity. Molecular genetic diagnosis is available.

Prenatal diagnosis is available for fetuses at risk by measurement of cystathionine β-synthase enzyme activity assayed in cultured amniocytes but not in chorionic villi, since this tissue has very low activity of the enzyme

Management. Challenge all patients with pyridoxine (vitamin B6) before starting treatment. Treat those who are responsive with pyridoxine, approximately 200 mg/day. Those that are not responsive still receive doses of 100–200 mg daily. All patients also require a protein-restricted diet, but B6-nonresponsive neonates also require frequent metabolic monitoring. Continue the diet indefinitely. Identification of disease in newborn screening yields the best results. Treatment with betaine, 5–10 g/day in two divided doses, provides an alternate remethylation pathway to convert excess homocysteine to methionine and may help prevent thrombosis. Folate and vitamin B12 optimize the conversion of homocysteine to methionine and help to decrease homocysteine levels.

Maple Syrup Urine Disease (Intermediate)

The three major branched-chain amino acids (BCAA) are leucine, isoleucine, and valine. In the course of their metabolism, they are first transaminated to α-ketoacids and then further catabolized by oxidative decarboxylation (see Figure 1-1). Branched-chain ketoacid (BCKA) dehydrogenase is the enzyme responsible for oxidative decarboxylation. Mutations in three different genes cause maple syrup urine disease (MSUD). These genes encode the catalytic components of the branched-chain alpha-keto acid dehydrogenase complex (BCKD), which catalyzes the catabolism of the branched-chain amino acids, leucine, isoleucine, and valine.

Clinical Features. Deficiency is associated with several different phenotypes (Strauss et al, 2009). Three recognized clinical phenotypes are *classic*, *intermittent*, and *intermediate*. An acute encephalopathy with ketoacidosis characterizes the classic and intermittent forms (see Chapters 1 and 10). The levels of dehydrogenase enzyme activity in the intermediate and intermittent forms are approximately the same (5–40 %), whereas activity in the classic form is 0–2 % of normal.

The onset of the intermediate form is late in infancy, often in association with a febrile illness or a large protein intake. In the absence of vigorous early therapeutic intervention, moderate cognitive impairment results. Ataxia and failure to thrive are common. Infants with intermediate MSUD are slow in achieving milestones and hyperactive. As children, they generally function in the moderately cognitively impaired range of intelligence. Physical development is normal except for coarse, brittle hair. The urine may have the odor of maple syrup. Acute mental changes, seizures, and focal neurological deficits do not occur.

Some infants with the intermediate form are thiamine responsive. In such children, cognitive impairment is moderate.

Diagnosis. BCAA and BCKA concentrations are elevated, though not as high as in the classic disease. A presumptive diagnosis requires the demonstration of BCAA in the urine by a ferric chloride test or the 2,4-dinitrophenylhydrazine test. Quantitative measurement of blood and urine BCAA and BCKA is diagnostic.

Treatment. Treatment of MSUD includes dietary leucine restriction, high-calorie BCAA-free formulas, and frequent monitoring. Correct metabolic decompensation by treating the precipitating stress and delivering sufficient calories, insulin, free amino acids, isoleucine,

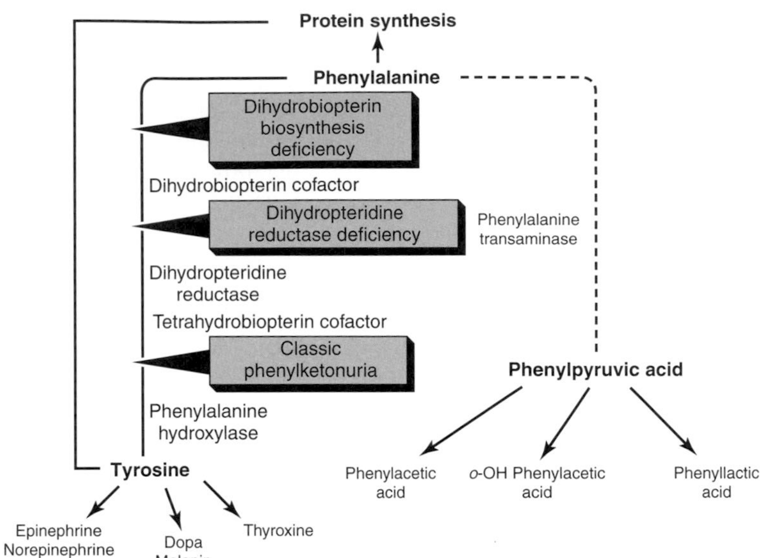

FIGURE 5-3 ■ Phenylalanine metabolism. 1. Phenylalanine hydroxylase. 2. Dihydropteridine reductase. 3. Tetrahydrobiopterin. 4. Phenylalanine transaminase. 5. Tyrosine transaminase. (Reproduced with permission from Swaiman KF. Aminoacidopathies and organic acidemias resulting from deficiency of enzyme activity and transport abnormalities. In: Swaiman KF, Ashwal S, eds. *Pediatric Neurology*, 3rd ed, vol 1. St Louis: Mosby; 1999.)

and valine, and, in some centers, hemodialysis/hemofiltration, to establish net positive protein accretion.

A protein-restricted diet is the main treatment of infants with intermediate MSUD. In addition, a trial of thiamine, 100 mg/day, tests if the biochemical error is thiamine responsive. If 100 mg is not effective, try daily dosages up to 1 g of thiamine before designating the condition as thiamine refractory. Brain edema, a common potential complication of metabolic decompensation, requires immediate therapy in an intensive care setting.

Orthotopic liver transplantation is an effective therapy for classic MSUD. Frequent monitoring of plasma amino acid concentrations and fetal growth is necessary to avoid essential amino acid deficiencies during pregnancy.

Phenylketonuria

Phenylketonuria is a disorder of phenylalanine metabolism caused by partial or total deficiency of the hepatic enzyme phenylalanine hydroxylase (PAH) (Mitchell & Scriver, 2010). Genetic transmission is autosomal recessive and occurrence is approximately 1 per 16 000 live births. Failure to hydroxylate phenylalanine to tyrosine leads to further metabolism by transamination to phenylpyruvic acid (Figure 5-3). Oxidation of phenylpyruvic acid to phenylacetic acid causes a musty odor in the urine.

The completeness of deficiency produces three categories of PAH deficiency; these are classic phenylketonuria (PKU), non-PKU hyperphenylalaninemia (HPA), and variant PKU. In *classic PKU*, PAH deficiency is complete or near complete. Affected children tolerate less than 250–350 mg of dietary phenylalanine per day to keep plasma phenylalanine concentration below a safe level of 300 µmol/L (5 mg/dL). If untreated, plasma phenylalanine concentrations are greater than 1000 µmol/L and dietary phenylalanine tolerance is less than 500 mg/day. Classic PKU has a high risk of severely impaired cognitive development.

Children with *non-PKU hyperphenylalaninemia* have plasma phenylalanine concentrations between 120 µmol/L and 1000 µmol/L on a normal diet and a lower risk of impaired cognitive development without treatment. *Variant PKU* includes individuals who do not fit the description for either PKU or non-PKU HPA.

HPA may also result from the impaired synthesis or recycling of tetrahydrobiopterin (BH4). BH4 is the cofactor in the phenylalanine, tyrosine, and tryptophan hydroxylation reactions. Inheritance of HPA caused by BH4 deficiency is as an autosomal recessive trait and accounts for 2 % of patients with HPA.

Clinical Features. Because affected children are normal at birth, early diagnosis requires compulsory mass screening. The screening test detects HPA, which is not synonymous with PKU (Box 5-6). Blood phenylalanine and tyrosine concentrations must be precisely determined in every newborn detected by the screening test in order to differentiate classic PKU from other conditions. In newborns with classic PKU, HPA develops 48 to 72 hours after initiation of milk feeding. Blood phenylalanine concentrations are 20 mg/dL or greater, and serum tyrosine levels are less than 5 mg/dL. When blood phenylalanine concentrations

BOX 5-6 Differential Diagnosis of Hyperphenylalaninemia

CLASSIC PHENYLKETONURIA

Complete hydroxylase deficiency (0–6 %)

BENIGN VARIANTS

Other
Partial hydroxylase deficiency (6–30 %)
Phenylalanine transaminase deficiency
Transitory hydroxylase deficiency

MALIGNANT VARIANTS

Dihydropteridine reductase deficiency
Tetrahydrobiopterin synthesis deficiency

TYROSINEMIA

Transitory tyrosinemia
Tyrosinosis

LIVER DISEASE

Galactose-l-phosphate uridylyl transferase deficiency

reach 15 mg/dL, phenylalanine spills over into the urine and the addition of ferric chloride solution (5–10 drops of FeCl to 1 mL of urine) produces a green color.

During the first months, the skin may have a musty odor because of phenylacetic acid in the sweat. Developmental delay is sometimes obvious by the third month and always before the end of the first year. By the beginning of the second year, developmental regression is evident. Behavioral disturbances characterized by hyperactivity and aggressiveness are common; focal neurological deficits are unusual. Approximately 25 % of affected infants have seizures. Some have infantile spasms and hypsarrhythmia; others have tonic-clonic seizures. Infants with phenylketonuria frequently have blond hair, pale skin, and blue eyes owing to diminished pigment production. Eczema is common. These skin changes are the only non-neurological features of phenylketonuria.

Diagnosis. Newborn screening detects all cases of PKU. The screening test detects the presence of HPA. Plasma phenylalanine concentrations above 1000 µmol/L in the untreated state are diagnostic. The use of molecular genetic testing is primarily for genetic counseling and prenatal testing. Blood phenylalanine levels less than 25 mg/dL and a normal concentration of tyrosine characterize benign variants of phenylketonuria. Disturbances in tetrahydrobiopterin underlie the malignant forms of phenylketonuria. Seizures are the initial symptom and cognitive impairment and motor deficits come later. Progressive calcification of the basal ganglia occurs in untreated children.

Transitory tyrosinemia occurs in 2 % of full-term newborns and in 25 % of premature newborns. The cause is a transitory deficiency of the enzyme *p*-hydroxyphenylpyruvic acid. It is a benign condition and can be distinguished from PKU because the blood concentrations of both tyrosine and phenylalanine are elevated.

Management. In classic PKU, initiate a low-protein diet and use of a phenylalanine-free medical formula as soon as possible after birth to achieve plasma phenylalanine concentrations of 120–360 µmol/L (2–6 mg/dL) or 40–240 µmol/L (1–4 mg/dL). Dietary supplementation with 6*R*-BH4 stereoisomer in doses up to 20 mg/kg daily depends on individual needs. Treatment of infants with non-PKU HPA with plasma phenylalanine concentrations consistently less than 600 µmol/L is uncertain.

BH4 is a cofactor for phenylalanine hydroxylase, tyrosine hydroxylase, and tryptophan hydroxylase. Defective recycling or synthesis causes deficiency. In infants with cofactor deficiency, a phenylalanine-restricted diet reduces the blood phenylalanine concentration but does not prevent neurological deterioration. For these children, BH4 administration is the therapy of choice.

Disorders of Lysosomal Enzymes

Lysosomes are cytoplasmic vesicles containing hydrolytic enzymes that degrade the products of cellular catabolism. The causes of lysosomal enzyme disorders are impaired enzyme synthesis, abnormal enzyme targeting, or a defective accessory factor needed for enzymatic processing. When lysosomal enzymes are impaired, abnormal storage of materials occurs, causing cell injury and death. One or several organs may be affected, and the clinical features depend on the organ(s) involved. Cognitive impairment and regression are features of many lysosomal enzyme storage diseases. In some diseases, such as acid lipase deficiency (Wolman disease) and ceramide deficiency (Farber lipogranulomatosis), cognitive impairment occurs, but is neither a prominent nor an initial feature. These disorders are not included for discussion

Gaucher Disease Type II (Glucosylceramine Lipidosis)

Transmission of Gaucher disease is by autosomal recessive inheritance. The abnormal gene is located on chromosome 1q21. Deficiency of the enzyme glucocerebrosidase (glucosylceramide β-glucosidase) causes the lysosomal storage of glucocerebrosides. Deficiency of saposin C, an enzymatic cofactor, is a rare cause.

While Gaucher disease encompasses a continuum of clinical findings, the identification of five clinical subtypes is useful in determining prognosis and management (Pastores et al, 2011). Type I is a perinatal lethal form that does not affect the brain. Age at onset distinguishes types II and III. Neurovisceral storage characterizes both types. Type II has onset before age 2 years, limited psychomotor development, and a rapidly progressive course with death by age 2 to 4 years. Type III begins after age 2 years and has a more slowly progressive course with longer survival. The other two types include a perinatal-lethal form and a cardiovascular form.

Clinical Features. Symptom onset in infants with Gaucher disease type II is usually before 6 months of age and frequently before 3 months of age. The initial features are motor regression and cranial nerve dysfunction. Children are first hypotonic and then spastic. Head retraction, an early and characteristic sign, probably is due to meningeal irritation. Difficulties in sucking and swallowing, trismus, and oculomotor palsies are typical. Mental deterioration is rapid, but seizures are uncommon. Splenomegaly is more prominent than hepatomegaly, and jaundice is not expected. Hypersplenism results in anemia, thrombocytopenia, and leukopenia. Death usually occurs during the first year and always by the second.

Diagnosis. Assay of acid β-glucosylceramidase enzyme activity in peripheral blood leukocytes or other nucleated cells is reliable for diagnosis. Glucosylceramidase enzyme activity in peripheral blood leukocytes is 0–15 % of normal. Carrier detection and prenatal diagnosis are available.

Management. Symptomatic treatment for Gaucher disease includes partial or total splenectomy for massive splenomegaly and thrombocytopenia, transfusion of blood for severe anemia and bleeding, analgesics for bone pain, joint replacement surgery for relief from chronic pain and restoration of function, and supplemental treatment such as oral bisphosphonates for severe osteopenia.

Patients with type III disease may benefit from bone marrow transplantation to correct the metabolic defect. Enzyme replacement therapy, using imiglucerase, is effective in reversing the hematological and liver/spleen involvement.

Globoid Cell Leukodystrophy (Krabbe Disease)

Krabbe disease (galactosylceramide lipidosis) is a rapidly progressive demyelinating disorder of infants caused by deficient activity of the enzyme galactosylceramide β-galactosidase (Wenger, 2011). A juvenile and an adult form of the disease also occur. Transmission is by autosomal recessive inheritance, and the gene maps to chromosome 14. Galactosylceramide is stored within multinucleated macrophages of the white matter of the CNS, forming globoid cells.

Clinical Features. The median age of onset is 4 months, with a range of 1 to 7 months. Initial symptoms are irritability and hyper-reactivity to stimuli. Progressive hypertonicity in the skeletal muscles follows. Unexplained low-grade fever is common. Psychomotor development arrests and then regresses. Within 2 to 4 months, the infant is in a permanent position of opisthotonos and all previously achieved milestones are lost. Tendon reflexes become hypoactive and disappear. Startle myoclonus and seizures develop. Blindness occurs, and before 1 year 90 % of these infants are either dead or in a chronic vegetative state.

Several variant forms of globoid leukodystrophy with different clinical features exist: infantile spasm syndrome (see Chapter 1), focal neurological deficits (see Chapters 10 and 11), and polyneuropathy (see Chapter 7). Discussion of the juvenile form is later in this chapter.

Diagnosis. MRI shows diffuse demyelination of the cerebral hemispheres (see Figure 5-1). Motor nerve conduction velocity of peripheral nerves is usually prolonged, and the protein content of CSF elevated. Deficient activity of galactosylceramide β-galactosidase in leukocytes or cultured fibroblasts establishes the diagnosis. The use of molecular genetic testing is only for carrier detection.

Management. Hematopoietic stem cell transplantation slows the course of disease in children with infantile-onset Krabbe disease diagnosed before symptom onset. Neurological manifestations may reverse.

Glycoprotein Degradation Disorders

Glycoproteins are complex molecules composed of oligosaccharides attached to protein. Disorders of glycoprotein degradation are uncommon and resemble mild forms of mucopolysaccharidoses. Genetic transmission is autosomal recessive. The main forms are deficiency of the enzyme α-mannosidase coded on chromosome 19cen-q12 and deficiency of the lysosomal enzyme α-fucosidase coded on chromosome 1q34.

Clinical Features. The clinical features are either a Hurler phenotype (Box 5-7) or a myoclonus-dementia complex. Some patients have macular degeneration (cherry-red spot).

BOX 5-7 The Hurler Phenotype

Abdominal hernia
Coarse facial features
Corneal opacity
Deafness
Dysostosis multiplex
Cognitive impairment
Stiff joints
Visceromegaly

Angiokeratoma can be present. These disorders are indistinguishable from other lysosomal storage diseases by clinical features alone.

Diagnosis. The urine shows excessive excretion of oligosaccharides or glycoasparagines but not mucopolysaccharides. Biopsy of the skin and other tissues shows membrane-bound vacuoles containing amorphous material. Tissue concentrations of glycoproteins, and often glycolipids, are increased.

Management. Treatment is supportive.

GM_1 Gangliosidosis

Deficiency of the lysosomal enzyme β-galactosidase causes GM_1 gangliosidosis. The amount and type of residual activity determine whether the phenotype is a generalized gangliosidosis, as in GM_1 gangliosidosis, or visceral storage of mucopolysaccharides with little brain disease, as in Morquio B disease. The β-galactosidase gene is located on chromosome 3p21 and disease transmission is autosomal.

Clinical Features. The onset is between 6 and 18 months. Weakness and incoordination are early features. Spasticity, cognitive impairment, and seizures follow. Psychomotor development is first slow and then regresses. Affected newborns are poorly responsive, hypotonic, and hypoactive. The Hurler phenotype is present (see Box 5-7), except that the cornea is clear and a cherry-red spot of the macula is present in 50% of patients (Box 5-8). Death occurs between the ages of 3 and 7 years.

Diagnosis. The absence of mucopolysacchariduria and the presence of a cherry-red spot distinguish infantile GM_1 gangliosidosis from Hurler syndrome. Showing enzyme deficiency in leukocytes, cultured fibroblasts, or serum establishes the diagnosis.

Management. Treatment is supportive.

GM_2 Gangliosidosis

These are a group of related disorders in which GM_2 gangliosides are stored because of deficiency of hexosaminidase A, hexosaminidase B, or the GM_2 activator of hexosaminidase A or B. The abnormal gene, transmitted by autosomal recessive inheritance, may be a mutation in the gene for the α-subunit on chromosome 15, the β-subunit on chromosome 5, or the glycoprotein activator for hexosaminidase (AB variant) on chromosome 5.

BOX 5-8 Lysosomal Enzyme Disorders with a Cherry-Red Spot

Cherry-red spot myoclonus (see Chapter 1)
Farber lipogranulomatosis
GM_1 gangliosidosis
GM_2 gangliosidosis
Metachromatic leukodystrophy
Niemann-Pick disease
Sialidosis type III

Sandhoff Disease. In Sandhoff disease, both hexosaminidase A and B are severely deficient. Disease transmission is by autosomal recessive inheritance. Globosides and GM_2 gangliosides accumulate in brain and viscera.

Clinical Features. The clinical features and course of Sandhoff disease are identical with those of Tay-Sachs disease. The only difference is that organs other than the CNS are sometimes involved. Moderate hepatosplenomegaly may be present, and occasionally patients have bony deformities similar to those of infantile GM_1 gangliosidosis.

Diagnosis. Suspect the disease in every non-Jewish infant with a Tay-Sachs phenotype. Peripheral lymphocytes are not vacuolated, but foamy histiocytes may be present in the bone marrow. Hexosaminidase deficiency in leukocytes, cultured fibroblasts, or serum establishes the diagnosis in patients and carriers. Prenatal diagnosis is available by the detection of *N*-acetylglucosaminyl oligosaccharides in amniotic fluid.

Management. Treatment is supportive.

Tay-Sachs Disease. Hexosaminidase A deficiency causes a group of neurodegenerative disorders caused by intralysosomal storage of the specific glycosphingolipid GM_2 ganglioside. Complete deficiency of hexosaminidase A causes Tay-Sachs disease (*infantile GM_2 gangliosidosis*). The gene frequency is 1:30 in Ashkenazi Jews and 1:300 in gentiles. The CNS is the only affected organ. Partial deficiencies of hexosaminidase A cause the juvenile and adult forms of GM_2 gangliosidosis (Kaback & Desnick, 2011).

Clinical Features. The typical initial symptom, between 3 and 6 months of age, is an abnormal startle reaction (Moro reflex) to noise or light. Motor regression begins between 4 and 6 months of age. The infant comes to medical attention because of either delayed achievement of motor milestones or loss of milestones previously attained. A cherry-red spot of the macula is present in almost every patient but is not specific for Tay-Sachs disease, because it also is present in several storage diseases and in central retinal artery occlusion (see Box 5-8). The cherry-red spot develops as retinal ganglion cells in the parafoveal region accumulate stored material, swell, and burst. The red color of the normal fundus is then enhanced. Optic atrophy and blindness follow.

By 1 year of age, the infant is severely cognitively impaired, unresponsive, and spastic. During the second year, the head enlarges and seizures develop. Most children die by 5 years of age.

Diagnosis. Suspect the diagnosis in any Jewish child with psychomotor retardation and a cherry-red spot of the macula. The diagnosis of hexosaminidase A deficiency relies upon the demonstration of absent to near-absent β-hexosaminidase A enzymatic activity in the serum or white blood cells of a symptomatic child in the presence of normal or elevated activity of the β-hexosaminidase B isoenzyme. Mutation analysis identifies the carrier state.

Management. Treatment is supportive.

I-Cell Disease

Deficiency or dysfunction of the enzyme *N*-acetylglucosamine phosphotransferase causes I-cell disease (mucolipidosis II). Lysosomal storage of several mucolipids occurs. Transmission is by autosomal recessive inheritance. The gene maps to chromosome 4q21-23.

Clinical Features. I-cell disease resembles Hurler syndrome except that symptoms appear earlier, the neurological deterioration is more rapid, and mucopolysacchariduria is not present. Affected newborns are small for gestational age and may have hyperplastic gums. Coarsening of facial features and limitation of joint movements occur within the first months. The complete Hurler phenotype is present within the first year, except that corneal opacification is not always present. Gingival hypertrophy is quite striking. Death from congestive heart failure usually occurs before age 5.

Diagnosis. Consider I-cell disease in infants with the Hurler phenotype and negative screening for mucopolysacchariduria. Showing a specific pattern of lysosomal enzyme deficiency in fibroblasts establishes the diagnosis.

Management. Treatment is supportive.

Mucopolysaccharidoses

Deficiency of the lysosomal enzymes responsible for catalyzing the degradation of glycosaminoglycans (mucopolysaccharides) causes the mucopolysaccharidoses (MPS). Mucopolysaccharides are a normal component of cornea, cartilage, bone, connective tissue, and the reticuloendothelial system. Excessive storage may occur in all these tissues. Transmission of all MPS except type II is by autosomal recessive inheritance. Type II is an X-linked trait.

Mucopolysaccharidosis Type I (MPS I; Hurler Syndrome). Absence of the lysosomal hydrolase α-L-iduronidase causes the Hurler syndrome. The gene maps to chromosome 4p16.3. Dermatan sulfate and heparan sulfate cannot be fully degraded and appear in the urine. Mucopolysaccharides are stored in the cornea, collagen, and leptomeninges, and gangliosides are stored in cortical neurons (Clarke, 2011).

Clinical Features. MPS I is a progressive multisystem disorder with mild to severe features. The traditional classification of *Hurler* syndrome, *Hurler-Scheie* syndrome, or *Scheie* syndrome is now discarded in favor of the terms *severe MPS I* or *attenuated MPS I.* Individuals with MPS I appear normal at birth. Coarsening of the facial features occurs within the first 2 years. Progressive skeletal dysplasia (dysostosis multiplex) involving all bones occurs in all children with severe MPS I. Linear growth stops by age 3 years, hearing loss occurs, and all develop progressive and profound cognitive impairment. Death, caused by cardiorespiratory failure, usually occurs within the first 10 years of life.

The greatest variability occurs in individuals with the attenuated MPS I. Onset is usually between ages 3 and 10 years. Although psychomotor development may be normal in early childhood, individuals with attenuated MPS I may have learning disabilities. The rate of disease progression and severity ranges from death in the second to third decades to a normal life span with significant disability from progressive severe restriction in range of motion of all joints. Hearing loss and cardiac valvular disease are common.

Diagnosis. The physical and radiographic appearance suggests the diagnosis. Deficiency of the enzyme α-L-iduronidase in peripheral blood leukocytes or cultured fibroblasts establishes the diagnosis. Mutation analysis is available for prenatal diagnosis.

Management. In addition to symptomatic treatment, hematopoietic stem cell transplantation in selected children with severe MPS I can increase survival, reduce facial coarseness and hepatosplenomegaly, improve hearing, and maintain normal heart function. Enzyme replacement therapy with Aldurazyme®, licensed for treatment of the non-CNS manifestations of MPS I, improves liver size, growth, joint mobility, breathing, and sleep apnea in those with attenuated disease.

MPS III (Sanfilippo Disease). MPS III is distinct from other MPS types because only heparan sulfate is stored in viscera and appears in the urine. Gangliosides are stored in neurons. Four different, but related, enzyme deficiencies cause similar phenotypes. All are transmitted by autosomal recessive inheritance.

Clinical Features. The Hurler phenotype is not prominent, but hepatomegaly is present in two-thirds of cases. Dwarfism does not occur. The major feature is neurological deterioration characterized by delayed motor development beginning toward the end of the second year, followed by an interval of arrested mental development and progressive dementia. Hyperactivity and sleep disorders are relatively common between the ages of 2 and 4 years. Cognitive impairment in most affected children is severe by age 11 years and death occurs before age 20 years. However, considerable variability exists, and MPS III is a consideration even when the onset of cognitive regression occurs after age 5 years.

Diagnosis. Suspect the diagnosis in infants and children with progressive psychomotor regression and a screening test positive for mucopolysacchariduria. The presence of heparan sulfate, but not dermatan sulfate, in the urine is presumptive evidence of the disease. Definitive diagnosis requires the demonstration of enzyme deficiency in cultured fibroblasts.

Management. Bone marrow transplantation is an experimental therapy.

Niemann-Pick Disease Type A (Sphingomyelin Lipidosis)

The traditional classification of acid sphingomyelinase (ASM) deficiency is either neuronopathic (Niemann-Pick disease type A), with death in early childhood, or non-neuronopathic (Niemann-Pick disease type B) (McGovern & Schuchman, 2009). While intermediate forms exist, this section only deals with type A.

Clinical Features. The onset of the acute infantile form occurs in the first months of life. The features are feeding difficulty, failure to thrive, and hepatosplenomegaly. With time the liver and spleen become massive. A cherry-red spot is present in half of cases (see Box 5-8). Psychomotor regression, characterized by postural hypotonia and loss of reactivity to the environment, occurs during the first year but is often overlooked because of the child's failure to thrive. With time, emaciation, a tendency toward opisthotonos, exaggerated tendon reflexes, and blindness develop. Seizures are uncommon. Interstitial lung disease caused by storage of sphingomyelin in pulmonary macrophages results in frequent respiratory infections and, often, respiratory failure. Most children succumb before the third year.

Diagnosis. The clinical course suggests the diagnosis. Vacuolated histiocytes are present in the bone marrow and vacuolated lymphocytes in the peripheral blood. The diagnosis of ASM deficiency is established when residual ASM enzyme activity in peripheral blood lymphocytes or cultured skin fibroblasts is less than 10% of controls. *SMPD1* is the only gene associated with ASM deficiency and genetic analysis detects mutations in almost all individuals with enzymatically confirmed ASM deficiency.

Management. Treatment is supportive.

Carbohydrate-Deficient Glycoprotein Syndromes

The carbohydrate-deficient glycoprotein (CDG) syndromes are a group of genetic, multisystem diseases with major nervous system involvement (Sparks & Krasnewich, 2011). The underlying defect is abnormal glycosylation of *N*-linked oligosaccharides. Thirteen different enzymes in the *N*-linked oligosaccharide synthetic pathway are defective in individual types of CDG. Deficiency of the carbohydrate moiety of secretory glycoproteins, lysosomal enzymes, and membrane glycoproteins is characteristic of the group. They occur mainly in northern Europeans and transmission is by autosomal recessive inheritance.

Clinical Features. Affected newborns with CDG syndrome type I seem normal except for the appearance of dysmaturity. Failure to thrive, developmental delay, hypotonia, and multisystem failure occur early in infancy. Neurological deterioration follows. The main features are mental deficiency, ataxia, retinitis pigmentosa, hypotonia, and weakness. Characteristic features in childhood and adolescence are short stature, failure of sexual maturation, skeletal abnormalities, liver dysfunction, and polyneuropathy.

Children with CDG syndrome type II have a more profound mental retardation but no cerebellar ataxia or peripheral neuropathy, and those with CDG syndrome types III and IV have severe neurological impairment and seizures from birth.

Diagnosis. The diagnostic test for all types of CDG is analysis of serum transferrin glycoforms.

Management. Treatment is supportive.

Hypothyroidism

Congenital hypothyroidism secondary to thyroid dysgenesis occurs in 1 per 4000 live births. Mutations in the genes encoding thyrotropin, thyrotropin-releasing hormone, thyroid transcription factor 2, and other factors are causative. Early diagnosis and treatment are imperative to ensure a favorable outcome. Fortunately, newborn screening is universal in the United States and detects virtually all cases.

Clinical Features. Affected infants are usually asymptomatic at birth. Clinical features evolve insidiously during the first weeks postpartum, and their significance is not always appreciated. Frequently gestation lasts for more than 42 weeks, and birth weight is greater than 4 kg. Early clinical features include a wide-open fontanelle, constipation, jaundice, poor temperature control, and umbilical hernia. Macroglossia may interfere with feedings. Edema of the eyes, hands, and feet may be present at birth but is often unrecognized in early infancy.

Diagnosis. Radiographs of the long bones show delayed maturation, and radiographs of the skull show excessive numbers of wormian bones. A low serum concentration of thyroxine (T_4) and a high serum concentration of thyroid-stimulating hormone establish the diagnosis.

Management. Initial treatment with levothyroxine at doses of 10–15 μg/kg/day is indicated as soon as detected. Early treatment prevents most, if not all, of the sequelae of congenital hypothyroidism. Each month of delay reduces the ultimate intelligence of the infant.

Mitochondrial Disorders

Mitochondrial disorders involve pyruvate metabolism, the Krebs cycle, and respiratory complexes. Figure 8-2 depicts the five respiratory complexes, and Box 8-6 lists the disorders assigned to abnormalities in each of these complexes.

Mitochondrial diseases arise from dysfunction of the mitochondrial respiratory chain (Chinnery, 2010). Mutations of either nuclear or mitochondrial (mtDNA) are causative. Some mutations affect a single organ, but most involve multiple organ systems and neurological dysfunction is prominent. In general, nuclear defects present in childhood and mtDNA defects present in late childhood or adult life. Many individuals show a cluster of clinical features that fall into a discrete clinical syndrome, but considerable clinical variability exists and many individuals do not fit into one particular category. Common clinical features of mitochondrial disease include ptosis, retinitis pigmentosa, external ophthalmoplegia, myopathy, exercise intolerance, cardiomyopathy, sensorineural deafness, optic atrophy, seizures, and diabetes mellitus. Serial cranial MRI may show migrating or fluctuating white matter changes. Children tend to decompensate with glucose loads, acute illnesses or use of valproic acid (contraindicated).

Alexander Disease

Alexander disease is a rare disorder caused by a mutation in the gene encoding NADH: ubiquinone oxidoreductase flavoprotein-1 (Gorospe, 2010). Disease transmission is autosomal dominant. Most affected newborns represent new mutations. The abnormal gene maps to chromosome 17q21 and encodes glial fibrillary acidic protein (GFAP). Rosenthal fibers, the pathological hallmark of disease, are rod-shaped or round bodies that stain red with hematoxylin and eosin and black with myelin stains. They appear as small granules within the cytoplasm of astrocytes. Rosenthal fibers are scattered diffusely in the cerebral cortex and the white matter but have a predilection for the subpial, subependymal, and perivascular regions.

Clinical Features. In the past, diagnosis depended on autopsy. Expansion of the clinical features expanded with accuracy of antemortem diagnosis. Infantile, juvenile, and adult forms are recognized. The infantile form is the most common. It accounts for 70 % of cases with an identifiable GFAP mutation. The onset is any time from birth to early childhood. Affected infants show arrest and regression of psychomotor development, enlargement of the head secondary to megalencephaly, spasticity, and seizures. Megalencephaly may be the initial feature. Optic atrophy does not occur. Death by the second or third year is the rule.

Diagnosis. Four of the five following criteria establish an MRI-based diagnosis of Alexander disease: (1) extensive cerebral white matter abnormalities with a frontal preponderance; (2) a periventricular rim of decreased signal intensity on T_2-weighted images and elevated signal intensity on T_1-weighted images; (3) abnormalities of the basal ganglia and thalami; (4) brainstem abnormalities, particularly involving the medulla and midbrain; and (5) contrast enhancement of one or more of the following: ventricular lining, periventricular rim, frontal white matter, optic chiasm, fornix, basal ganglia, thalamus, dentate nucleus, brainstem (van der Knaap et al, 1995). Genetic testing confirms the diagnosis.

Management. Treatment is supportive.

Progressive Infantile Poliodystrophy (Alpers-Huttenlocher Syndrome)

The original description of Alpers disease was a progressive degeneration of cerebral gray matter, with intractable seizures, and associated with cirrhosis of the liver. It probably encompassed several disease processes with ophthalmoplegia as a prominent feature. One cause is a mutation in the nuclear gene encoding mitochondrial DNA polymerase gamma *(POLG)*. Autosomal recessive and dominant forms exist.

Clinical Features. The onset of symptoms is during either infancy or childhood. The disorder with infantile onset tends to be sporadic and characterized by early convulsions. Seizures usually manifest as progressive myoclonic epilepsy very refractory to treatment. A progressive neurological disorder follows with spasticity, myoclonus, and dementia. Status epilepticus is often the terminating development. Although clinical signs of liver disease often appear later in the course, biochemical evidence of liver disease may predate the onset of seizures. Most patients die before the age of 3 years.

Diagnosis. Postmortem examination establishes the definitive diagnosis. However, an elevated blood lactate concentration should suggest disturbed pyruvate utilization and prompt investigation of mitochondrial enzymes in liver and skeletal muscle.

Management. Treatment is supportive. Zonisamide with titration from 2 to 20 mg/kg/day targeting levels between 10 and 40 µg/mL or levetiracetam with doses from 20 to 60 mg/kg/day targeting levels around 10–40 µg/mL are the best treatments for myoclonic epilepsies. Valproic acid may be effective, but should be used with caution as mitochondrial disease is a possibility.

Subacute Necrotizing Encephalomyelopathy (Leigh Disease) and NARP

mtDNA-associated Leigh syndrome and NARP (**N**eurogenic muscle weakness, **A**taxia, and **R**etinitis **P**igmentosa) are part of a continuum of progressive neurodegenerative disorders caused by abnormalities of mitochondrial energy generation. Subacute necrotizing encephalomyelopathy (SNE) is a progressive disorder primarily affecting neurons of the brainstem, thalamus, basal ganglia, and cerebellum. Several different abnormalities in mtDNA cause SNE. Transmission is usually by autosomal recessive inheritance, but X-linked inheritance occurs as well (Thorburn & Rahman, 2011).

Clinical Features. Onset of SNE is typically between 3 and 12 months of age. Decompensation, often with lactic acidosis, occurs during an intercurrent illness. Features may include psychomotor regression with hypotonia, spasticity, movement disorders (including chorea), cerebellar ataxia, and peripheral neuropathy. Extraneurologic manifestations may include hypertrophic cardiomyopathy.

Most individuals have a progressive course with episodic deterioration interspersed with variable periods of stability during which development may be quite stable or even show some progress. Death typically occurs by 2 to 3 years of age, most often due to respiratory or cardiac failure. In undiagnosed cases, death may appear to be sudden and unexpected. Later onset of SNE, i.e., after 1 year of age, including presentation in adulthood, and slower progression occur in up to 25 % of individuals.

The features comprising NARP are neuropathy, ataxia, and pigmentary retinopathy. Onset of symptoms, particularly ataxia and learning difficulties, is often in early childhood. Episodic deterioration interrupts periods of stability, often in association with illnesses.

Diagnosis. Lactate concentrations increased in blood and/or CSF. Lactic acidemia is usually more common in postprandial samples. An oral glucose load causes blood lactate concentrations to double after 60 minutes and is more consistent in CSF samples than in blood samples. Blood concentrations of lactate and pyruvate are usually elevated and rise even higher at the time of clinical exacerbation. MRI greatly increases diagnostic accuracy. MRI features include bilateral symmetrical hyperintense signal abnormality in the brainstem (periaqueductal) and/or basal ganglia on T_2-weighted images.

Approximately 10–20 % of individuals with SNE have detectable abnormalities on molecular genetic testing.

Management. Treatment is supportive and includes use of sodium bicarbonate or sodium citrate for acidosis and antiepileptic drugs for seizures. Dystonia can be treated with benzhexol, baclofen, and tetrabenazine, or by injections of botulinum toxin.

Neurocutaneous Syndromes

Neurofibromatosis Type 1

The neurofibromatoses (NF) are divisible into a peripheral type (type 1) and a central type (type 2). Transmission of both is by autosomal dominant inheritance with considerable variation in expression. The abnormal gene for neurofibromatosis type 1 *(NF1)* is located on chromosome 17q, and its abnormal protein product is neurofibromin. Approximately 100 mutations of *NF1* have been identified in various regions of the gene. NF1 is the most common of the neurocutaneous syndromes, occurring in approximately 1 in 3000 individuals. Almost 50% of patients with NF1 are new mutations. New mutations are associated with increased paternal age.

Neurofibromatosis type 2 (NF2) is characterized by bilateral acoustic neuromas as well as other intracranial and intraspinal tumors (see Chapter 17).

Clinical Features. The clinical manifestations are highly variable (Stevenson, 2011). In mild cases, café au lait spots and subcutaneous neurofibromas are the only features. Axillary freckles are common. Macrocephaly is common.

Severely affected individuals have developmental and neoplastic disorders of the nervous system. The main CNS abnormalities are optic pathway glioma, intraspinal neurofibroma, dural ectasia, and aqueductal stenosis. Acoustic neuromas are not part of NF1. The usual cognitive defect is a learning disability, not mental retardation.

Diagnosis. Two or more of the following features are considered diagnostic: (1) six café au lait spots more than 5 mm in diameter in prepubertal individuals or more than 15 mm in postpubertal individuals; (2) two or more neurofibromas or one plexiform neurofibroma; (3) freckling in the axillary or inguinal region; (4) optic glioma; (5) two or more iris hamartomas (Lisch nodules); (6) a distinctive osseous lesion such as sphenoid dysplasia or thinning of long bones; and (7) a first-degree relative with NF1. Only about half of children with NF1 with no known family history of NF meet the above criteria for diagnosis by age 1 year, but almost all do by age 8 years.

MRI may provide additional diagnostic information (Figure 5-4). Areas of increased T_2 signal intensity are often present in the basal ganglia, cerebellum, brainstem, and subcortical white matter. The histology of these areas is not established, and they tend to disappear with age. However, the total burden of such areas correlates with intellectual impairment. DNA-based testing is available but rarely needed. MRI surveillance at regular intervals is not recommended as it is unlikely to modify the management. Yearly examinations, on the other hand, provide guidance regarding management and the need for imaging studies.

Management. Management is primarily supportive: anticonvulsant drugs for seizures, surgery for accessible tumors, and orthopedic procedures for bony deformities. Routine MRI studies to screen for optic gliomas in nonsymptomatic children are unnecessary. Surgical procedures are recommended when gliomas or fibromas are symptomatic, causing mass effect, medically intractable pain or cosmetic problems. Neuropathic pain associated with spinal neurofibromas may be treated with gabapentin 20–60 mg/kg/day or pregabalin 2–8 mg/kg/day. Pregabalin is a more effective drug that can be used twice a day. Both medications may cause increased appetite, edema, and sedation. The sedative effect, when present, may provide hypnotic benefit with larger nighttime doses.

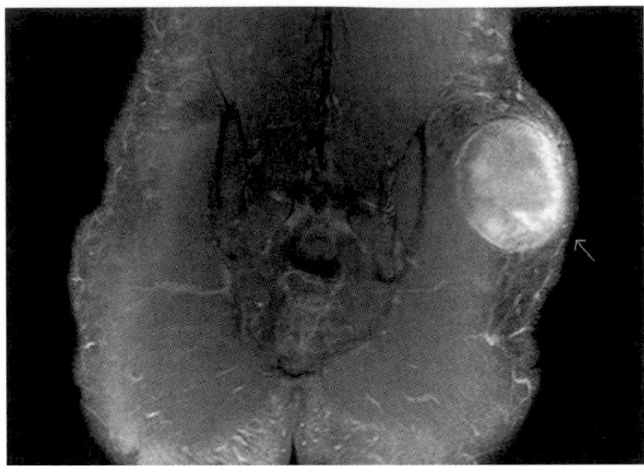

FIGURE 5-4 ■ Neurofibromatosis. Pelvic MRI shows a large single neurofibroma within the subcutaneous tissue of the left superior gluteal region with heterogeneous contrast enhancement.

Tuberous Sclerosis

Transmission of the tuberous sclerosis complex (TSC) is by autosomal dominant inheritance and has variable phenotypic expression (Northrup et al, 2011). Two genes are responsible for TSC. One gene *(TSC1)* is located at chromosome 9q34, and the other *(TSC2)* is near the gene for adult polycystic kidney disease at chromosome 16p13.3. *TSC1* is more likely than *TSC2* to account for familial cases and is generally a less severe phenotype. As a group, patients with *TSC1* were younger at seizure onset, more cognitively impaired, and had a greater tuber burden (Jansen et al, 2008).

Clinical Features. The most common initial symptom of neurological dysfunction during infancy is seizures, especially infantile spasms (see Chapter 1). Some infants have evidence of developmental delay before the onset of seizures. The delay is often insufficient to prompt medical consultation. Most children with tuberous sclerosis who have cognitive impairment eventually have seizures, and all infants with intractable seizures will later function

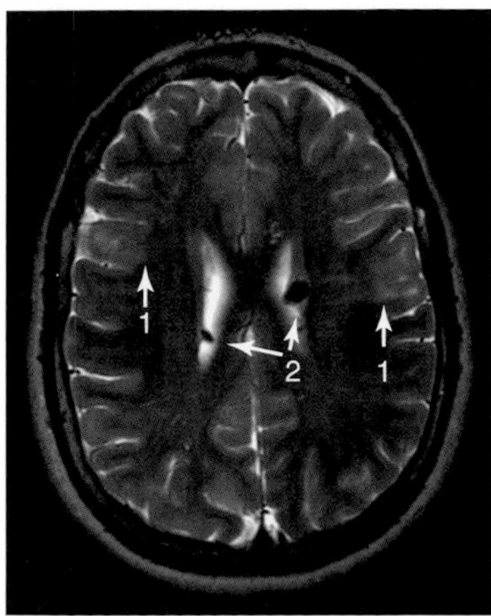

FIGURE 5-5 ■ Tuberous sclerosis. T_2 axial MRI shows (1) cortical tubers and (2) subependymal nodules.

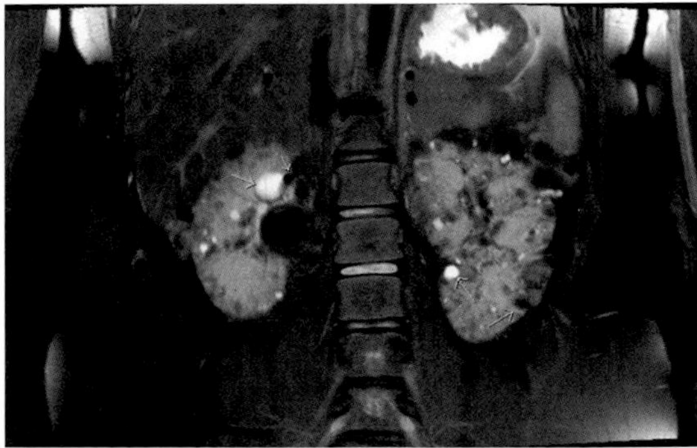

FIGURE 5-6 ■ Tuberous sclerosis. T_2 fat suppression coronal MRI of abdomen shows kidney cysts and angiomyolipomas.

in the cognitive impaired range. Seizures and cognitive impairment are due to disturbed histogenesis of the brain, which contains decreased numbers of neurons and bizarrely shaped astrocytes. Subependymal hamartomas are common and tend to calcify with age and only rarely cause obstructive hydrocephalus. Subependymal giant cell astrocytoma (SEGA) is a possible complication in these children (Figure 5-5).

Hypomelanotic macules are the most common dermatologic manifestation. In late infancy and early childhood, raised plaques of thicker skin may develop (*Shagreen patches*) and are present by 15 years in 50% of affected children. During childhood, adenomata sebaceum (actually angiokeratomas) appear on the face, usually in a butterfly distribution. Other organ involvement includes retinal tumors, rhabdomyoma of the heart, renal tumors, and cysts of the kidney, bone, and lung (Figure 5-6). Rhabdomyomas of the heart may manifest as prenatal arrhythmias and are detected by ultrasound. These lesions tend to decrease in size with time.

A shortened life expectancy results from renal disease, cardiovascular disorders, pleural involvement, brain tumors (SEGA) and status epilepticus.

Diagnosis. The NIH Consensus Development Conference (2001) diagnostic criteria for TSC have been revised (Roach & Sparagana, 2004). The revised diagnostic criteria for TSC recognize that individuals with lymphangiomyomatosis who have associated renal angiomyolipomas do not have TSC (Box 5-9). The new criteria have eliminated nonspecific features (e.g., infantile spasms and myoclonic, tonic, or atonic seizures) and have made certain features more specific (e.g., nontraumatic ungual or periungual fibroma; three or more hypomelanotic macules).

Complicating molecular genetic testing of the *TSC1* and the *TSC2* genes are the large size of the two genes, the large number of disease causing mutations, and a 10–25% rate of somatic mosaicism. However, molecular testing for both genes is available.

Management. The recommended evaluations in children with TSC are renal ultrasonography every 1 to 3 years followed by renal CT/MRI if large or numerous renal tumors are detected; cranial CT/MRI every 1 to 3 years; echocardiography if cardiac symptoms indicate the need; and chest CT if pulmonary symptoms indicate the need.

Anticonvulsant drugs are helpful in reducing seizure frequency, but when compared with other epilepsies a larger percentage of patients remain incompletely controlled. Vigabatrin is a good option for children with infantile spasms, starting at 50 mg/kg/day (divided twice a day) and increasing every 5 to 7 days up to 250 mg/kg/day or cessation of spasms and correction of hypsarrhythmia. The concern of possible retinal injury from vigabatrin and associated loss of peripheral vision should not stop its use, since hypsarrhythmia often causes cortical visual impairment and progressive decline in all functions. Transition to a different anticonvulsant should be considered after a few months of correction of hypsarrhythmia and control of infantile spasms to minimize the possibility of retinal or MRI changes.

The hamartin–tuberin complex regulates the activity of the target of rapamycin complex 1, which lies downstream of cellular pathways controlling cell growth and proliferation. Medications such as sirolimus (Rapamune®) and everolimus (Afinitor®) are known as mTOR (mammalian target of rapamycin) inhibitors and

BOX 5-9 Clinical Diagnosis of Tuberous Sclerosis

Definite TSC: Two major features or one major feature plus two minor features
Probable TSC: One major feature plus one minor feature
Possible TSC: One major feature or two or more minor features

MAJOR FEATURES

- Cardiac rhabdomyoma, single or multiple
- Cortical tuber[1]
- Facial angiofibromas or forehead plaque
- Hypomelanotic macules (three or more)
- Lymphangiomyomatosis[2]
- Multiple retinal nodular hamartomas
- Nontraumatic ungual or periungual fibromas
- Renal angiomyolipoma[2]
- Shagreen patch (connective tissue nevus)
- Subependymal nodule
- Subependymal giant cell astrocytoma

MINOR FEATURES

- Bone cysts[3]
- Cerebral white matter radial migration lines[1,3,4]
- "Confetti" skin lesions
- Gingival fibromas
- Hamartomatous rectal polyps[5]
- Multiple randomly distributed pits in dental enamel
- Multiple renal cysts[5]
- Nonrenal hamartoma[5]
- Retinal achromic patch

1. Cerebral cortical dysplasia and cerebral white matter migration tracts occurring together are counted as one rather than two features of TSC.
2. When both lymphangiomyomatosis and renal angiomyolipomas are present, other features of tuberous sclerosis must be present before TSC is diagnosed.
3. Radiographic confirmation is sufficient.
4. White matter migration lines and focal cortical dysplasia are often seen in individuals with TSC; however, because these lesions can be seen independently and are relatively nonspecific, they are considered a minor diagnostic criterion for TSC.
5. Histological confirmation is suggested.

have a positive effect controlling the growth of affected tissues in patients with tuberous sclerosis. Everolimus received an FDA indication for the treatment of SEGA. In one study everolimus therapy was associated with marked reduction in the volume of SEGA and seizure frequency and was felt to represent an alternative to neurosurgical resection (Krueger et al 2010). In another small study, oral rapamycin caused regression of SEGAs (Franz et al, 2006). Another study with sirolimus showed regression of angiomyolipomas that tended to increase in volume after the therapy was stopped. Some patients with lymphangioleiomyomatosis had improvement in spirometric measurements and gas trapping that persisted after treatment (Bissler et al, 2008). Cognitive impairment is not reversible. Genetic counseling is an important aspect of patient management. Although disease transmission is autosomal dominant, gene expression is so variable that neither parent may appear affected. One-quarter of parents without a personal or family history of tuberous sclerosis are shown to be affected by a careful history and physical examination, including fundoscopic examination, skin examination with the Wood's light, renal ultrasound, and cranial MRI. Rapamune as a compounded cream seems to decrease the size and number of facial angiofibromas.

Other Disorders of Gray Matter

Early Infantile Neuronal Ceroid Lipofuscinosis (Santavuori-Haltia Disease)

The neuronal ceroid lipofuscinoses (NCLs) are a group of inherited, lysosomal-storage disorders characterized by progressive mental and motor deterioration, seizures, and early death. Visual loss is a feature of most forms. Classification of these disorders had been by age at onset and rapidity of progression, but now by mutation analysis (Mole & Williams, 2010). The two infantile forms are infantile (INCL) and late-infantile (LINCL). INCL occurs primarily in Finnish people. The responsible mutation occurs in the palmitoyl protein thioesterase *(PPT)* gene on chromosome 1. This site has been designated NCL1.

The more common NCL types occur after age 2 years (see section on Progressive Encephalopathies with Onset after Age 2 later in this chapter) and are caused by mutations at other sites.

Clinical Features. Children with INCL are normal at birth and usually develop symptoms between 6 and 24 months of age. The initial signs include delayed development, myoclonic jerks and/or seizures, and progressive cognitive impairment.

LINCL begins between 2 and 4 years of age with seizures followed by mental decline, ataxia, spasticity, and movement disorders. Visual impairment begins between 4 and 6 years and rapidly progresses to blindness. Life expectancy ranges from age 6 to greater than 40 years of age.

Diagnosis. Molecular genetic testing is available. EEG is useful in LINCL, since photic stimulation at 1 Hz produces giant evoked potentials in the form of a spike followed by a slow wave. Otherwise the EEG shows an encephalopathic pattern with myoclonic seizures.

Management. Treatment of seizures and myoclonus is with a combination of anticonvulsant drugs (see Chapter 1). No treatment for the underlying metabolic error is available. Zonisamide and levetiracetam are the best choices in the treatment of progressive myoclonic epilepsies.

Infantile Neuroaxonal Dystrophy

Infantile neuroaxonal dystrophy (*Seitelberger disease*) is a disorder of axon terminals transmitted by autosomal recessive inheritance. Many infants with this disorder have a mutation in the *PLA2G6* gene. It shares many pathological features with Hallervorden-Spatz disease (see Chapter 14) and may be an infantile form.

Clinical Features. Affected children usually develop normally during the first year, but most children never walk. Facial dysmorphism includes prominent forehead, strabismus, small nose, wide mouth, micrognathia, and large, low-set ears (Seven et al, 2002). Motor regression occurs at the end of the first year as clumsiness and frequent falling. The infant is first hypotonic and hyporeflexic. Muscle atrophy may be present as well. At this stage, suspect a peripheral neuropathy, but motor nerve conduction velocity and the protein content of the CSF are normal.

After the initial phase of hypotonia, symptoms of cerebral degeneration become prominent. Increasing spastic quadriparesis, optic atrophy, involuntary movements, and cognitive regression are evident. By 2 years of age, most children are severely handicapped. Deterioration to a vegetative state follows, and death usually occurs by age 10 years.

Diagnosis. The CSF is usually normal. Electromyography shows a denervation pattern consistent with anterior horn cell disease. Motor nerve conduction velocities are normal. MRI shows high iron in the globus pallidus, and the diagnosis is therefore a consideration in the differential diagnosis of neurodegeneration with high brain iron (Morgan et al, 2006).

A definitive diagnosis requires evidence of neuroaxonal spheroids in peripheral nerve endings, conjunctiva, or brain. Neuroaxonal spheroids are large eosinophilic spheroids, caused by axonal swelling, throughout the gray matter. They are not unique to neuroaxonal dystrophy and are seen in pantothenate kinase deficiency (Hallervorden-Spatz disease), infantile GM_2 gangliosidosis, Niemann-Pick disease type C, and several other neurodegenerative conditions.

Management. Treatment is supportive.

Lesch-Nyhan Disease

Lesch-Nyhan disease results from deficiency of the enzyme hypoxanthine guanine phosphoribosyltransferase (Nyhan et al, 2010). The gene map locus is chromosome Xq26-q27.2.

Clinical Features. Affected newborns appear normal at birth, except for mild hypotonia. Delayed motor development and poor head control are present during the first 3 months. Progressive limb rigidity and torticollis or retrocollis follow. The progression of neurological disturbance is insidious, and cerebral palsy is often misdiagnosed. During the second year, facial grimacing, corticospinal tract dysfunction, and involuntary movements (usually chorea but sometimes athetosis) develop.

It is not until after age 2 years, and sometimes considerably later, that affected children begin biting their fingers, lips, and cheeks. Compulsive self-mutilation is characteristic, but not constant, and causes severe disfigurement. Often wrapping the hands or removing teeth is necessary to prevent further harm. In addition to self-directed aggressive behavior, aggressive behavior toward caretakers may be present. Cognitive impairment is constant but of variable severity. Intelligence is difficult to evaluate because of behavioral and motor disturbances.

Diagnosis. Uric acid concentrations in the blood and urine are elevated. Indeed, some parents note a reddish discoloration of diapers caused by uric acid. The demonstration that hypoxanthine guanine phosphoribosyltransferase activity is less than 1.5 % in erythrocytes or cultured fibroblasts establishes the diagnosis. Molecular genetic testing of *HPRT1* (chromosome Xq26-q27.2) is used for determination of status in at-risk females.

Management. Allopurinol decreases the urinary concentration of uric acid and prevents the development of nephropathy. Levodopa or tetrabenazine may abate the self-mutilatory behavior. However, no treatment is available to prevent progressive degeneration of the nervous system.

Rett Syndrome

Classic Rett syndrome occurs only in girls (Christodoulou, 2009). The estimated prevalence is 1:10 000–1:20 000. Mutations in the gene encoding methyl-CpG-binding protein-2 (MECP2), chromosome Xq28, cause the disease.

Males meeting the clinical criteria have a 47, XXY phenotype and postzygotic *MECP2* mutations. Males with a 46,XY karyotype and a *MECP2* mutation have such a severe phenotype that they do not survive.

Clinical Features. Affected girls are normal during the first year. Developmental arrest usually begins at 12 months, but may appear as early as 5 months or as late as 18 months. The initial features are deceleration of head growth leading to microcephaly, lack of interest in the environment, and hypotonia. Within a few months, rapid developmental regression occurs characterized by loss of language skills, gait ataxia, seizures, and autistic behavior. A characteristic feature of the syndrome is loss of purposeful hand movements before the age of 3 years. Stereotyped activity develops that looks like hand wringing or washing. Repetitive blows to the face are another form of stereotyped hand movement.

Following the initial rapid progression is a continued slower progression of neurological deterioration. Spastic paraparesis and quadriparesis are frequent endpoints. Dementia is usually severe. Stimulation produces an exaggerated, stereotyped reaction consisting of jerking movements of the trunk and limbs with episodes of disorganized breathing and apnea, followed by tachypnea. Seizures occur in most children before age 3 years. After the period of rapid deterioration, the disease becomes relatively stable, but dystonia may develop later. Females with Rett syndrome usually survive into early adulthood, but have an increased incidence of sudden, unexplained death.

Diagnosis. The clinical features are the initial basis for diagnosis. Confirmation by molecular genetic testing is available.

Management. Seizures often respond to standard anticonvulsant drugs. Treatment is otherwise supportive.

Trichopoliodystrophy (Menkes Syndrome) and Occipital Horn Syndrome

Characteristic of Menkes syndrome and occipital horn syndrome is low tissue concentrations of copper due to impaired intestinal copper absorption, accumulation of copper in other tissues, and reduced activity of copper-dependent enzymes such as dopamine β-hydroxylase and lysyl oxidase (Kaler, 2010). The gene defect maps to chromosome Xq13.

Clinical Features. Affected infants are healthy until 2 months of age and then show loss of developmental milestones, hypotonia, and seizures. The appearance of the scalp hair and eyebrows is almost pathognomonic. The hair is sparse, poorly pigmented, and wiry. The shafts break easily, forming short stubble (kinky hair). Radiographs of the long bones suggest osteogenesis imperfecta. Other facial abnormalities include abnormal fullness of the cheeks, a high-arched palate, and micrognathia. Temperature instability and hypoglycemia may be present in the neonatal period. Death usually occurs by 3 years of age.

Occipital horns are distinctive wedge-shaped calcifications at the sites of attachment of the trapezius muscle and the sternocleidomastoid muscle to the occipital bone. Occipital horns may be clinically palpable or observed on skull imaging. Other features of the syndrome are lax skin and joints, bladder diverticula, inguinal hernias, and vascular tortuosity. Intellect is normal or slightly reduced. Autonomic dysfunction including temperature instability and hypoglycemia may be present in the neonatal period. Death occurs by age 3 years.

Infants with occipital horn syndrome show developmental arrest and regression by age 3 months. The infant becomes lethargic and less reactive. Myoclonic seizures, provoked by stimulation, are an early and almost constant feature. By the end of the first year, the infant is in a chronic vegetative state, and most die before 18 months.

Diagnosis. Low plasma concentrations of ceruloplasmin and copper suggest the diagnosis. A protocol of mutation analysis, mutation scanning, and sequence analysis detects mutations in >95 % of patients. Such testing is clinically available. Prenatal diagnosis is possible.

Management. Subcutaneous injections of copper histidine or copper chloride before 10 days of age normalize developmental outcome in some individuals but not in others.

Other Disorders of White Matter

Aspartoacylase Deficiency (Canavan Disease)

The inheritance of Canavan disease (also called *spongy degeneration of infancy*) is autosomal recessive. Deficiency of aspartoacylase underlies the disease. Different mutations account for Jewish and non-Jewish cases, but the variability of the clinical course cannot be explained by genetic heterogeneity alone (Matalon & Michals-Matalon, 2011).

Clinical Features. Psychomotor arrest and regression occur during the first 6 months postpartum. Clinical features include decreased awareness of the environment, difficulty in feeding, irritability, and hypotonia. Eventually, spasticity replaces the initial flaccidity. A characteristic posture, with leg extension, arm flexion, and head retraction, occurs, especially when the child is stimulated. Macrocephaly is evident by 6 months of age. The head continues to enlarge throughout infancy, and this growth reaches a plateau by the third year. Optic atrophy leading to blindness evolves between 6 and 10 months. Life expectancy is the second decade.

Diagnosis. Molecular genetic testing is not commercially available. Abnormal excretion of *N*-acetylaspartic acid is detectable in the urine, and aspartoacylase activity in cultured fibroblasts is less than 40 % of normal. MRI shows diffuse symmetric leukoencephalopathy even before neurological symptoms are evident. Demyelination of peripheral nerves does not occur, and the cerebrospinal fluid is normal. Molecular diagnosis is available for the mutation in Ashkenazi Jews.

Management. Treatment is supportive.

Galactosemia: Transferase Deficiency

Three separate inborn errors of galactose metabolism produce galactosemia in the newborn, but only galactose-1-phosphate uridyltransferase (GALT) deficiency produces mental deficits. Transmission of the defect is by autosomal recessive inheritance, and the gene map locus is 9p13 (Elsas, 2010).

Clinical Features. Affected newborns appear normal, but cataracts are already developing. The first milk feeding provokes the initial symptoms. These include failure to thrive, vomiting, diarrhea, jaundice, and hepatomegaly. During this time, some newborns have clinical features of increased intracranial pressure, probably resulting from cerebral edema. The combination of a tense fontanelle and vomiting suggests a primary intracranial disturbance and can delay the diagnosis and treatment of the metabolic error.

Diagnosis. Newborn screening detects galactosemia. However, it is a consideration in any newborn with vomiting and hepatomegaly, especially when cataracts are present. The best time to test the urine for reducing substances is after feeding. Measurement of erythrocyte GALT activity and by isoelectric focusing of GALT establishes the diagnosis. Molecular genetic testing is available for carrier detection and genetic counseling.

Management. Immediate dietary intervention requires replacement of all milk and milk products with a formula that is free of bioavailable galactose. However, long-term results of treatment have been disappointing (Ridel et al, 2005); IQ is low in many cases despite early and seemingly adequate therapy. Delayed achievement of developmental milestones occurs during the first year. Intellectual function is only in the moderately impaired range by age 5 years. After age 5, truncal ataxia develops and progresses in severity. Associated with ataxia is a coarse resting tremor of the limbs. Because of the restricted diet, cataracts and hepatomegaly are not present.

Pelizaeus-Merzbacher Disease

Pelizaeus-Merzbacher disease (PMD) is a demyelinating disorder transmitted by X-linked recessive inheritance. The gene maps to chromosome Xq22. Defective biosynthesis of a proteolipid protein (PLP1) that comprises half of the myelin sheath protein causes the disorder (Garbern et al, 2010). Mutations in the *PLP1* gene are also responsible for one form of hereditary spastic paraplegia (see Chapter 12). An infantile, a neonatal, and a transitional phenotype of Pelizaeus-Merzbacher disease exist.

Clinical Features. Disorders related to PLP1 are a continuum of neurological findings from severe CNS involvement (PMD) to spastic paraplegia. Disease characteristics are usually consistent within families. The first symptoms of the neonatal form suggest spasmus nutans (see Chapter 15). The neonate has an intermittent nodding movement of the head and pendular nystagmus. Chorea or athetosis develops, psychomotor development arrests by the third month, and regression follows. Limb movements become ataxic and tone becomes spastic, first in the legs and then in the arms. Optic atrophy and seizures are late occurrences. Death occurs by 5 to 7 years of age.

The later the disease onset, the slower the progression of the disease and the more prolonged the course. Survival to adult life is relatively common.

Diagnosis. MRI shows diffuse demyelination of the hemispheres with sparing of scattered small areas. Molecular genetic testing is available for diagnosis and carrier detection.

Management. Treatment is supportive.

Progressive Cavitating Leukoencephalopathy

Progressive cavitating leukoencephalopathy describes a progressive degenerative disorder of early childhood characterized by progressive cystic degeneration of the white matter (Naidu et al, 2005). The term encompasses mutations in any of the five genes encoding subunits of the translation initiation factor.

Clinical Features. Age at onset is between 2 months and 3.5 years. The initial features are episodes of irritability or focal neurological deficits. Steady clinical deterioration follows often with spasticity and bulbar dysfunction leading to death.

Diagnosis. MRI shows a patchy leukoencephalopathy with cavity formation first affecting the corpus callosum and centrum semiovale. Later, large cystic lesions appear in the brain and spinal cord. Elevated levels of lactate in brain, blood, and CSF suggest a mitochondrial disturbance.

Management. Management is supportive.

Progressive Hydrocephalus

Clinical Features. Progressive dilatation of the ventricular system may be a consequence of congenital malformations, infectious diseases, intracranial hemorrhage, or connatal tumors. Whatever the cause, the clinical features of increasing intracranial pressure are much the same. Head circumference enlarges, the anterior fontanelle feels full, and the child becomes lethargic, has difficulty feeding, and vomits. Ataxia and a spastic gait are common.

Diagnosis. Progressive hydrocephalus is often insidious in premature newborns with intraventricular hemorrhage, especially when delayed progression follows initial arrest. Hydrocephalus is always suspect in newborns and infants with excessive head growth. Head ultrasound, CT or MRI confirm the diagnosis.

Management. Ventriculoperitoneal shunt is the usual procedure to relieve hydrocephalus in newborns and small infants with primary dilatation of the lateral ventricles (see Chapter 18).

PROGRESSIVE ENCEPHALOPATHIES WITH ONSET AFTER AGE 2

Disorders of Lysosomal Enzymes

GM_2 Gangliosidosis (Juvenile Tay-Sachs Disease)

Deficiency of *N*-acetyl-β-hexosaminidase (HEX A) underlies both the infantile and juvenile forms of Tay-Sachs disease (Kaback & Desnick, 2011). Different mutations underlie the acute and chronic forms. No ethnic predilection exists.

Clinical Features. HEX A deficiency often begins with ataxia and uncoordination between 2 and 10 years of age. Speech, life skills, and cognition decline. Spasticity and seizures are present by the end of the first decade of life. Loss of vision occurs much later than in the acute infantile form of the disease, and a cherry-red spot is not a consistent finding. Instead, optic atrophy may occur late in the course. A vegetative state with decerebrate rigidity develops by 10 to 15 years of age, followed within a few years by death, usually due to infection. In some cases, the disease pursues a particularly aggressive course, culminating in death in 2 to 4 years.

Diagnosis. Serum, leukocytes, and fibroblasts are deficient in HEX A activity.

Management. Treatment is supportive.

Gaucher Disease Type III (Glucosylceramide Lipidosis)

As in other types, the cause of late-onset Gaucher disease is deficiency of the enzyme glucocerebrosidase (Pastores et al, 2011). Transmission is by autosomal recessive inheritance.

Clinical Features. The range of age at onset is from early childhood to adult life. Hepatosplenomegaly usually precedes neurological deterioration. The most common neurological manifestations are seizures and mental regression. Mental regression varies from mild memory loss to severe dementia. Myoclonus and myoclonic seizures develop in many patients. Some combination of spasticity, ataxia, and cranial nerve dysfunction may be present as well. Vertical oculomotor apraxia, as described in Niemann-Pick disease, may occur in late-onset Gaucher disease as well.

Diagnosis. Gaucher cells are present in the bone marrow and are virtually diagnostic. Confirmation requires the demonstration of deficient glucocerebrosidase activity in hepatocytes or leukocytes.

Management. Patients with chronic neurological involvement benefit from bone marrow transplant. Transplantation corrects the metabolic defect, improves blood counts, and reduces increased liver volume. However, the associated morbidity and mortality limits its usefulness. Enzyme replacement therapy utilizes imiglucerase (Cerezyme®), a recombinant glucosylceramidase enzyme preparation. Regular intravenous infusions of imiglucerase are safe and effective in reversing hematological and visceral involvement, but not neurological disease.

Globoid Cell Leukodystrophy (Late-Onset Krabbe Disease)

Deficiency of the enzyme galactosylceramide β-galactosidase causes globoid cell leukodystrophy

(Wenger, 2011). Transmission is by autosomal recessive inheritance. The onset of symptoms in late infancy and in adolescence can occur in the same family. The severity of the enzyme deficiency is similar in all phenotypes from early infancy to adolescence.

Clinical Features. Neurological deterioration usually begins between the ages of 2 and 6 years, but may start as early as the second year or as late as adolescence. The major features are mental regression, cortical blindness, and generalized or unilateral spasticity. The initial feature may be progressive spasticity rather than dementia. Unlike the infantile form, peripheral neuropathy is not a feature of the juvenile form, and the protein content of the CSF is normal. Progressive neurological deterioration results in a vegetative state.

Diagnosis. MRI shows diffuse demyelination of the cerebral hemispheres. Showing the enzyme deficiency in leukocytes or cultured fibroblasts establishes the diagnosis.

Management. Hematopoietic stem cell transplantation slows the course of disease in children with infantile-onset Krabbe disease diagnosed before symptom onset. Neurological manifestations may reverse. Treatment is supportive.

Metachromatic Leukodystrophy (Late-Onset Lipidosis)

Deficiency of the enzyme arylsulfatase A causes the juvenile and infantile forms of sulfatide lipidosis (Fluharty, 2011). The late-infantile metachromatic leukodystrophy (MLD) comprises 50–60 % of cases; juvenile MLD comprises about 20–30 %, and remainder have adult onset. Genetic transmission of both is autosomal recessive inheritance. Two groups of mutations in the gene encoding arylsulfatase A are identified as I and A. Patients with I mutations generate no active enzyme, and those with A mutations generate small amounts. Late-onset disease is associated with I-A genotype, and the adult form with an A-A genotype.

Clinical Features. Age of onset within a family is usually similar. All individuals eventually lose motor and intellectual functions. The disease course may be from 3 to 10 or more years in the late infantile-onset form and up to 20 years or more in the juvenile- and adult-onset forms. Death most commonly results from pneumonia or other infection.

In *late-infantile MLD*,onset is between 1 and 2 years of age. Typical presenting symptoms include clumsiness, frequent falls, toe walking, and slurred speech. Weakness and hypotonia are initially observed. Later signs include inability to stand, difficult speech, deterioration of mental function, increased muscle tone, pain in the arms and legs, generalized or partial seizures, compromised vision and hearing, and peripheral neuropathy. The final stages include tonic spasms, decerebrate posturing with rigidly extended extremities, feeding by gastrostomy tube, blindness, and general unawareness of surroundings. Expected lifespan is about 3.5 years after onset of symptoms but can be up to 10 or more years with current treatment approaches. The onset of symptoms is generally between 5 and 10 years but may be delayed until adolescence or occur as early as late infancy. The early onset juvenile form is clinically different from the infantile form despite the age overlap. No clinical symptoms of peripheral neuropathy occur, progression is slow, and the protein content of the cerebrospinal fluid is normal.

Mental regression, speech disturbances, and clumsiness of gait are the prominent initial features. The dementia usually progresses slowly over a period 3 to 5 years but sometimes progresses rapidly to a vegetative state. A delay of several years may separate the onset of dementia from the appearance of other neurological disturbances. Ataxia may be an early and prominent manifestation. A spastic quadriplegia eventually develops in all affected children, and most have seizures. Death usually occurs during the second decade.

Diagnosis. The juvenile form can overlap in age with a late-onset form, which usually manifests as psychosis or dementia. MRI shows demyelination in the cerebral hemispheres with sparing of the U-fibers (Figure 5-7). Motor nerve conduction velocities may be normal early in the course. Showing deficiency of arylsulfatase A in leukocytes or cultured fibroblasts establishes the diagnosis.

Management. Treatment is supportive.

Mucopolysaccharidoses

The MPS result from deficiencies of enzymes involved in the catabolism of dermatan sulfate, heparan sulfate, or keratin sulfate. At least seven major types of MPS are recognized. Four of these, types I, II, III, and VII, affect the nervous system and cause cognitive impairment/regression. The onset of types I and III are in infancy and discussed in the prior section. Types II and VII ordinarily have their onset in childhood following two or more years of normal development.

MPS II (Hunter Syndrome). This is the only MPS transmitted by X-linked inheritance (Scarpa, 2011). The gene maps to chromosome Xq28.

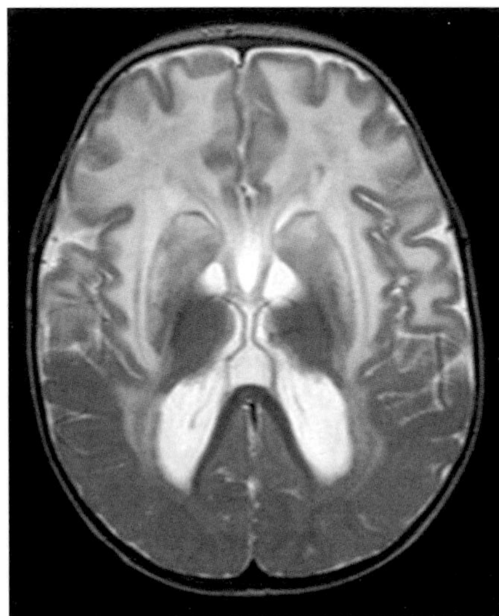

FIGURE 5-7 ■ Metachromatic leukodystrophy.

Clinical Features. Patients with the Hunter syndrome have a Hurler phenotype (see Box 5-7), but lack corneal clouding. Iduronate sulfatase is the deficient enzyme; dermatan sulfate and heparan sulfate are stored in the viscera and appear in the urine.

The Hurler phenotype may develop rapidly or evolve slowly during childhood and not be recognized until the second decade or later. A prominent feature is the appearance of a nodular, ivory-colored lesion on the back, usually around the shoulders and upper arms. Affected children have short stature, macrocephaly, with or without communicating hydrocephalus, macroglossia, hoarse voice, conductive and sensorineural hearing loss, hepatomegaly and/or splenomegaly, dysostosis multiplex, and joint contractures which include ankylosis of the temporomandibular joint, spinal stenosis, and carpal tunnel syndrome.

Mental regression caused by neuronal storage of gangliosides is slowly progressive, but many patients come to medical attention because of chronic hydrocephalus. Affected children survive into adult life. The accumulation of storage materials in collagen causes the entrapment of peripheral nerves, especially the median and ulnar nerves.

Diagnosis. The presence of mucopolysacchariduria with equal excretion of dermatan sulfate and heparan sulfate suggests the diagnosis. Establishing the diagnosis requires showing enzyme deficiency in cultured fibroblasts or serum. The detection of iduronate sulfatase activity in amniotic fluid is useful for prenatal diagnosis.

Management. Treatment is supportive.

MPS VII (Sly Disease). Sly disease is a rare disorder caused by deficiency of the enzyme β-glucuronidase. Transmission is by autosomal recessive inheritance.

Clinical Features. The patient has an incomplete Hurler phenotype, with hepatosplenomegaly, inguinal hernias, and dysostosis multiplex as the major features. Corneal clouding does not occur, and the face, although unusual, is not typical of the Hurler phenotype. Psychomotor retardation develops after age 2 years but not in all cases.

Diagnosis. Both dermatan sulfate and heparan sulfate are present in the urine, causing a screening test to be positive for mucopolysacchariduria. Specific diagnosis requires the demonstration of β-glucuronidase deficiency in leukocytes or cultured fibroblasts.

Management. Treatment is supportive.

Niemann-Pick Disease Type C (Sphingomyelin Lipidosis)

The chronic neuronopathic form of Niemann-Pick disease type C is similar to the acute infantile form except that onset is usually after age 2 years, progression is slower, and there is no specific racial predilection. The biochemical defect is deficient esterification of cholesterol. Transmission of the defect is autosomal recessive inheritance, and the gene maps to chromosome 18q11-12 (Patterson, 2008).

Clinical Features. Age at onset and predominant symptoms distinguish three phenotypes. Characteristic of the early-onset form is organomegaly and rapidly progressive hepatic dysfunction during the first year, often in the first 6 months. Developmental delay occurs during the first year, and neurological deterioration (ataxia, vertical gaze apraxia, and dementia) occurs between 1 and 3 years of age.

The delayed-onset form is more common than the other two and has the most stereotyped clinical features. Early development is normal. Cerebellar ataxia or dystonia is the initial feature (mean age, 3 years), and apraxia of vertical gaze and cognitive difficulties follow (mean age, 6 years). Oculomotor apraxia, in which the eyes move reflexively but not voluntarily, is unusual in children (see Chapter 15). Vertical gaze apraxia is particularly uncommon and always suggests Niemann-Pick disease type C. Progressive neurological degeneration is relentless. Dementia, seizures, and spasticity cause severe disability during the second decade. Organomegaly is seldom prominent early in the course.

The late-onset form begins in adolescence or adult life and is similar to the delayed-onset form except that the progression is considerably slower.

Diagnosis. Biochemical testing that demonstrates impaired cholesterol esterification and positive filipin staining in cultured fibroblasts confirms the diagnosis.

Management. Treatment is supportive. Bone marrow transplantation, combined bone marrow and liver transplantation, and cholesterol-lowering therapy are not effective.

Infectious Diseases

Infectious diseases are an uncommon cause of progressive dementia in childhood. Several fungal species may cause chronic meningitis characterized by personality change and some decline in higher intellectual function. *Cryptococcus* infection is especially notorious for its indolent course. However, the major features of these infections are fever and headache. Chronic meningitis is not a serious consideration in the differential diagnosis of isolated psychomotor regression.

In contrast, chronic viral infections, especially HIV (see the previous discussion of AIDS encephalopathy), may produce a clinical picture similar to that of many genetic disorders in which dementia is a prominent feature.

Subacute Sclerosing Panencephalitis

Subacute sclerosing panencephalitis (SSPE) is a form of chronic measles encephalitis that was once endemic in several parts of the world but has almost disappeared in countries that require routine measles immunization (Honarmand et al, 2004). In a nonimmunized population, the average age at onset is 8 years. As a rule, children with SSPE have experienced natural infection with the rubeola virus at an early age, half before age 2 years. A concomitant infection with a second virus at the time of initial exposure to measles and immunosuppression are additional risk factors for SSPE. In the United States, incidence rates were highest in rural areas, especially in the southeastern states and the Ohio River Valley.

Clinical Features. The first symptoms of disease are personality change and declining school performance. Personality change may consist of aggressive behavior or withdrawal, and parents may seek psychological rather than medical services. However, retinal examination during this early stage shows pigmentary changes in the macula. Generalized seizures, usually myoclonic, develop next. An EEG at this time shows the characteristic pattern of periodic bursts of spike-wave complexes (approximately every 5 to 7 seconds) occurring synchronously with the myoclonic jerk. We treated a 12-year-old boy with SSPE who presented with acute encephalopathy and myoclonus. His EEG showed characteristic generalized periodic discharges and the use of levetiracetam produced dramatic improvement in both myoclonus and encephalopathy and also appeared to improve the EEG pattern. We suggested that the generalized periodic discharges associated with the myoclonus contributed to the patient's encephalopathy (Becker et al, 2009). After the onset of seizures, the child shows rapid neurological deterioration characterized by spasticity, dementia, and involuntary movements. Within 1 to 6 years from the onset of symptoms, the child is in a chronic vegetative state.

Diagnosis. Suspicion of the diagnosis comes from the clinical course and an EEG characterized by periodic high amplitude sharp and slow-wave bursts associated with myoclonic jerks. Confirmation requires demonstration of an elevated antibody titer against rubeola, usually associated with elevated gamma-globulin concentrations, in the CSF. The CSF is otherwise normal. The rubeola antibody titer in blood is also markedly elevated.

A similar progressive disorder of the nervous system may occur in children who were born with rubella embryopathy (chronic rubella panencephalitis).

Management. Some patients have improved or stabilized after several 6-week treatments of intraventricular α-interferon, starting at 105 U/m^2 body surface area per day combined with oral isoprinosine, 100 mg/kg/day. Repeat courses up to six times at 2- to 6-month intervals. The use of levetiracetam may improve the myoclonus and encephalopathy (Becker et al, 2009).

Other Disorders of Gray Matter

Ceroid Lipofuscinosis

Several neurodegenerative disorders characterized by dementia and blindness are forms of ceroid lipofuscinosis (Mole & Williams, 2010). When first described, the classification relied on eponyms depending on the age at onset (Table 5-2). The common pathological feature is the accumulation of autofluorescent lipopigments, ceroid and lipofuscin within the brain, retina, and some visceral tissues. Genetic transmission of all neuronal lipofuscinoses is by autosomal recessive inheritance except for one adult form.

TABLE 5-2 **The Neuronal Ceroid Lipofuscinoses**

	Infantile (INCL)	Late Infantile (cLINCL)	Early Juvenile (JNCL)	Late Juvenile
Other names	Santavuori-Haltia disease	Jansky-Bielschowsky disease	Batten or Spielmeyer-Vogt disease	Batten or Spielmeyer-Vogt disease
Age of onset	6–12 months	2–3 years	4–10 years	8–12 years
Chromosome location	1p *(CLN1)*	11p15.5 *(CLN2)*	16p12.1 *(CLN3)*	16p12.1 *(CLN3)*

Description of the early-infantile form is in the previous section. The early and late juvenile disorders are allelic. The early infantile, late infantile, and juvenile forms map to different chromosomes.

Late Infantile Neuronal Ceroid Lipofuscinois (Jansky-Bielschowsky Disease)

Clinical Features. Visual failure begins between 2 and 3 years of age and progresses slowly. The onset of seizures and dementia is at 2 to 4 years. The seizures are myoclonic, akinetic, and tonic-clonic and are usually refractory to anticonvulsant drugs. Severe ataxia develops, owing in part to seizures and in part to motor system deterioration. Myoclonus, involuntary movements, and dementia follow. Dementia sometimes precedes the first seizure.

Ophthalmoscopic findings are abnormal before visual symptoms occur. They include attenuation of vessels, early optic atrophy, and pigmentary degeneration of the macula. The loss of motor, mental, and visual function is relentlessly progressive, and within months the child is in a chronic vegetative state. Death is usually between 10 and 15 years.

Diagnosis. The finding of diminished CLN2 protease activity in blood leads to molecular genetic testing, which accomplishes antemortem and prenatal diagnosis.

Management. Seizures are difficult to control but may respond in part to a combination of anticonvulsant drugs (see Chapter 1). No treatment is available for the underlying metabolic error.

Early Juvenile Ceroid Lipofuscinosis (Batten)

Clinical Features. Onset of visual failure is between 4 and 5 years, and the onset of seizures and dementia is between 5 and 9 years. Macular degeneration and pigmentary aggregation are present on ophthalmoscopic examination. Loss of ambulation occurs during the second decade. Myoclonus is prominent. Death occurs between 10 and 20 years.

Diagnosis. Molecular genetic testing is available.

Management. Treatment is the same as for the late infantile form.

Late Juvenile Ceroid Lipofuscinosis (Spielmeyer-Vogt Disease)

Clinical Features. The mean age at onset of the juvenile disease is 5 years, with a range from 4 to 10 years. Decreasing visual acuity is the most prominent feature. Time to blindness is shorter than in the early juvenile form. Ophthalmoscopic examination shows attenuation of retinal vessels, a patchy retinal atrophy that resembles retinitis pigmentosa, mild optic atrophy, and a granular discoloration of the macula that may have a bull's-eye appearance with a dull red spot in the center.

Declining school performance and behavioral disturbances are characteristic. Delusions and hallucinations are common. Blindness and dementia are the only symptoms for many years. Late in the course, speech becomes slurred and Parkinson-like rigidity develops. Myoclonic jerks and tonic-clonic seizures begin some years after onset but are not usually severe. Death usually occurs within 15 years of onset.

Diagnosis. Antemortem diagnosis is reasonably certain because of the characteristic retinal changes and confirmed by skin and conjunctival biopsy or by molecular genetic testing. Fingerprint bodies are present in the cytoplasm of several cell types. The electroretinogram shows depression or absence of retinal potentials early in the course. Leukocytes in the peripheral blood are frequently abnormal. Translucent vacuoles are present in lymphocytes, and azurophilic granules occur in neutrophils.

Management. Treatment is not available for the underlying metabolic defect. Seizures usually respond to standard anticonvulsant drugs.

Huntington Disease

Huntington disease (HD) is a chronic degenerative disease of the nervous system transmitted by autosomal dominant inheritance. The HD gene maps to chromosome 4p16.3 and codes a protein known as *huntingtin*. The function of huntingtin is unknown. The gene contains an expanded trinucleotide (CAG) repeat sequence. The normal number of repeats is less than 29. Adult-onset HD patients usually have more than 35 repeats, while juvenile-onset patients often have 50 or more (Warby et al, 2010).

Clinical Features. The age of onset is usually between 35 and 55 years but may be as early as 2 years. Approximately 10 % of affected children show symptoms before 20 years of age and 5 % before 14 years of age. When HD begins in childhood, the father is the affected parent in 83 % of cases and may be asymptomatic when the child is born.

The initial features are usually progressive dementia and behavioral disturbances. Declining school performance often brings the child to medical attention. Rigidity, with loss of facial expression and associative movements, is more common than choreoathetosis and hyperkinesia in early-onset cases. Cerebellar dysfunction occurs in approximately 20 % of cases and can be a major cause of disability. Ocular motor apraxia may also be present (see Chapter 15). Seizures, which are rare in adult-onset cases, are present in 50 % of affected children. The course in childhood is relentlessly progressive, and the average duration from onset to death is 8 years.

Diagnosis. Reliable molecular testing is available to determine the size of the expanded CAG repeat.

Management. Rigidity may be temporarily relieved with levodopa, bromocriptine, and amantadine. Neuroleptics are useful for behavioral control, but treatment is not available for the dementia.

Mitochondrial Encephalomyopathies

The mitochondrial encephalomyopathies are a diverse group of disorders with defects of oxidative metabolism. Descriptions of three such disorders are in the section on progressive encephalopathies of infancy. Progressive external ophthalmoplegia or myopathy is characteristic on the later-onset mitochondrial disorders. However, childhood dementia occurs in a syndrome of myoclonic epilepsy associated with ragged-red fibers in skeletal muscle. Genetic transmission is by maternal inheritance.

Myoclonic Epilepsy and Ragged-Red Fibers. Point mutations in mtDNA cause the syndrome of myoclonic epilepsy and ragged-red fibers. Ragged-red fibers usually indicate a combined defect of respiratory complexes I and IV (Sarnat & Marin-Garcia, 2005). Mutation in more than one mitochondrial gene produces the phenotype. The severity of the clinical phenotype is proportional to the amount of mutant mtDNA (DiMauro & Hirano, 2009).

Clinical Features. Clinical heterogeneity is common even among members of the same family and ranges from severe CNS dysfunction to myopathy. The four cardinal features are myoclonus, myoclonic epilepsy, ataxia, and ragged-red fiber in muscle biopsy. Onset may be anytime during childhood or up until the fourth decade. An insidious decline in school performance is often the initial feature, but generalized tonic-clonic seizures or myoclonus may be the symptoms that first prompt medical consultation. Flickering light or watching television may induce seizures. Brief myoclonic twitching develops, often induced by action (action myoclonus), which may interfere with hand movement and posture. Ataxia is a constant feature as the disease progresses, and this may be due to action myoclonus rather than cerebellar dysfunction. Some patients have hearing loss, short stature, and exercise intolerance.

Neurological deterioration is progressive and may include spasticity, sensory loss, and central hypoventilation. Clinical evidence of myopathy is not always present.

Diagnosis. Molecular genetic testing is available. The most common mutation, present in over 80 % of individuals with typical findings, is an A-to-G transition at nucleotide 8344 in the mitochondrial DNA gene *MT-TK*. Serum concentrations of pyruvate and lactate may be elevated. EEG shows slowing of the background rhythms and a photoconvulsive response. Muscle specimens of weak muscles show ragged-red fibers (see Figure 8-3) and increased punctuate lipid within myofibers. Unaffected muscles do not contain ragged red fibers.

Management. Anticonvulsant therapy may provide seizure control early in the course but often fails as the disease progresses. Avoid glucose loads. Treatment is not available for the underlying defect but coenzyme Q10 (100 mg) and L-carnitine (1000 mg) given three times a day are often used in hopes of improving mitochondrial function.

Xeroderma Pigmentosum

Xeroderma pigmentosum (XP) is a group of uncommon neurocutaneous disorders characterized by susceptibility to sun-induced skin disorders and progressive neurological deterioration

(Kraemer, 2012). Genetic transmission is autosomal recessive. Several different gene mutations have been associated with these disorders. In the United States, the most common form is termed *XPAC* and the gene maps to chromosome 9q34.

Clinical Features. A photosensitive dermatitis develops during the first year, and skin cancer may develop as well. After age 3 years, progressive psychomotor retardation and poor head growth lead to microcephaly. Sensorineural hearing loss and spinocerebellar degeneration may develop after age 7 years. Approximately one-third of patients are short in stature and some have a phenotype suggesting Cockayne syndrome, which is a separate genetic error (see Chapter 7) but also involves defective DNA repair.

Diagnosis. The typical skin rash and neurological deterioration in both the central and peripheral nervous systems suggest the diagnosis. Molecular genetic testing is available on a research basis but abnormal DNA repair is demonstrable in cultured fibroblasts.

Management. Treatment is supportive. Radiation is contraindicated.

Other Diseases of White Matter

Adrenoleukodystrophy

Adrenoleukodystrophy is a progressive demyelination of the CNS associated with adrenal cortical failure (Steinberg et al, 2012) Genetic transmission is X-linked. Affected children have an impaired ability to oxidize very-long-chain fatty acids, especially hexacosanoic acid, because of deficiency of a peroxisomal acyl coenzyme A (CoA) synthetase. Very-long-chain fatty acids accumulate in tissues and plasma. Many cases previously designated as *Schilder disease* were probably the juvenile form of adrenoleukodystrophy.

Four phenotypes may coexist in the same family. The cerebral form accounts for approximately 56% of cases and is discussed in this section; a slowly progressive adrenomyeloneuropathy accounts for 25% of cases (see Chapter 12), and the remainder have only Addison disease or are asymptomatic.

Clinical Features. The onset of the cerebral form is usually between 4 and 8 years of age. The first symptoms are usually an alteration in behavior ranging from a withdrawn state to aggressive outbursts. Poor school performance follows invariably and may lead parents to seek psychological services. Neurological deterioration is then relentlessly progressive and includes disturbances of gait and coordination, loss of vision and hearing, and ultimate deterioration to a vegetative state. Seizures are a late manifestation. The average interval from onset to a vegetative state or death is 3 years.

Diagnosis. T_2-weighted MRI shows high signal intensity in the periventricular white matter even in asymptomatic individuals. Adrenal insufficiency, as evidenced by a subnormal response to stimulation by adrenocorticotropic hormone, may be demonstrable even in asymptomatic children.

The level of very-long-chain fatty acids in plasma is elevated in males of all ages, even in those who are asymptomatic, and in 85% of female carriers. Molecular-based diagnosis is available but is used primarily for genetic counseling.

Management. Assessment of adrenal function and corticosteroid replacement therapy can be lifesaving but have no effect on nervous system involvement. Bone marrow transplantation is an option for boys and adolescents who are in the early clinical stages and have MRI evidence of brain involvement. Dietary therapy has no established benefit.

Cerebrotendinous Xanthomatosis

Cerebrotendinous xanthomatosis is a rare lipid storage disease (Federico et al, 2011).

Clinical Features. Affected infants have diarrhea. Dementia begins in early childhood but is insidious in its progression so that affected children seem mildly cognitively impaired rather than actively deteriorating. By age 15 years, cataracts are present and tendinous xanthomas begin to form. They are small at first and may go unnoticed until adult life. Progressive spasticity and ataxia develop during adolescence, and the patient becomes incapacitated in early adult life. A demyelinating neuropathy may be present as well. Speech and swallowing are impaired, and death occurs from brainstem dysfunction or myocardial infarction.

Diagnosis. The symptom complex of diarrhea, cataracts, tendon xanthomas, and progressive neurological deterioration establishes the diagnosis, but complete expression of all features occurs late in the course. The presence of cataracts or Achilles tendon xanthoma is an indication for biochemical screening. Elevated plasma concentrations of cholestanol or xanthomas establish the diagnosis. MRI shows a progressive cerebral atrophy and demyelination. Molecular genetic testing is clinically available.

Management. Long-term treatment with chenodeoxycholic acid (CDCA) normalizes bile acid synthesis, normalizes plasma and CSF concentration of cholestanol, and improves neurophysiologic findings. However, CDCA is only available in Italy. Inhibitors of HMG-CoA reductase alone or in combination with CDCA are also effective in decreasing cholestanol concentration and improving clinical signs; however, they may induce muscle damage.

REFERENCES

Becker D, Patel A, Abou-Khalil BW, et al. Successful treatment of encephalopathy and myoclonus with levetiracetam in a case of subacute sclerosing panencephalitis. Journal of Child Neurology 2009;24:763–7.

Bissler JJ, McCormack FX, Young LR, et al. Sirolimus for angiomyolipoma in tuberous sclerosis complex or lymphangioleiomyomatosis. New England Journal of Medicine 2008;358:140–51.

Bonthius DJ, Wright R, Tseng B, et al. Congenital lymphocytic choriomeningitis virus infection: Spectrum of disease. Annals of Neurology 2007;62:347–55.

Caldeira AH, Smit W, Verhoeven NM, et al. Guanidinoacetate methyltransferase deficiency identified in adults and children with mental retardation. American Journal of Medical Genetics 2005;133A:122–7.

Chinnery PF. Mitochondrial disorders. In: GeneClinics: Medical Genetics Knowledge Base [database online]. Seattle: University of Washington. Available at http://www.geneclinics.org. PMID: 20301403. Last updated September 16, 2010.

Christodoulou J. MECP2-related disorders. In: GeneClinics: Medical Genetics Knowledge Base [database online]. Seattle: University of Washington. Available at http://www.geneclinics.org. PMID: 20301670. Last updated April 2, 2009.

Clarke LA. Mucopolysaccharidoses type I. In: GeneClinics: Medical Genetics Knowledge Base [database online]. Seattle: University of Washington. Available at http://www.geneclinics.org. PMID: 20301341. Last updated July 21, 2011.

DiMauro S, Hirano M. MERRF. In: GeneClinics: Medical Genetics Knowledge Base [database online]. Seattle: University of Washington. Available at http://www.geneclinics.org. PMID: 20301693. Last updated August 18, 2009.

Elsas LJ. Galactosemia. In: GeneClinics: Medical Genetics Knowledge Base [database online]. Seattle: University of Washington. Available at http://www.geneclinics.org. PMID: 20301691. Last updated October 26, 2010.

Federico A, Dotti MT, Gallus GN. Cerebrotendinous xanthomatosis. In: Pagon RA, Bird TD, Dolan CR, et al., eds. GeneReviews™. Seattle: University of Washington. Available at http://www.geneclinics.org. PMID: 20301583. Last updated October 20, 2011.

Fluharty AL. Arylsulfatase A deficiency. In: Pagon RA, Bird TD, Dolan CR, et al., eds. GeneReviews™. Seattle: University of Washington. Available at http://www.geneclinics.org. PMID: 20301309. Last updated August 25, 2011.

Franz DN, Leonard J, Tudor C, et al. Rapamycin causes regression of astrocytomas in tuberous sclerosis complex. Annals of Neurology 2006;59:490–8.

Galli L, de Martino M, Tovo PA, et al. Predictive value of the HIV paediatric classification system for the long-term course of perinatally infected children. International Journal of Epidemiology 2000;29:573–8.

Garbern JY, Hobson GM. PLP1-related disorders. In: Pagon RA, Bird TD, Dolan CR, et al., eds. GeneReviews™. Seattle: University of Washington. Available at http://www.geneclinics.org. PMID: 20301361. Last updated March 16, 2010.

Gorospe JR. Alexander disease. In: Pagon RA, Bird TD, Dolan CR, et al., eds. GeneReviews™. Seattle: University of Washington. Available at http://www.geneclinics.org. PMID: 20301351. Last updated April 22, 2010.

Honarmand S, Glaser CA, Chow E, et al. Subacute sclerosing panencephalitis in the differential diagnosis of encephalitis. Neurology 2004;63:1489–93.

Jansen EE, Braams O, Vincken KL, et al. Overlapping neurologic and cognitive phenotypes in patients with TSC1 or TSC2 mutations. Neurology 2008;70:908–15.

Kaback MM, Desnick RJ. Hexosaminidase A deficiency. In: Pagon RA, Bird TD, Dolan CR, et al., eds. GeneReviews™. Seattle: University of Washington. Available at http://www.geneclinics.org. PMID: 20301397. Last updated August 11, 2011.

Kaler SG. ATP7A-related copper transport disorders. In: Pagon RA, Bird TD, Dolan CR, et al., eds. GeneReviews™. Seattle: University of Washington. Available at http://www.geneclinics.org. PMID: 20301586. Last updated October 14, 2010.

Kraemer KH, DiGiovanna JJ. Xeroderma pigmentosum. In: Pagon RA, Bird TD, Dolan CR, et al., eds. GeneReviews™. Seattle: University of Washington. Available at http://www.geneclinics.org. PMID: 20301571. Last updated March 15, 2012.

Krueger DA, Care MM, Holland K, et al. Everolimus for subependymal giant-cell astrocytomas in tuberous sclerosis. New England Journal of Medicine 2010;363:1801–11.

Matalon R, Michals-Matalon K. Canavan disease. In: Pagon RA, Bird TD, Dolan CR, et al., eds. GeneReviews™. Seattle: University of Washington. Available at http://www.geneclinics.org. PMID: 20301412. Last updated August 11, 2011.

McGovern MM, Schuchman EH. Acid sphingomyelinase deficiency. In: Pagon RA, Bird TD, Dolan CR, et al., eds. GeneReviews™. Seattle: University of Washington. Available at http://www.geneclinics.org. PMID: 20301544. Last updated June 25, 2009.

Mitchell JJ, Scriver CR. Phenylalanine hydroxylase deficiency. In: Pagon RA, Bird TD, Dolan CR, et al., eds. GeneReviews™. Seattle: University of Washington. Available at http://www.geneclinics.org. PMID: 20301677. Last updated May 4, 2010.

Mole SE, Williams RE. Neuronal ceroid-lipofuscinoses. In: Pagon RA, Bird TD, Dolan CR, et al., eds. GeneReviews™. Seattle: University of Washington. Available at http://www.geneclinics.org. PMID: 20301601. Last updated March 2, 2010.

Morgan NV, Westaway SK, Morton JEV, et al. PLA2G6, encoding a phospholipase A2, is mutated in neurodegenerative disorders with high brain iron. Nature Genetics 2006;38:752–4.

Naidu S, Bibat G, Lin D, et al. Progressive cavitating leukoencephalopathy: A novel childhood disease. Annals of Neurology 2005;58:929–38.

NIH Consensus Development Conference Statement. Phenylketonuria: diagnosis and management. Pediatrics 2001;108:972–82.

Northrup H, Koenig MK, Au KS. Tuberous Sclerosis Complex. In: Pagon RA, Bird TD, Dolan CR, et al., eds. GeneReviews™. Seattle: University of Washington. Available at http://www.geneclinics.org. PMID: 20301399. Last updated November 23, 2011.

Nyhan WL, O'Neill JP, Jinnah HA, et al. Lesch-Nyhan syndrome. In: Pagon RA, Bird TD, Dolan CR, et al., eds. GeneReviews™. Seattle: University of Washington. Available at http://www.geneclinics.org. PMID: 20301328. Last updated June 10, 2010.

Pastores GM, Hughes DA. Gaucher disease. In: Pagon RA, Bird TD, Dolan CR, et al., eds. GeneReviews™. Seattle: University of Washington. Available at http://www.geneclinics.org. PMID: 20301446. Last updated July 21, 2011.

Patterson M. Niemann-Pick disease type C. In: Pagon RA, Bird TD, Dolan CR, et al., eds. GeneReviews™. Seattle: University of Washington. Available at http://www.geneclinics.org. PMID: 20301473. Last updated July 22, 2008.

Picker JD, Levy HL. Homocystinuria caused by cystathionine beta-synthase deficiency. In: Pagon RA, Bird TD, Dolan CR, et al., eds. GeneReviews™. Seattle: University of Washington. Available at http://www.geneclinics.org. PMID: 20301697. Last updated April 26, 2011.

Rapin I. The autistic-spectrum disorders. New England Journal of Medicine 2002;347:302–3.

Roach ES, Sparagana SP. Diagnosis of tuberous sclerosis complex. Journal of Child Neurology 2004;19:643–9.

Ridel KR, Leslie ND, Gilbert DL. An updated review of the long-term neurological effects of galactosemia. Pediatric Neurology 2005;33:153–61.

Sarnat HB, Marin-Garcia J. Pathology of mitochondrial encephalomyopathies. Canadian Journal of Neurological Science 2005;32:152–66.

Saul RA, Tarleton JC. FMR1-related disorders. In: Pagon RA, Bird TD, Dolan CR, et al., eds. GeneReviews™. Seattle: University of Washington. Available at http://www.geneclinics.org. PMID: 20301558. Last updated April 26, 2012.

Scarpa M. Mucopolysaccharidosis type II. In: Pagon RA, Bird TD, Dolan CR, et al., eds. GeneReviews™. Seattle: University of Washington. Available at http://www.geneclinics.org. PMID: 20301451. Last updated February 22, 2011.

Schellenberg GD, Dawson G, Sung YJ, et al. Evidence for multiple loci from a genome scan of autism kindreds. Molecular Psychiatry 2006;11:1049–60.

Seven M, Ozkilic A, Yuksel A. Dysmorphic face in two siblings with infantile neuroaxonal dystrophy. Genetic Counseling 2002;13:465–73.

Shevell M, Ashwal S, Donley D, et al. Practice parameter: Evaluation of the child with global developmental delay. Report of the Quality Standards Committee of the American Academy of Neurology and the Practice Committee of the Child Neurology Society. Neurology 2003;60:367–80.

Sparks SE, Krasnewich DM. Congenital disorders of glycosylation. Overview. In: Pagon RA, Bird TD, Dolan CR, et al., eds. GeneReviews™. Seattle: University of Washington. Available at http://www.geneclinics.org. PMID: 20301507. Last updated August 11, 2011.

Steinberg SJ, Moser AB, Raymond GV. X-linked adrenoleukodystrophy. In: Pagon RA, Bird TD, Dolan CR, et al., eds. GeneReviews™. Seattle: University of Washington. Available at http://www.geneclinics.org. PMID: 20301491. Last updated April 19, 2012.

Stevenson D, Viskochil D, Mao R, et al. Legius syndrome. In: Pagon RA, Bird TD, Dolan CR, et al., eds. GeneReviews™. Seattle: University of Washington. Available at http://www.geneclinics.org. PMID: 20945555. Last updated May 12, 2011.

Strauss KA, Puffenberger EG, Morton DH. Maple syrup urine disease. In: Pagon RA, Bird TD, Dolan CR, et al., eds. GeneReviews™. Seattle: University of Washington. Available at http://www.geneclinics.org. PMID: 20301495. Last updated December 15, 2009.

Thorburn DR, Rahman S. Mitochondrial DNA-associated Leigh syndrome and NARP. In: Pagon RA, Bird TD, Dolan CR, et al., eds. GeneReviews™. Seattle: University of Washington. Available at http://www.geneclinics.org. PMID: 20301352. Last updated May 3, 2011.

van der Knaap MS, Valk J, Barth PG, et al. Leukoencephalopathy with swelling in children and adolescents: MRI patterns and differential diagnosis. Neuroradiology 1995;37:679–86.

Volkmar F, Chawarska K, Klin A. Autism in infancy and early childhood. Annual Review of Psycholology 2005;56:315–36.

Warby SC, Graham RK, Hayden MR. Huntington disease. In: Pagon RA, Bird TD, Dolan CR, et al., eds. GeneReviews™. Seattle: University of Washington. Available at http://www.geneclinics.org. PMID: 20301482. Last updated April 22, 2010.

Wenger DA. Krabbe disease. In: Pagon RA, Bird TD, Dolan CR, et al., eds. GeneReviews™. Seattle: University of Washington. Available at http://www.geneclinics.org. PMID: 20301416. Last updated March 31, 2011.

CHAPTER 6

THE HYPOTONIC INFANT

Tone is the resistance of muscle to stretch. Clinicians test two kinds of tone: phasic and postural. *Phasic tone* is a rapid contraction in response to a high-intensity stretch (deep tendon reflexes). Striking the patellar tendon briefly stretches the quadriceps muscle. The spindle apparatus, sensing the stretch, sends an impulse through the sensory nerve to the spinal cord. This information is transmitted to the alpha motor neuron, and the quadriceps muscle contracts (the *monosynaptic reflex*). *Postural tone* is the prolonged contraction of antigravity muscles in response to the low-intensity stretch of gravity. When postural tone is depressed, the trunk and limbs cannot maintain themselves against gravity and the infant appears hypotonic.

The maintenance of normal tone requires intact central and peripheral nervous systems. Not surprisingly, hypotonia is a common symptom of neurological dysfunction and occurs in diseases of the brain, spinal cord, nerves, and muscles (Box 6-1). One anterior horn cell and all the muscle fibers that it innervates make up a *motor unit*. The motor unit is the unit of force. Therefore, weakness is a symptom of all motor unit disorders. A primary disorder of the anterior horn cell body is a *neuronopathy*, a primary disorder of the axon or its myelin covering is a *neuropathy*, and a primary disorder of the muscle fiber is a *myopathy*. In infancy and childhood, cerebral disorders are far more common than motor unit disorders. The term *cerebral hypotonia* encompasses all causes of postural hypotonia caused by cerebral diseases or defects.

THE APPEARANCE OF HYPOTONIA

When lying supine, all hypotonic infants look much the same, regardless of the underlying cause or location of the abnormality within the nervous system. Spontaneous movement may be decreased, full abduction of the legs places the lateral surface of the thighs against the examining table, and the arms lie either extended at the sides of the body or flexed at the elbow with the hands beside the head. Pectus excavatum is present when the infant has long-standing weakness in the chest wall muscles. Infants who lie motionless eventually develop flattening of the occiput and loss of hair on the portion of the scalp that is in constant contact with the crib sheet. When placed in a sitting posture, the head falls forward, the shoulders droop, and the limbs hang limply.

Newborns that are hypotonic and weak in utero may be born with hip dislocation, multiple joint contractures (*arthrogryposis*), or both, due to lack of mobility. Hip dislocation is a common feature of intrauterine hypotonia. The forceful contraction of muscles pulling the femoral head into the acetabulum is a requirement of normal hip joint formation. Arthrogryposis varies in severity from isolated clubfoot, the most common manifestation, to symmetric flexion deformities of all limb joints. Joint contractures are a nonspecific consequence of intrauterine immobilization. However, among the several disorders that equally decrease fetal movement, some commonly produce arthrogryposis and others never do. Box 6-2 summarizes the differential diagnosis of arthrogryposis. As a rule, newborns with arthrogryposis who require respiratory assistance do not survive extubation unless the underlying disorder is myasthenia. The traction response, vertical suspension, and horizontal suspension further evaluate tone in infants who appear hypotonic at rest.

The Traction Response

The traction response is the most sensitive measure of postural tone and is testable in premature newborns within an incubator. Grasping the hands and pulling the infant towards a sitting position initiates the response. A normal term infant lifts the head from the surface immediately with the body (Figure 6-1). When attaining the sitting position, the head is erect in the midline for a few seconds. During traction, the examiner should feel the infant pulling back against traction and observe flexion at the elbow, knee, and ankle. The traction response is not present in premature newborns of less than 33 weeks' gestation. After 33 weeks, the

BOX 6-1 Differential Diagnosis of Infantile Hypotonia

CEREBRAL HYPOTONIA
- Benign congenital hypotonia*
- Chromosome disorders
  - Prader-Willi syndrome
  - Trisomy
- Chronic nonprogressive encephalopathy
  - Cerebral malformation
  - Perinatal distress*
  - Postnatal disorders*
- Peroxisomal disorders
  - Cerebrohepatorenal syndrome (Zellweger syndrome)
  - Neonatal adrenoleukodystrophy
- Other genetic defects
  - Familial dysautonomia
  - Oculocerebrorenal syndrome (Lowe syndrome)
- Other metabolic defects
  - Acid maltase deficiency* (see Metabolic Myopathies)
  - Infantile GM_1 gangliosidosis (see Chapter 5)
  - Pyruvate carboxylase deficiency

SPINAL CORD DISORDERS

SPINAL MUSCULAR ATROPHIES
- Acute infantile
  - Autosomal dominant
  - Autosomal recessive
  - Cytochrome c oxidase deficiency
  - X-linked
- Chronic infantile
  - Autosomal dominant
  - Autosomal recessive
  - Congenital cervical spinal muscular atrophy
  - Infantile neuronal degeneration
  - Neurogenic arthrogryposis

POLYNEUROPATHIES
- Congenital hypomyelinating neuropathy
- Giant axonal neuropathy (see Chapter 7)
- Hereditary motor-sensory neuropathies (see Chapter 7)

DISORDERS OF NEUROMUSCULAR TRANSMISSION
- Familial infantile myasthenia
- Infantile botulism
- Transitory myasthenia gravis

FIBER-TYPE DISPROPORTION MYOPATHIES
- Central core disease
- Congenital fiber-type disproportion myopathy
- Myotubular (centronuclear) myopathy
  - Acute
  - Chronic
- Nemaline (rod) myopathy
  - Autosomal dominant
  - Autosomal recessive

METABOLIC MYOPATHIES
- Acid maltase deficiency
- Cytochrome c oxidase deficiency

MUSCULAR DYSTROPHIES
- Bethlem myopathy (see Chapter 7)
- Congenital dystrophinopathy (see Chapter 7)
- Congenital muscular dystrophy
  - Merosin deficiency primary
  - Merosin deficiency secondary
  - Merosin positive
- Congenital myotonic dystrophy

*Denotes the most common conditions and the ones with disease modifying treatments

BOX 6-2 Differential Diagnosis of Arthrogryposis

- Cerebral malformations
- Cerebrohepatorenal syndrome
- Chromosomal disorders
- Fetal, nonnervous system causes
- Motor unit disorders
  - Congenital benign spinal muscular atrophy
  - Congenital cervical spinal muscular atrophy
  - Congenital fiber-type disproportion myopathy
  - Congenital hypomyelinating neuropathy
  - Congenital muscular dystrophy
  - Genetic myasthenic syndromes
  - Infantile neuronal degeneration
  - Myotonic dystrophy
  - Neurogenic arthrogryposis
  - Phosphofructokinase deficiency
  - Transitory neonatal myasthenia
- Nonfetal causes

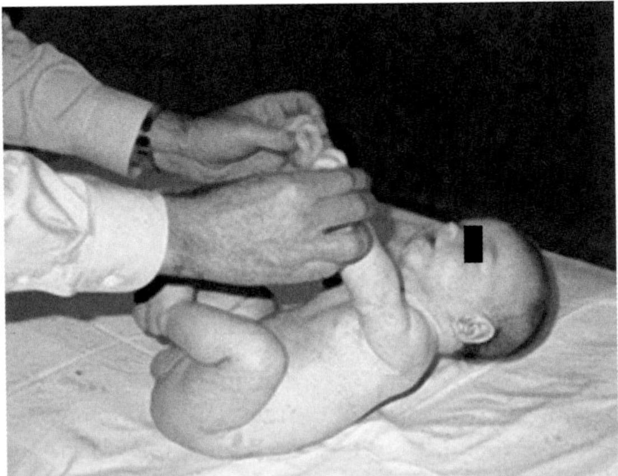

FIGURE 6-1 ■ Normal traction response. The lift of the head is almost parallel to the body and there is flexion in all limb joints. (Reprinted with permission from Fenichel GM. *Neonatal Neurology*, 4th ed. Philadelphia: Elsevier; 2007.)

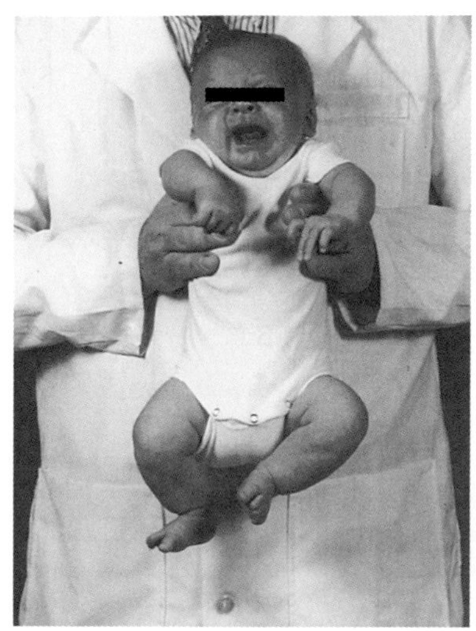

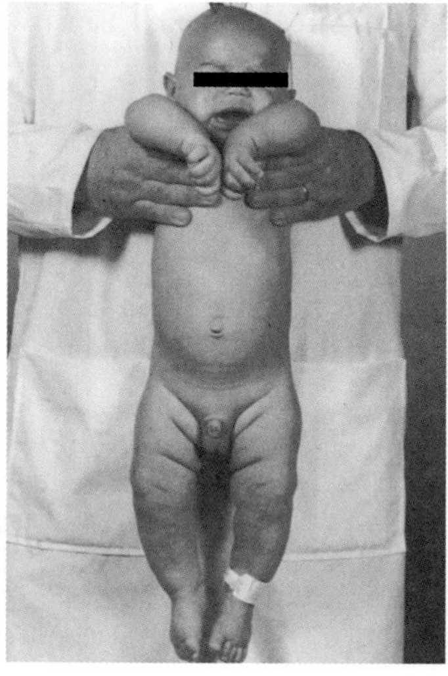

FIGURE 6-2 ■ Normal vertical suspension. The head is in the midline and the legs flex against gravity. (Reprinted with permission from Fenichel GM. *Neonatal Neurology*, 4th ed. Philadelphia: Elsevier; 2007.)

neck flexors show increasing success in lifting the head. At term, only minimal head lag is present; after attaining the sitting posture, the head may continue to lag or may erect briefly and then fall forward. The presence of more than minimal head lag and failure to counter traction by flexion of the limbs in the term newborn is abnormal and indicates weakness and hypotonia.

Vertical Suspension

To perform vertical suspension, the examiner places both hands in the infant's axillae and, without grasping the thorax, lifts straight up. The muscles of the shoulders should have sufficient strength to press down against the examiner's hands and allow the infant to suspend vertically without falling through (Figure 6-2). While in vertical suspension, the head is erect in the midline with flexion at the knee, hip, and ankle joints. When suspending a weak and hypotonic infant vertically, the head falls forward, the legs dangle, and the infant may slip through the examiner's hands because of weakness in the shoulder muscles.

Horizontal Suspension

When suspended horizontally, a normal infant keeps the head erect, maintains the back straight, and flexes the elbow, hip, knee, and ankle joints (Figure 6-3). A healthy full-term newborn makes intermittent efforts to maintain the head erect, the back straight, and the limbs flexed against gravity. Hypotonic and weak newborns and infants drape over the examiner's hands, with the head and legs hanging limply.

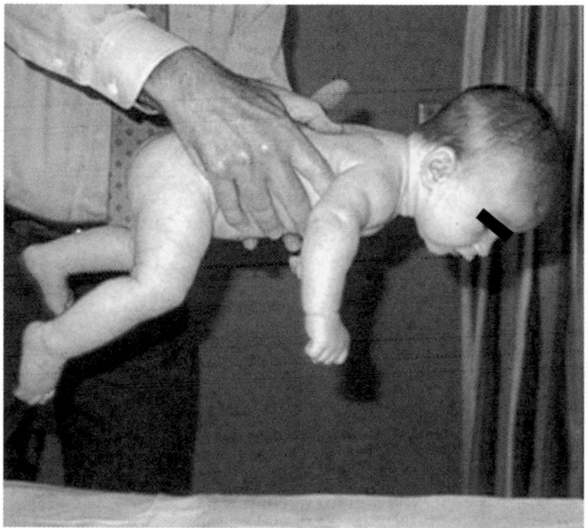

FIGURE 6-3 ■ Normal horizontal suspension. The head rises intermittently and the head and limbs resist gravity. (Reprinted with permission from Fenichel GM. *Neonatal Neurology*, 4th ed. Philadelphia: Elsevier; 2007.)

APPROACH TO DIAGNOSIS

The first step in diagnosis is to determine whether the disease location is in the brain, spine, or motor unit. More than one site may be involved (Box 6-3). The brain and the peripheral nerves are concomitantly involved in some lysosomal and mitochondrial disorders. Both brain and skeletal muscles are abnormal in infants with acid maltase deficiency and congenital myotonic dystrophy. Newborns with severe hypoxic-ischemic encephalopathy may have hypoxic injury to the spinal cord as well as the brain. Several motor unit disorders produce sufficient hypotonia at birth to impair respiration and cause perinatal asphyxia (Box 6-4). Such infants may then have cerebral hypotonia as well.

BOX 6-3 Combined Cerebral and Motor Unit Hypotonia

Acid maltase deficiency*
Familial dysautonomia
Giant axonal neuropathy
Hypoxic-ischemic encephalomyopathy
Infantile neuronal degeneration
Lipid storage diseases
Mitochondrial (respiratory chain) disorders
Neonatal myotonic dystrophy
Perinatal asphyxia secondary to motor unit disease

*Denotes the most common conditions and the ones with disease modifying treatments

BOX 6-4 Motor Unit Disorders with Perinatal Respiratory Distress

Acute infantile spinal muscular atrophy
Congenital hypomyelinating neuropathy*
Congenital myotonic dystrophy
Familial infantile myasthenia*
Neurogenic arthrogryposis
X-linked myotubular myopathy

*Denotes the most common conditions and the ones with disease modifying treatments

Newborns with spinal cord injuries are frequently the product of long, difficult deliveries in which brachial plexus injuries and hypoxic-ischemic encephalopathy are concomitant problems.

The etiology of hypotonia in neonates may be obtained in 67–85 % of newborns. Central hypotonia (60–80 %) is more common than peripheral hypotonia (15–30 %). Sixty percent of the cases are due to genetic/metabolic disease (Prasad & Prasad, 2011).

The assessment of the floppy infant should look into the following: three-generation pedigree, history of drug or teratogen exposure (alcohol, solvents, drugs), breech presentation, reduced fetal movements, history of polyhydramnios, family history of recurrent infantile deaths, parental age, consanguinity, history of neuromuscular disease, perinatal asphyxia, Apgar scores, dysmorphism, arthrogryposis, DTRs and fasciculations (Prasad & Prasad, 2011).

Testing of the hypotonic infant may include brain imaging and karyotype. Array comparative genomic hybridization (CGH) shows abnormalities in 5–17 % of floppy infants with normal karyotype. Array CGH is a very sensitive technique that may reveal variants of unclear significance (Prasad & Prasad, 2011).

Inborn errors of metabolism are divided into: (1) toxic encephalopathies due to accumulation of toxic metabolites; (2) energy-deficient encephalopathies due to lack of energy production or utilization; and (3) disorders affecting the intracellular processing of complex molecules. Testing may include ammonia (elevated in urea cycle defects, organic acidemias or fatty acid oxidation disorders), high lactate levels in blood and CSF (cerebrospinal fluid) or magnetic resonance spectroscopy in disorders of carbohydrate metabolism and mitochondrial disease. Other tests include quantitative analysis of amino acids in blood and urine (aminoacidopathies), urine organic acids, acylcarnitine profiles in the plasma (organic acidemias, fatty acid oxidation defects), very-long-chain fatty acids (VLCFAs) in plasma (peroxisomal disorders), uric acid (normal in sulfite oxidase deficiency and low in molybdenum cofactor deficiency), isoimmune electrophoresis for transferrin (abnormal pattern in disorders of congenital disorders of glycosylation) and 7-dehydrocholesterol (elevated in Smith-Lemli-Opitz syndrome) (Prasad & Prasad, 2011).

BOX 6-5 Clues to Cerebral Hypotonia

Abnormalities of other brain functions
Dysmorphic features
Fisting of the hands
Malformations of other organs
Movement through postural reflexes
Normal or brisk tendon reflexes
Scissoring on vertical suspension

Clues to the Diagnosis of Cerebral Hypotonia

Cerebral or central hypotonia in newborns usually does not pose diagnostic difficulty. The history and physical examination identifies the problem. Many clues to the diagnosis of cerebral hypotonia exist (Box 6-5). Most important is the presence of other abnormal brain functions such as decreased consciousness and seizures. Cerebral malformation is the likely explanation for hypotonia in an infant with dysmorphic features or with malformations in other organs.

A tightly fisted hand in which the thumb is constantly enclosed by the other fingers and does not open spontaneously (*fisting*), and adduction of the thigh so that the legs are crossed when the infant is suspended vertically (*scissoring*), are early signs of spasticity and indicate cerebral dysfunction. Eliciting postural reflexes in newborns and infants when spontaneous movement is lacking indicates cerebral hypotonia. In some acute encephalopathies, and especially in metabolic disorders, the Moro reflex may be exaggerated. The tonic neck reflex is

BOX 6-6 Clues to Motor Unit Disorders

Absent or depressed tendon reflexes
Failure of movement on postural reflexes
Fasciculations
Muscle atrophy
No abnormalities of other organs

an important indicator of cerebral abnormality if the responses are excessive, obligatory, or persist beyond 6 months of age. When hemispheric damage is severe but the brainstem is intact, turning the head produces full extension of both ipsilateral limbs and tight flexion on the contralateral side. An obligatory reflex is one in which these postures are maintained as long as the head is kept rotated. Tendon reflexes are generally normal or brisk, and clonus may be present.

Clues to Motor Unit Disorders

Disorders of the motor unit are not associated with malformations of other organs except for joint deformities and the maldevelopment of bony structures. The face sometimes looks dysmorphic when facial muscles are weak or when the jaw is underdeveloped.

Tendon reflexes are absent or depressed. Loss of deep tendon reflexes that is out of proportion to weakness is more likely caused by neuropathy than myopathy, whereas diminished reflexes that are consistent with the degree of weakness are more often caused by myopathy than neuropathy (Box 6-6). Muscle atrophy suggests motor unit disease but does not exclude the possibility of cerebral hypotonia. Failure of growth and even atrophy can be considerable in infants with brain insults. The combination of atrophy and fasciculations is strong evidence of denervation. However, the observation of fasciculations in newborns and infants is often restricted to the tongue, and distinguishing fasciculations from normal random movements of an infant's tongue is difficult unless atrophy is present.

Postural reflexes, such as the tonic neck and Moro reflex, are not imposable on weak muscles. The motor unit is the final common pathway of tone; limbs that will not move voluntarily cannot move reflexively.

CEREBRAL HYPOTONIA

Hypotonia is a feature of almost every cerebral disorder in newborns and infants. This section does not deal with conditions in which the major symptoms are states of decreased consciousness, seizures, and progressive psychomotor retardation. Rather, the discussion focuses on conditions in which hypotonia is sufficiently prominent that the examining physician may consider the possibility of motor unit disease.

Benign Congenital Hypotonia

The term benign congenital hypotonia is retrospective and refers to infants who are hypotonic at birth or shortly thereafter and later have normal tone. This diagnosis should be reserved for patients that besides recovering normal tone exhibit no other evidence of cerebral dysfunction; however, the majority of children with cerebral hypotonia without clear etiology may later exhibit cognitive impairment, learning disabilities, and other sequelae of cerebral abnormality, despite the recovery of normal muscle tone.

Chromosomal Disorders

Despite considerable syndrome diversity, common characteristics of autosomal chromosome aberrations in the newborn are dysmorphic features of the hands and face and profound hypotonia. For this reason, any hypotonic newborn with dysmorphic features of the hands and face, with or without other organ malformation, requires chromosome studies.

MECP2 Duplication Syndrome

The *MECP2* duplication syndrome occurs only in males; inheritance is as an X-linked trait. Occasionally females have been described with a *MECP2* duplication and related clinical findings, often associated with concomitant X-chromosomal abnormalities that prevent inactivation of the duplicated region (Van Esch, 2010).

Clinical Features. Characteristic of the syndrome is infantile hypotonia, severe cognitive impairment with absence of speech, progressive spasticity, recurrent respiratory infections, and seizures. During the first weeks of life, feeding difficulties resulting from hypotonia becomes evident. The child may exhibit difficulty with swallowing and extensive drooling. In some cases, nasogastric tube feeding is required. Dysmorphic features include brachycephaly, midfacial hypoplasia, large ears, and flat nasal bridge.

Generalized tonic-clonic, atonic and absence seizures are common (50%). Almost 50% die before age 25 years, presumably from complications of recurrent infection. Growth measurements at birth, including head circumference, are usually normal.

Because of hypotonia, delayed motor developmental is the rule. Walking is late, some individuals have an ataxic gait, and one-third never walk independently. Most never develop speech and some individuals who attained limited speech lose it in adolescence. Hypotonia gives way to spasticity in childhood. The spasticity is greatest in the legs; mild contractures may develop over time. Often the use of a wheelchair is necessary in adulthood.

Diagnosis. Duplications of *MECP2* ranging from 0.3 to 8 Mb are observable in all affected males and identified by commercially available genetic testing.

Management. Treatment is symptomatic and genetic counseling. The vast majority of affected males inherit the *MECP2* duplication from a carrier mother; however, spontaneous mutations have been reported. If the mother of the proband has an *MECP2* duplication, the chance of transmitting it in each pregnancy is 50%. Males who inherit the *MECP2* duplication will be affected; females who inherit the *MECP2* duplication are usually asymptomatic carriers

Prader-Willi Syndrome

Hypotonia, hypogonadism, cognitive impairment, short stature, and obesity characterize the Prader-Willi syndrome (Cassidy & Schwartz, 2009). Approximately 70% of children with this syndrome have an interstitial deletion of the paternally contributed proximal long arm of chromosome 15(q11-13). The basis for the syndrome in most patients who do not have a deletion is *maternal disomy* (both chromosomes 15 are from the mother). Paternal disomy of the same region of chromosome 15 causes *Angelman syndrome*.

Clinical Features. Decreased fetal movement occurs in 75% of pregnancies, hip dislocation in 10%, and clubfoot in 6%. Hypotonia is profound at birth and tendon reflexes are absent or greatly depressed. Feeding problems are invariable, and prolonged nasogastric tube feeding is common (Box 6-7). Cryptorchidism is present in 84% and hypogenitalism in 100%. However, some newborns lack the associated features and only show hypotonia (Miller et al, 1999).

Both hypotonia and feeding difficulty persist until 8 to 11 months of age and are then replaced by relatively normal muscle tone and insatiable hunger. Delayed developmental milestones and later cognitive impairment are constant features. Minor abnormalities that become more obvious during infancy include a narrow bifrontal diameter of the skull, strabismus, almond-shaped eyes, enamel hypoplasia, and small hands and feet. Obesity is the rule during childhood. The combination of obesity and minor abnormalities of the face and limbs produces a resemblance among children with this syndrome.

BOX 6-7 Difficulty of Feeding in the Alert Newborn

- Congenital myotonic dystrophy
- Familial dysautonomia
- Genetic myasthenic syndromes
- Hypoplasia of bulbar motor nuclei (see Chapter 17)
- Infantile neuronal degeneration
- Myophosphorylase deficiency
- Neurogenic arthrogryposis
- Prader-Willi syndrome
- Transitory neonatal myasthenia*

*Denotes the most common conditions and the ones with disease modifying treatments

Major and minor clinical criteria are established (Box 6-8). Weighting of major criteria is one point each; minor criteria are one half-point each. For children under 3 years of age, five points are required for diagnosis, four of which must be major criteria. For individuals 3 years of age and older, eight points are required for diagnosis, at least five of which must be major criteria. Supportive findings only increase or decrease the level of suspicion of the diagnosis.

Diagnosis. The mainstay of diagnosis is DNA-based testing to detect abnormal parent-specific imprinting within the Prader-Willi critical region on chromosome 15. This testing determines whether the region is maternally inherited only (the paternally contributed region is absent) and detects more than 99% of individuals.

Management. In infancy, special nipples or gavage feeding assures adequate nutrition. Physical therapy may improve muscle strength. Strabismus and cryptorchidism require surgical treatment. Growth hormone replacement therapy normalizes height and increases lean body mass. Medication for behavior modification is a consideration. Replacement of sex hormones produces adequate secondary sexual characteristics.

Chronic Nonprogressive Encephalopathy

Cerebral dysgenesis may be due to known or unknown noxious environmental agents, chromosomal disorders, or genetic defects. In the absence of an acute encephalopathy, hypotonia may be the only symptom at birth or during early infancy. Hypotonia is usually worse at birth and improves with time. Suspect cerebral dysgenesis

BOX 6-8 Criteria for the Clinical Diagnosis of Prader-Willi Syndrome

MAJOR CRITERIA

- Neonatal and infantile central hypotonia with poor suck and improvement with age
- Feeding problems and/or failure to thrive in infancy, with need for gavage or other special feeding techniques
- Onset of rapid weight gain between 12 months and 6 years of age, causing central obesity
- Hyperphagia
- Characteristic facial features: narrow bifrontal diameter, almond-shaped palpebral fissures, down-turned mouth
- Hypogonadism
  - Genital hypoplasia: small labia minora and clitoris in females; hypoplastic scrotum and cryptorchidism in males
  - Incomplete and delayed puberty
  - Infertility
- Developmental delay/mild to moderate cognitive impairment/multiple learning disabilities

MINOR CRITERIA

- Decreased fetal movement and infantile lethargy, improving with age
- Typical behavior problems, including temper tantrums, obsessive-compulsive behavior, stubbornness, rigidity, stealing, and lying
- Sleep disturbance/sleep apnea
- Short stature for the family by 15 years of age
- Hypopigmentation
- Small hands and feet for height age
- Narrow hands with straight ulnar border
- Esotropia, myopia
- Thick, viscous saliva
- Speech articulation defects
- Skin picking

SUPPORTIVE FINDINGS

- High pain threshold
- Decreased vomiting
- Scoliosis and/or kyphosis
- Early adrenarche
- Osteoporosis
- Unusual skill with jigsaw puzzles
- Normal neuromuscular studies (e.g., muscle biopsy, electromyography, nerve conduction velocity)

(Data from: Cassidy SB, Schwartz S. Prader-Willi syndrome. In: GeneClinics. Medical Genetic Knowledge Base [database online]. Seattle: University of Washington. Available at http://www.geneclinics.org. PMID: 20301505. Last updated September 3, 2009.)

when hypotonia associates with malformations in other organs or abnormalities in head size and shape. Magnetic resonance imaging (MRI) of the brain is advisable when suspecting a cerebral malformation. The identification of a cerebral malformation provides useful information not only for prognosis but also on the feasibility of aggressive therapy to correct malformations in other organs.

Brain injuries occur in the perinatal period and, less commonly, throughout infancy secondary to anoxia, hemorrhage, infection, and trauma. The sudden onset of hypotonia in a previously well newborn or infant, with or without signs of encephalopathy, always suggests a cerebral cause. The premature newborn showing a decline in spontaneous movement and tone may have an intraventricular hemorrhage. Hypotonia is an early feature of meningitis in full-term and premature newborns. Tendon reflexes may be diminished or absent during the acute phase.

Genetic Disorders

Familial Dysautonomia

Familial dysautonomia, the *Riley-Day syndrome*, is a genetic disorder transmitted by autosomal recessive inheritance in Ashkenazi Jews (Shohat & Halpern, 2010). The abnormality is in the *IKBKAP* gene, located on chromosome 9q31-q33, which encodes the elongator complex protein 1. Similar clinical syndromes also occur in non-Jewish infants that are often sporadic and with an unknown pattern of inheritance.

Clinical Features. In the newborn, the important clinical features are meconium aspiration, poor or no sucking reflex, and hypotonia. The causes of hypotonia are disturbances in the brain, the dorsal root ganglia, and the peripheral nerves. Tendon reflexes are hypoactive or absent. The feeding difficulty is usual and provides a diagnostic clue. Sucking and swallowing are normal separately but cannot be coordinated for effective feeding. Other noticeable clinical features of the newborn or infants are pallor, temperature instability, absence of fungiform papillae of the tongue, diarrhea, and abdominal distention. Poor weight gain and lethargy, episodic irritability, absent corneal reflexes, labile blood pressure, and failure to produce overflow tears completes the clinical picture.

Diagnosis. Mutation analysis is diagnostic. Two mutations account for more than 99% of mutant genes in individuals with familial dysautonomia of Ashkenazi descent. Ophthalmological examination is useful to detect the signs of postganglionic parasympathetic denervation: supersensitivity of the pupil, shown by a positive miotic response to 0.1 % pilocarpine or 2.5 % methacholine, corneal insensitivity, and absence of tears.

Management. Treatment is symptomatic; improved treatment of symptoms has increased longevity.

Oculocerebrorenal Syndrome (Lowe Syndrome)

Lowe syndrome is caused by markedly reduced activity of the enzyme inositol polyphosphate 5-phosphatase OCRL-1. Transmission is by X-linked recessive inheritance. Female carriers show partial expression in the form of minor lenticular opacities (Lewis et al, 2012).

Clinical Features. Lowe syndrome involves the eyes, central nervous system (CNS), and kidneys. All affected boys have dense cataracts and half have glaucoma. Box 6-2 lists the differential diagnosis of cataracts in newborns and infants. Corrected acuity is rarely better than 20/100. Hypotonia is present at birth and the tendon reflexes are usually absent. Hypotonia may improve, but tone never is normal. Motor milestones are achieved slowly and all boys have some degree of intellectual impairment. All boys have some degrees of proximal renal tubular dysfunction of the Fanconi type, including bicarbonate wasting and renal tubular acidosis, phosphaturia with hypophosphatemia and renal rickets, aminoaciduria, low-molecular weight proteinuria, sodium and potassium wasting, and polyuria. Slowly progressive chronic renal failure is the rule, resulting in end-stage renal disease after age 10 to 20 years.

Diagnosis. Diagnosis depends on recognition of the clinical constellation. MRI shows diffuse and irregular foci of increased signal consistent with demyelination. The diagnosis is established by demonstrating reduced (<10 % of normal) activity of inositol polyphosphate 5-phosphatase OCRL-1 in cultured skin fibroblasts. Such testing is available clinically.

Management. Symptomatic treatment includes early removal of cataracts, nasogastric tube feedings or feeding gastrostomy to achieve appropriate nutrition, occupational or speech therapy to address feeding problems, standard measures for gastroesophageal reflux, and programs to promote optimal psychomotor development.

Peroxisomal Disorders

Peroxisomes are subcellular organelles that participate in the biosynthesis of ether phospholipids and bile acids, the oxidation of VLCFAs, prostaglandins, and unsaturated long-chain fatty acids, and the catabolism of phytanate, pipecolate, and glycolate. Hydrogen peroxide is a product of several oxidation reactions, and catabolized by the enzyme catalase. Mutations in eleven different *PEX* genes cause this spectrum of disorders. *PEX* genes encode the proteins required for peroxisomal assembly.

The infantile syndromes of peroxisomal dysfunction are all disorders of peroxisomal biogenesis; the intrinsic protein membrane is identifiable, but all matrix enzymes are missing. The clinical spectrum of disorders of peroxisomal biogenesis includes the prototype, cerebrohepatorenal or Zellweger syndrome, as well as neonatal adrenoleukodystrophy and infantile Refsum disease (see Chapter 16). The latter two disorders are milder variants. Infantile hypotonia is a prominent feature of peroxisomal biogenesis disorders (Steinberg et al, 2012).

Clinical Features. Affected newborns are poorly responsive and have severe hypotonia, arthrogryposis, and dysmorphic features. Sucking and crying are weak. Tendon reflexes are hypoactive or absent. Characteristic craniofacial abnormalities include a pear-shaped head owing to a high forehead and an unusual fullness of the cheeks, widened sutures, micrognathia, a high-arched palate, flattening of the bridge of the nose, and hypertelorism. Organ abnormalities include biliary cirrhosis, polycystic kidneys, retinal degeneration, and cerebral malformations secondary to abnormalities of neuronal migration.

Limited extension of the fingers and flexion deformities of the knee and ankle characterize the arthrogryposis. Neonatal seizures are common. Bony stippling (chondrodysplasia punctata) of the patella and other long bones may occur. Older children have retinal dystrophy, sensorineural hearing loss, developmental delay with hypotonia, and liver dysfunction. Infants with Zellweger syndrome are significantly impaired and usually die during the first year of life, usually having made no developmental progress. The clinical courses of neonatal adrenoleukodystrophy and infantile Refsum disease are variable; while children can be very hypotonic, others learn to walk and talk. These conditions are often slowly progressive.

Difficult to control seizures often begin shortly after birth but may commence any time during infancy. Death from aspiration, gastrointestinal bleeding, or liver failure usually occurs within 6 months and usually within 1 year.

Diagnosis. Biochemical assay definitively establishes the diagnosis. Confirm biochemical abnormalities detected in blood and/or urine with cultured fibroblasts. Measurement of plasma VLCFA levels is the most commonly used and most informative. Elevation of C26:0 and C26:1 and the ratios C24/C22 and C26/C22 are consistent with a defect in peroxisomal fatty acid metabolism.

Management. Treatment is symptomatic, anticonvulsants for seizures, vitamin K for bleeding disorders, hearing aids, cataract removal in infancy, and other initiatives as needed.

Pyruvate Carboxylase Deficiency

The initial features of pyruvate carboxylase deficiency are neonatal hypotonia, tachypnea, and movement disorders (Garcia-Cazorla et al, 2006).

Clinical Features. All affected newborns are conscious, but hypotonic and tachypneic during the first hours after birth. High amplitude tremor of the limbs is the rule, and bizarre eye movements are present in some affected infants. Seizures are uncommon. A rapid fatal outcome is the rule.

Diagnosis. Hypoglycemia, lactic acidosis, and hypercitrullinemia are constant findings. Brain MRI shows cystic periventricular leukomalacia.

Treatment. Diet therapy, in the first hours postpartum, with triheptanoin and citrate reverses the biochemical errors. The long-term outcome is not established.

Other Metabolic Defects

Infantile hypotonia is rarely the only manifestation of inborn errors of metabolism. Acid maltase deficiency causes a severe myopathy and is discussed with other metabolic myopathies. Hypotonia may be the only initial feature of generalized GM_1 gangliosidosis (see Chapter 5).

SPINAL CORD DISORDERS

Hypoxic-Ischemic Myelopathy

Hypoxic-ischemic encephalopathy is an expected outcome in severe perinatal asphyxia (see Chapter 1). Affected newborns are hypotonic and areflexic. The main cause of hypotonia is the cerebral injury but spinal cord dysfunction also contributes. Concurrent ischemic necrosis of gray matter occurs in the spinal cord as well as in the brain. The spinal cord component is evident on postmortem examination and by electromyography (EMG) in survivors.

Spinal Cord Injury

Only in the newborn does spinal cord injury enter the differential diagnosis of hypotonia. Injuries to the cervical spinal cord occur almost exclusively during vaginal delivery; approximately 75 % are associated with breech presentation and 25 % with cephalic presentation. Because the injuries are always associated with a difficult and prolonged delivery, decreased consciousness is common and hypotonia falsely attributed to asphyxia or cerebral trauma. Loss of response to sensory modalities below the midchest should suggest myelopathy.

Injuries in Breech Presentation

Traction injuries to the lower cervical and upper thoracic regions of the cord occur almost exclusively when the angle of extension of the fetal head exceeds 90 %. Indeed, the risk of spinal cord injury to a fetus in breech position whose head is hyperextended is greater than 70 %. In such cases, delivery should always be by cesarean section. The tractional forces applied to the extended head are sufficient not only to stretch the cord but also to cause herniation of the brainstem through the foramen magnum. In addition, the hyperextended position compromises the vertebral arteries as they enter the skull.

The spectrum of pathological findings varies from edema of the cord without loss of anatomical continuity to massive hemorrhage (epidural, subdural, and intramedullary). Hemorrhage is greatest in the lower cervical and upper thoracic segments but may extend the entire length of the cord. Concurrent hemorrhage in the posterior fossa and laceration of the cerebellum may be present as well.

Clinical Features. Mild tractional injuries, which cause cord edema but not intraparenchymal hemorrhage or loss of anatomical continuity, produce few clinical features. The main feature is hypotonia, often falsely attributed to asphyxia.

Hemorrhage into the posterior fossa accompanies severe tractional injuries. Affected newborns are unconscious and atonic at birth with flaccid quadriplegia and diaphragmatic breathing. Few survive the neonatal period. Injuries restricted to the low cervical and high thoracic segments produce near-normal strength in the biceps muscles and weakness of the triceps muscles. The result is flexion of the arms at the elbows and flaccid paraplegia. Spontaneous movement and tendon reflexes in the legs are absent, but foot withdrawal from pinprick may occur as a spinal reflex. The infant has a distended bladder and dribbling of urine. Absence of sweating below the injury marks the sensory level, which is difficult to measure directly.

Diagnosis. Radiographs of the vertebrae show no abnormalities because bony displacement does not occur. MRI of the spine shows intraspinal edema and hemorrhage. Unconscious newborns are generally thought to have intracerebral hemorrhage or asphyxia (see Chapter 2), and the diagnosis of spinal cord injury may not be considered until consciousness is regained and the typical motor deficits are observed. Even then, the suspicion of a neuromuscular disorder may exist until disturbed bladder function and the development of progressive spastic paraplegia alert the physician to the correct diagnosis.

Management. The treatment of spinal cord traction injuries of the newborn is similar to the management of cord injuries in older children (see Chapter 12).

Injuries in Cephalic Presentation

Twisting of the neck during midforceps rotation causes high cervical cord injuries in cephalic presentation. The trunk fails to rotate with the head. The risk is greatest when amniotic fluid is absent because of delay from the time of membrane rupture to the application of forceps. The spectrum of injury varies from intraparenchymal hemorrhage to complete transection. Transection usually occurs at the level of a fractured odontoid process, with atlantoaxial dislocation.

Clinical Features. Newborns are flaccid and fail to breathe spontaneously. Those with milder injuries may have shallow, labored respirations, but all require assisted ventilation at birth. Most are unconscious at birth owing to edema in the brainstem. When conscious, eye movements, sucking, and the withdrawal reflex are the only movements observed. Tendon reflexes are at first absent but later become exaggerated if the child survives. Bladder distention and overflow incontinence occur. Priapism may be present. Sensation is difficult to assess because the withdrawal reflex is present.

Death from sepsis or respiratory complications generally occurs in the first week. Occasionally children have survived for several years.

Diagnosis. The appearance of children with high cervical cord injuries suggests a neuromuscular disorder, especially infantile spinal muscular atrophy, because the limbs are flaccid but the eye movements are normal. EMG of the limbs should exclude that possibility. Radiographs of the cervical vertebrae usually do not show abnormalities, but MRI shows marked thinning or disruption of the cord at the site of injury.

Management. Intubation and respiratory assistance commence prior to diagnosis. Chapter 12 discusses management of spinal cord transection.

MOTOR UNIT DISORDERS

Evaluation of Motor Unit Disorders

In the diagnosis of cerebral hypotonia in infants, the choice of laboratory tests varies considerably, depending on the disease entity. This is not the case with motor unit hypotonia. The available battery of tests readily defines the anatomy and cause of pathological processes affecting the motor unit (Box 6-9). DNA-based testing is now commercially available for many disorders and preferable to muscle or nerve biopsy.

Serum Creatine Kinase

Increased serum concentrations of creatine kinase (CK) reflect skeletal or cardiac muscle necrosis. Obtain blood for CK determination before the performance of EMG or muscle biopsy. Both transiently elevate the serum concentration of CK. The basis for laboratory reference values for normal serum concentration is nonambulatory adults. Normal values tend to be higher in an ambulatory population, especially after exercise. The serum concentration of CK in severely asphyxiated newborns is as high as 1000 IU/L secondary to acidosis. Even normal newborns have a higher than normal concentration during the first 24 hours postpartum. A normal CK level in a hypotonic infant is strong evidence against a rapidly progressive myopathy, but it does not exclude fiber-type disproportion myopathies and some metabolic myopathies. Conversely, expect mild elevations in CK concentration in rapidly progressive spinal muscular atrophies.

BOX 6-9 Evaluation of Motor Unit Disorders

- DNA-based testing
- Edrophonium chloride (Tensilon test)
- Electrodiagnosis
  - Electromyography
  - Nerve conduction studies
  - Repetitive stimulation
- Muscle biopsy
- Nerve biopsy
- Serum creatine kinase

Electrodiagnosis

EMG is extremely useful in the diagnosis of infantile hypotonia when an experienced physician performs the study. It enables the prediction of the final diagnosis in most infants younger than 3 months of age with hypotonia of motor unit origin. Hypotonic infants with normal EMG findings rarely show abnormalities on muscle biopsy. The needle portion of the study helps to distinguish myopathic from neuropathic processes. The appearance of brief, small-amplitude, polyphasic potentials characterize myopathies, while the presence of denervation potentials at rest (fibrillations, fasciculations, sharp waves) and motor unit potentials that are large, prolonged, and polyphasic characterize denervation. Studies of nerve conduction velocity are useful in distinguishing axonal from demyelinating neuropathies; demyelinating neuropathies cause greater slowing of conduction velocity. Repetitive nerve stimulation studies demonstrate disturbances in neuromuscular transmission.

Muscle Biopsy

The muscle selected for biopsy should be weak but still able to contract. Histochemical analysis is essential for the complete evaluation of muscle histology. The demonstration of fiber types, muscle proteins, and storage materials is required. The intensity of the reaction to myosin adenosine triphosphatase (ATPase) at pH 9.4 arbitrarily divides skeletal muscle into two fiber types. Type I fibers react weakly to ATPase, are characterized by oxidative metabolism and serve a tonic function. Type II fibers react intensely to ATPase, utilize glycolytic metabolism and serve a phasic function. Type I and II fibers are generally equal in number and randomly distributed in each fascicle. Abnormalities in fiber type number, fiber type size, or both characterize some disorders.

Chapter 7 describes and illustrates the structural proteins of muscle. Merosin is the main protein associated with congenital muscular dystrophy. The important storage materials identified in skeletal muscle are glycogen and lipid. In most storage disorders, vacuoles are present in the fibers that contain the abnormal material. Light microscopy reveals the vacuoles and histochemical reactions identify the specific material.

Nerve Biopsy

Sural nerve biopsy has limited value in the diagnosis of infantile hypotonia and it is only an option when EMG shows sural neuropathy. Its main utility is in the diagnosis of vasculitis, although abnormalities such as onion bulb formations are present with Dejerine-Sottas syndrome (see Chapter 7). The latter diagnosis is associated with abnormal nerve conduction studies, and may be confirmed by genetic testing.

The Tensilon Test

Edrophonium chloride (*Tensilon*™) is a rapidly acting anticholinesterase that temporarily reverses weakness in patients with myasthenia. Clear deficits such as ptosis or oculomotor paresis are essential to increase the reliability on this test. Rare patients are supersensitive to edrophonium chloride and may stop breathing because of depolarization of endplates or an abnormal vagal response. Equipment for mechanical ventilation should always be available when performing the test. In newborns, a subcutaneous injection of 0.15 mg/kg produces a response within 10 minutes. In infants, administer the drug intravenously at a dose of 0.2 mg/kg and reverse weakness within 1 minute.

We discourage the use of this test. The danger of causing apnea is real and the measure of response is very subjective. EMG, antibody testing and response to oral medications are good alternatives.

Spinal Muscular Atrophies

The spinal muscular atrophies (SMAs) are genetic disorders in which anterior horn cells in the spinal cord and motor nuclei of the brainstem are progressively lost. The mechanism is probably a defect in programmed cell death where the deletion of cells, a normal process during gestation, continues after birth. The onset of weakness may be at any age from birth to adult life. Some SMAs show a generalized distribution of weakness, and others affect specific muscle groups. Those with onset in infancy usually cause generalized weakness and hypotonia. Infantile SMA is one of the more common motor unit disorders causing infantile hypotonia.

Infantile Spinal Muscular Atrophy (SMA I)

The clinical subtypes of autosomal recessive of SMA are a continuum of disease. Discussion of the severe type (SMA I), which always begins before 6 months, follows. Discussion of the intermediate (SMA II) and juvenile (SMA III) types is in Chapter 7. *SMN1* (survival motor neuron) on 5q12.2-q13.3 is the primary SMA disease-causing gene (Prior & Russman, 2011). Normal individuals have both *SMN1* and a variable number of copies of *SMN2*, an almost identical copy of the *SMN1* gene, except for a single substitution that results in a partially functioning protein, on the same chromosome. The overlap in clinical features between the three types is considerable, and two different clinical phenotypes can occur in a single family. The course among siblings is usually the same, but sometimes both SMA I and SMA II phenotypes occur in siblings, and is then attributed to the number of copies of the *SMN2* gene.

Clinical Features. The age at onset is birth to 6 months. Reduced fetal movement may occur when neuronal degeneration begins in utero. Affected newborns have generalized weakness involving proximal more than distal muscles, hypotonia, and areflexia. Newborns that are hypotonic in utero and weak at birth may have difficulty adapting to extrauterine life and experience postnatal asphyxia and encephalopathy. Most breathe adequately at first and appear alert despite the generalized weakness because facial expression is relatively well preserved and extraocular movement is normal. Some newborns have paradoxical respiration because intercostal paralysis and thoracic collapse occur before diaphragmatic movement is impaired, while others have diaphragmatic paralysis as an initial feature. Despite intrauterine hypotonia, arthrogryposis is not present. Neurogenic arthrogryposis may be a distinct entity and is described separately in this chapter.

When weakness begins in infancy, the decline in strength can be sudden or decremental. At times, the child seems to improve because of normal cerebral development, but the progression of weakness is relentless. The tongue may show atrophy and fasciculations but these are difficult to see in newborns. After the gag reflex is lost, feeding becomes difficult and death results from aspiration and pneumonia. When weakness is present at birth, death usually occurs by 6 months of age, but the course is variable when symptoms develop after 3 months of age. Some infants will attain sitting balance but will not walk. Survival time is not predictable.

Diagnosis. Molecular genetic testing of the *SMN1* gene is available. About 95 % of individuals with SMA are homozygous for the absence of exons 7 and 8 of *SMN1*, and about 5 % are compound heterozygotes for absence of exons 7 and 8 of one *SMN1* allele and a point mutation in the other *SMN1* allele (Prior & Russman, 2011). The serum concentration of CK is usually normal but may be mildly elevated in infants with rapidly progressive weakness. EMG studies show fibrillations and fasciculations at rest, and the mean amplitude of motor unit potentials is increased. Motor nerve conduction velocities are usually normal.

Muscle biopsy is unnecessary because of the commercial availability of DNA-based testing. The pathological findings in skeletal muscle are characteristic. Routine histological stains show groups of small fibers adjacent to groups of normal-sized or hypertrophied fibers. When the myosin ATPase reaction is applied, all hypertrophied fibers are type I, whereas medium-sized and small fibers are a mixture of types I and II (Figure 6-4). Type grouping, a sign of reinnervation in which large numbers of fibers of the same type are contiguous, replaces the normal random arrangement of fiber types. Some biopsy specimens show uniform small fibers of both types.

DNA analysis of chorionic villus biopsies provides prenatal diagnosis.

Management. Treatment is supportive. Noninvasive ventilation and feeding gastrostomy has markedly increased survival (Oskoui et al, 2007). Agents that inhibit histone deacetylase were shown in in vitro experiments to increase production of SMN2 mRNA, but clinical trials of a number of these agents were either discontinued due to adverse events, or failed to show clinical efficacy. A more recently developed therapeutic approach, which is the subject of an ongoing clinical trial, is to deliver to the intrathecal space an antisense oligonucleotide designed to restore

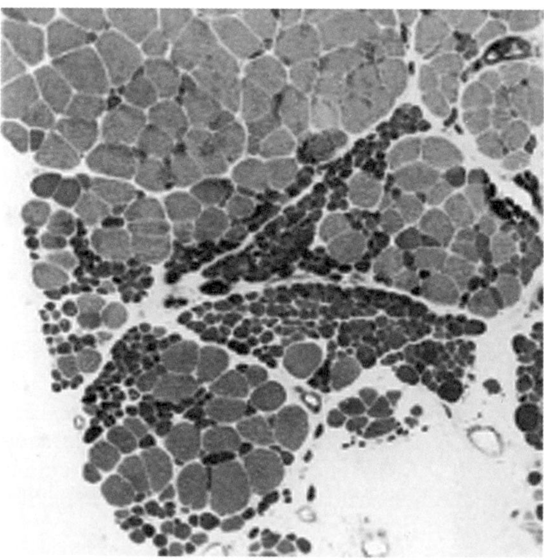

FIGURE 6-4 ■ Infantile spinal muscular atrophy (ATPase reaction). The normal random distribution pattern of fiber types is lost. Groups of large type I fibers (light shade) are adjacent to groups of small type II fibers (dark shade).

expression of-full length SMN2 mRNA in anterior horn cells, thereby improving motor neuron survival.

Infantile Spinal Muscular Atrophy with Respiratory Distress Type 1 (SMARD1)

Originally classified as a variant of SMA I, SMARD1 is a distinct genetic disorder resulting from mutations in the gene encoding the immunoglobulin μ-binding protein 2 (IGHMBP2) on chromosome 11q13 (Grohmann et al, 2003).

Clinical Features. Intrauterine growth retardation, weak cry, and foot deformities are the initial features. Most infants come to attention between 1 and 6 months because of respiratory distress secondary to diaphragmatic weakness, weak cry, and progressive distal weakness of the legs. Sensory and autonomic nerve dysfunction accompanies the motor weakness. Sudden infant death occurs without respiratory support.

Diagnosis. Consider the diagnosis in infants with an SMA I phenotype lacking the 5q gene abnormality, and those with distal weakness and respiratory failure.

Management. Treatment is supportive.

Congenital Cervical Spinal Muscular Atrophy

This is a rare sporadic disorder characterized by severe weakness and wasting confined to the arms. Contractures of the shoulder, elbow, and wrist joints are present at birth. The legs are normal. Postnatal progression of weakness does not occur. CNS function is normal. This cervical distribution of weakness usually occurs as a progressive disorder with onset in adolescence (see Chapter 7).

Neurogenic Arthrogryposis

The original use of the term neurogenic arthrogryposis was to denote the association of arthrogryposis with infantile spinal muscular atrophy. Transmission occurs by autosomal recessive inheritance in some families and by X-linked inheritance in others. Some individuals with autosomal recessive inheritance have deletions in the *SMN* gene. We are aware of two sets of identical twins in which one twin was born with neurogenic arthrogryposis and the other remained normal. This suggests that some sporadic cases may have nongenetic causes.

Families with X-linked neurogenic arthrogryposis tend to have clinical or pathological features that distinguish them from others. Arthrogryposis may not occur in every affected family member, weakness or joint deformity may be limited to the legs or arms, and progression is minimal.

Clinical Features. In neurogenic arthrogryposis, the most active phase of disease occurs in utero. Severely affected newborns have respiratory and feeding difficulties, and some die of aspiration. The less severely affected ones survive and have little or no progression of their weakness. Indeed, the respiratory and feeding difficulties lessen with time. Contractures are present in both proximal and distal joints. Micrognathia and a high-arched palate may be associated features, and a pattern of facial anomalies suggesting trisomy 18 is present in some newborns. Newborns with respiratory distress at birth may not have a fatal course. Limb weakness may be minimal, and long intervals of stability occur.

Diagnosis. Suspect the diagnosis in newborns with arthrogryposis, normal serum concentrations of CK, and EMG findings compatible with a neuropathic process. Muscle histological examination reveals the typical pattern of denervation and reinnervation. Cranial MRI investigates cerebral malformations in children with microcephaly.

Management. Initiate an intensive program of rehabilitation immediately after birth. Surgical release of contractures is often required.

Cytochrome c Oxidase Deficiency

Cytochrome c oxidase (COX) deficiency is clinically heterogeneous. Phenotypes range from isolated myopathy to a fatal infantile cardioencephalomyopathy. A boy with a marked spinal muscular atrophy presented with hypotonia, severe axial and limb weakness, and normal bulbar muscle strength (Rubio-Gozalbo et al, 1999). He died at the age of 5 months from respiratory failure. Electrodiagnosis revealed positive sharp waves and fibrillation potentials with normal motor nerve conduction velocities. Muscle biopsy showed a preponderance of type I fibers, with atrophy of both fiber types. COX activity was absent from all but intrafusal muscle fibers, and the activity was reduced in cultured skin fibroblasts. Western blot analysis showed decreased levels of all COX subunits. Analysis of mitochondrial DNA and the *SMN* gene was unrevealing.

Polyneuropathies

Polyneuropathies are uncommon in childhood and are even less common during infancy. Box 6-10 lists the polyneuropathies with onset in infancy. They divide into those that primarily

BOX 6-10 Polyneuropathies with Possible Onset in Infancy

Axonal

- Familial dysautonomia
- Hereditary motor-sensory neuropathy type II (see Chapter 7)
- Idiopathic with encephalopathy (see Chapter 7)
- Infantile neuronal degeneration
- Subacute necrotizing encephalopathy (see Chapters 5 and 10)

Demyelinating

- Acute inflammatory demyelinating polyneuropathy (Guillain-Barré syndrome) (see Chapter 7)
- Chronic inflammatory demyelinating polyneuropathy (see Chapter 7)
- Congenital hypomyelinating neuropathy
- Globoid cell leukodystrophy (see Chapter 5)
- Hereditary motor-sensory neuropathy type I (see Chapter 7)
- Hereditary motor-sensory neuropathy type III (see Chapter 7)
- Metachromatic leukodystrophy (see Chapter 5)

affect the myelin (demyelinating) or those that affect the axon (axonal). In newborns and infants, the term demyelinating also refers to disorders in which myelin has failed to form (hypomyelinating). Only with congenital hypomyelinating neuropathy is infantile hypotonia the initial feature. The others are more likely to start as progressive gait disturbance or psychomotor retardation. Chapter 7 provides a complete discussion of the clinical approach to neuropathy.

Congenital Hypomyelinating Neuropathy

The term congenital hypomyelinating neuropathy (CHN) encompasses several disorders with similar clinical and pathological features. Sporadic occurrence is the rule, but autosomal recessive inheritance occurs in some families. CHN results from a congenital impairment in myelin formation and can be caused by mutation in the early growth response 2 (*EGR2*) gene (Warner et al., 1998) or the myelin protein zero (*MPZ*) gene (Kochanski et al, 2004).

Clinical Features. The clinical features are indistinguishable from those of acute infantile spinal muscular atrophy. Arthrogryposis may be present. Newborns have progressive flaccid weakness and atrophy of the skeletal muscles, a bulbar palsy that spares extraocular motility, and areflexia. Respiratory insufficiency causes death during infancy.

In some children, failure to meet motor milestones is the initial manifestation. Examination shows diffuse weakness, distal atrophy, and areflexia. Weakness progresses slowly and is not life threatening during childhood. Sensation remains intact.

Diagnosis. The serum concentration of CK is normal, EMG findings are consistent with denervation, and motor nerve conduction velocities are usually less than 10 m/sec. The protein concentration of the cerebrospinal fluid is markedly elevated in almost every case. Screening for mutations in the peripheral myelin protein and *MPZ* genes is essential to separate the genetic causes of this syndrome from those of chronic demyelinating inflammatory demyelinating polyneuropathies.

Management. Some infants with hypomyelinating neuropathies respond to treatment with oral prednisone. One prednisone-treated newborn in our practice became normal, both clinically and electrophysiologically, by 1 year of age. He relapsed several times later in childhood and then responded to prednisone and to intravenous immunoglobulin. Such children may have a connatal form of chronic inflammatory demyelinating neuropathy (see Chapter 7). Whatever the mechanism, treat every affected child with a course of oral prednisone, 2 mg/kg/day. Those who respond become stronger within 4 weeks of starting therapy. Following the initial response, maintain alternate-day therapy, 0.5 mg/kg, for at least 1 year.

Disorders of Neuromuscular Transmission

Infantile Botulism

Human botulism ordinarily results from eating food contaminated by preformed exotoxin of the organism *Clostridium botulinum*. The exotoxin prevents the release of acetylcholine, causing a cholinergic blockade of skeletal muscle and end organs innervated by autonomic nerves. Infantile botulism is an age-limited disorder in which ingested *C. botulinum* colonizes the intestinal tract and produces toxin in situ. Dietary contamination with honey or corn syrup accounts for almost 20% of cases, but in most the source is not defined (Cherington, 1998).

Clinical Features. The clinical spectrum of infantile botulism includes asymptomatic carriers of organisms, mild hypotonia and failure to thrive, severe, progressive, life-threatening paralysis, and sudden infant death. Infected infants are between 2 and 26 weeks of age and usually live in a dusty environment adjacent to construction or agricultural soil disruption. The highest incidence is between March and October. A prodromal syndrome of constipation and poor feeding is common. Progressive bulbar and skeletal muscle weakness and loss of tendon reflexes develop 4 to 5 days later. Typical features on examination include diffuse hypotonia, ptosis, dysphagia, weak cry, and dilated pupils that react sluggishly to light.

Infantile botulism is a self-limited disease generally lasting for 2 to 6 weeks. Recovery is complete, but relapse occurs in as many as 5 % of babies.

Diagnosis. The syndrome suggests acute inflammatory demyelinating polyradiculoneuropathy (Guillain-Barré syndrome), infantile spinal muscular atrophy, or generalized myasthenia gravis. Clinical differentiation of infantile botulism from Guillain-Barré syndrome is difficult, and some reported cases of Guillain-Barré syndrome during infancy might actually have been infantile botulism. Infantile botulism differs from infantile spinal muscular atrophy by the early appearance of facial and pharyngeal weakness, the presence of ptosis and dilated pupils, and the occurrence of severe constipation. Infants with generalized myasthenia do not have dilated pupils, absent reflexes, or severe constipation.

Electrophysiological studies provide the first clue to the diagnosis. Repetitive stimulation between 20 and 50 Hz reverses the presynaptic block and produces a gradual increase in the size of the motor unit potentials in 90 % of cases. The EMG shows short-duration, low-amplitude motor unit potentials. The isolation of organisms from the stool is diagnostic.

Management. Intensive care is necessary throughout the period of profound hypotonia, and many infants require ventilator support. Sudden apnea and death are a constant danger. Early use of immune globulin reduces the length of hospitalization and shortens the duration of intensive care, mechanical ventilation, and intravenous or tube feedings (Arnon et al, 2006; Underwood et al, 2007). Avoid aminoglycoside antibiotics such as gentamicin as they produce presynaptic neuromuscular blockade and may worsen the condition.

Congenital Myasthenic Syndromes

Several genetic defects causing myasthenic syndromes have been identified (Abicht et al, 2012). All are autosomal recessive traits except for the slow channel syndrome, which is an autosomal dominant trait. All genetic myasthenic syndromes are seronegative for antibodies that bind the acetylcholine receptor (AChR). Both the genetic and clinical features are the basis for classifying congenital myasthenic syndromes.

Clinical Features. Respiratory insufficiency and feeding difficulty may be present at birth. Many affected newborns require mechanical ventilation. Ptosis and generalized weakness are present either at birth or develop during infancy (Mullaney et al, 2000). Arthrogryposis may also be present. Although facial and skeletal muscles are weak, extraocular motility is usually normal. Within weeks, many infants become stronger and no longer need mechanical ventilation. However, episodes of weakness and life-threatening apnea occur repeatedly throughout infancy and childhood, sometimes even into adult life.

Diagnosis. The basis for the diagnosis of a congenital myasthenic syndrome is the clinical findings, a decremental EMG response of the compound muscle action potential on low frequency (2–3 Hz) stimulation, negative tests for anti-AChR and anti-MuSK (muscle-specific tyrosine kinase) antibodies in the serum, and lack of improvement of clinical symptoms with immunosuppressive therapy. The intravenous or subcutaneous injection of edrophonium chloride, 0.15 mg/kg, is safe in intubated newborns, and usually establishes the diagnosis. The weakness and the respiratory distress reverse almost immediately after intravenous injection and within 10 minutes of subcutaneous injection. Several genes encoding proteins expressed at the neuromuscular junction are associated with congenital myasthenic syndrome.

Management. Long-term treatment with neostigmine or pyridostigmine prevents sudden episodes of apnea at the time of intercurrent illness. The weakness in some children responds to a combination of pyridostigmine and diaminopyridine. Diaminopyridine was granted an orphan designation by the FDA in the United States for its use in Lambert Eaton myasthenic syndrome in 2009. Thymectomy and immunosuppressive therapy are not beneficial.

Transitory Neonatal Myasthenia

A transitory myasthenic syndrome occurs in approximately 15 % of newborns of myasthenic mothers (Hoff et al, 2003). The passive transfer of antibody directed against fetal AChR from the myasthenic mother to her normal fetus is the presumed cause. Fetal AChR is structurally different from adult AChR. The severity of symptoms in the newborn correlates with the ratio of fetal to adult AChR antibodies in the mother but does not correlate with the severity or duration of weakness in the mother.

Clinical Features. Women with myasthenia have a higher rate of complications of delivery. Difficulty feeding and generalized hypotonia are the major clinical features in the infant. Affected children are eager to feed, but the ability to suck fatigues quickly and nutrition is inadequate. Symptoms usually arise within hours of birth but delay until the third day occurs. Some newborns are hypotonic in utero and born with arthrogryposis. Weakness of cry and lack of facial expression is present in 50 % of affected newborns, but only 15 % have limitation of extraocular movement and ptosis. Respiratory insufficiency is uncommon. Weakness becomes progressively worse in the first few days and then improves. The mean duration of symptoms is 18 days, with a range of 5 days to 2 months. Recovery is complete, and transitory neonatal myasthenia does not develop into myasthenia gravis later in life.

Diagnosis. High serum concentrations of AChR-binding antibody in the newborn and temporary reversal of weakness by the subcutaneous or intravenous injection of edrophonium chloride, 0.15 mg/kg, establishes the diagnosis.

Management. Treat newborns with severe generalized weakness and respiratory distress with plasma exchange. For those less impaired, 0.1% neostigmine methylsulfate by intramuscular injection before feeding sufficiently improves sucking and swallowing to allow adequate nutrition. Progressively reduce the dose as symptoms remit. An alternative route for neostigmine is by nasogastric tube at a dose 10 times the parenteral dose.

Congenital Myopathies

Congenital myopathies are developmental disorders of skeletal muscle. The main clinical feature is infantile hypotonia and weakness. Muscle biopsy is usual for diagnosis. The common histological feature is that type I fibers are greater in number, but smaller than type II fibers (Figure 6-5). Many infants with hypotonia and type I fiber predominance are later shown to have a cerebral abnormality; cerebellar aplasia is particularly common.

The term congenital fiber-type disproportion (CFTD) myopathy describes newborns with hypotonia, and sometimes arthrogryposis, whose muscle biopsy specimens show type I predominance as the only histological abnormality. The biopsy specimens in some infants have not only a type I fiber predominance but also a unique histological feature that names the condition (*central core disease, multi-minicore disease, myotubular myopathy, and nemaline myopathy*). Not discussed are several other congenital myopathies, reported in one child or one family.

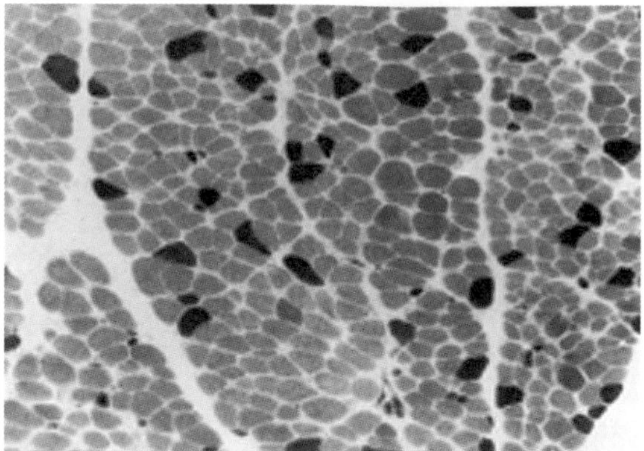

FIGURE 6-5 ■ Fiber-type disproportion myopathy (ATPase reaction). Type I fibers (light shade) are more numerous than type II fibers (dark shade). Type II fibers are generally larger in diameter than type I fibers.

Central Core Disease

Central core disease is a rare but distinct genetic entity transmitted primarily by autosomal dominant inheritance, although recessive and sporadic cases occur. Mutations in the ryanodine receptor-1 gene (*RYR1*) on chromosome 19q13 are responsible for central core disease and malignant hyperthermia (Malicdan & Nishino, 2011).

Clinical Features. Mild hypotonia is present immediately after birth or during infancy. Congenital dislocation of the hips is relatively common. Slowly progressive weakness begins after the age of 5 years. Weakness is greater in proximal than in distal limb muscles and is greater in the arms than in the legs. Tendon reflexes of weak muscles are depressed or absent. Extraocular motility, facial expression, and swallowing are normal. Some children become progressively weaker, have motor impairment, and develop kyphoscoliosis. In others, weakness remains mild and never causes disability.

Most children with central core disease are assumed to be at risk of malignant hyperthermia and should not be administered anesthetics without appropriate caution (see Chapter 8).

Diagnosis. The serum concentration of CK is normal, and the EMG findings may be normal as well. More frequently, the EMG suggests a myopathic process. The basis for diagnosis is the characteristic histopathological finding of sharply demarcated cores of closely packed myofibrils undergoing varying degrees of degeneration in the center of all type I fibers (Figure 6-6). Because of the tight packing of myofibrils, the cores are deficient in sarcoplasmic reticulum, glycogen, and mitochondria. Approximately 90 % of children with central

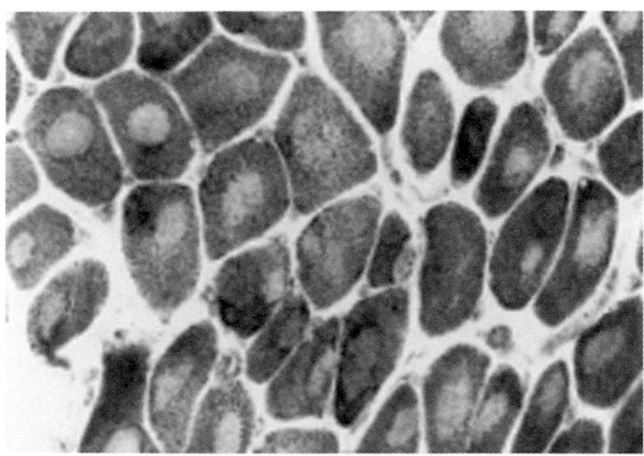

FIGURE 6-6 ■ Central core disease (DPNH reaction). The center of every fiber has a central core that appears clear when oxidative enzyme reactions are applied.

core disease have mutations in *RYR1*, the gene encoding the ryanodine receptor 1 (Wu et al, 2006). Sequence analysis identifies about 50% of affected individuals.

Management. Treatment is supportive.

Congenital Fiber-Type Disproportion Myopathy

The CFTD myopathies are a heterogeneous group of diseases that have a similar pattern of muscle histology. The initial feature of all these diseases is infantile hypotonia. Both genders are involved equally. Most cases are sporadic; genetic transmission may be autosomal dominant, autosomal recessive, or X-linked (Clarke et al, 2005). The largest group of inherited cases is associated with mutations in the *TPM3* gene, which encodes the slow isoform of skeletal muscle α-tropomyosin (Clarke et al, 2008). Despite the label "congenital," an identical pattern of fiber-type disproportion may be present in patients who are asymptomatic at birth and first have weakness during childhood.

Clinical Features. The severity of weakness in the newborn varies from mild hypotonia to respiratory insufficiency. Many had intrauterine hypotonia and show congenital hip dislocation, dysmorphic features, and joint contractures. Proximal muscles are weaker than distal muscles. Facial weakness, high-arched palate, ptosis, and disturbances of ocular motility may be present. When axial weakness is present in infancy, kyphoscoliosis often develops during childhood. Tendon reflexes are depressed or absent. Intellectual function is normal. Weakness is most severe during the first 2 years and then becomes relatively stable or progresses slowly.

Diagnosis. Type I fiber predominance and hypotrophy are the essential histological features. Type I fibers are 15% smaller than type II fibers. Other laboratory studies are not helpful. The serum concentration of CK may be slightly elevated or normal, and the EMG may be consistent with a neuropathic process, a myopathic process, or both. Nerve conduction velocities are normal.

Management. Physical therapy should be initiated immediately, not only to relieve existing contractures but also to prevent new contractures from developing.

Multi-Minicore Disease

The presence of multiple small zones of sarcomeric disorganization with lack of oxidative activity defines multi-minicore disease (Ferreiro et al, 2000). The clinical features associated with the defining pathology are variable. Inheritance is probably autosomal recessive. Some cases are associated with *RYR1* mutations (Ferreiro et al, 2002a), while others are caused by mutations in the selenoprotein 1 gene (*SEPN1*) (Ferreiro et al, 2002b).

Clinical Features. Both genders are equally affected. Onset is at birth or during infancy. Affected newborns are hypotonic. Delayed achievement of motor milestones characterizes infantile onset. Axial weakness is typical, as evidenced by scoliosis and neck flexor weakness. Proximal limb muscles weakness is common and distal weakness rare. Limb contractures are uncommon.

Diagnosis. Muscle biopsy specimens show zones of sarcomeric disorganization in both muscle fiber types that do not run the entire length of the fiber. Not every fiber contains a minicore. Type I fibers predominate in number.

Management. Treatment is supportive.

Myotubular (Centronuclear) Myopathy

Several clinical syndromes are included in the category of myotubular (centronuclear) myopathy. Transmission of some is by X-linked inheritance, others by autosomal dominant inheritance, and still others by autosomal recessive inheritance. The autosomal dominant form has a later onset and a milder course. The common histological feature on muscle biopsy is an apparent arrest in the morphogenesis of the muscle fiber at the myotube stage.

Severe/Infantile Myotubular Myopathy. The abnormal gene that causes acute myotubular myopathy (MTM) maps to the long arm of the X chromosome (Xq28) and is designated *MTM1*. *Myotubularin* is the protein encoded by the *MTM1* gene (Das et al 2011).

Clinical Features. Newborns with severe MTM1 are hypotonic and require respiratory assistance. The face has a myopathic appearance, motor milestones are delayed, and most fail to walk. Death in infancy is common. Those with forms that are more moderate achieve motor milestones more quickly and about 40 % require no ventilator support. In the mildest forms, ventilatory support is only required in the newborn period; delay of motor milestones is mild, walking is achieved, and facial strength is normal. Weakness is not progressive and may improve slowly over time. Female carriers are generally asymptomatic.

Diagnosis. The serum concentration of CK is normal. The EMG may suggest a neuropathic process, a myopathic process, or both. Muscle biopsy shows type I fiber predominance and hypotrophy, the presence of many internal nuclei, and a central area of increased oxidative enzyme and decreased myosin ATPase activity. Molecular genetic testing is available.

Management. Treatment is supportive.

Intermediate/Mild Myotubular Myopathy. Inheritance of milder forms of myotubular myopathy may be either autosomal or X-linked inheritance. Some forms are associated with mutations in the myogenic factor-6 gene (Kerst et al, 2000), while others are caused by mutations in the dynamin-2 gene (Bitoun et al, 2005).

Clinical Features. In general, age at onset of the recessive form is later than the X-linked form and earlier than the dominant form. Some children with the disease have hypotonia at birth; others come to attention because of delayed motor development. The pattern of limb weakness may be proximal or distal. The axial and neck flexor muscles are weak as well. Ptosis, but not ophthalmoplegia, is sometimes present at birth. The course is usually slowly progressive. Possible features include ophthalmoplegia, loss of facial expression, and continuing weakness of limb muscles. Some have seizures and cognitive impairment.

Diagnosis. The serum concentration of CK is normal, and EMG findings are abnormal but do not establish the diagnosis. Muscle biopsy is essential for diagnosis, and the histological features are identical to those of the acute form.

Management. Treatment is supportive.

Nemaline (Rod) Myopathy

Transmission of nemaline myopathy (NM) is either as an autosomal dominant or recessive trait. Approximately 20 % of cases are recessive, 30 % dominant, and 50 % are sporadic (North & Ryan, 2012). Several different genetic abnormalities cause the same histological features that define the disorder.

Clinical Features. NM is characterized by weakness and hypotonia with depressed or absent deep tendon reflexes. Muscle weakness is usually most severe in the face, the neck flexors, and the proximal limb muscles. Significant differences exist in survival between patients classified as having severe, intermediate, and typical NM. The severity of neonatal respiratory disease and the presence of arthrogryposis multiplex congenita are associated with death in the first year of life. Independent ambulation before 18 months of age is predictive of survival. Most children with typical NM are eventually able to walk.

At least three different phenotypes occur in children. Transmission of two congenital types is by autosomal recessive inheritance: (1) a severe neonatal form that causes immediate respiratory insufficiency and neonatal death; and (2) a milder form in which affected newborns often appear normal or are mildly hypotonic and not brought to medical attention until motor milestones are delayed. This form tends to be slowly progressive, with greater weakness in proximal than distal muscles. Weakness of facial muscles causes a dysmorphic appearance in which the face appears long and narrow and the palate is high and arched. Axial weakness leads to scoliosis.

Transmission of the childhood-onset form is by autosomal dominant inheritance. Onset of ankle weakness occurs late in the first or early in the second decade. The weakness is slowly progressive, and affected individuals may be wheelchair confined as adults.

Diagnosis. The term nemaline myopathy refers to a group of genetically distinct disorders linked by common morphologic features observed on muscle histology. Electrophysiological studies may suggest a myopathic process but are not specific, and the concentration of serum CK is usually normal or minimally elevated.

Muscle biopsy is essential for diagnosis. Within most fibers are multiple small rod-like particles, thought to be derived from lateral expansion of the Z disk. The greatest concentration of particles is under the sarcolemma (Figure 6-7). Type I fiber predominance is a prominent feature. Mutations in five genes encoding components of the sarcomeric thin filaments are associated with disease. The incidence of each of the genetic subgroups has not been established.

Management. Treatment is supportive. Parents who have the abnormal gene but are not weak may have rod bodies and fiber-type predominance in their muscles.

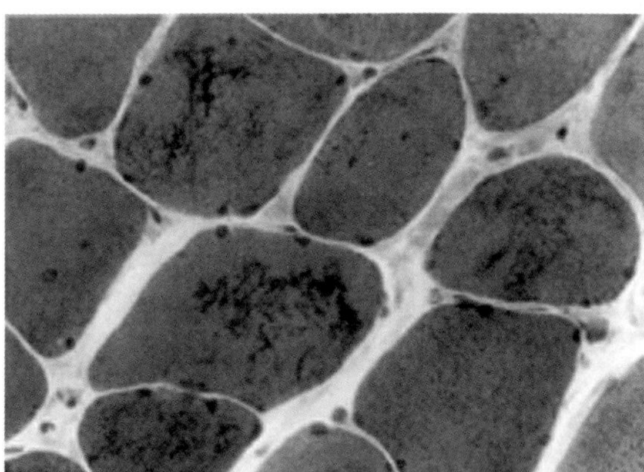

FIGURE 6-7 ■ Nemaline (rod) myopathy (trichrome). A spectrum of fiber sizes is present. The small fibers are all type I and contain rod-like bodies in a subsarcolemmal position.

Muscular Dystrophies

Congenital Dystrophinopathy

Dystrophinopathies occasionally cause weakness at birth. In such cases, dystrophin is completely absent. Immunofluorescence reactions for all three domains of dystrophin are essential for diagnosis. See Chapter 7 for a complete discussion of dystrophinopathies.

Congenital Muscular Dystrophy

The congenital muscular dystrophies (CMDs) are a group of myopathies characterized by hypotonia at birth or shortly thereafter, the early formation of multiple joint contractures, and diffuse muscle weakness and atrophy (Sparks et al, 2011). Inheritance of all CMDs is autosomal recessive. CMDs are divisible into syndromic and nonsyndromic forms. In syndromic CMD, both muscle and brain are abnormal. In nonsyndromic forms, muscular disease occurs without cerebral involvement.

An alternative classification of CMD is by the absence or presence of *merosin* (laminin α2) in muscle. Merosin, located in the extracellular matrix, is the linking protein for the dystroglycan complex (see Figure 7-2). Merosin-deficiency may be primary or secondary. Primary merosin deficiency only affects muscle while secondary merosin deficiencies occur in the syndromic CMD.

Merosin-Positive Nonsyndromic Congenital Muscular Dystrophy. The phenotype associated with merosin-positive CMD is not homogeneous. Transmission is by autosomal recessive inheritance with considerable genetic heterogeneity. One form, characterized by early rigidity of the spine, scoliosis, and reduced vital capacity, is associated with mutations in the *SEPN1* gene (Moghadaszadeh et al, 2001), and is allelic with a form of multi-minicore disease. *Ullrich disease*, caused by mutations in the collagen VI gene, is a form of CMD in which muscle fiber necrosis is secondary to loss of collagen links (Ishikawa et al, 2002).

Clinical Features. Approximately half of affected individuals are abnormal at birth because of some combination of hypotonia, poor ability to suck, and respiratory distress. Delayed achievement of motor milestones is usual. Limb-girdle weakness is the rule, generalized weakness may be present, and about half of the individuals have facial weakness. Joint deformities may be present at birth or develop during infancy.

Diagnosis. The serum concentration of CK is mildly elevated, and muscle biopsy shows fiber necrosis and regeneration. Brain MRI is normal.

Management. Physical therapy is important to prevent and reduce contractures.

Primary Merosin-Deficient Congenital Muscular Dystrophy. The abnormal gene site for primary merosin-deficient CMD is chromosome 6q22-23. The abnormal protein is laminin. The phenotypes associated with merosin deficiency are generally more severe than the phenotypes with merosin present. Merosin deficiency is also associated with later-onset muscular dystrophies (Jones et al, 2001).

Clinical Features. Hypotonia, arthrogryposis, and respiratory insufficiency are severe at birth. The infant has generalized limb weakness, with proximal muscles affected earlier and more severely than distal muscles. Facial and neck weakness is common, but extraocular motility is normal. Tendon reflexes may be present or absent and are often difficult to test because of joint contractures. Contractures at birth may involve any joint, but torticollis and clubfoot are particularly common, and congenital dislocation of the hips is often an associated feature.

Muscle hypertrophy is not present. Weakness and contractures delay motor development. The best motor achievement is the ability to sit unsupported. Intelligence is either normal or borderline subnormal. Chronic hypoventilation leading to respiratory failure is the usual cause of death.

Diagnosis. The serum concentration of CK is high in the newborn and tends to decline with age. Asymptomatic siblings and parents may have elevated serum concentrations of CK. EMG findings are consistent with a myopathic process. The muscle histological appearance is characteristic. Features include a variation in fiber size with occasional central nucleation, extensive fibrosis, and proliferation of adipose tissue, fibers undergoing regeneration and degeneration, and thickening of the muscle spindle capsule. A mononuclear infiltrate surrounding muscle fibers is often present early in the course. Cases of "neonatal polymyositis" are actually merosin-deficient CMD. Molecular genetic diagnosis is available.

Infants who are merosin deficient have an abnormal T_2 MRI signal in the cerebral white matter indicating hypomyelination mainly in the occipital horns. Structural disturbances of the occipital cortex may be associated (Philpot et al, 1999).

Management. Physical therapy is important to prevent further contractures.

Syndromic Congenital Muscular Dystrophy. In at least three disorders, CMD coexists with involvement of the CNS. These are *Fukuyama CMD* (FCMD), *muscle-eye-brain disease* (MEBD), and the *Walker-Warburg syndrome* (WWS). FCMD occurs almost exclusively in Japan, MEBD occurs mainly in Finland, and WWS has wide geographical distribution. Each has a different gene abnormality.

The major feature is a disturbance of cellular migration to the cortex between the fourth and fifth gestational months, resulting in polymicrogyria, lissencephaly, and heterotopia. Other abnormalities may include fusion of the frontal lobes, hydrocephalus, periventricular cysts, optic nerve atrophy, hypoplasia of the pyramidal tracts, reduction in the number of anterior horn cells, and inflammation of the leptomeninges.

WWS and FCMD show reduced but not absent merosin expression. MEBD has normal merosin expression. An abnormal MRI T_2 signal in the centrum semiovale that resembles hypomyelination is a marker of abnormal merosin expression.

Clinical Features. FCMD is the most common form of muscular dystrophy in Japan. One-quarter of mothers with an affected child have a history of spontaneous abortion. Affected newborns are normal at birth but soon develop hypotonia, an expressionless face, a weak cry, and an ineffective suck. Weakness affects proximal more than distal limb muscles. Mild contractures of the elbow and knee joints may be present at birth or develop later. Tendon reflexes are usually absent. Pseudohypertrophy of the calves develops in half of cases. Affected children may achieve sitting balance, but never stand.

Symptoms of cerebral involvement are present early in infancy. Febrile or nonfebrile generalized seizures are usually the first manifestation. Delayed development is always global and microcephaly is the rule. Cognitive impairment is severe. Weakness and atrophy are progressive and result in severe disability, cachexia, and death before 10 years of age.

Neonatal hypotonia, developmental delay, and ocular abnormalities characterize MEBD. Most affected children walk by age 4 years and then decline in all psychomotor skills. Specific eye abnormalities include glaucoma, progressive myopia, progressive retinal atrophy, and juvenile cataracts. The cerebral and muscle abnormalities of WWS are similar to those in MEBD. Ocular abnormalities include corneal clouding, cataracts, retinal dysplasia or detachment, and optic nerve hypoplasia.

Diagnosis. Molecular genetic testing is available for all three syndromes. The serum concentration of CK is generally elevated, and the EMG indicates a myopathy. Muscle biopsy specimens show excessive proliferation of adipose tissue and collagen out of proportion to the degree of fiber degeneration. Typical MRI abnormalities are dilatation of the cerebral ventricles and subarachnoid space and lucency of cerebral white matter.

Management. Treatment is supportive.

Congenital Myotonic Dystrophy

Myotonic dystrophy is a multisystem disorder transmitted by autosomal dominant inheritance (Bird, 2011). Symptoms usually begin in the second decade (see Chapter 7). An unstable DNA triplet in the *DMPK* gene (chromosome 19q13.2-13.3) causes the disease. Repeats may increase 50 to several thousand times in successive generations. The number of repeats correlates with the severity of disease, but repeat size alone does not predict phenotype. Repeat size changes from mother to child are greater than from father to child, and for this reason the mother is usually the affected parent when a child has CMD. A mother with repeats of 100 units has a 90 % chance that her child will have repeats of 400 units or more.

The main features during pregnancy are reduced fetal movement and polyhydramnios. Fifty percent of babies are born prematurely. Inadequate uterine contraction may prolong labor and forceps assistance is common. Severely affected newborns have inadequate diaphragmatic and intercostal muscle function and are incapable of spontaneous respiration. In the absence of prompt intubation and mechanical ventilation, many will die immediately after birth.

Prominent clinical features in the newborn include facial diplegia, in which the mouth is oddly shaped so that the upper lip forms an inverted V (Figure 6-8); generalized muscular hypotonia; joint deformities ranging from bilateral clubfoot to generalized arthrogryposis; and gastrointestinal dysfunction, including choking, regurgitation, aspiration, swallowing difficulties, and gastroparesis. Limb weakness in the newborn is more often proximal than distal. Tendon reflexes are usually absent in weak muscles. Percussion does not elicit myotonia in newborns, nor is EMG a reliable test.

Neonatal mortality is 16 %, a frequent cause of death being cardiomyopathy. Survivors usually gain strength and are able to walk; however, a progressive myopathy similar to the late-onset form occurs eventually. Severe cognitive impairment is the rule, and may result from a combination of early respiratory failure and a direct effect of the mutation on the brain.

Diagnosis. Suspicion of the diagnosis of CMD in the newborn requires examination of the mother. She is likely to have many clinical features of the disease and show myotonia on EMG. Showing DNA amplification on chromosome 19 in both mother and child confirms the diagnosis. Carrier testing is available on at-risk, non-symptomatic family members.

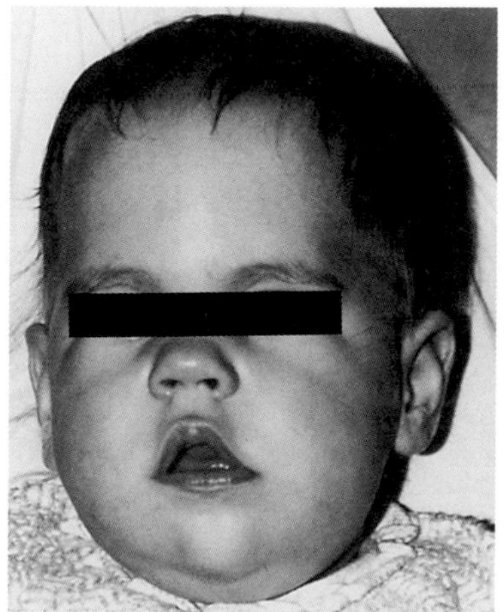

FIGURE 6-8 ■ Infantile myotonic dystrophy. The mouth has an inverted V position. (Reprinted with permission from Amato AA, Brook MH. Disorders of skeletal muscle. In: Bradley WG, Daroff RB, Fenichel GM, Jankovic J, eds. *Neurology in Clinical Practice*, 5th ed. Philadelphia: Elsevier, 2008.)

Management. The immediate treatment is intubation and mechanical ventilation. Joint contractures respond to physical therapy and casting. Metoclopramide alleviates gastroparesis.

Metabolic Myopathies

Acid Maltase Deficiency (Pompe Disease)

Acid maltase is a lysosomal enzyme, present in all tissues, that hydrolyzes maltose and other branches of glycogen to yield glucose (Tinkle & Leslie, 2010). It has no function in maintaining blood glucose concentrations. Three distinct clinical forms of deficiency are recognized: infantile, childhood (see Chapter 7), and adult. Transmission of all forms is by autosomal recessive inheritance. The defective gene site is chromosome 17q25.2-25.3.

Clinical Features. The infantile form may begin immediately after birth but usually appears during the second month. Profound generalized hypotonia without atrophy and congestive heart failure are the initial symptoms. Hypotonia is the result of glycogen storage in the brain, spinal cord, and skeletal muscles, causing mixed signs of cerebral and motor unit dysfunction: decreased awareness and depressed tendon reflexes. The mixed signs may be confusing, but the presence of cardiomegaly is almost diagnostic. The electrocardiogram shows abnormalities, including short PR intervals and high QRS complexes on all leads. Most patients die of cardiac failure by 1 year of age.

Characteristic of a second, milder subtype of the infantile form is less severe cardiomyopathy, absence of left ventricular outflow obstruction, and less than 5 % of residual acid maltase activity. Longer survival is possible with assisted ventilation and intubation.

Diagnosis. Measurement of acid α-glucosidase enzyme activity is diagnostic. Muscle biopsy reveals muscle fibers with large vacuoles packed with glycogen. Acid maltase activity is deficient in fibroblasts and other tissues. Molecular genetic testing is available.

Management. Individualized care of cardiomyopathy is required. Begin enzyme replacement therapy with Myozyme® (alglucosidase alfa) as soon as possible. Most infants treated before age 6 months and before requiring ventilatory assistance showed improved survival, ventilator-independent survival, acquisition of motor skills, and reduced cardiac mass compared to untreated controls. Improvements of skeletal muscle functions also occurred.

REFERENCES

Abicht A, Müller J, Lochmüller H. Congenital myasthenic syndromes. In: GeneClinics: Medical Genetic Knowledge Base [database online]. University of Washington. Available at http://www.geneclinics.org. PMID: 20301347. Last updated March 22, 2012.

Arnon SS, Shechter R, Maslanka SE, et al. Human botulism immune globulin for the treatment of infant botulism. New England Journal of Medicine 2006;354:462–71.

Bird TD. Myotonic dystrophy type 1. In: GeneClinics: Medical Genetic Knowledge Base [database online]. University of Washington. Available at http://www.geneclinics.org. PMID: 20301344. Last updated February 8, 2011.

Bitoun M, Maugenre S, Jeannet PY, et al. Mutations in dynamin 2 cause dominant centronuclear myopathy. Nature Genetics 2005;37:1207–9.

Cassidy SB, Schwartz S. Prader-Willi syndrome. In: GeneClinics. Medical Genetic Knowledge Base [database online]. University of Washington. Available at http://www.geneclinics.org. PMID: 20301505. Last updated September 3, 2009.

Cherington M. Clinical spectrum of botulism. Muscle and Nerve 1998;21:701–10.

Clarke NF, Smith RLL, Bahlo M, North KN. A novel X-linked form of congenital fiber-type disproportion. Annals of Neurology 2005;58:767–72.

Clarke NF, Kolski H, Dye DE, et al. Mutations in TPM3 are a common cause of congenital fiber type disproportion. Annals of Neurology 2008;63:329–37.

Das S, Dowling J, Pierson CR. X linked myotubular myopathy. In: GeneClinics: Medical Genetic Knowledge Base [database online]. University of Washington. Available at http://www.geneclinics.org. PMID: 20301605. Last updated October 6, 2011.

Ferreiro A, Estounet B, Chareau D, et al. Multi-minicore disease – searching for boundaries: Phenotype analysis of 38 cases. Annals of Neurology 2000;48:745–57.

Ferreiro A, Monnier N, Romero NB, et al. A recessive form of central core disease, transiently presenting as multi-minicore disease, is associated with a homozygous recessive mutation in the ryanodine receptor type 1 gene. Annals of Neurology 2002a;51:750–9.

Ferreiro A, Quijano-Roy S, Pichereau C, et al. Mutations of the selenoprotein N gene, which is implicated in rigid spine muscular dystrophy, cause the classical phenotype of multiminicore disease: reassessing the nosology of early-onset myopathies. American Journal of Human Genetics 2002b;71:739–49.

Garcia-Cazorla A, Rabier D, Touati G, et al. Pyruvate carboxylase deficiency: Metabolic characteristics and new neurological aspects. Annals of Neurology 2006;59:121–7.

Grohmann K, Varon R, Stolz P, et al. Infantile spinal muscular atrophy with respiratory distress type 1 (SMARD). Annals of Neurology 2003;54:719–24.

Hoff JM, Daltveit AK, Gilhus NE. Myasthenia gravis. Consequences for pregnancy, delivery, and the newborn. Neurology 2003;61:1362–6.

Ishikawa H, Sugie K, Murayama K, et al. Ullrich disease: Collagen VI deficiency: EM suggests a new basis for molecular weakness. Neurology 2002;59:920–3.

Jones KJ, Morgan G, Johnston H, et al. The expanding phenotype of laminin α2 chain (merosin) abnormalities: case series and review. Journal of Medical Genetics 2001;38:649–57.

Kerst B, Mennerich D, Schuelke M, et al. Heterozygous myogenic factor 6 mutation associated with myopathy and severe course of Becker muscular dystrophy. Neuromuscular Disorders 2000;10:572–7.

Kochanski A, Drac H, Kabzinska D, et al. A novel MPZ gene mutation in congenital neuropathy with hypomyelination. Neurology 2004;8:2122–3.

Lewis RA, Nussbaum RL, Brewer ED. Lowe disease. In: GeneClinics: Medical Genetic Knowledge Base [database online]. University of Washington. Available at http://www.geneclinics.org. PMID: 20301653. Last updated February 23, 2012.

Malicdan MCV, Nishino I. Central core disease. In: GeneClinics: Medical Genetic Knowledge Base [database online]. University of Washington. Available at http://www.geneclinics.org. PMID: 20301565. Last updated May 11, 2011.

Miller SP, Riley P, Shevell MI. The neonatal presentation of Prader-Willi syndrome revisited. Journal of Pediatrics 1999;134:226–8.

Moghadaszadeh B, Petit N, Jaillard C, et al. Mutations in SEPN1 cause congenital muscular dystrophy with spinal rigidity and restrictive respiratory syndrome. Nature Genetics 2001;29:17–8.

Mullaney P, Vajsar J, Smith R, et al. The natural history and ophthalmic involvement in childhood myasthenia gravis at The Hospital for Sick Children. Ophthalmology 2000;107:504–10.

North K, Ryan MM. Nemaline myopathy. In: GeneClinics: Medical Genetic Knowledge Base [database online]. University of Washington. Available at http://www.geneclinics.org. PMID: 20301465. Last updated March 15, 2012.

Oskoui M, Levy G, Garland CJ, et al. The changing natural history of spinal muscular atrophy type 1. Neurology 2007;69:1–2.

Philpot J, Cowan F, Pennock J, et al. Merosin-deficient muscular dystrophy: The spectrum of brain involvement on magnetic resonance imaging. Neuromuscular Disorders 1999;9:81–5.

Prasad AN, Prasad C. Genetic evaluation of the floppy infant. Seminars in Fetal & Neonatal Medicine 2011;16:99–108.

Prior TW, Russman BS. Spinal muscular atrophy. In: GeneClinics: Medical Genetic Knowledge Base [database online]. University of Washington. Available at http://www.geneclinics.org. PMID: 20301526. Last updated January 27, 2011.

Rubio-Gozalbo MD, Smeitink JAM, Ruitenbeek W, et al. Spinal muscular atrophy-like picture, cardiomyopathy, and cytochrome-c-oxidase deficiency. Neurology 1999;52:383–6.

Shohat M, Halpern GJ. Familial dysautonomia. In: GeneClinics: Medical Genetic Knowledge Base [database online]. University of Washington. Available at http://www.geneclinics.org. PMID: 20301359. Last updated June 1, 2010.

Sparks S, Quijano-Roy S, Harper A, et al. Congenital muscular dystrophy overview. In: GeneClinics: Medical Genetic Knowledge Base [database online]. University of Washington. Available at http://www.geneclinics.org. PMID: 20301468. Last updated January 4, 2011.

Steinberg SJ, Raymond GV, Braverman NE, et al. Peroxisome biogenesis disorders: Zellweger syndrome spectrum. In: GeneClinics: Medical Genetic Knowledge Base [database online]. Seattle: University of Washington. Available at http://www.geneclinics.org. PMID: 20301621. Last updated May 10, 2012.

Tinkle BT, Leslie N. Glycogen storage disease type II (Pompe disease). In: GeneClinics: Medical Genetic Knowledge Base [database online]. Seattle: University of Washington. Available at http://www.geneclinics.org. PMID: 20301438. Last updated August 12, 2010.

Underwood K, Rubin S, Deakers T, et al. Infant botulism: A 30-year experience spanning the introduction of botulism Immune Globuline Intravenous in the Intensive care unit at Children's Hospital Los Angeles. Pediatrics 2007;120:e1380–5.

Van Esch H. MECP2 duplication syndrome. In: GeneClinics: Medical Genetic Knowledge Base [database online]. Seattle: University of Washington. Available at http://www.geneclinics.org. PMID: 20301461. Last updated June 24, 2010.

Warner LE, Mancians P, Butler IJ, et al. Mutations in the early growth response 2 (EGR2) gene are associated with hereditary myelinopathies. Nature Genetics 1998;18:382–4.

Wu S, Ibarra CA, Malicdan MCV, et al. Central core disease is due to RYR1 mutations in more than 90% of patients. Brain 2006;129:1470–80.

CHAPTER 7

Flaccid Limb Weakness in Childhood

The majority of children with flaccid limb weakness have a motor unit disorder. Flaccid leg weakness may be the initial feature of disturbances in the lumbosacral region, but other symptoms of spinal cord dysfunction are usually present. Also, consult Box 12-1 when considering the differential diagnosis of flaccid leg weakness without arm impairment. Cerebral disorders may cause flaccid weakness, but dementia (see Chapter 5) or seizures (see Chapter 1) are usually concomitant features.

CLINICAL FEATURES OF NEUROMUSCULAR DISEASE

Weakness is decreased strength, as measured by the force of a maximal contraction. Fatigue is an inability to maintain a less than maximal contraction, as measured by exercise tolerance. Weak muscles are always more easily fatigued than normal muscles, but fatigue may occur in the absence of weakness. Chapter 8 discusses conditions in which strength is normal at rest but muscles fatigue or cramp on exercise.

The Initial Complaint

Limb weakness in children is usually noted first in the legs and then in the arms (Box 7-1). This is because the legs are required to bear weight and are subject to continuous testing while standing or walking. Delayed development of motor skills is often an initial or prominent feature in the history of children with neuromuscular disorders. Marginal motor delay in children with otherwise normal development rarely raises concern, and is often considered part of the spectrum of normal development. Prompts for neurological consultation in older children with neuromuscular disorders are failure to keep up with peers, frequent falls or easy fatigability.

An abnormal gait can be the initial symptom of either proximal or distal leg weakness. With proximal weakness, the pelvis fails to stabilize and waddles from side to side as the child walks. Running is especially difficult and accentuates the hip waddle. Descending stairs is particularly difficult in children with quadriceps weakness; the knee cannot lock and stiffen. Difficulty with ascending stairs suggests hip extensor weakness. Rising from the floor or a deep chair is difficult, and the hands help to push off.

Stumbling is an early complaint when there is distal leg weakness, especially weakness of the evertors and dorsiflexors of the foot. Falling is first noted when the child walks on uneven surfaces. The child is thought to be clumsy, but after a while parents realize that the child is "tripping on nothing at all." Repeated ankle spraining occurs because of lateral instability. Children with foot drop tend to lift the knee high in the air so that the foot will clear the ground. The weak foot then comes down with a slapping motion (*steppage gait*).

Toe walking is commonplace in Duchenne muscular dystrophy (DMD) because the pelvis thrusts forward to shift the center of gravity and the gastrocnemius muscle is stronger than the peroneal muscles. Toe walking occurs also in upper motor neuron disorders that cause spasticity and in children who have tight heel cords but no identifiable neurological disease. Muscular dystrophy is usually associated with hyporeflexia and spasticity with hyperreflexia. However, the ankle tendon reflex may be difficult to elicit when the tendon is tight for any reason. Rarely toe walking is part of a compulsive gait in children with obsessive-compulsive behaviors.

BOX 7-1 Symptoms of Neuromuscular Disease

Abnormal Gait
- Steppage
- Toe walking
- Waddling

Easy Fatigability

Frequent Falls

Slow Motor Development

Specific Disability
- Arm elevation
- Climbing stairs
- Hand grip
- Rising from floor

Adolescents, but usually not children, with weakness complain of specific disabilities. A young woman with proximal weakness may have difficulty keeping her arms elevated to groom her hair or rotating the shoulder to get into and out of garments that have a zipper or hook in the back. Weakness of hand muscles often comes to attention because of difficulty with handwriting. Adolescents may notice difficulty in unscrewing jar tops or working with tools. Teachers report to parents when children are slower than classmates in climbing stairs, getting up from the floor, and skipping and jumping. Parents may report a specific complaint to the physician, but more often they define the problem as inability to keep up with peers.

A child whose limbs are weak also may have weakness in the muscles of the head and neck. Specific questions should be asked about double vision, drooping eyelids, difficulty chewing and swallowing, change of facial expression and strength (whistling, sucking, chewing, blowing), and the clarity and tone of speech. Weakness of neck muscles is frequently noticed when the child is a passenger in a vehicle that suddenly accelerates or decelerates, as it is normal in the first couple of months of life. The neck muscles are unable to stabilize the head, which snaps backward or forward.

Physical Findings

The examination begins by watching the child sit, stand, and walk. A normal child sitting cross-legged on the floor can rise to a standing position in a single movement without using the hands. This remarkable feat is lost sometime after age 15 years in most children, in which case rising from a low stool is a better test of proximal leg strength. The child with weak pelvic muscles uses the hands for assistance (Figure 7-1), and with progressive weakness the hands are used to climb up the legs (*Gower sign*).

After normal gait is observed, the child is asked to walk first on the toes and then on the heels (Box 7-2). Inability to walk on the toes indicates gastrocnemius muscle weakness, and inability to walk on the heels indicates weakness of the anterior compartment muscles. Push-ups are a quick test of strength in almost all arm muscles. Most normal children can do at least one push-up. Then ask the child to touch the tip of the shoulder blade with the ipsilateral thumb. This is an impossible task when the rhomboids are weak.

Finally, face and eye movements are tested. The best test of facial strength is to blow out the cheeks and hold air against compression. Normally the lips are smooth. Wrinkling of the perioral tissues and failure to hold air indicate facial weakness. During this period of observation and again during muscle strength testing, the physician should look for atrophy or hypertrophy. Wasting of muscles in the shoulder causes bony prominences to stand out even further. Wasting of hand muscles flattens the thenar and hypothenar eminences. Wasting of the quadriceps muscles causes a tapering appearance of the thigh that exaggerates when the patient tenses the thigh by straightening the knee. Atrophy of the anterior tibial and peroneal muscles gives the anterior border of the tibia a sharp appearance, and atrophy of the gastrocnemius muscle diminishes the normal contour of the calf.

Loss of tendon reflexes occurs early in denervation, especially when sensory nerves are involved, but parallels the degree of weakness in myopathy. Tendon reflexes are usually normal even during times of weakness in patients with

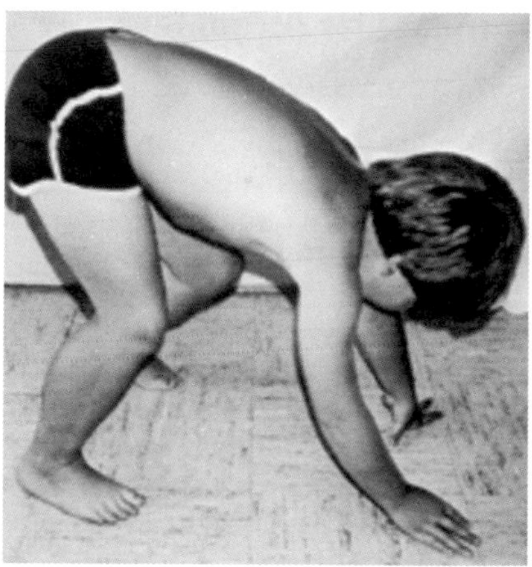

FIGURE 7-1 ■ Gower sign. The child rises from the floor by pushing off with the hands to overcome proximal pelvic weakness.

BOX 7-2 Signs of Neuromuscular Disease

Observation
- Atrophy and hypertrophy
- Fasciculations
- Functional ability

Palpation
- Muscle texture
- Tenderness

Examination
- Joint contractures
- Myotonia
- Strength
- Tendon reflexes

myasthenia gravis and may be normal between episodes of recurrent weakness in those with metabolic myopathies. The description of myotonia, a disturbance in muscle relaxation following contraction, is in the section on myotonic dystrophy.

PROGRESSIVE PROXIMAL WEAKNESS

Progressive proximal weakness in childhood is most often due to myopathy, usually a muscular dystrophy (Box 7-3). Juvenile spinal muscular atrophy (SMA) is the only chronic denervating disease in which weakness is more proximal than distal. Electromyography (EMG) and muscle biopsy readily distinguishes it from myopathic disorders. Limb-girdle myasthenia is rare but is an important consideration because specific treatment is available (Table 7-1).

BOX 7-3 Progressive Proximal Weakness

SPINAL CORD DISORDERS (SEE CHAPTER 12)

JUVENILE SPINAL MUSCULAR ATROPHIES
- Autosomal dominant
- Autosomal recessive

GM_2 GANGLIOSIDOSIS (HEXOSAMINIDASE A DEFICIENCY)

MYASTHENIC SYNDROMES
- Acquired limb-girdle myasthenia
- Slow-channel syndrome

MUSCULAR DYSTROPHIES
- Bethlem myopathy
- Dystrophinopathies
- Facioscapulohumeral syndrome
- Severe childhood autosomal recessive muscular dystrophy

INFLAMMATORY MYOPATHIES
- Dermatomyositis*
- Polymyositis*

METABOLIC MYOPATHIES
- Acid maltase deficiency*
- Carnitine deficiency*
- Debrancher enzyme deficiency* (see Chapter 8)
- Lipid storage myopathies
- Mitochondrial myopathies (see Chapter 8)
- Myophosphorylase deficiency (see Chapter 8)

ENDOCRINE MYOPATHIES
- Adrenal cortex*
- Parathyroid*
- Thyroid*

*Denotes the most common conditions and the ones with disease modifying treatments

Spinal Muscular Atrophies

Autosomal Recessive Type

Spinal muscular atrophy (SMA) is the most common inherited disorder of the spinal cord resulting in hypotonia and weakness in infants with an incidence of approximately 1 in 10 000 live births per year. It is an autosomal recessive disorder with a molecular defect leading to increased apoptosis in anterior horn cells and in motor nuclei of lower cranial nerves. In approximately 95 % of cases, the genetic defect is homozygous deletion of the survival motor neuron 1 gene (*SMN1*), which is located on the telomeric region of chromosome 5q13 (Ogino & Wilson, 2002; Prior & Russman, 2011). A virtually identical centromeric gene on 5q13, referred to as *SMN2*, encodes a similar but less active product (Swoboda et al, 2005). The protein product of *SMN2* partially appears to rescue the SMA phenotype such that a larger SMN2 copy number generally results in a milder disease. While age at onset distinguishes three subtypes of SMA, the subtypes are actually a continuum. The severe type (SMA I) always begins during before 6 months of age (see Chapter 6), the intermediate type (SMA II) begins between 6 and 18 months, and the juvenile type (SMA III) begins after 18 months.

Clinical Features. In SMA II, fetal movements are normal and the child is normal at birth. The initial feature of SMA II is delayed motor development. As a rule, affected children achieve sitting balance, but are unable to stand unsupported and are wheelchair confined. A fine hand tremor is often present. Contractures of the hips and knees and scoliosis eventually develop. Some of those affected die in childhood because of respiratory failure, but most survive into adult life. An unusual form of SMA II is one that begins with head drop followed by generalized weakness and respiratory insufficiency. This variant causes death by 3 years of age.

The initial feature of SMA III is gait instability caused by proximal weakness. Similar to SMA II, a fine action tremor is common. Disease progression is very slow, sometimes in a stepwise fashion, and often seems arrested. Weakness may progress either to the distal muscles of the legs or to the proximal muscles of the arms. The hands are the last parts affected. Facial muscles may be weak, but extraocular motility is always normal. Tendon reflexes are hypoactive or absent. The sensory examination is normal.

TABLE 7-1 **Distinguishing Features in Proximal Weakness**

	Neuronopathy	Myopathy	Myasthenia
Tendon reflexes	Absent	Depressed or absent	Normal
Electromyography	Fasciculations; denervation potentials; high-amplitude polyphasic motor potentials	Brief, small-amplitude polyphasic motor units	Normal
Nerve conduction	Normal or mildly slow	Normal	Abnormal repetitive stimulation
Creatine kinase concentration	Normal or mildly elevated	Elevated	Normal
Muscle biopsy	Group atrophy; group typing	Fiber necrosis; fatty replacement; excessive collagen	Normal

Cases with ophthalmoplegia are probably genetically distinct.

Some children have more profound weakness of the arms than of the legs and are likely to have facial weakness as well. Within a family, some children may have predominant leg weakness, whereas their siblings may have predominant arm weakness.

Diagnosis. Showing the gene abnormality on chromosome 5 establishes the diagnosis. EMG and muscle biopsy are unnecessary if genetic analysis shows the appropriate mutation. The findings on both tests are similar to those described for SMA I in Chapter 6. The serum concentration of creatine kinase (CK) may be two to four times the upper limit of normal, and the increase in concentration correlates directly with the duration of illness.

Management. Proper management of SMA in children increases longevity and decreases disability. The goals are to maintain function and prevent contractures. Children who quickly take to a wheelchair develop disuse atrophy. Dietary counseling prevents obesity, which only increases the strain on weak muscles. The prevention of contractures usually requires range of motion exercise and the early use of splints, especially at night. Families need genetic counseling for this autosomal recessive illness with a 25 % risk for future children from same parents.

Autosomal Dominant Type

Several childhood autosomal dominant types of SMA exist. Genetic linkage is not on chromosome 5. The onset of weakness is from childhood into adult life. A new dominant mutation would be difficult to distinguish from the autosomal recessive form.

Clinical Features. A more generalized pattern of weakness is more prominent in the autosomal dominant type than in the autosomal recessive type, but proximal muscles are weaker than distal muscles. The weakness is slowly progressive and may stabilize after adolescence. Most patients walk and function well into middle and late adult life. Bulbar weakness is unusual and mild when present. Extraocular muscles are not affected. Tendon reflexes are depressed or absent in weak muscles. Joint contractures are uncommon.

Diagnosis. The serum concentration of CK is normal or only mildly elevated. The EMG is the basis for diagnosis.

Management. Treatment for the dominant type is the same as for the recessive type. Antenatal diagnosis is not available. When the family has no history of SMA, genetic counseling is difficult, but autosomal dominant inheritance is a consideration if the onset is after 3 years of age.

X-Linked Type

This rare X-linked anterior horn cell degenerative disorder shares a considerable degree of phenotypic overlap with SMN-related SMA. Polyhydramnios secondary to impaired fetal swallowing and arthrogryposis are common. The diagnosis should be considered in any case of a male infant with an SMA phenotype and normal *SMN1* genetic test. The only known causative gene encodes the ubiquitin-activating enzyme 1 (UBE1), for which testing is available on a research basis only (Ramser et al, 2008). This condition is also discussed in Chapter 6.

GM_2 Gangliosidosis

The typical clinical expression of hexosaminidase A deficiency is *Tay-Sachs disease* (see Chapter 5). Several phenotypic variants of the enzyme deficiency with onset throughout childhood and adult life exist. Transmission of all variants is by autosomal recessive inheritance. The initial features of the juvenile-onset type mimic those of juvenile SMA (Navon et al, 1997).

Clinical Features. Weakness, wasting, and cramps of the proximal leg muscles begin after infancy and frequently not until adolescence. Distal leg weakness, proximal and distal arm weakness, and tremor follow. Symptoms of cerebral degeneration (personality change, intermittent psychosis, and dementia) become evident after motor neuron dysfunction is established.

Examination shows a mixture of upper and lower motor neuron signs. The macula is usually normal and the cranial nerves are intact, with the exception of atrophy and fasciculations in the tongue. Fasciculations also may be present in the limbs. Tendon reflexes are absent or exaggerated, depending on the relative severity of upper and lower motor neuron dysfunction. Plantar responses are sometimes extensor and sometimes flexor. Tremor, but not dysmetria, is present in the outstretched arms, and sensation is intact.

Some children never develop cerebral symptoms and have only motor neuron disease; some adults have only dementia and psychosis. The course is variable and compatible with prolonged survival.

Diagnosis. The serum concentration of CK is normal or only mildly elevated. Motor and sensory nerve conduction velocities are normal, but needle EMG shows neuropathic motor units. Showing a severe deficiency or absence of hexosaminidase-A activity in leukocytes or cultured fibroblasts establishes the diagnosis.

Management. No treatment is available. Heterozygote detection is possible because enzyme activity is partially deficient. Prenatal diagnosis is available.

Myasthenic Syndromes

Proximal weakness and sometimes wasting may occur in acquired immune-mediated myasthenia and in a genetic myasthenic syndrome.

Limb-Girdle Myasthenia

Limb-girdle myasthenia is immune-mediated myasthenia gravis that begins as progressive proximal weakness of the limbs and affects ocular motility later. This entity is very uncommon.

Clinical Features. Onset is after 10 years of age, and girls are more often affected than are boys. Weakness does not fluctuate greatly with exercise. Muscles of facial expression may be affected, but other bulbar function is not. Tendon reflexes are usually present but may be hypoactive. The clinical features suggest limb-girdle dystrophy or polymyositis.

Diagnosis. The diagnosis of limb-girdle myasthenia is possible in every child with proximal weakness and preserved tendon reflexes. Repetitive nerve stimulation shows a decremental response, and the serum concentration of antibodies that bind the acetylcholine receptor is increased. Some reports of families with limb-girdle myasthenia affecting two or more siblings have appeared recently. Some of these families may have had the slow-channel syndrome or another genetic myasthenia.

Management. The treatment is the same as for other forms of antibody-positive myasthenia (see Chapter 15).

Slow-Channel Syndrome

The slow-channel syndrome is a genetic disorder of the skeletal muscle acetylcholine receptor (Croxen et al, 2002). Genetic transmission is by autosomal dominant inheritance.

Clinical Features. No symptoms are present at birth. Onset is usually during infancy but delay until adult life occurs. Weakness of the cervical and scapular muscles is often the initial feature. Other common features are exercise intolerance, ophthalmoparesis, and muscle atrophy. Ptosis, bulbar dysfunction, and leg weakness are unusual. The syndrome progresses slowly, and many patients do not come to medical attention until after the first decade.

Diagnosis. Weakness does not respond either to injection or to oral administration of anticholinesterase medication. Two patients were hypersensitive to edrophonium (Tensilon™) and responded with muscarinic side effects. Repetitive nerve stimulation at a rate of 3 stimuli per second causes an abnormal decremental response, and single-nerve stimulation causes a repetitive muscle potential. Muscle biopsy shows type I fiber predominance. Group atrophy, tubular aggregates, and an abnormal endplate configuration are present in some specimens.

Management. Cholinesterase inhibitors, thymectomy, and immunosuppression are not effective. Quinidine sulfate improves strength and fluoxetine is equally beneficial in patients who do not tolerate quinidine (Harper et al, 2003).

Muscular Dystrophies

No agreed upon definition of muscular dystrophy exists. I prefer to use the term to embrace *all genetic myopathies caused by a defect in a structural protein of the muscle* (Figure 7-2). Enzyme deficiencies, such as acid maltase deficiency, are not dystrophies, but rather *metabolic myopathies.*

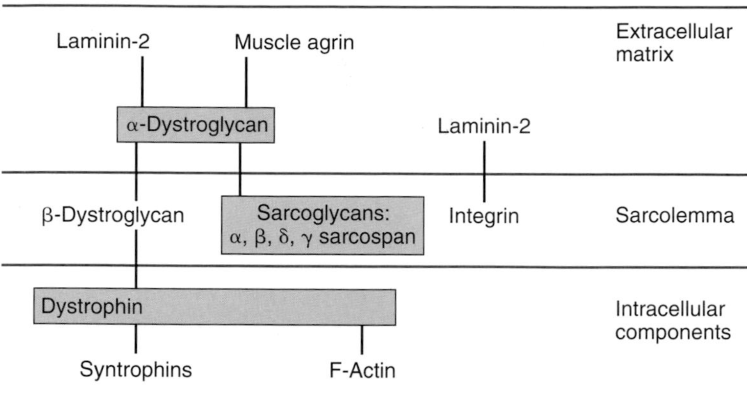

FIGURE 7-2 ■ The structural proteins of muscle fibers.

TABLE 7-2 Autosomal Recessive Limb-Girdle Muscular Dystrophies

LGMD type	Location	Gene product	Clinical features
LGMD-2A	15q	Calpain 3	Onset at 8–15 years, progression variable
LGMD-2B	2p13-16	Dysferlin	Onset at adolescence, mild weakness; gene site is the same as for Miyoshi myopathy
LGMD-2C	13q12	Sarcoglycan	Duchenne-like, severe childhood autosomal recessive muscular dystrophy (SCARMD1)
LGMD-2D	17q21	A-Sarcoglycan (adhalin)	Duchenne-like, severe childhood autosomal recessive muscular dystrophy (SCARMD2)
LGMD-2E	4q12	B-Sarcoglycan	Phenotype between Duchenne and Becker muscular dystrophies
LGMD-2F	5q33-34	Sarcoglycan	Slowly progressive, growth retardation

For most dystrophies, the abnormal gene and gene product is established.

The term *limb-girdle muscular dystrophy* (LGMD) encompasses several muscular dystrophies characterized by progressive proximal muscle weakness (Gordon et al, 2009). The discussion of LGMD transmitted by X-linked inheritance is in the section on Duchenne and Becker Muscular Dystrophy. Not discussed is *Danon disease*, an X-linked cardiomyopathy and skeletal myopathy with onset in late adolescence (Sugie et al, 2002).

The more common forms of LGMD transmitted by autosomal dominant inheritance are facioscapulohumeral dystrophy (FSHD; see Chapter 17), the dominant form of Emery-Dreifuss dystrophy, Bethlem myopathy, and the myopathies associated with caveolinopathies. The caveolinopathies are uncommon and not discussed.

Autosomal recessive types may begin in childhood or adult life. These are distinguishable by the location of the abnormal gene and in some cases by the abnormal gene product (Table 7-2). Deficiencies in the dystrophin-associated glycoprotein complex called the sarcoglycan cause many. Some of the phenotypes are similar to DMD and explain most cases of affected females with a DMD phenotype (see the later section on Severe Childhood Autosomal Recessive Muscular Dystrophy).

Bethlem Myopathy

Bethlem myopathy is a slowly progressive limb-girdle muscular dystrophy transmitted by autosomal dominant inheritance. The abnormal gene links to the collagen type VI gene located on chromosome 21 (Lampe et al, 2007).

Clinical Features. The onset of contractures or weakness is always in the first 2 years. Diminished fetal movements and congenital hypotonia may be present. The usual initial features are congenital flexion contractures of the elbows, ankles, and interphalangeal joints of the last four fingers, but sparing the spine. The contractures are at first mild and unrecognized by parents. Mild proximal weakness and delayed motor development are common. Both the contractures and the weakness progress slowly and produce disability in middle life but

BOX 7-4 Phenotypes Associated with the Xp21 Gene Site

Becker muscular dystrophy
Dilated cardiomyopathy without skeletal muscle weakness
Duchenne muscular dystrophy
Familial X-linked myalgia and cramps (see Chapter 8)
McLeod syndrome (elevated serum creatine kinase concentration, acanthocytosis, and absence of Kell antigen)
Mental retardation and elevated serum creatine kinase
Quadriceps myopathy

do not shorten the life span. Tendon reflexes are normal or depressed. Cardiomyopathy does not occur.

Diagnosis. Molecular genetic testing is available. The serum concentration of CK is normal or slightly elevated, EMG usually shows myopathy, and muscle biopsy shows a nonspecific myopathy.

Management. Physical therapy for contractures is the main treatment.

Dystrophinopathies: Duchenne and Becker Muscular Dystrophy

Duchenne Muscular Dystrophy (DMD) and Becker Muscular Dystrophy (BMD) are variable phenotypic expressions of a gene defect at the Xp21 site (Darras et al, 2011). Several different phenotypes are associated with abnormalities at the Xp21 site (Box 7-4). The abnormal gene product in both DMD and BMD is a reduced muscle content of the structural protein dystrophin. In DMD, the dystrophin content is 0–5 % of normal, and in BMD the dystrophin content is 5–20 % of normal. DMD has a worldwide distribution with a mean incidence of 1 per 3500 male births. The traditional phenotypic difference between the two dystrophies is that BMD has a later age of onset (after age 5 years), unassisted ambulation after age 15 years, and survival into adult life. However, a spectrum of intermediate phenotypes exists depending on dystrophin content.

Among the spectrum of dystrophinopathy phenotypes are *quadriceps myopathy* and *cramps on exercise*. The characteristic features of quadriceps myopathy are slowly progressive weakness of the quadriceps muscle, calf enlargement, and an elevated serum concentration of CK.

Clinical Features. The initial feature in most boys with DMD is a gait disturbance; onset is always before age 5 years and is often before age 3 years. Toe walking and frequent falling are typical complaints. Often, one obtains a retrospective history of delayed achievement of motor milestones. Early symptoms are insidious and likely dismissed by both parents and physicians. Only when proximal weakness causes difficulty in rising from the floor and an obvious waddling gait is medical attention sought. At this stage, mild proximal weakness is present in the pelvic muscles and the Gower sign is present (Figure 7-1). The calf muscles are often large (Figure 7-3). The ankle tendon is tight, and the heels do not quite touch the floor. Tendon reflexes may still be present at the ankle and knee but are difficult to obtain.

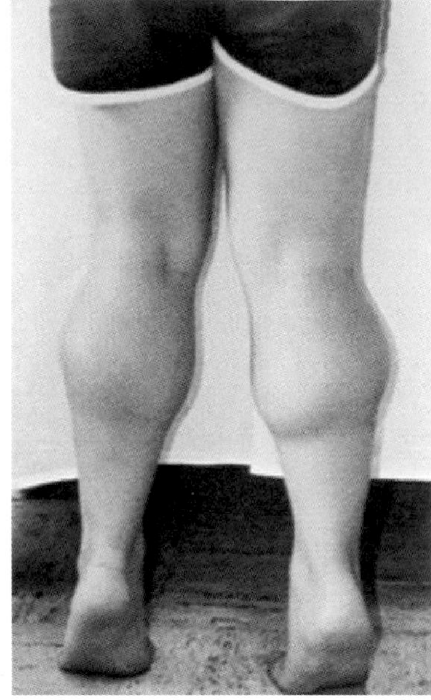

FIGURE 7-3 ■ Enlarged calf muscles in DMD. Enlarged calves also occur in other neuromuscular disorders.

The decline in motor strength is linear throughout childhood. Motor function usually appears static between the ages of 3 and 6 years because of cerebral maturation. Most children maintain their ability to walk and climb stairs until 8 years of age. Between ages 3 and 8, the child shows progressive contractures of the ankle tendons and the iliotibial bands, increased lordosis, a more pronounced waddling gait, and increased toe walking. Gait is more precarious, and the child falls more often. Tendon reflexes at the knees and ankles are lost, and proximal weakness develops in the arms. Considerable variability of expression occurs even within the DMD phenotype. On average, functional ability declines rapidly after 8 years of age because of increasing muscle weakness and contractures. By 9 years of age, some children require a wheelchair, but most can remain ambulatory until age 12 and may continue to stand in braces until age 16.

The range of intelligence scores in boys with DMD shifts downward. While most of these boys function in the normal range, the percentage of those with learning disabilities and cognitive impairment is increased.

Scoliosis occurs in some boys and early use of a wheelchair is not the cause. Deterioration of vital capacity to less than 20 % of normal leads to symptoms of nocturnal hypoventilation. The child awakens frequently and is afraid to sleep. The immediate cause of death is usually a combination of respiratory insufficiency and cardiomyopathy. In some patients with chronic hypoxia, intercurrent infection or aspiration causes respiratory arrest.

Diagnosis. Before 5 years of age, the serum concentration of CK is 10 times the upper limit of normal. The concentration then declines with age at an approximate rate of 20 % per year.

Mutation analysis is the standard for diagnosis, carrier detection, and fetal diagnosis. Intragenic deletions occur in 60 % of affected boys and duplications in another 6 %. Dystrophin analysis of muscle is useful to distinguish DMD from BMD. However, muscle biopsy is not essential when molecular diagnosis is positive.

Management. Although DMD is not curable, it is treatable. Prednisone, 0.75 mg/kg/day, increases strength and function. Treatment goals are to maintain function, prevent contractures, and provide psychological support not only for the child but also for the family. The child must be kept standing and walking as long as possible. Passive stretching exercises prevent contractures, lightweight plastic ankle-foot orthoses maintain the foot in a neutral position during sleep, and long-leg braces maintain walking. Scoliosis is neither preventable nor reversible by external appliances; only surgery is effective to straighten the spine.

Facioscapulohumeral Dystrophy

Although the classification of progressive facioscapulohumeral (FSH) weakness is as a muscular dystrophy, patients with genetic FSH weakness may have histological evidence of myopathy, neuropathy, and inflammation. The FSH syndrome is associated with a deletion within a repeat motif named D4Z4 at chromosome 4q35 (Lemmers 2009). The size of the deletion correlates with the severity of disease. Considerable interfamily and intrafamily heterogeneity exists. A negative family history may result because affected family members are unaware that they have a problem.

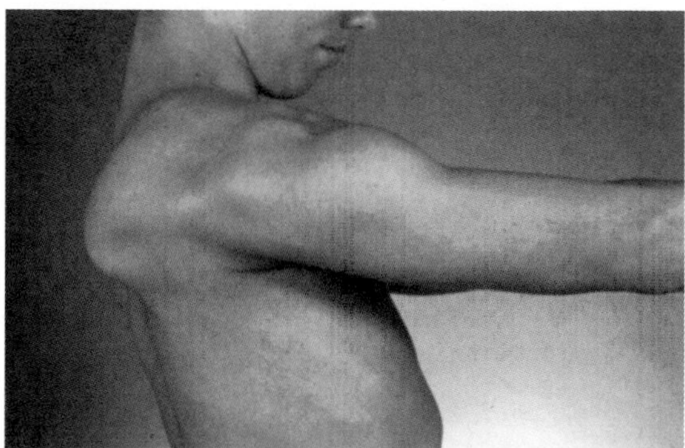

FIGURE 7-4 ■ Asymmetrical scapular winging in facioscapulohumeral dystrophy. (Reproduced with permission from Preston DC, Shapiro BA, Robinson JA: Proximal, distal, and generalized weakness. In: Bradley WG, Daroff R, Fenichel G, Jankovic J, eds. *Neurology in Clinical Practice*, 5th ed. Philadelphia: Elsevier; 2008.)

Clinical Features. Weakness usually begins in the second decade. Initial involvement is often in the shoulder girdle (Figure 7-4), with subsequent spread to the humeral muscles. The deltoid is never affected. Facial weakness is present but often overlooked until late in the course. The progression of weakness is insidious, and delays the diagnosis. Late in the course, leg muscles may be involved. Anterior tibial weakness is most prominent, but proximal weakness may occur as well.

The course of FSH syndrome is variable. Many patients do not become disabled, and their life expectancy is normal. Others are wheelchair-confined in adult life. In the infantile form, progression is always rapid and disability is always severe (see Chapter 17). Deafness and retinal vascular abnormalities are part of the phenotype. The most severe manifestations are retinal telangiectasia, exudation, and detachment (*Coates disease*).

Diagnosis. Molecular genetic testing is the standard for diagnosis. The serum concentration of CK can be normal or increased to five times normal. The EMG may show denervation potentials, myopathic motor units, or both. Histological changes are minimal in many limb muscles and are never diagnostic. Occasional fibers are myopathic, some appear denervated, and inflammatory cells may be present.

Management. No treatment for the weakness is available. Retinal examination for Coates disease is required. Coagulation of retinal telangiectasia prevents blindness.

Proximal Myotonic Dystrophy

Myotonic dystrophy 2 (DM2) or proximal myotonic dystrophy is genetically distinct from the more common distal form (DM1). A CCTG repeat expansion is present at locus 3q21. Unlike DM1, a congenital form does not exist (Day et al, 2003). Onset of symptoms is usually between the third and fourth decade of life, although myotonia may be present in childhood. Therefore, discussion of the disorder is inappropriate for this text except that molecular genetic testing is available for children at risk.

Severe Childhood Autosomal Recessive Muscular Dystrophy

A deficiency of any of the subunits of the sarcoglycan complex of proteins associated with dystrophin causes severe childhood autosomal recessive muscular dystrophy (SCARMD) (see Table 7-2). Sarcoglycan complex defects account for 11 % of children with Duchenne phenotypes.

Clinical Features. SCARMD affects both genders equally. The clinical features are identical to those described for the dystrophinopathies.

Diagnosis. SCARMD is a likely diagnosis in all girls with a Duchenne phenotype and in boys who appear to have DMD but show normal dystrophin content in muscle. Immunohistochemical reagents applied to muscle sections show the absence or presence of the sarcoglycan components. Mutation analysis is available for diagnosis.

Management. Management is similar as for DMD.

Inflammatory Myopathies

The inflammatory myopathies are a heterogeneous group of disorders whose causes are infectious, immune-mediated, or both. A progressive proximal myopathy occurs in adults, but not in children, with acquired immune deficiency syndrome (AIDS). However, the concentration of serum CK is elevated in children with AIDS treated with zidovudine. The description of *acute infectious myositis* is in the section on acute generalized weakness. The conditions discussed in this section are immune-mediated.

Dermatomyositis

Dermatomyositis is a systemic angiopathy in which vascular occlusion and infarction account for all pathological changes observed in muscle, connective tissue, skin, gastrointestinal tract, and small nerves. More than 30 % of adults with dermatomyositis have an underlying malignancy, but cancer is not a factor before the age of 16. The childhood form of dermatomyositis is a relatively homogeneous disease.

Clinical Features. Peak incidence is generally between the ages of 5 and 10 years, but onset may be as early as 4 months. The initial features may be insidious or fulminating. Characteristic of the insidious onset is fever, fatigue, and anorexia in the absence of rash or weakness. These symptoms may persist for weeks or months and suggest an underlying infection. Dermatitis precedes myositis in most children. An erythematous discoloration and edema of the upper eyelids that spread to involve the entire periorbital and malar regions is characteristic. Erythema and edema of the extensor surfaces overlying the joints of the knuckles, elbows, and knees develop later. With time, the skin appears atrophic and scaly. In chronic, long-standing dermatomyositis of childhood, the skin changes may be more disabling than the muscle weakness.

Proximal weakness, stiffness, and pain characterize the myopathy. Weakness generalizes, and flexion contractures develop rapidly and cause joint deformities. Tendon reflexes become increasingly difficult to obtain and finally disappear.

Calcinosis of subcutaneous tissue, especially under discolored areas of skin, occurs in 60 % of children. When severe, it produces an armor-like appearance, termed *calcinosis universalis*, on radiographs. In some children, stiffness is the main initial feature, and skin and muscle symptoms are only minor. In the past, gastrointestinal tract infarction was a leading cause of death. The mortality rate is less than 5 % with modern treatment.

Diagnosis. The combination of fever, rash, myalgia, and weakness is compelling evidence for the diagnosis of dermatomyositis. The serum concentration of CK is usually elevated early in the course. During the time of active myositis, the resting EMG shows increased insertional activity, fibrillations, and positive sharp waves; muscle contraction produces brief, small-amplitude polyphasic potentials. The diagnostic feature on muscle biopsy is perifascicular atrophy (Figure 7-5). Capillary necrosis usually starts at the periphery of the muscle fascicle and causes ischemia in the adjacent muscle fibers. The most profound atrophy occurs in fascicular borders that face large connective tissue septae.

Management. The inflammatory process is active for approximately 2 years. Corticosteroids may suppress the inflammatory response and provide symptomatic relief but do not cure the underlying disease. The best results are obtained when corticosteroids are started early in high doses and are maintained for long periods.

Initiate prednisone at 2 mg/kg/day, not to exceed 100 mg/day. The response follows a predictable pattern. Temperature returns to normal

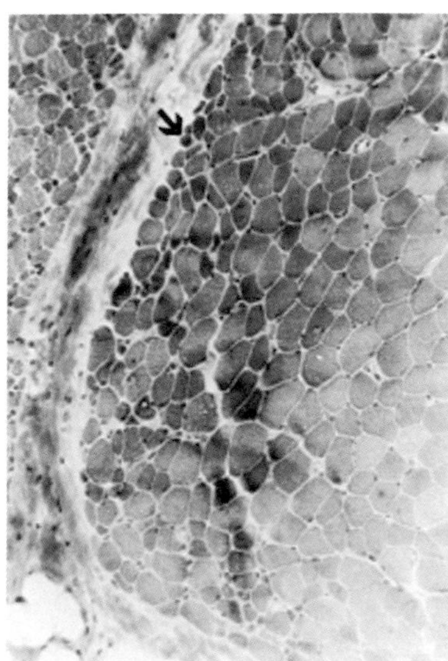

FIGURE 7-5 ■ Perifascicular atrophy in childhood dermatomyositis (trichrome stain). The muscle fibers at the edge of each fascicle are atrophied (arrow).

within 48 hours. The serum CK concentration returns to normal by the second week, and muscle strength increases simultaneously. When these events occur, reduce the prednisone dosage to alternate day therapy to reduce the frequency and severity of corticosteroid-induced side effects. Alternate-day or every-day therapy is equally effective if the doses are large and the treatment maintained. As muscle strength increases, taper the original dosage of alternate-day prednisone by 10 % per month for 5 months. Further reductions are at a rate of 5 % per month. For most children the alternate-day maintenance dosage needed for normal muscle strength and a normal serum CK concentration is 25 % of the starting dosage. When the response is inadequate, add methotrexate. The response of the skin rash to prednisone is variable; in some children, the rash heals completely, but most will have some permanent scarring from the disease.

Although most children show a dramatic improvement and seem normal within 3 months, continue prednisone for a full 2 years. Relapse invariably follows premature discontinuation of treatment. Calcinosis and contractures are more likely to develop in children treated intermittently. Corticosteroids also are useful in the treatment of calcinosis universalis. In addition to prednisone, a well-structured program of physical therapy prevents contractures.

Eighty percent of children with dermatomyositis have a favorable outcome after initiating high-dose prednisone within 4 months of the onset of symptoms. Start oral methotrexate, 10–20 mg/m^2, twice weekly to children who do not respond to high-dose prednisone. Regular monitoring of liver function and the white blood cell count is required.

Plasmapheresis or courses of intravenous immunoglobulin are a valuable adjunct in children whose condition is refractory to corticosteroids. Once the disease becomes inactive, reactivation is unlikely. However, late progression or recurrence may occur and require treatment with an additional 1-year course of corticosteroids.

Polymyositis

Polymyositis without evidence of other target organ involvement is uncommon before puberty. Children with systemic lupus erythematosus may have myalgia and arthralgia as early symptoms, but rarely have muscle weakness at onset. Skin, joint, and systemic manifestations usually precede the onset of myopathy. Polymyositis in children is similar to the disorder in adult life except that malignancy is not a causative factor.

Clinical Features. Polymyositis begins as a symmetric proximal weakness that develops insidiously and progresses to a moderate handicap within weeks to months. The patient may have prolonged periods of stability or even remission that suggest the diagnosis of LGMD because of the slow progress. Tendon reflexes are present early in the course but are less active as muscle bulk is lost. Cardiorespiratory complications are less common in childhood than in adult polymyositis.

Diagnosis. The serum CK concentration is not always increased, but EMG usually shows both myopathic and neuropathic features. Muscle biopsy may show several different patterns of abnormality, and perivascular inflammation may not be present. Instead, one observes features of myopathy, denervation, or both.

Management. The same treatment schedule suggested for childhood dermatomyositis is useful for children with polymyositis. Unfortunately, the response to corticosteroids is far less predictable in polymyositis than in dermatomyositis. Treat those who fail to respond to corticosteroids with methotrexate. Plasmapheresis and intravenous immunoglobulins are reasonable alternatives when other therapies fail.

Metabolic Myopathies

Acid Maltase Deficiency (Pompe Disease)

Acid maltase deficiency is an autosomal recessive deficiency of the lysosomal enzyme acid α-1,4-glucosidase (acid maltase) characterized by skeletal and cardiac myopathy and sometimes encephalopathy. The initial features of acid maltase deficiency may occur in infancy, childhood, or adult life depending on the percentage of residual enzyme deficiency. The enzyme defect is the same regardless of the age of onset, and different ages of onset may occur within the same family. The speed of progression is variable, but the severity of cardiorespiratory involvement correlates with the amount of residual enzyme activity.

Clinical Features. Infants with acid maltase deficiency have glycogen storage in both skeletal and cardiac muscles. Death occurs from cardiac failure during infancy (see Chapter 6). In the childhood form, only skeletal muscle is involved and the main clinical feature is slowly progressive proximal limb weakness. Tendon reflexes are hypoactive or unobtainable. Some children have mild hypertrophy of the calves simulating DMD. The weakness is steadily progressive and leads to disability and respiratory insufficiency by 20 years of age. A late age at onset predicts a more benign course.

Diagnosis. Routine histochemical stains show accumulation of glycogen in lysosomal vacuoles and within the sarcoplasm. The diagnosis is confirmed with biochemical assay of enzyme (acid maltase) activity in muscle or in cultured skin fibroblasts. Complete deficiency is associated with classic infantile onset, while residual activity produces later-onset disease.

Management. Recombinant human enzyme is approved by the United States FDA for replacement therapy, which can prolong survival (Kishnani et al, 2006). The most recent information indicates that α-glucosidase is safe and effective in treating infant onset Pompe disease (Kishnani et al, 2007). Begin enzyme replacement therapy with Myozyme® (alglucosidase alfa) as soon as the diagnosis is established. Myozyme, initiated before age 6 months and before the need for ventilatory assistance, improves ventilator-independent survival and acquisition of motor skills.

Other Carbohydrate Myopathies

Slowly progressive proximal weakness is sometimes the initial features of McArdle disease and debrancher enzyme deficiency. Both disorders are considerations in the differential diagnosis. The initial symptom of these disorders is usually exercise intolerance and is discussed in Chapter 8.

Carnitine Deficiency

Carnitine is an essential cofactor in the transfer of long-chain fatty acids across the inner mitochondrial membrane and modulates the ratio of acyl to acyl-coenzyme A. For this reason, carnitine is one of the supplements often given in cases of suspected mitochondrial disease. Its deficiency causes a failure in the production of energy for metabolism and the storage of triglycerides. It occurs (1) in newborns receiving total parenteral alimentation; (2) in several systemic disorders; (3) as the result of several genetic disorders of organic acid metabolism; (4) in children treated with valproate; (5) as primary genetic defects that cause deficiency of the cellular carnitine transporter; and (6) may occur if not supplemented while receiving ketogenic diet therapy. The myopathic and systemic forms are caused by different genetic loci.

Transmission of the primary genetic defect on chromosome 5q33.1 is by autosomal recessive inheritance. The clinical features may be restricted to skeletal muscle or may include systemic symptoms resembling those of Reye syndrome (see Chapter 2).

Clinical Features. The main clinical feature of muscle carnitine deficiency is the childhood onset of slowly progressive proximal weakness, affecting the legs before, and more severely than, the arms. Sudden exacerbations or fluctuations are superimposed. Occasionally patients have recurrent attacks of myoglobinuria and cardiomyopathy. The cardiomyopathy is usually asymptomatic but is demonstrable on electrocardiography (ECG) and echocardiography.

Diagnosis. The serum concentration of CK is elevated. EMG findings are nonspecific. Muscle biopsy specimens show a vacuolar myopathy with lipid storage mainly in type I fibers. The biochemical measurement of carnitine, both free and total, establishes the diagnosis.

Management. Dietary therapy with L-carnitine is usually effective. Diarrhea and a fishy odor are the most common side effects. The usual dosage is 100 mg/kg/day in three or four divided doses.

Other Lipid Myopathies

Children with progressive proximal weakness associated with lipid storage in muscle and normal carnitine content usually have a disturbance of mitochondrial fatty acid oxidation. These disorders are genetically heterogeneous and difficult to distinguish from other mitochondrial myopathies.

Clinical Features. Progressive proximal weakness begins any time from early childhood to adolescence. The legs are affected first and then the arms. Exercise intolerance is noted, and, in some cases, the ingestion of fatty foods leads to nausea and vomiting. The pattern and progression of weakness may simulate those of DMD even to the presence of calf hypertrophy. Limb weakness is steadily progressive, and cardiomyopathy may develop.

Diagnosis. The serum concentration of CK is markedly elevated. EMG findings are abnormal and are consistent with a myopathic process. Muscle biopsy is critical to diagnosis. Type I muscle fibers contain fatty droplets. Carnitine and carnitine palmitoyl transferase concentrations are normal.

Management. Patients with fat intolerance may show improvement on a diet free of long-chain fatty acids.

Endocrine Myopathies

Progressive proximal limb weakness may occur in children with hyperthyroidism, hypothyroidism, hyperparathyroidism, hypoparathyroidism, hyperadrenalism, and hypoadrenalism.

Clinical Features. Systemic features of endocrine disease usually predate the onset of weakness. However, weakness may be the initial feature in primary or secondary hypoparathyroidism and in thyroid disorders. Weakness is much more prominent in the legs than in the arms. Tendon reflexes, even in weak muscles, are normal or diminished but generally are not absent.

Diagnosis. The serum concentration of CK is typically normal. EMG is not useful for diagnosis. Many endocrinopathies produce both neuropathy and myopathy. In Cushing disease and in hyperparathyroidism, muscle histological studies show type II fiber atrophy. Other endocrinopathies show nonspecific myopathic changes that vary with the severity of disease.

Management. These disorders should be evaluated in cases of weakness of unknown etiology as they are correctable causes of weakness. Treating the underlying endocrinopathy corrects the weakness.

PROGRESSIVE DISTAL WEAKNESS

Neuropathy is the most common cause of progressive distal weakness (Box 7-5). Among the slowly progressive neuropathies of childhood, hereditary disorders are far more common than acquired disorders. The only common acquired neuropathy is acute inflammatory demyelinating polyradiculoneuropathy (Guillain-Barré syndrome), in which weakness evolves rapidly.

BOX 7-5 Progressive Distal Weakness

SPINAL CORD DISORDERS (SEE CHAPTER 12)

MOTOR NEURON DISEASES

- Juvenile amyotrophic lateral sclerosis
- Monomelic (see Chapter 13)
- Spinal muscular atrophies
  - Autosomal dominant forms
  - Autosomal recessive forms

NEUROPATHIES

- Hereditary motor sensory neuropathies
  - Charcot-Marie-Tooth disease
  - Familial amyloid neuropathy (see Chapter 9)
  - Giant axonal neuropathy (16q24)
  - Other genetic neuropathies
  - Other lipid neuropathies
  - Pyruvate dehydrogenase deficiency (see Chapter 10)
  - Refsum disease
  - Sulfatide lipidoses: metachromatic leukodystrophy
- Neuropathies with systemic diseases
  - Drug-induced*
  - Systemic vasculitis*
  - Toxins*
  - Uremia*
- Idiopathic neuropathy
  - Chronic axonal neuropathy*
  - Chronic demyelinating neuropathy*

MYOPATHIES

- Autosomal dominant childhood myopathy
- Autosomal dominant infantile myopathy
- Autosomal recessive distal (Miyoshi) myopathy
- Inclusion body myopathies
- Myotonic dystrophy

SCAPULO (HUMERAL) PERONEAL SYNDROME

- Emery-Dreifuss muscular dystrophy type 1
- Emery-Dreifuss muscular dystrophy type 2
- Scapuloperoneal myopathy
- Scapuloperoneal neuronopathy

*Denotes the most common conditions and the ones with disease modifying treatments

Diagnosis in Neuropathy and Neuronopathy

The initial feature of neuropathy in children is progressive symmetric distal weakness affecting the legs and then the arms. When sensation is disturbed, dysesthesias are experienced. These consist of tingling, "pins and needles," or a burning sensation in the feet. Dysesthesias usually occur in acquired but not in hereditary neuropathies. The progression of weakness and sensory loss are in a distal to proximal direction (glove and

TABLE 7-3 **Electrodiagnosis in Neuropathy**

	Neuronopathy	Axonal	Demyelinating
Fasciculations	+++	+++	+
Denervation potentials	+++	+++	+
Reduced number of motor units	+++	+++	0
High-amplitude potentials	+++	+++	0
Slow motor velocity	0	+	+++
Reduced sensory potentials	0	+	+++

0, absent; +, rare; +++, common.

stocking distribution). Tendon reflexes are lost early, especially when sensory fibers are affected.

An important first step in diagnosis is to determine the primary site of the disorder: cell body (anterior horn cell), nerve axon, or myelin. Electrodiagnosis accomplishes localization (Table 7-3). In primary disorders of the cell body (neuronopathy), resting muscle shows fibrillations and fasciculations, which is a sign of denervation. Voluntary contraction activates reduced numbers of motor unit potentials whose amplitude is normal or increased because of collateral reinnervation. Motor conduction nerve velocity is normal or only slightly diminished, and the amplitude of sensory action potentials is normal. In axonopathies, the EMG shows fibrillations at rest and a reduced number of motor unit potentials that are normal or increased in amplitude. High-amplitude potentials may be polyphasic. Motor nerve conduction velocity slows and sensory action potentials have reduced amplitude. Marked slowing of motor conduction velocity and reduced amplitude of sensory evoked potentials characterize demyelinating neuropathies. EMG findings may be normal early in the course.

Neuronopathy

Juvenile Amyotrophic Lateral Sclerosis

Amyotrophic lateral sclerosis 2 (ALS2)-related disorders are a group of motor neuron diseases affecting mainly the upper motor neuron but include forms with lower motor neuron involvement (Bertini et al, 2011).

Clinical Features. ALS2-related disorders involve retrograde degeneration of the upper motor neurons of the pyramidal tracts and comprise a clinical spectrum that includes pure upper motor neuron disease (*infantile ascending hereditary spastic paraplegia*) to juvenile forms without lower motor neuron disease involvement (*juvenile primary lateral sclerosis*). Characteristic of juvenile amyotrophic lateral sclerosis is onset of spasticity with increased reflexes and sustained clonus of the legs in the first 2 years, progressive weakness and spasticity of the arms by age 8 years, followed by wheelchair dependence and progressive severe spastic tetraparesis and a pseudobulbar palsy.

Diagnosis. Molecular genetic testing is available.

Management. Only supportive therapy is available.

Spinal Muscular Atrophy, Distal

The distal form of spinal muscular atrophy is also called Charcot-Marie-Tooth neuropathy type 2D (Bird, 2012).

Clinical Features. Onset is in adolescence. The earliest features in many individuals are transitory cramping and pain in the hands on exposure to cold and cramping in calf muscles on exertion. Bilateral weakness and atrophy of thenar and first dorsal interosseus muscles follows with sparing of the hypothenar eminence until later. The atrophy usually arrests, but may progress to involve the legs.

Diagnosis. Molecular genetic testing is not readily available and electrodiagnosis is critical to distinguish these disorders from peripheral neuropathies. Motor nerve conduction velocity is normal despite total denervation of the small muscles of the foot. Sensory evoked potentials are also normal. The serum concentration of CK is usually normal but may be mildly elevated. Muscle biopsy specimens show nonspecific changes of denervation, and the sural nerve is normal.

Management. Hand and leg braces may help to prolong function.

Neuropathy

Charcot-Marie-Tooth Disease

The terms *Charcot-Marie-Tooth* (CMT) disease and *hereditary motor and sensory neuropathy* (HMSN) are interchangeable terms (Bird, 2011).

Each encompasses several genetic neuropathies that are further divisible based on molecular and linkage findings. The typical patient has progressive distal weakness, mild to moderate sensory loss, depressed or absent tendon reflexes, and high-arched feet.

Charcot-Marie-Tooth 1 (CMT1): Demyelinating Type. CMT1 (HMSN-I) is an autosomal dominant form of demyelinating neuropathy. It accounts for up to 50% of all CMT cases (Bird, 2012). The genetic abnormality may consist of cases with DNA duplications of the peripheral myelin protein gene (*PMP2*) on chromosome 17p (CMT1A) or an abnormality of the *MPZ* gene on chromosome 1q22 (CMT1B). The 17p11 duplication causes trisomic expression of the peripheral myelin protein, PMP-22. Deletion in the 17p11 region with monosomic expression of PMP-22 is the cause of *hereditary polyneuropathy with liability to pressure palsies* (see Chapter 13).

Clinical Features. The subtypes are clinically indistinguishable and the molecular findings are the sole basis of designation.

CMT1 is not usually a severe disorder in childhood. The main early features are pes cavus, weakness of the peroneal muscles, and diminished reactivity of the ankle tendon reflex. With time the anterior tibial as well as the peroneal muscles become weak, producing foot drop. The calf muscles become weak in some families but may hypertrophy in some families with the 17p duplication. Eventually, usually after 20 years of age, weakness spreads to the proximal muscles of the legs and hands. Scoliosis is unusual. Cramps with exercise are present in weak muscles. Position sense becomes impaired in the fingers and toes. Dysesthesias are never a problem. Hip dysplasia may be an associated feature.

Peripheral nerve enlargement occurs in adults but not in children. Repeated episodes of demyelination and remyelination are the cause of enlargement.

Diagnosis. Diagnosis relies on characteristic clinical findings and a family history of the disease. Motor nerve conduction velocities are less than 50% of normal in affected individuals. The cerebrospinal fluid protein content is usually normal in children but may be elevated in adults. A DNA-based test is available for CMT1A that detects more than 95% of cases. Persons with CMT1A have three copies of the *PMP-22* gene.

Management. No specific treatment is available, but proper foot care may minimize discomfort and maximize function. Shoes should be roomy and soft to prevent rubbing against bony prominences. Footwear molded to the shape of the foot is especially useful. When foot drop is present, a lightweight plastic ankle-foot orthosis that fits into the patient's own shoe not only lifts the foot but also prevents turning and injury of the ankle.

Charcot-Marie-Tooth 2 (CMT2): Neuronal Type. Genetic transmission of CMT2 is by autosomal dominant inheritance. CMT2 accounts for 20–40% of CMT cases. The phenotype clinically resembles CMT1, except that the nerve conduction velocity is either normal or mildly abnormal. Several subtypes are recognized and several different genetic abnormalities are associated with a similar phenotype.

Clinical Features. The clinical features of CMT2 overlap with those of CMT1. In general, patients with CMT2 are less disabled and have less sensory loss than do patients with CMT1. Distal weakness begins in the legs and can be asymmetric. Later, the hands are affected. Tendon reflexes are obtainable to a later age in CMT2 as compared to CMT1. Progression of symptoms is slow, and disability does not occur until middle adult life.

Prominent vocal cord and respiratory (intercostal and diaphragmatic) muscle paralysis occurs in CMT2C. The onset is insidious and difficult to date precisely. The initial symptom may be hoarseness or frequent tripping, but neonatal respiratory disturbance also occurs. The course is one of progressive peroneal atrophy with minimal sensory deficit. CMT2D includes prominent weakness and atrophy of the hands.

Diagnosis. The cerebrospinal fluid protein content is normal, as is the serum concentration of CK. Because the pathological process is primarily axonal rather than demyelinating, motor nerve conduction velocities are either normal or only mildly slowed (60% or more of normal). The EMG shows a denervation pattern in affected muscles. DNA-based testing is clinically available for almost all forms.

Management. Management is the same as for CMT1.

Charcot-Marie-Tooth 4 (CMT4). CMT4 comprises several different disorders characterized by progressive motor and sensory neuropathy and autosomal recessive inheritance. Genetic identification of all loci and most gene products is complete.

Clinical Features. Affected people have the typical CMT phenotype. Distal muscle weakness develops in the second year, and proximal muscles are involved by age 10 years. Associated findings may include mild sensory loss, absent tendon reflexes, skeletal deformities, and scoliosis.

Diagnosis. All members of the CMT4 group are demyelinating neuropathies with normal protein concentrations in the spinal fluid. Nerve conduction velocities are slow (15–17 m/sec). Molecular genetic diagnosis is clinically available for all forms.

Management. The treatment plan is similar to that for other CMTs.

Charcot-Marie-Tooth X (CMTX). Inheritance of CMTX is as an X-linked dominant trait. Mutations in the connexin 32 genes are associated.

Clinical Features. Affected males have a moderate to severe peripheral neuropathy that tends to be more severe than that seen in CMT1A. Females have a mild neuropathy or are asymptomatic. Symptoms develop in males during the first decade. The initial physical findings are depressed or absent tendon reflexes and foot drop. Mild to moderate sensory loss in the feet and hearing loss may be associated.

Diagnosis. Detection of CMTX is by a DNA-based test of the connexin 32 gene. The test detects 100 % of cases and is commercially available.

Management. The treatment plan is similar to that for other CMTs.

Other Genetic Neuropathies

Giant Axonal Neuropathy. Giant axonal neuropathy (GAN) is a rare disorder transmitted by autosomal recessive inheritance (Kuhlenbäumer & Timmerman, 2009). The cause is in the *GAN* gene encoding gigaxonin. The gene maps to chromosome 16q24.1. The underlying defect is one of generalized intermediate filament organization, with neurofilaments predominantly affected. Central and peripheral axons are both affected.

Clinical Features. Patients with GAN have a severe early-onset peripheral motor and sensory neuropathy and characteristic tightly curled hair that differs markedly from that of the parents. Patients often show signs of central nervous system involvement including cognitive impairment, cerebellar signs (ataxia, nystagmus, dysarthria), and pyramidal tract signs.

Both genders are at equal risk and many are from consanguineous marriages. Affected children are pale and thin and have a chronic polyneuropathy accompanied by kinky pale hair. Gait impairment usually begins by 3 years of age but can appear later. Symmetric distal atrophy of leg muscles is a constant early feature. Impairment of vibratory and proprioceptive sensations in the legs is profound and diminished or absent tendon reflex response is the rule. Central involvement may result in cerebellar dysfunction, dementia, optic atrophy, and cranial neuropathies.

Diagnosis. Genetic diagnosis is only on a research basis. Sural nerve biopsy shows enlarged axons filled with disrupted neurofilaments surrounded by thin or fragmented myelin sheaths. Large myelinated nerve fibers are mainly affected. Magnetic resonance imaging (MRI) of the brain may show increased signal intensity of the white matter.

Management. Treatment is symptomatic.

Sulfatide Lipidosis: Metachromatic Leukodystrophy. Metachromatic leukodystrophy (MLD) is an autosomal recessive inherited disorder of myelin metabolism caused by deficient activity of the enzyme arylsulfatase A (Fluharty, 2011). Infantile, juvenile, and adult forms are recognized. This section only discusses the late infantile form.

Clinical Features. After a period of normal development, gait disturbances develop, usually before 2 years of age but sometimes not until age 4. Initial features may be spasticity, ataxia, or distal weakness of the feet with loss of the ankle tendon reflex. Progressive weakness of all limbs results in generalized hypotonia and hyporeflexia. Weakness, dementia, and optic atrophy are progressive. Death occurs within several years of onset.

Diagnosis. At the time of initial leg weakness, the protein content of the cerebrospinal fluid is elevated and motor nerve conduction velocities reduced. Head MRI shows subcortical demyelination with a posterior predominance of white matter abnormalities and sparing of the subcortical U-fibers. MLD is suggested by arylsulfatase A enzyme activity in leukocytes that is less than 10 % of normal controls using the Baum-type assay. Molecular genetic testing confirms the diagnosis.

Management. Bone marrow transplantation early in the course of disease may slow its progress.

Other Lipid Disorders. Peripheral neuropathy occurs in globoid cell leukodystrophy (Krabbe disease), but is not as prominent a feature as in metachromatic leukodystrophy. The usual initial features are psychomotor retardation and irritability rather than flaccid weakness (see Chapter 5). Tendon reflexes may be absent or hyperactive, and half of cases show slowing of motor nerve conduction velocity. The cerebrospinal fluid protein concentration is always elevated.

Progeria, small stature, ataxia, retinitis pigmentosa, deafness, and cognitive decline are characteristic of *Cockayne syndrome* (see Chapter 16). A primary segmental demyelinating neuropathy is present in 10–20 % of cases but is not an initial symptom. The main features are hyporeflexia and reduced motor nerve conduction velocity. Other disorders of lipid metabolism in which demyelinating neuropathy is present, but not an important feature, include Niemann-Pick disease, Gaucher disease, and Farber disease.

Idiopathic Axonal Neuropathy

Clinical Features. Most axonal neuropathies are either hereditary or toxic. Glue sniffing is an example of a toxic cause. Some children have a progressive axonal neuropathy for which no cause can be determined. Progressive weakness of the feet, with or without sensory impairment, is often the initial feature. Electrodiagnostic studies in parents and siblings sometimes establish a hereditary basis.

Diagnosis. The EMG shows fibrillations and fasciculations, but motor nerve conduction velocity is normal or only mildly delayed. The protein content of the cerebrospinal fluid is normal.

Management. Children with idiopathic axonal neuropathies usually have a slowly progressive weakness unresponsive to corticosteroids. However, occasional patients do respond, and patients with a subacute progression deserve a 2-month trial of prednisone. These responsive cases may be variants of chronic inflammatory demyelinating neuropathy, in which both axonal involvement and demyelination are present.

Neuropathies with Systemic Disease

Drug-Induced Neuropathy. Several medications can cause neuropathy. Such neuropathies are often subclinical and detected only by electrodiagnosis or because of loss of the ankle tendon reflex. Drugs that commonly produce clinical evidence of motor and sensory neuropathy are isoniazid, nitrofurantoin, vincristine, and zidovudine. Vitamin B6 (pyridoxine) has been implicated as a potential cause of neuropathy in several case reports; however, it was often being used in patients with tuberculosis on isoniazid therapy, or with other emaciating conditions, which may have been the true underlying cause of the neuropathy. I have not seen the development of neuropathy in cases of pyridoxine-dependent epilepsy (which requires high doses of pyridoxine for treatment), or when pyridoxine is used empirically to treat irritability.

Isoniazid

Clinical Features. The initial symptoms are numbness and paresthesias of the fingers and toes. If treatment is continued, superficial sensation diminishes in a glove-and-stocking pattern. Distal limb weakness follows and is associated with tenderness of the muscles and burning dysesthesias. Reduced or absent ankle tendon reflexes are expected.

Diagnosis. Suspect isoniazid neuropathy whenever neuropathy develops in children taking the drug.

Management. Isoniazid interferes with pyridoxine metabolism and produces neuropathy by causing a pyridoxine deficiency state. The administration of pyridoxine along with isoniazid prevents neuropathy without interfering with antituberculous activity. The longer the symptoms progress, the longer the time until recovery. Although pyridoxine can prevent the development of neuropathy, it has little effect on the speed of recovery once neuropathy is established.

Nitrofurantoin

Clinical Features. Nitrofurantoin neuropathy most often occurs in patients with impaired renal function. A high blood concentration of nitrofurantoin causes an axonal neuropathy. The initial features are usually paresthesias, followed within a few days or weeks by glove-and-stocking sensory loss and weakness of distal muscles. Pure motor neuropathy is occasionally present.

Diagnosis. Suspect nitrofurantoin neuropathy in any child with neuropathy taking the drug. It may be difficult to distinguish from uremic neuropathy.

Management. Complete recovery usually follows complete cessation of the drug. Occasional patients have developed complete paralysis and death despite discontinuation of nitrofurantoin.

Vincristine

Clinical Features. Neuropathy is an expected complication of vincristine therapy. The ankle tendon reflex is lost first; later, other tendon reflexes become less reactive and may be lost. The first symptoms are paresthesias, often starting in the fingers rather than the feet and progressing to mild loss of superficial sensation but not position sense. Weakness follows sensory loss as evidenced by clumsiness in the hands and cramps in the feet. Distal muscles are affected more than proximal muscles and extensors more than flexors. Weakness may progress rapidly, with loss of ambulation in a few weeks. The initial weakness may be asymmetric and suggests mononeuropathy multiplex.

Diagnosis. Electrodiagnostic features are consistent with axonal neuropathy, fibrillations and fasciculations on needle EMG, but with normal motor nerve conduction velocity.

Management. The neuropathy is dose related, and usually the patient recovers 1 to 3 months after discontinuing drug.

Toxins. Several heavy metals, inorganic chemicals, and insecticides produce polyneuropathies in children. In adults, industrial exposure, agricultural exposure, or attempted homicide are the usual causes of heavy metal poisoning. Small children who have a single accidental ingestion are more likely to have acute symptoms of systemic disease or central nervous system dysfunction than a slowly progressive neuropathy. Sometimes, progressive distal weakness is an early sign in older children addicted to sniffing glue or gasoline. Even in these cases, symptoms of central nervous system dysfunction are usually present.

Uremia. Some degree of neuropathy occurs at some time or in many children undergoing long-term periodic hemodialysis. Uremic neuropathy is more common in males than in females, but the reason for the gender bias is unknown.

Clinical Features. The earliest symptoms may be muscle cramps in the hands and feet, burning feet or restless legs, and loss of the ankle tendon reflex. After the initial sensory symptoms, the disorder progresses to a severe distal, symmetric, mixed motor and sensory polyneuropathy affecting the legs more than the arms. The rate of progression is variable and may be fulminating or may evolve over several months.

A pure motor neuropathy develops in some children with uremia. Symptoms begin after starting hemodialysis. The rapid progression of distal weakness in all limbs does not respond to dialysis but may reverse after renal transplantation.

Diagnosis. Uremia causes an axonal neuropathy, but chronic renal failure causes segmental demyelination that is out of proportion to axonal changes. Therefore, repeated measures of motor nerve conduction velocity are a useful way to monitor neuropathy progression. Slow conduction velocities are present even before clinical symptoms occur. Reduced creatine clearance correlates with slowing of the conduction velocity.

Management. Dialysis reverses early neuropathy. Patients with severe neuropathy rarely recover fully despite adequate treatment.

Vasculitis and Vasculopathy. Polyneuropathy and mononeuropathy multiplex are relatively common neurological complications of vasculitis in adults, but not in children. Children with lupus erythematosus are generally sicker than are adults, but peripheral neuropathy is neither an initial nor a prominent feature of their disease. Motor and sensory neuropathies occur in children with chronic juvenile rheumatoid arthritis.

Myopathies

Hereditary Distal Myopathies

The hereditary distal myopathies, as a group, are uncommon except for myotonic dystrophy (Saperstein et al, 2001). Not discussed here are forms that usually have an adult onset.

Autosomal Dominant Childhood-Onset Distal Myopathy. This clinical phenotype most resembles the syndromes described by Gower and later by Laing. The gene site is on chromosome 14q11 and encodes the heavy chain of myosin (Laing et al, 1995).

Clinical Features. Characteristics common to reported families are onset in the second or third year of life and selective wasting and weakness of the anterior tibial and extensor digitorum longus muscles (Hedera et al, 2003; Mastaglia, 2002). The course is slowly progressive, and involves the hand extensors, neck flexor, and abdominal muscles at later stages. Some patients develop tremor.

Age at onset is after 4 years and may delay to the third decade. The initial weakness is in the toe and ankle extensors and the neck flexors. Weakness of the finger extensors develops years later, with relative sparing of the finger flexors and intrinsic hand muscles. Some proximal limb muscles become weak late in life without impairing walking.

Diagnosis. EMG findings are consistent with a myopathic process. Muscle biopsy specimens show variation in fiber size, nuclear clumps, moth-eaten type I fibers, and small-angulated type II fibers. The serum concentration of CK is one to three times the upper limit of normal.

Management. Treatment is symptomatic.

Autosomal Recessive Distal (Dysferlin) Myopathy. Two main phenotypes characterize the dysferlinopathies, one with limb-girdle weakness, and the other with distal weakness (Aoki, 2010). *Miyoshi myopathy* is the distal weakness phenotype and LGMD type 2B (LGMD2B) is the proximal weakness phenotype.

The two disorders are allelic and both phenotypes occur in members of the same family.

Clinical Features. Age at onset of Miyoshi myopathy is in adolescence. The initial weakness is in the distal parts of the legs, especially the gastrocnemius and soleus muscles. Over a period of years, the weakness and atrophy spread to the thighs and gluteal muscles. The forearms may become mildly atrophic with decrease in grip strength, but sparing the small muscles of the hands. Ambulation is usually preserved.

Diagnosis. The peculiar pattern of calf atrophy is almost diagnostic. The serum CK concentration is at least five times the upper limit of normal; this distinguishes Miyoshi myopathy from the other distal myopathies. Molecular genetic testing is available

Management. Most patients are not greatly impaired and do not require assistive devices.

Inclusion Body Myopathy 2. The presence of vacuolar degeneration of muscle fibers, accompanied by intrafiber clusters of paired helical filaments (*inclusion bodies*), defines inclusion body myopathies. When inflammation is an associated feature, the term *inclusion body myositis* is applied. In general, inclusion body myositis is a sporadic disorder with onset after age 30 years, whereas *inclusion body myopathy* is hereditary, transmitted by autosomal recessive inheritance, with onset during adolescence. *Nonaka myopathy* is the term applied in hereditary inclusion body myopathy in Japan.

Clinical Features. The onset of weakness is in the second or third decade. The initial symptom is difficulty with gait due to foot drop. The weakness progresses to involve the thigh and hand muscles within several years. Neck flexor and shoulder girdle weakness, with relative sparing of the triceps, is a late feature. Quadriceps sparing, even at advanced stages, is common but not constant.

Diagnosis. The serum concentration of CK is normal or only mildly elevated. Light microscopy characteristically shows muscle fibers with single or multiple vacuoles rimmed with basophilic material. Electron microscopy shows the filamentous inclusions, usually adjacent to vacuoles. Molecular genetic testing is available.

Management. The weakness does not respond to corticosteroid or immunosuppressive therapy. Treatment is symptomatic.

Myotonic Dystrophy. Myotonic dystrophy (DM1) is a multisystem disorder transmitted by autosomal dominant inheritance with variable penetrance. An unstable DNA region on chromosome 19 that can amplify 50 to several thousand times causes the disease (Bird, 2011). Amplification (increasing size of trinucleotide repeats) occurs in successive generations and correlates with more severe disease with earlier onset (anticipation). A neonatal form occurs in children born to mothers with myotonic dystrophy (see Chapter 6).

A proximal form of myotonic dystrophy (DM2) is a distinct genetic disorder and considered in the section on distal weakness.

Clinical Features. The onset of symptoms is usually during adolescence or later. The major features are myotonia (a disturbance characterized by decreased muscle relaxation after contraction), weakness in the face and distal portion of the limbs, cataracts, frontal baldness, and multiple endocrinopathies. The pattern of muscle atrophy in the face is so stereotypical that all patients with the disease have a similar facies. The face is long and thin because of wasting of the temporal and masseter muscles, and the neck is thin because of atrophy of the sternocleidomastoid muscles. The eyelids and corners of the mouth droop and the lower part of the face sags, producing the appearance of sadness.

Although seeking medical treatment is rare before adolescence, myotonia is usually present in childhood and is detectable by EMG, if not by clinical examination. Percussion of muscle demonstrates myotonia. When percussed, the thenar eminence dimples and remains dimpled at the site of percussion. In addition, the thumb adducts and remains in that position for several seconds. The physician can also detect myotonia by shaking hands with the patient, who has difficulty letting go and releases the grip in part by flexing the wrist to force the finger flexors to open.

Some patients have little or no evidence of muscle weakness, only cataracts, frontal baldness, or endocrine disturbances. However, the presence of muscle weakness before age 20 years is likely to be relentlessly progressive, causing severe distal weakness in the hands and feet by adult life. Smooth and cardiac muscle involvement may be present. Disturbed gastrointestinal motility is characteristic. Endocrine disturbances include testicular atrophy, infertility in women, hyperinsulinism, diabetes, hypothyroidism, adrenal atrophy, and disturbances in growth hormone secretion.

Diagnosis. The basis for the diagnosis of myotonic dystrophy is usually the clinical features, the family history, and molecular genetic studies. EMG and muscle biopsy are unnecessary. Studies to show the presence and number of trinucleotide repeats are commercially available and are the best method to detect asymptomatic individuals and for prenatal diagnosis.

Management. Myotonia frequently responds to drugs that stabilize membranes: mexiletine is probably the most effective; procainamide, phenytoin, and carbamazepine are also useful. However, weakness and not myotonia disable the patient. Braces for foot drop are usually required as the disease progresses.

Scapulo (Humeral) Peroneal Syndromes

Progressive weakness and atrophy affecting the proximal muscles of the arms and the distal muscles of the legs may result from neuronopathy or myopathy. Some patients with dominantly inherited scapulo (humeral) peroneal syndromes are a variant phenotype of FSH syndrome, whereas others do not show linkage to the FSH locus on chromosome 4q35.

Emery-Dreifuss Muscular Dystrophy Type 1 (EDMD1). Genetic transmission of EDMD1 is by X-linked recessive inheritance. The abnormal gene product is emerin (Bonne et al, 2010).

Clinical Features. The onset of symptoms is between 5 and 15 years of age. The earliest feature of the disease is the development of contractures in the flexors of the elbows, the ankle tendon, and the extensors of the hand. This is followed by muscle weakness and wasting in the biceps and triceps muscles and then in the deltoid and other shoulder muscles. The peroneal muscles are severely affected. Calf hypertrophy does not occur. The progression of symptoms is slow, and the condition usually stabilizes by 20 years of age. In some patients, however, weakness progresses into adult life and ambulation is eventually lost.

All patients develop a cardiomyopathy that leads to permanent atrial paralysis. Bradycardia and syncope may precede muscle weakness or be delayed until the third decade. The earliest symptom is pathological fatigue on minor activity. A permanent pacemaker is required at the first sign of cardiac involvement. Sudden death is common. Female heterozygotes develop a cardiomyopathy late in life and require a pacemaker. They do not develop skeletal muscle weakness.

Diagnosis. Neither EMG nor muscle biopsy is diagnostic. Molecular genetic testing establishes the diagnosis.

Management. Treatment is for the skeletal muscle weakness is symptomatic. Early implantation of a permanent pacemaker is lifesaving.

Emery-Dreifuss Muscular Dystrophy Types 2 and 3 (EDMD2 and EDMD3). Transmission of EDMD2 is by autosomal dominant inheritance and transmission of EDMD3 is by autosomal recessive inheritance. The responsible gene encodes lamins A and C (Bonne et al, 2010). The phenotype is the same as for EDMD1.

BOX 7-6 Acute Generalized Weakness

INFECTIOUS DISORDERS

- Acute infectious myositis
- Acute inflammatory polyradiculoneuropathy* (Guillain-Barré syndrome)
- Acute axonal neuropathies
- Chronic inflammatory polyradiculoneuropathy* (CIDP)
- Enterovirus infections

METABOLIC DISORDERS

- Acute intermittent porphyria (see Chapter 9)
- Hereditary tyrosinemia (see Chapter 9)

NEUROMUSCULAR BLOCKADE

- Botulism*
- Corticosteroid-induced quadriplegia*
- Intensive Care Unit weakness
- Tick paralysis*

PERIODIC PARALYSIS

- Andersen-Tawil syndrome
- Familial hypokalemic* (FPPI)
- Familial hyperkalemic* (FPPII)
- Familial normokalemic (FPPIII)

*Denotes the most common conditions and the ones with disease modifying treatments

ACUTE GENERALIZED WEAKNESS

The sudden onset or rapid evolution of generalized flaccid weakness, in the absence of symptoms of encephalopathy, is always due to disorders of the motor unit (Box 7-6). Among these disorders, acute inflammatory demyelinating polyradiculoneuropathy (Guillain-Barré syndrome) is by far the most common.

The combination of acute weakness and rhabdomyolysis, as evidenced by myoglobinuria, indicates that muscle is degenerating rapidly. This may occur in some disorders of carbohydrate and fatty acid metabolism (see Chapter 8), after intense and unusual exercise, in some cases of infectious and idiopathic polymyositis, and in intoxication with alcohol and cocaine. Death from renal failure is a possible outcome in patients with rhabdomyolysis. Intravenous fluids are needed to prevent this outcome.

Infectious Disease

Acute Infectious Myositis

Acute myositis in children most often follows influenza or other respiratory infections (Mackay et al, 1999). Boys are more often affected than are girls.

Clinical Features. Ordinarily, prodromal respiratory symptoms persist for 3 to 8 days before the onset of severe symmetric muscle pain and weakness, which may cause severe disability within 24 hours. Pain and tenderness are most severe in the calf muscles. Tendon reflexes are present.

Diagnosis. The serum concentration of CK is elevated, usually more than 10 times the upper limit of normal.

Management. Spontaneous resolution of the myositis occurs almost immediately. Bed rest is required for 2 to 7 days until pain subsides, after which the patient recovers completely. Intravenous fluids at rates higher than maintenance are needed to prevent renal failure when rhabdomyolysis with high CK levels is detected.

Acute Inflammatory Demyelinating Polyradiculoneuropathy (AIDP)

AIDP, more commonly called Guillain-Barré syndrome (GBS), is an acute monophasic demyelinating neuropathy. Peripheral nerves are the target of an abnormal immune response. More than half of patients describe an antecedent viral infection. Respiratory tract infections are more common than gastrointestinal infections (Paradiso et al, 1999). Enteritis caused by specific strains of *Campylobacter jejuni* 19 is more often the inciting disease in the acute axonal form of GBS than in the demyelinating form.

Clinical Features. The natural history of AIDP in children is substantially the same as in adults. The clinical features are sufficiently stereotypical that establishing the diagnosis usually does not require laboratory confirmation. This is especially important because the characteristic laboratory features may not be present at the onset of clinical symptoms. The two essential features are progressive motor weakness involving more than one limb and areflexia. Frequently, insidious sensory symptoms, usually ignored, precede the onset of weakness. These consist of fleeting dysesthesias and muscle tenderness in limbs that are soon to become paralytic. Weakness progresses rapidly, and approximately 50 % of patients will reach a nadir by 2 weeks, 80 % by 3 weeks, and the rest by 4 weeks. The weakness is usually ascending and relatively symmetric qualitatively, if not quantitatively. Tendon reflexes are absent in all weak muscles and are absent even before the muscle is weak. Bilateral facial weakness occurs in as many as half. Autonomic dysfunction (arrhythmia, labile blood pressure, and gastrointestinal dysfunction) is commonly associated, and a syndrome of acute autonomic dysfunction without paralysis may be a variant.

Recovery of function usually begins 2 to 4 weeks after progression stops. In children, recovery is usually complete. The prognosis is best when recovery begins early. Respiratory paralysis is unusual, but by supporting respiratory function during the critical time of profound paralysis, complete recovery is expected.

Diagnosis. Examination of the cerebrospinal fluid was once critical in distinguishing GBS from acute poliomyelitis. In the absence of poliomyelitis, this examination is less important. A physician first sees most children during the second week of symptoms. At that time, the concentration of protein may be normal or elevated and the number of mononuclear leukocytes per cubic millimeter may be 10 or fewer.

Electrophysiological studies are more important than cerebrospinal fluid analysis for diagnosis, especially to distinguish AIDP from acute axonal neuropathy. AIDP has a better prognosis than acute axonal neuropathy.

Management. Careful monitoring of respiratory function is critical. Intubation is essential if vital capacity falls rapidly to less than 50 % of normal. Adequate control of respiration prevents death from the disorder. Corticosteroids are not helpful because, although they may produce some initial improvement, they tend to prolong the course. Plasma exchange or the use of intravenous immune globulin hastens recovery from GBS (Hughes et al, 2003).

Acute Motor Axonal Neuropathy (AMAN)

The axonal form of GBS occurs more often in rural and economically deprived populations than does AIDP and often follows enteritis (Paradiso et al, 1999).

Clinical Features. The clinical features are indistinguishable from the AIDP except that sensation is not usually affected. Maximal weakness, symmetric quadriparesis, and respiratory failure usually occur in 1 week. Tendon reflexes are absent early in the course. Distal atrophy occurs. Recovery is slow, and the mean time to ambulation is 5 months.

Diagnosis. The cerebrospinal fluid cell count is normal, but the protein concentration increases after 1 or 2 weeks. Electrophysiological studies are consistent with an axonopathy rather than a demyelinating neuropathy, and sensory nerve action potentials are normal.

Management. Respiratory support is often required. Specific treatment is not available, but most children recover spontaneously.

Chronic Inflammatory Demyelinating Polyradiculoneuropathy

Acquired demyelinating polyradiculoneuropathies occur in both an acute and a chronic form. The acute form is the GBS described in the section above. The chronic form is *chronic inflammatory demyelinating polyradiculoneuropathy* (CIDP). The acute and chronic forms may be difficult to distinguish from each other at the onset of symptoms but their distinguishing feature is the monophasic or recurrent course (Ryan et al, 2000).

CIDP, like GBS, is immune-mediated. The preceding infection is more often a respiratory illness than a gastrointestinal illness. However, both are so common in all school-age children that the cause and effect relationship is difficult to establish.

Clinical Features. CIDP is more common in adults than in children. The usual initial features are weakness and paresthesias in the distal portions of the limbs causing a gait disturbance. Cranial neuropathies are unusual. Mandatory criteria for diagnosis are: (1) progressive or relapsing motor and sensory dysfunction of more than one limb, of a peripheral nerve nature, developing over at least 2 months; and (2) areflexia or hyporeflexia, usually affecting all four limbs. The course is monophasic in a quarter of children and has a relapsing course in the remainder. Three-quarters have residual weakness.

Diagnosis. Exclusionary criteria in establishing the diagnosis of CIDP are a family history of a similar disorder, a pure sensory neuropathy, other organ involvement, or abnormal storage of material in nerves. The protein content of the cerebrospinal fluid is always greater than 0.45 g/L, and a small number of mononuclear cells may be present. Motor nerve conduction velocity is less than 70 % of the lower limit of normal in at least two nerves. Sural nerve biopsy is not mandatory but shows features of demyelination, cellular infiltration of the nerve, and no evidence of vasculitis.

Electrodiagnosis differentiates acquired demyelinating neuropathies from familial demyelinating neuropathies. Acquired neuropathies show a multifocal disturbance of conduction velocity, whereas slowing of conduction velocity is uniform throughout the length of the nerve in hereditary disorders.

Management. An ideal treatment protocol is not established (Ropper, 2003). Immediate and chronic use of prednisone and intravenous immuneglobulin or plasma exchange is effective in most children. As a rule, long-term therapy is essential, and relapse may follow discontinuation of therapy. The outcome is more favorable in children than in adults.

Viral Infections

Enterovirus Infections. Poliovirus, coxsackievirus, and the echovirus group are RNA viruses that inhabit the intestinal tract of humans. They are neurotropic and produce paralytic disease by destroying the motor neurons of the brainstem and spinal cord. Of this group, poliovirus causes the most severe and devastating disease. Coxsackievirus and echoviruses are more likely to cause aseptic meningitis, although they can cause an acute paralytic syndrome similar to that of poliomyelitis.

Clinical Features. Enterovirus infections occur in epidemics during the spring and summer. The most common syndrome associated with poliovirus infection is a brief illness characterized by fever, malaise, and gastrointestinal symptoms. Aseptic meningitis occurs in more severe cases. The extreme situation is paralytic poliomyelitis. Initial symptoms are fever, sore throat, and malaise lasting for 1 to 2 days. After a brief period of apparent well-being, fever recurs in association with headache, vomiting, and signs of meningeal irritation. Pain in the limbs or over the spine is an antecedent symptom of limb paralysis. Flaccid muscle weakness develops rapidly thereafter. The pattern of muscle weakness varies, but is generally asymmetric. One arm or leg is often weaker than the other limbs.

Bulbar polio occurs with or without spinal cord disease. It is often life threatening. Affected children have prolonged episodes of apnea and require respiratory assistance. Several motor cranial nerves may be involved as well, but sparing the extraocular muscle.

The introduction of inactivated poliomyelitis vaccine in 1954, followed by the use of live-attenuated vaccine in 1960, has abolished the disease in the Western hemisphere and Europe. Vaccine-associated poliomyelitis is rare since inactivated polio vaccine replaced the live-attenuated vaccine.

Diagnosis. Suspect the diagnosis from the clinical findings. Isolation and viral typing from stool and nasopharyngeal specimens provide confirmation. The cerebrospinal fluid initially shows a polymorphonuclear reaction, with the cell count ranging from $50/mm^3$ to $200/mm^3$.

After 1 week, lymphocytes predominate; after 2 to 3 weeks, the total cell count decreases. The protein content is elevated early and remains elevated for several months.

Management. Treatment is supportive.

West Nile Virus. West Nile Virus has spread across the United States since arriving in New York in 1999 (Li et al, 2003). It is now the most important cause of arboviral meningitis, encephalitis, and acute flaccid paralysis in the continental United States (Davis et al, 2006). Almost all transmission occurs from the bite of an infected mosquito. Rare person-to-person transmission occurs through organ transplantation, blood and blood product transfusion, and intrauterine spread.

Clinical Features. Within 3–14 days of a mosquito bite, a flu-like illness occurs. An acute, severe, asymmetric paralysis follows. It may affect only one limb and may involve the face. Sensory features are minimal and encephalopathy does not occur. Neurological disease is rare in infants and children. Clinical features may include movement disorders and severe weakness of a lower motor neuron type.

Diagnosis. EMG indicates severe denervation in affected muscles. Both EMG and MRI studies localize the abnormality to the motor neuron or ventral horn.

Management. Treatment is supportive.

Neuromuscular Blockade

Children treated for prolonged periods with neuromuscular blocking agents for assisted ventilation may remain in a flaccid state for days or weeks after discontinuing the drug. This is especially true in newborns receiving several drugs that block the neuromuscular junction.

Botulism. *Clostridium botulinum* produces a toxin that interferes with the release of acetylcholine at the neuromuscular junction. Chapter 6 describes the infantile form, but most cases occur after infancy in people who eat food, usually preserved at home, contaminated with the organism.

Clinical Features. The first symptoms are blurred vision, diplopia, dizziness, dysarthria, and dysphagia, which have their onset 12 to 36 hours after the ingestion of toxin. Some patients have only bulbar signs; in others, flaccid paralysis develops in all limbs. Patients with generalized weakness always have ophthalmoplegia with sparing of the pupillary response. Tendon reflexes may be present or absent.

Diagnosis. Repetitive supermaximal nerve stimulation at a rate of 20–50 stimuli per second produces an incremental response characteristic of a presynaptic defect. The electrical abnormality evolves with time and may not be demonstrable in all limbs on any given day.

Management. Botulism can be fatal because of respiratory depression. Treatment relies primarily on supportive care, which is similar to the management of GBS. Antitoxin is recommended in confirmed cases.

Corticosteroid-Induced Quadriplegia. The administration of high-dose intravenous corticosteroids, especially in combination with a neuromuscular blocking agent, may cause acute generalized weakness.

Clinical Features. Most patients with this syndrome receive corticosteroids to treat asthma. The onset of weakness is 4 to 14 days after starting treatment. The weakness is usually diffuse at onset but may be limited to proximal or distal muscles. Tendon reflexes are usually preserved. Complete recovery is the rule.

Diagnosis. The serum CK concentration may be normal or elevated. EMG shows brief, small-amplitude polyphasic potentials, and the muscle is electrically inexcitable to direct stimulation.

Management. Respiratory assistance may be required. Cessation of the offending drugs usually ends the disorder and allows the patient to recover spontaneously.

Tick Paralysis. In North America, the female tick of the species *Dermacentor andersoni* and *D. variabilis* elaborates a salivary gland toxin that induces paralysis. The mechanism of paralysis is unknown (Vednarayanan et al, 2002).

Clinical Features. Affected children are usually less than 5 years of age. The clinical syndrome is similar to GBS, except that ocular motor palsies and pupillary abnormalities are more common. A severe generalized flaccid weakness, usually first affecting the legs, develops rapidly and is sometimes associated with bifacial palsy. Respiratory paralysis requiring assisted ventilation is common. Tendon reflexes are usually absent or greatly depressed. Dysesthesias may be present at the onset of weakness, but examination fails to show loss of sensation.

Diagnosis. The cerebrospinal fluid protein concentration is normal. Nerve conduction studies may be normal or may show mild slowing of motor nerve conduction velocities. Decreased amplitude of the compound muscle action potentials is common. High rates of repetitive stimulation may show a normal result or an abnormal incremental response.

Management. Strength returns quickly once removing the causative tick in North America.

However, the tick may be hard to find, because it hides in body hair. In contrast, paralysis is more severe in Australia and may worsen over 1 to 2 days after removal of the tick before improvement begins.

Intensive Care Unit Weakness. Almost 2 % of children admitted to critical care units develop muscle weakness (Banwell et al, 2003). Most were organ transplant recipients treated with neuromuscular blocking agents, corticosteroids, and aminoglycoside antibiotics. The usual clinical feature is failure to wean from a respirator. Some exemplify "corticosteroid-induced quadriplegia" described above. Corticosteroid myopathy accounts for some. These show increased blood concentrations of CK and histological evidence of myofiber necrosis. A third possible cause is the depletion of myosin from muscle. Muscle biopsy distinguishes the several types of prolonged weakness that may occur in people with severe illness requiring intensive care.

PERIODIC PARALYSES

The usual classification of periodic paralyses is in relation to serum potassium: hyperkalemic, hypokalemic, or normokalemic. In addition, periodic paralysis may be primary (genetic) or secondary. The cause of secondary hypokalemic periodic paralysis is by urinary or gastrointestinal loss of potassium. Urinary loss accompanies primary hyperaldosteronism, licorice intoxication, amphotericin B therapy, and several renal tubular defects. Gastrointestinal loss most often occurs with severe chronic diarrhea, prolonged gastrointestinal intubation and vomiting, and a draining gastrointestinal fistula. Either urinary or gastrointestinal loss, or both, may occur in children with anorexia nervosa who overuse diuretics or induce vomiting. Thyrotoxicosis is an important cause of hypokalemic periodic paralysis, especially in Asians. Secondary hyperkalemic periodic paralysis is associated with renal or adrenal insufficiency.

Familial Hypokalemic Periodic Paralysis

Genetic transmission of familial hypokalemic periodic paralysis is by autosomal dominant inheritance with decreased penetrance in women. In as many as 70 % of cases, the responsible mutation links to a gene encoding a dihydropyridine receptor on chromosome 1q (Venance et al, 2006). This channel functions as the voltage sensor of the ryanodine receptor and plays an important role in excitation-contraction coupling in skeletal muscle.

Clinical Features. The onset of symptoms occurs before 16 years of age in 60 % of cases and by 20 years of age in the remainder. Attacks of paralysis are at first infrequent but then may occur several times a week. Factors that trigger an attack include rest after exercise (therefore many attacks occur early in the morning), a large meal with high carbohydrate content (pizza is the trigger of choice in adolescents), emotional or physical stress, alcohol ingestion, and exposure to cold. Before and during the attack the patient may have excessive thirst and oliguria. The weakness begins with a sensation of aching in the proximal muscles. Sometimes, only the proximal muscles are affected; at other times, there is complete paralysis so that the patient cannot even raise the head. Facial muscles are rarely affected, and extraocular motility is always normal. Respiratory distress does not occur. When the weakness reaches extreme, the muscles feel swollen and the tendon reflexes are absent. Most attacks last for 6 to 12 hours and some for the whole day. Strength recovers rapidly, but after several attacks residual weakness may be present.

Diagnosis. Molecular genetic testing is available but the clinical features usually establish the diagnosis. During the attack, the serum concentration of potassium ranges from 0.9 to 3.0 mL (normal range 3.5–5 mL) and ECG changes occur, including bradycardia, flattening of T waves, and prolongation of the PR and Q-T intervals. The muscle is electrically silent and not excitable. The oral administration of glucose, 2 g/kg, with 10 to 20 units of crystalline insulin given subcutaneously provokes attacks. The serum potassium concentration falls, and paralysis follows within 2 to 3 hours.

Management. Treatment of attacks in patients with good renal function is with repeated oral doses of potassium. Intravenous infusions cannot raise the serum potassium concentration. In adolescents, 5–10 g is used. Consider smaller amounts for younger children. Daily use of carbonic anhydrase inhibitors, dichlorphenamide 100 mg/day), is beneficial in many families to prevent attacks (Tawil et al, 2000).

Familial Hyperkalemic Periodic Paralysis Type 1

Genetic transmission of familial hyperkalemic periodic paralysis type 1 is by autosomal dominant inheritance. The frequency is the same in both genders. The cause is a defect of the gene encoding the sodium channel (Jurkat-Rott & Lehmann-Horn, 2011).

Clinical Features. The onset of weakness is in early childhood and sometimes in infancy. As in hypokalemic periodic paralysis, resting after exercise may provoke attacks. However, only moderate exercise is required. Weakness begins with a sensation of heaviness in the back and leg muscles. Sometimes the patient can delay the paralysis by walking or moving about. In infants and small children, characteristic attacks are episodes of floppiness in which the child lies around and cannot move. In older children and adults, both mild and severe attacks may occur. Factors causing attacks are potassium rich foods, rest after exercise, a cold environment, emotional stress, glucocorticoids, and pregnancy. Mild attacks last for less than an hour and do not produce complete paralysis. More than one mild attack may occur in a day. Severe attacks are similar to the complete flaccid paralysis seen in hypokalemic periodic paralysis and may last for several hours. Residual weakness may persist after several severe attacks. Mild myotonia of the eyelids, face, and hands may be present between attacks. Older patients may develop a progressive myopathy.

Diagnosis. Molecular genetic testing is commercially available for several of the mutations that cause disease. Between attacks, the serum concentration of potassium is normal but increases at least 1.5 mM/L during attacks. When the potassium concentration is high, ECG changes are consistent with hyperkalemia. The oral administration of potassium chloride just after exercise in the fasting state provokes an attack. During the attack, the muscles are electrically silent. Myotonia in patients with hyperkalemic periodic paralysis is mild and may occur only on exposure to cold.

Management. Acute attacks seldom require treatment because they are brief. Prophylactic measures include avoidance of meals rich in potassium (grapefruit juice) and cold exposure. Daily low dosages (25–50 mg) of hydrochlorothiazide may prevent attacks by decreasing serum potassium concentrations.

Familial Normokalemic Periodic Paralysis

Several families have experienced an autosomal dominant inherited periodic paralysis in which no alteration in the serum concentration of potassium could be detected (FPPIII). These cases may represent a variant of hyperkalemic periodic paralysis due to a mutation in the muscle specific sodium gene (Chinnery et al, 2002).

Andersen-Tawil Syndrome

Andersen-Tawil syndrome is a distinct channelopathy affecting both skeletal and cardiac muscles (Tawil & Venance, 2010). The genetic defect involves the α-subunit of the skeletal muscle sodium channel and the cardiac muscle potassium channel responsible for most long Q-T intervals.

Clinical Features. The main features are short stature, dysmorphic features, periodic paralysis, and a prolonged Q-T interval. The dysmorphic features include a broad nose, low-set ears, a small mandible, and syndactyly. The periodic paralysis may be associated with hyperkalemia, hypokalemia, or normokalemia. The prolonged Q-T interval may be the only feature in some individuals. The initial feature may be an arrhythmia, especially ventricular tachycardia, or attacks of paralysis.

Diagnosis. Suspect the diagnosis in any dysmorphic child with a prolonged Q-T interval or a periodic paralysis.

Management. The arrhythmias associated with prolonged Q-T interval are life threatening and must be treated. Affected members with periodic paralysis are responsive to oral potassium.

REFERENCES

Aoki M. Dysferlinopathy. In: GeneClinics: Medical Genetic Knowledge Base [database online]. Seattle: University of Washington. Available at www.geneclinics.org. PMID: 20301480. Last updated April 22, 2010.

Banwell BL, Mildner RJ, Hassall AC, et al. Muscle weakness in critically ill children. Neurology 2003;61:1779–82.

Bertini ES, Eymard-Pierre E, Boespflug-Tanguy O, et al. ALS2 related disorders. In: GeneClinics: Medical Genetic Knowledge Base [database online]. Seattle: University of Washington. Available at www.geneclinics.org. PMID: 20301421. Last updated February 10, 2011.

Bird TD. Myotonic dystrophy type 1. In: Pagon RA, Bird TD, Dolan CR, et al., eds. GeneReviews™. Seattle: University of Washington. Available at www.geneclinics.org. PMID: 20301344. Last updated February 8, 2011.

Bird TD. Charcot-Marie-Tooth hereditary neuropathy overview. In: Pagon RA, Bird TD, Dolan CR, et al., eds. GeneReviews™. Seattle: University of Washington. Available at www.geneclinics.org. PMID: 20301532. Last updated February 9, 2012.

Bonne G, Leturcq F, Ben Yaou R. Emery-Dreifuss muscular dystrophy. In: Pagon RA, Bird TD, Dolan CR, et al., eds. GeneReviews™. Seattle: University of Washington. Available at www.geneclinics.org. PMID: 20301609. Last updated August 24, 2010.

Chinnery PF, Walls TJ, Hanna MG, et al. Normokalemic periodic paralysis revisited: Does it really exist? Annals of Neurology 2002;52:251–2.

Croxen R, Hatton C, Shelley C, et al. Recessive inheritance and variable penetrance of slow-channel congenital myasthenic syndromes. Neurology 2002;59:162–8.

Darras BT, Miller DT, Urion DK. Dystrophinopathies. In: Pagon RA, Bird TD, Dolan CR, et al., eds. GeneReviews™. Seattle: University of Washington. Available at www.geneclinics.org. PMID: 20301298. Last updated November 23, 2011.

Davis LE, DeBiasi R, Goade DE, et al. West Nile virus neuroinvasive disease. Annals of Neurology 2006;60:286–300.

Day JW, Ricker K, Jacobson JF, et al. Myotonic dystrophy type 2: Molecular, diagnostic and clinical spectrum. Neurology 2003;60:657–64.

Fluharty AL. Arylsulfatase A deficiency. In: Pagon RA, Bird TD, Dolan CR, et al., eds. GeneReviews™. Seattle: University of Washington. Available at www.geneclinics.org. PMID: 20301309. Last updated August 25, 2011.

Gordon E, Pegoraro E, Hoffman EP. Limb-girdle muscular dystrophy overview. In: Pagon RA, Bird TD, Dolan CR, et al., eds. GeneReviews™. Seattle: University of Washington. Available at www.geneclinics.org. PMID: 20301582. Last updated July 23, 2009.

Harper CM, Fukodome T, Engel AG. Treatment of slow-channel congenital myasthenic syndrome with fluoxetine. Neurology 2003:1710–3.

Hedera P, Petty EM, Bui MR, et al. The second kindred with autosomal dominant distal myopathy linked to chromosome 14q: Genetic and clinical analysis. Archives of Neurology 2003;60:1321–5.

Hughes RAC, Wijdicks EFM, Barohn R, et al. Practice parameter: Immunotherapy for Guillain-Barré syndrome. Report of the quality standards committee of the American Academy of Neurology. Neurology 2003;61:736–40.

Jurkat-Rott K, Lehmann-Horn F. Hyperkalemic periodic paralysis type 1. In: Pagon RA, Bird TD, Dolan CR, et al., eds. GeneReviews™. Seattle: University of Washington. Available at www.geneclinics.org. PMID: 20301669. Last updated May 31, 2011.

Kishnani PS, Nicolino M, Voit T, et al. Chinese hamster ovary cell-derived recombinant human acid alpha-glucosidase in infantile-onset Pompe disease. Journal of Pediatrics 2006;149:89–97.

Kishnani PS, Corzo D, Nicoloini M, et al. Recombinant human acid α-glucosidase. Major clinical benefits in infantile onset Pompe disease. Neurology 2007;68:99–109.

Kuhlenbäumer G, Timmerman V. Giant axonal neuropathy. In: Pagon RA, Bird TD, Dolan CR, et al., eds. GeneReviews™. Seattle: University of Washington. Available at www.geneclinics.org. PMID: 20301315. Last updated August 11, 2009.

Laing NG, Laing BA, Meredith C, et al. Autosomal dominant distal myopathy: Linkage to chromosome 14. American Journal of Human Genetics 1995;56:422–7.

Lampe AK, Flanigan KM, Bushby KM. Collagen type VI-related disorders. In: Pagon RA, Bird TD, Dolan CR, et al., eds. GeneReviews™. Seattle: University of Washington. Available at www.geneclinics.org. PMID: 20301676. Last updated April 6, 2007.

Lemmers RJLF, van der Maarel SM. Facioscapulohumeral muscular dystrophy. In: Pagon RA, Bird TD, Dolan CR, et al., eds. GeneReviews™. Seattle: University of Washington. Available at www.geneclinics.org. PMID: 20301616. Last updated July 9, 2009.

Li J, Loeb JA, Shy ME, et al. Asymmetric flaccid paralysis: A neuromuscular presentation of West Nile Virus infection. Annals of Neurology 2003;53:703–10.

Mackay MT, Kornberg AJ, Shield LK, et al. Benign acute childhood myositis. Laboratory and clinical features. Neurology 1999;53:2127–31.

Mastaglia FL, Phillips BA, Cala LA, et al. Early onset chromosome 14-linked distal myopathy (Laing). Neuromuscular Disorders 2002;12:350–7.

Navon R, Khosravi R, Melki J, et al. Juvenile-onset spinal muscular atrophy caused by compound heterozygosity for mutations in the HEXA gene. Annals of Neurology 1997;41:631–8.

Ogino S, Wilson RB. Genetic testing and risk assessment for spinal muscular atrophy. Human Genetics 2002;111:477–500.

Paradiso G, Tripoli J, Galicchio S, et al. Epidemiological, clinical, and electrodiagnostic findings in childhood Guillain-Barré syndrome: A reappraisal. Annals of Neurology 1999;46:701–7.

Prior TW, Russman BS. Spinal muscular atrophy. In: Pagon RA, Bird TD, Dolan CR, et al., eds. GeneReviews™. Seattle: University of Washington. Available at www.geneclinics.org. PMID: 20301526. Last updated January 27, 2011.

Ramser J, Ahearn ME, Lenski C, et al. Rare missense and synonymous variants in UBE1 are associated with X-linked infantile spinal muscular atrophy. American Journal of Human Genetics 2008;82:188–93.

Ropper AH. Current treatments for CIDP. Neurology 2003;60(Suppl 3):S16–22.

Ryan MM, Grattan-Smith PJ, Procopis PG, et al. Childhood chronic inflammatory demyelinating polyneuropathy: clinical course and long-term outcome. Neuromuscular Disorders 2000;10:398–406.

Saperstein DS, Amato AA, Barohn RJ. Clinical and genetic aspects of distal myopathies. Muscle and Nerve 2001;24:1440–50.

Sugie K, Yamamoto A, Murayama K, et al. Clinicopathological features of genetically confirmed Danon disease. Neurology 2002;58:1773–8.

Swoboda KJ, Prior TW, Scott CB, et al. Natural history of denervation in SMA: Relation to age, SMN2 copy number, and function. Annals of Neurology 2005;57:704–12.

Tawil R, McDermott MP, Brown Jr R, et al. Randomized trials of dichlorphenamide in the periodic paralyses. Annals of Neurology 2000;47:46–53.

Tawil R, Venance SL. Andersen-Tawil syndrome. In: Pagon RA, Bird TD, Dolan CR, et al., eds. GeneReviews™. Seattle: University of Washington. Available at www.geneclinics.org. PMID: 20301441. Last updated May 13, 2010.

Vednarayanan VV, Evans OB, Subramony SH. Tick paralysis in children. Electrophysiology and possibility of misdiagnosis. Neurology 2002;59:1088–90.

Venance SL, Cannon SC, Fialho D, et al. The primary periodic paralyses: diagnosis, pathogenesis and treatment. Brain 2006;129:8–17.

CHAPTER 8

CRAMPS, MUSCLE STIFFNESS, AND EXERCISE INTOLERANCE

A cramp is an involuntary painful contraction of a muscle or part of a muscle. Cramps can occur in normal children during or after vigorous exercise, and after excessive loss of fluid or electrolytes. The characteristic electromyography (EMG) finding for such cramps is the repetitive firing of normal motor unit potentials. Stretching the muscle relieves the cramp. Partially denervated muscle is particularly susceptible to cramping not only during exercise but also during sleep. Night cramps may awaken patients with neuronopathies, neuropathies, or root compression. Cramps during exercise occur also in patients with several different disorders of muscle energy metabolism. The EMG characteristic of these cramps is electrical silence.

Muscle stiffness and spasms are not cramps, but are actually prolonged contractions of several muscles that are able to impose postures. Such contractions may or may not be painful. When painful, they lack the explosive character of cramps. Prolonged contractions occur when muscles fail to relax (myotonia) or when motor unit activity is continuous (Box 8-1). Prolonged, painless muscle contractions occur also in dystonia and in other movement disorders (see Chapter 14).

Many normal children, especially preadolescent boys, complain of pain in their legs at night and sometimes during the day, especially after a period of increased activity. These pains are not true cramps. The muscle is not in spasm, the pain is diffuse, and aching in quality and the discomfort lasts for an hour or longer. Stretching the muscle does not relieve the pain. This is not a symptom of neuromuscular disease and is called *growing pains*, for want of better understanding. One-third of the cases are associated with abdominal pain or headaches, which suggest a common ground with migraines (Abu-Arafeh &Russel, 1996). Mild analgesics or heat, relieve symptoms.

Exercise intolerance is a relative term for an inability to maintain exercise at an expected level. The causes of exercise intolerance considered in this chapter are fatigue and muscle pain. Fatigue is a normal consequence of exercise and occurs in everyone at some level of activity. In general, weak children become fatigued more quickly than children who have normal strength. Many children with exercise intolerance and cramps, but no permanent weakness, have a defect in an enzyme needed to produce energy for muscular contraction (Box 8-2). A known mechanism underlies several such inborn errors of metabolism. However, even when the full spectrum of biochemical tests is available, identification of a metabolic defect is not possible in some children with cramps during exercise.

Myasthenia gravis is a disorder characterized by fatigability and exercise intolerance, but not covered in this chapter because the usual initial symptoms are either isolated cranial nerve disturbances (see Chapter 15) or limb weakness (see Chapters 6 and 7).

Conditions that produce some combination of cramps and exercise intolerance are divisible into three groups: diseases with abnormal muscle activity, diseases with decreased energy for muscle contraction, and myopathies. As a rule, the first and third groups are symptomatic at all times, whereas the second group is symptomatic

BOX 8-1 Diseases with Abnormal Muscle Activity

CONTINUOUS MOTOR UNIT ACTIVITY

- Neuromyotonia
- Paroxysmal ataxia and myokymia (see Chapter 10)
- Schwartz-Jampel syndrome
- Stiff man syndrome
- Thyrotoxicosis*

CRAMPS-FASCICULATION SYNDROME

MYOTONIA

- Myotonia congenita
- Myotonia fluctuans

SYSTEMIC DISORDERS

- Hypoadrenalism*
- Hypocalcemia* (tetany)
- Hypothyroidism*
- Strychnine poisoning*
- Uremia*

*Denotes the most common conditions and the ones with disease modifying treatments

BOX 8-2 Diseases with Decreased Muscle Energy

DEFECTS OF CARBOHYDRATE UTILIZATION
- Lactate dehydrogenase deficiency
- Myophosphorylase deficiency
- Phosphofructokinase deficiency
- Phosphoglycerate kinase deficiency
- Phosphoglycerate mutase deficiency

DEFECTS OF FATTY ACID OXIDATION
- Carnitine palmitoyl transferase 2 deficiency
- Very-long-chain acyl coenzyme A dehydrogenase deficiency

MITOCHONDRIAL (RESPIRATORY CHAIN) MYOPATHIES

MYOADENYLATE DEAMINASE DEFICIENCY

only with exercise. The first group usually requires EMG for diagnosis. EMG is the initial diagnostic test in children with muscle stiffness that is not due to spasticity or rigidity. It usually leads to the correct diagnosis (Box 8-3).

BOX 8-3 Electromyography in Muscle Stiffness

NORMAL BETWEEN CRAMPS*
- Brody myopathy
- Defects of carbohydrate metabolism
- Defects of lipid metabolism
- Mitochondrial myopathies
- Myoadenylate deaminase deficiency
- Rippling muscle disease
- Tubular aggregates

SILENT CRAMPS
- Brody disease
- Defects of carbohydrate metabolism
- Rippling muscle disease
- Tubular aggregates

CONTINUOUS MOTOR ACTIVITY
- Neuromyotonia
- Myotonia
- Myotonia congenita
- Myotonic dystrophy
- Schwartz-Jampel syndrome
- Stiff man syndrome

MYOPATHY
- Emery-Dreifuss muscular dystrophy
- Rigid spine syndrome
- X-linked myalgia

*Or may be myopathic.

ABNORMAL MUSCLE ACTIVITY

Continuous Motor Unit Activity

The cause of continuous motor unit activity (CMUA) is the uncontrolled release of acetylcholine (ACh) packets at the neuromuscular junction. The EMG features of CMUA are repetitive muscle action potentials in response to a single nerve stimulus; high frequency bursts of motor unit potentials of normal morphology abruptly start and stop. Rhythmic firing of doublets, triplets, and multiplets occurs. During long bursts the potentials decline in amplitude. This activity is difficult to distinguish from normal voluntary activity. CMUA occurs in a heterogeneous group of disorders characterized clinically by some combination of muscle pain, fasciculations, myokymia, contractures, and cramps (Box 8-4).

BOX 8-4 Abnormal Muscle Activity

Fasciculations: Spontaneous, random twitching of a group of muscle fibers
Fibrillation: Spontaneous contraction of a single muscle fiber, not visible through the skin
Myotonia: Disturbance in muscle relaxation following voluntary contraction or percussion
Myokymia: Repetitive fasciculations causing a quivering or undulating twitch
Neuromyotonia: Continuous muscle activity characterized by muscle rippling, muscle stiffness, and myotonia

The primary defect in CMUA disorder may reside within the spinal cord (stiff man syndrome) or the peripheral nerve (neuromyotonia). The original name for neuromyotonia is *Isaac syndrome*. These disorders may be sporadic or familial in occurrence. When familial, the usual mode of transmission is autosomal dominant inheritance.

Neuromyotonia

The primary abnormality in neuromyotonia is decreased outward potassium current of voltage-gated potassium channel function. Most childhood cases are sporadic in occurrence, but some show a pattern of autosomal dominant inheritance. An autoimmune process directed against the potassium channel may account for some sporadic cases.

Clinical Features. The clinical triad includes involuntary muscle twitching (fasciculations or myokymia), muscle cramps or stiffness, and myotonia. Excessive sweating is frequently associated with the muscle stiffness. The age at onset is any time from birth to adult life.

The initial features are muscle twitching and cramps brought on by exercise. Later these symptoms occur also at rest and even during sleep. The cramps may affect only distal muscles, causing painful posturing of the hands and feet. As a rule, leg weakness is greater than arm weakness. These disorders are not progressive and do not lead to permanent disability. Attacks of cramping are less frequent and severe with age.

In some children, cramps and fasciculations are not as prominent as stiffness, which causes abnormal limb posturing associated frequently with excessive sweating. Leg involvement is more common than arm involvement, and the symptoms suggest dystonia (see Chapter 14). Limb posturing may begin in one foot and remain asymmetric for months. Most cases are sporadic.

Muscle mass, muscle strength, and tendon reflexes are normal. Fasciculations are sporadic and seen only after prolonged observation.

Diagnosis. Some adult-onset cases are associated with malignancy, but this is never the case in children. Muscle fibers fire repetitively at a rate of 100–300 Hz, either continuously or in recurring bursts, producing a pinging sound. The discharge continues during sleep and persists after procaine block of the nerve.

Management. Carbamazepine and phenytoin, at usual anticonvulsant doses, are both effective in reducing or abolishing symptoms. Intravenous immunoglobulin and plasmapheresis may be an option for patients refractory to symptomatic treatment with sodium channel blocking drugs (Van den Berg 1999).

Schwartz-Jampel Syndrome

The Schwartz-Jampel syndrome type 1 (SJS1) is a hereditary disorder, transmitted by autosomal recessive inheritance. Neonatal Schwartz-Jampel syndrome type 2 (SJS2), also known as *Stuve-Wiedemann syndrome*, is a genetically distinct disorder with a more severe phenotype. Characteristic features of SJS1 include short stature, skeletal abnormalities, and persistent muscular contraction and hypertrophy.

Clinical Features. SJS1 corresponds to the original description of Schwartz and Jampel. Bone deformities are not prominent at birth. CMUA of the face is the main feature producing a characteristic triad that includes narrowing of the palpebral fissures (blepharophimosis), pursing of the mouth, and puckering of the chin. Striking or even blowing on the eyelids induces blepharospasm. CMUA in the limbs produces stiffness of gait and exercise intolerance. Motor development during the first year is slow, but intelligence is normal.

Diagnosis. EMG shows CMUA. Initial reports suggested incorrectly that the abnormal activity seen on the EMG and expressed clinically was myotonia. Myotonia may be present, but CMUA is responsible for the facial and limb symptoms. The serum concentration of creatine kinase (CK) can be mildly elevated. The histological appearance of the muscle is usually normal but may show variation in fiber size and an increased number of central nuclei.

Management. Carbamazepine, phenytoin and possibly other sodium channel blockers such as lamotrigine, oxcarbazepine, and lacosamide may diminish the muscle stiffness. Early treatment with relief of muscle stiffness reduces the severity of subsequent muscle deformity. Botulinum toxin injections may help.

Myotonic Disorders

Myotonia Congenita

Myotonia congenita is a genetic disorder characterized by muscle stiffness and hypertrophy (Dunø & Colding-Jorgensen, 2011). Weakness is not prominent, but stiffness may impair muscle function. The disease can be transmitted as either an autosomal dominant (*Thomsen disease*) or autosomal recessive (*Becker disease*) trait. The overlap of clinical features is considerable, and the clinical features alone cannot always determine the pattern of genetic transmission. Abnormalities in the chloride channel underlie all cases.

Clinical Features. Age of onset is variable. In the dominant form, age at onset is usually in infancy or early childhood; in the recessive form, the age of onset is slightly older, but both may begin in adult life. The autosomal recessive form of myotonia congenita is often more severe than the dominant form. Individuals with the recessive form may have mild, progressive, distal weakness and transitory attacks of weakness induced by movement after rest.

Clinical features of the dominant form are stereotyped. After rest, muscles are stiff and difficult to move. With activity, the stiffness disappears and movement may be normal. One of our patients played Little League baseball and could not sit while he was waiting to bat for fear that he would be unable to get up. The myotonia may cause generalized muscle hypertrophy, giving the infant a herculean appearance. The tongue, face, and jaw muscles are sometimes involved. Cold exposure exacerbates stiffness, which is painless. Percussion myotonia is present. Strength and tendon reflexes are normal.

Diagnosis. EMG establishes the diagnosis. Repetitive discharges at rates of 20–80 cycles/sec are recorded when the needle is first inserted into the muscle and again on voluntary contraction. Two types of discharges occur: a biphasic spike potential of less than 5 msec and a positive wave of less than 50 msec. The waxing and waning of the amplitude and frequency of potentials produces a characteristic sound (dive-bomber). Dystrophy is not present. The serum concentration of CK is normal and muscle biopsy specimens do not contain necrotic fibers.

The *CLCN1* gene, encoding a chloride channel, is the only gene associated with myotonia congenita. Sequence analysis is commercially available.

Management. Myotonia does not always require treatment. Mexiletine is the most effective drug for treatment (Logigian, 2010).

Myotonia Fluctuans

Myotonia fluctuans is a distinct disorder caused by mutations of the muscle sodium channel (Colding-Jorgensen et al, 2006). Transmission is by autosomal dominant inheritance. Allelic disorders with overlapping clinical phenotypes include hyperkalemic periodic paralysis and paramyotonia congenita.

Clinical Features. The onset of stiffness is usually in the second decade and worsens with exercise or potassium ingestion. Cramps in the toes, fingers, and eyelids, especially when tired or cold, begin in childhood. Physical examination reveals mild myotonia but normal strength. Symptoms vary from day to day. Myotonia affects the extraocular muscles as well as the trunk and limbs. The severity of myotonia fluctuates on a day-by-day basis. "Warming up" usually relieves symptoms, but exercise may also worsen symptoms. A bad day may follow a day of exercise or potassium ingestion, but neither precipitant causes immediate worsening of myotonia. Cooling does not trigger or worsen myotonia.

Diagnosis. EMG shows myotonia, and a mild reduction in the amplitude of compound muscle action potential on cooling and administration of potassium. DNA analysis shows a mutation in the gene for the sodium channel subunit.

Management. Daily use of mexilitine or acetazolamide may relieve the stiffness (Meola, 2009).

Systemic Disorders

Hypoadrenalism

A small percentage of patients with Addison disease complain of cramps and pain in truncal muscles. At times, paroxysmal cramps occur in the lower torso and legs and cause the patient to double up in pain. Hormone replacement relieves the symptoms.

Hypocalcemia and Hypomagnesemia

Tetany caused by dietary deficiency of calcium is rare in modern times, except in newborns fed cows' milk. Hypocalcemic tetany is more likely to result from hypoparathyroidism or hyperventilation-induced alkalosis.

The initial symptom of tetany is tingling around the mouth and in the hands and feet. With time, the tingling increases in intensity and becomes generalized. Spasms in the muscles of the face, hands, and feet follow. The hands assume a typical posture in which the fingers extend, the wrists flex, and the thumb abducts. Fasciculations and laryngeal spasm may be present. Percussion of the facial nerve, either just anterior to the ear or over the cheek, produces contraction of the muscles innervated by that branch of the nerve. (Chvostek' sign)

A similar syndrome occurs with magnesium deficiency. In addition to the tetany, encephalopathy occurs. Restoring the proper concentration of serum electrolytes relieves the cramps associated with hypocalcemia and hypomagnesemia.

Thyroid Disease

Myalgia, cramps, and stiffness are the initial features in up to half of patients with hypothyroidism. Stiffness is worse in the morning, especially on cold days, and the probable cause is the slowing of muscular contraction and relaxation. This is different from myotonia, in which only relaxation is affected. Indeed, activity worsens the stiffness of hypothyroidism, which may be painful, whereas activity relieves myotonia and is painless. The slowing of muscular contraction and relaxation is sometimes demonstrated when tendon reflexes are tested. The response tends to "hang up."

Percussion of a muscle produces a localized knot of contraction called myoedema. This localized contraction lasts for up to 1 minute before slowly relaxing.

Myokymia, continuous motor unit activity of the face, tongue, and limbs, and muscle cramps develop occasionally in patients with thyrotoxicosis. Restoring the euthyroid state reverses all of the neuromuscular symptoms of hypothyroidism and hyperthyroidism.

Uremia

Uremia is a known cause of polyneuropathy (see Chapter 7). However, 50 % of patients complain of nocturnal leg cramps and flexion cramps of the hands even before clinical evidence of polyneuropathy is present. Excessive use of diuretics may be the triggering factor. Muscle cramps occur also in approximately one-third of patients undergoing hemodialysis. Monitoring with EMG during dialysis documents a build-up of spontaneous discharges. After several hours, usually toward the end of dialysis treatment, repetitive high-voltage discharges occur associated with clinical cramps. Because standard dialysis fluid is slightly hypotonic, many nephrologists have attempted to treat the cramps by administering hypertonic solutions. Either sodium chloride or glucose solutions relieve cramps in most patients. The cramps apparently result from either extracellular volume contraction or hypoosmolarity. Similar cramps occur in children with severe diarrhea or vomiting.

DECREASED MUSCLE ENERGY

Three sources for replenishing adenosine triphosphate (ATP) during exercise are available: the phosphorylation of adenosine diphosphate (ADP) to ATP by phosphocreatine (PCr) within the exercising muscles; glycogen and lipids within the exercising muscles; and glucose and triglycerides brought to the exercising muscles by the blood. A fourth and less efficient source derives from ADP via an alternate pathway using adenylate kinase and deaminase. PCr stores are the main source that replenishes ATP during intense activity of short duration. During the first 30 seconds of intense endurance exercise, PCr decrease 35 % and muscle glycogen stores reduce by 25 %. Exercise lasting longer than 30 seconds is associated with the mobilization of substantial amounts of carbohydrate and lipid.

The breakdown of muscle glycogen (glycogenolysis) and the anaerobic metabolism of glucose to pyruvate (glycolysis) provide the energy to sustain a prolonged contraction (Figure 8-1). Anaerobic glycolysis is an inefficient mechanism for producing energy and is not satisfactory for endurance exercise. Endurance requires the further aerobic metabolism in mitochondria of pyruvate generated in muscle by glycolysis. Oxidative metabolism provides high levels of energy for every molecule of glucose metabolized (Figure 8-1).

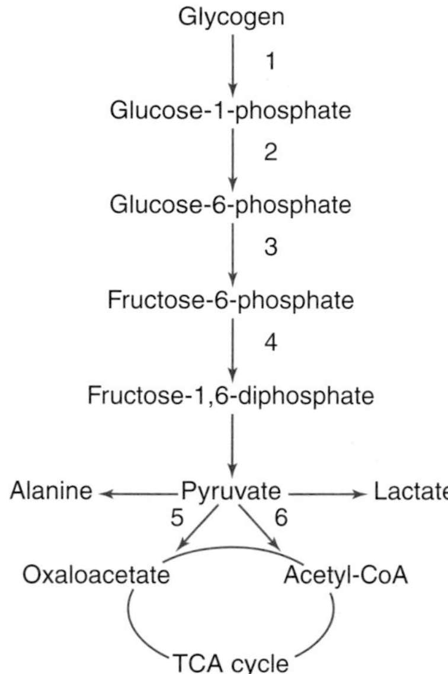

FIGURE 8-1 ■ Glycogen metabolism. 1. Myophosphorylase, initiates glycogen breakdown; 2. Phosphoglucomutase; 3. Phosphoglucose isomerase; 4. Phosphofructokinase; 5. Pyruvate carboxylase; 6. Pyruvate dehydrogenase complex.

The central compound of oxidative metabolism in mitochondria is acetyl-coenzyme A (acetyl-CoA). Acetyl-CoA derives from pyruvate, from fatty acids, and from amino acids. When exercise is prolonged, fatty acids become an important substrate to maintain muscular contraction. Oxidation of acetyl-CoA is through the Krebs cycle. Hydrogen ion release reduces nicotinamide adenine dinucleotide (NAD). These reduced compounds then enter a sequence of oxidation-reduction steps in the respiratory chain that liberate energy. Energy is stored as ATP. This process of releasing and storing energy is *oxidation-phosphorylation coupling*. Therefore, disorders that prevent the delivery of glucose or fatty acids, the oxidation process in the mitochondria, or the creation of ATP impair the production of energy for muscular contraction.

Clinical Features of Decreased Muscle Energy

Exercise intolerance is the invariable result of any disturbance in the biochemical pathways that support muscle contraction. The common symptom is fatigue. Other symptoms are myalgia and cramps. Muscle pain is the expected outcome from unaccustomed exercise. Muscle pain develops during exercise when the mechanisms to supply energy for contraction are impaired.

The ischemic exercise test had been the first step in the diagnosis of muscle energy disorders, but it has become less important with the ease of tissue diagnosis by muscle biopsy and the commercial availability of methods for measuring enzyme activity in fibroblasts. Further, ischemia is unnecessary to perform the test. We have stopped using the test. It is almost impossible to get a child to cooperate sufficiently to do the test properly.

Defects of Carbohydrate Utilization

Myophosphorylase Deficiency (McArdle Disease, Glycogen Storage Disease Type V)

Myophosphorylase deficiency exists in two forms: phosphorylase-a is the active form and phosphorylase-b is the inactive form. Phosphorylase-b kinase is the enzyme that converts the inactive form to the active form and is itself activated by a protein kinase. Deficiencies of either enzyme result in exercise intolerance.

Genetic transmission of myophosphorylase deficiency is by autosomal recessive inheritance. The gene encodes on chromosome 11q13. Reports of autosomal dominant inheritance may represent manifesting heterozygotes. Phosphorylase activity is deficient only in muscle. The deficiency blocks the first step of glycogenolysis and muscle glycogen is unavailable to produce glucose for energy. Liver phosphorylase concentrations are normal, and hypoglycemia does not occur.

Clinical Features. The severity of symptoms varies with the percentage of enzyme activity. Children with only mild deficiency states have few or no symptoms until adolescence. Aching becomes increasingly prominent and then, after an episode of vigorous exercise, severe cramps occur in exercised muscles. Myoglobinuria is sometimes present. The pain can last for hours. Thereafter, exercise leads to repeated bouts of cramps that cause a decline in the overall level of activity. Pain begins soon after initiating vigorous exercise and myoglobinuria several hours later. Some patients exercise through the pain by slowing down just before the time of fatigue. Once passing that point, exercise may continue unimpeded. This "second wind" phenomenon is probably due to an increase in cardiac output, the use of blood glucose and free fatty acids as a substrate for muscle metabolism, and the recruitment of more motor units.

Muscle mass, muscle strength, and the tendon reflexes are usually normal. Only adult patients develop weakness, and, even then, the tendon reflexes are normal.

An alternate presentation of myophosphorylase deficiency is a slowly progressive proximal weakness beginning during childhood or adult life. Affected individuals may never complain of cramps on exercise or of myoglobinuria. Tendon reflexes are present until late in the course of disease.

Diagnosis. EMG examination is usually normal. The serum concentration of CK is elevated, and myoglobin may appear in the urine coincidentally with the cramps.

Salient features of muscle biopsy specimens are histochemical evidence of subsarcolemmal vacuoles containing glycogen and the absence of phosphorylase. Muscle fiber degeneration and regeneration are present immediately after an episode of cramps and myoglobinuria. Definitive diagnosis requires the biochemical demonstration of decreased myophosphorylase activity.

Management. Creatine supplementation may increase muscle function (Vorgerd et al, 2002). Moderate aerobic conditioning improves exercise capacity (Haller et al, 2006). Ingestion of oral sucrose 30 to 40 minutes before aerobic exercise may also improve exercise tolerance (Vissing & Haller, 2003). Patients usually learn to live with their disorder by controlling their level of exercise.

Other Disorders of Glucose Utilization

Four other enzyme deficiencies associated with the anaerobic glycolysis of carbohydrates produce a syndrome identical with myophosphorylase deficiency, i.e., cramps on exercise and myoglobinuria (see Figure 8-1). They are muscle phosphofructokinase (PFK) deficiency (glycogen storage disease type VII, Tarui disease), muscle phosphoglycerate kinase (PFK) deficiency (glycogen storage disease type IX, muscle phosphoglycerate mutase deficiency (glycogen storage disease type X), and lactate dehydrogenase deficiency (glycogen storage disease type XI). All are autosomal recessive traits except phosphoglycerate kinase deficiency, which is an X-linked trait. PFK deficiency is the most common member of this group and causes infantile hypotonia as well (see Chapter 6). Attacks may be associated with nausea, vomiting, and muscle pain. The mutase deficiency occurs mainly in Afro-Americans.

Muscle biopsy results show subsarcolemmal collections of glycogen, but the histochemical reaction for phosphorylase is normal. Biochemical analysis correctly identifies the disorders.

Defects of Long-Chain Fatty Acid Metabolism

Long-chain fatty acids are the principal lipid oxidized to produce acetyl-CoA.

Carnitine Palmitoyl Transferase 2 Deficiency

The mitochondrial oxidation of fatty acids is the main source of energy for muscles during prolonged exercise and during fasting. The carnitine palmitoyl transferase (CPT) enzyme system is essential for the transfer of fatty acids across the mitochondrial membrane. This system includes CPT-1 in the outer mitochondrial membrane and CPT-2 and carnitine-acylcarnitine translocase in the inner mitochondrial membrane.

CPT-2 deficiency is an autosomal recessive trait (gene locus 1p32) with three main phenotypes (Deschauer et al, 2005). The most severe phenotype is a fatal nonketotic hypoglycemic encephalopathy of infants in which CPT-2 is deficient in several organs. Exercise intolerance with myoglobinuria characterizes the less severe phenotype of CPT-2 deficiency of muscle. CPT-2 deficiency is the most common metabolic disorder of skeletal muscle. The phenotypic variations in the muscle diseases caused by CPT-2 deficiency probably relate to the type of molecular defect, and to superimposed environmental factors, such as prolonged fasting, exercise, cold exposure, and intercurrent illness.

Clinical Features. Age at onset of symptoms ranges from 1 year to adult life. In 70%, the disease starts by age 12 years, and in most of the rest between 13 and 22 years. Performing heavy exercise of short duration poses no difficulty. However, pain, tenderness, and swelling of muscles develop after sustained aerobic exercise. Severe muscle cramps, as in myophosphorylase deficiency, do not occur. Associated with the pain may be actual muscle injury characterized by an increased serum concentration of CK and myoglobinuria. Muscle injury may also accompany periods of prolonged fasting, especially in patients on low-carbohydrate, high-fat diets.

In the interval between attacks, results of muscle examination, serum concentration of CK, and EMG are usually normal. People with CPT-2 deficiency are at risk for malignant hyperthermia.

Diagnosis. The clinical features suggest the diagnosis and measuring the concentration of CPT-2 in muscle provides confirmation. Muscle histology is usually normal between attacks.

Management. Frequent carbohydrate feedings and the avoidance of prolonged aerobic activity minimize muscle destruction.

Very-Long-Chain Acyl-Coenzyme A Dehydrogenase Deficiency

The chain length of their preferred substrates describes four mitochondrial acyl-CoA dehydrogenases: short, medium, long, and very long (VLCAD). The first three are located in the mitochondrial matrix, and deficiency causes recurrent coma (see Chapter 2). VLCAD is bound to the inner mitochondrial membrane, and deficiency causes exercise-induced myoglobinuria (Gregersen et al, 2001).

Clinical Features. Onset is usually in the second decade but can be as early as 4 years. Pain and myoglobinuria occur during or following prolonged exercise or fasting. Weakness may be profound. Carbohydrate ingestion before or during exercise reduces the intensity of pain. Examination between attacks is normal.

Diagnosis. The serum CK concentration is slightly elevated between attacks and increased further at the time of myoglobinuria. EMG is consistent with myopathy, and muscle biopsy shows lipid storage in type I fibers. Plasma-free fatty acids but not ketones, increase during a 24-hour fast, suggesting impaired ketogenesis.

Management. Frequent small carbohydrate feeds, dietary fat restriction, and carnitine supplementation reduce the frequency of attacks.

Mitochondrial (Respiratory Chain) Myopathies

The respiratory chain, located in the inner mitochondrial membrane, consists of five protein complexes: complex I (NADH–coenzyme Q reductase); complex II (succinate–coenzyme Q reductase); complex III (reduced coenzyme Q–cytochrome c reductase); complex IV (cytochrome c oxidase); and complex V (ATP synthase) (Figure 8-2).

Coenzyme Q is a shuttle between complexes I and II and complex III. One newborn with a defect of coenzyme Q had a clinical syndrome of seizures, abnormal ocular movements, and lactic acidosis. The clinical syndromes associated with mitochondrial disorders are continually expanding and revised. The organs affected are those highly dependent on aerobic metabolism: nervous system, skeletal muscle, heart, and kidney (Box 8-5). Exercise intolerance, either alone or in combination with symptoms of other organ failure, is a common feature of mitochondrial disorders. The several clinical syndromes defined do not correspond exactly with any one of the respiratory complexes (Box 8-6).

Clinical Features. The age at which mitochondrial myopathies begin ranges from birth to adult life but is before 20 years in most patients. Half of patients have ptosis or ophthalmoplegia, one-quarter has exertional complaints in the limbs, and one-quarter has cerebral dysfunction.

With time, considerable overlap occurs among the three groups. Seventy-five percent eventually have ophthalmoplegia, and 50% have exertional complaints. Pigmentary retinopathy occurs in 33% and neuropathy in 25%.

Exercise intolerance usually develops by 10 years of age. With ordinary activity, active muscles become tight, weak, and painful. Cramps and myoglobinuria are unusual but may occur. Nausea, headache, and breathlessness are sometimes associated features. During these episodes, the serum concentration of lactate and CK may increace. Generalized weakness with ptosis and ophthalmoplegia may follow prolonged periods of activity or fasting. Such symptoms may last for several days, but recovery is usually complete.

Diagnosis. A mitochondrial myopathy is a consideration in all children with exercise intolerance and ptosis or ophthalmoplegia. This combination of symptoms may also suggest myasthenia gravis. However, in myasthenia the ocular motor features fluctuate, while in mitochondrial myopathies they are constant.

Some children with mitochondrial myopathies have an increased concentration of serum lactate after exercise. An easy-to-perform test is the glucose-lactate tolerance test. During an ordinary oral glucose tolerance test, measure lactate and glucose concentrations simultaneously. In some children with mitochondrial disorders, lactic acidosis develops and glucose is slow to clear. We no longer use this test as it may precipitate a crisis in children with severe mitochondrial disease.

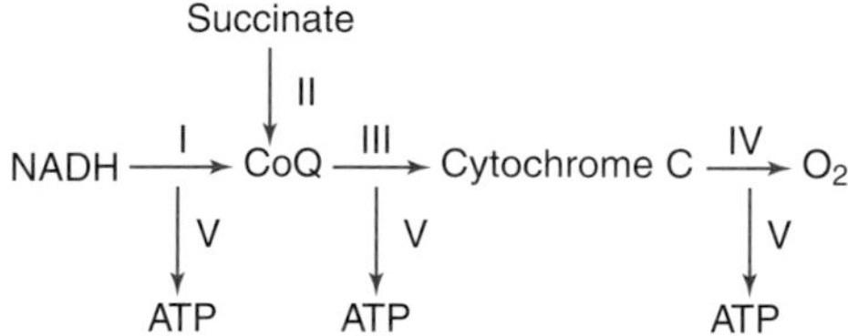

FIGURE 8-2 ■ Respiratory complexes: complex I (NADH:coenzyme Q reductase); complex II (succinate–coenzyme Q reductase); complex III (reduced coenzyme Q:cytochrome c reductase); complex IV (cytochrome c oxidase); and complex V (ATP synthase).

Muscle biopsy specimens, taken from a weak muscle, show a clumping of the mitochondria, which become red when the Gomorri trichrome stain is applied (Figure 8-3). These muscle cells are *ragged-red fibers*. Commercial laboratories can identify several specific respiratory complex disturbances.

Management. The following supplements are worth trying but often fail to provide benefits: coenzyme Q 10–20 mg/kg/day, riboflavin 100 mg/day, pyridoxine 30 mg/kg/day, biotin 5–20 mg/day and carnitine 50–100 mg/kg/day.

Myoadenylate Deaminase Deficiency

The muscle form of adenosine monophosphate deaminase encodes on chromosome 1p. Deficiency of myoadenylate deaminase is clearly a familial trait, and the mode of inheritance is autosomal recessive. The deficiency state occurs in infants with hypotonia, in children with progressive myopathies and recurrent rhabdomyolysis, in children and adults with exercise intolerance, and in asymptomatic individuals. Establishing a cause-and-effect relationship between myoadenylate deaminase deficiency and exercise intolerance in any particular individual is often difficult because most people with the deficiency state are asymptomatic.

Clinical Features. The typical history is one of intermittent muscle pain and weakness with

BOX 8-5 Clinical Features of Mitochondrial Disease

NERVOUS SYSTEM

- Ataxia
- Central apnea
- Cognitive impairment
- Deafness – sensorineural*
- Dementia
- Dystonia
- Hypotonia*
- Migraine-like headaches
- Neuropathy – sensorimotor
- Ophthalmoplegia*
- Optic atrophy
- Polyneuropathy
- Retinitis pigmentosa
- Seizures
- Spinal muscular atrophy

HEART

- Cardiomyopathy
- Conduction defects

KIDNEY

- Aminoaciduria
- Hyperphosphaturia

SKELETAL MUSCLE

- Exercise intolerance
- Myopathy*

*Denotes the most common conditions and the ones with disease modifying treatments

exercise. The pain varies from a diffuse aching to a severe cramping type associated with muscle tenderness and swelling. Between attacks, the children are normal. Symptoms last for 1 to 20 years, with a mean duration of less than 9 years.

Diagnosis. During attacks, the serum concentration of CK may be normal or markedly elevated. EMG and muscle histological studies are usually normal. The forearm ischemic exercise test suggests the diagnosis. Patients with myoadenylate deaminase deficiency fail to generate ammonia but show normal elevations of lactate. However, ammonia levels may fail to rise even in normal individuals, and enzyme analysis of muscle is required for diagnosis.

Obligate heterozygotes have a reduced concentration of myoadenylate deaminase in muscle but are capable of normal ammonia production and are asymptomatic.

Management. Treatment is not available.

MYOPATHIC STIFFNESS AND CRAMPS

This section deals with several conditions that cause muscle stiffness or cramps, or both, in which the primary abnormality is thought to be in skeletal muscle.

Brody Myopathy

The autosomal recessive, but not the autosomal dominant, form of Brody myopathy is caused by a mutation in the gene (16p12) that encodes the fast-twitch skeletal muscle calcium-activated ATPase (*SERCA1*) in sarcoplasmic reticulum (Odermatt et al, 1997). In one Italian family with autosomal dominant inheritance, the Brody phenotype cosegregated with a chromosome (2;7) (p11.2;p12.1) translocation (Novelli et al, 2004).

Clinical Features. The main clinical feature is difficulty of relaxation after contraction. EMG supports the diagnosis. Symptoms of exercise-induced stiffness and cramping begin in the first decade and become progressively worse with age. Unlike myotonia, stiffness becomes worse rather than better with continued exercise. Exercise resumes after a period of rest. Muscle strength and tendon reflexes are normal.

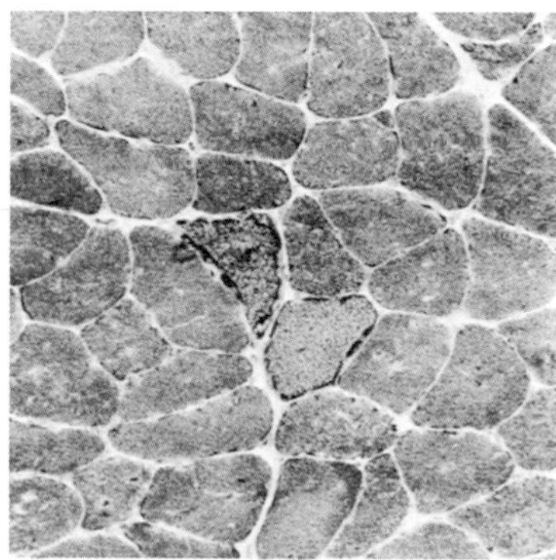

FIGURE 8-3 ■ Ragged-red fibers (trichrome stain). The mitochondria are enlarged and stain intensely with hematoxylin.

BOX 8-6 Mitochondrial Disorders

Complex I (NADH:Coenzyme Q Reductase)

- Congenital lactic acidosis, hypotonia, seizures, and apnea
- Exercise intolerance and myalgia
- Kearns-Sayre syndrome (see Chapter 15)
- Metabolic encephalopathy, lactic acidosis, and stroke (see Chapter 11)
- Progressive infantile poliodystrophy (see Chapter 5)
- Subacute necrotizing encephalomyelopathy (see Chapter 5)

Complex II (Succinate:Coenzyme Q Reductase)

- Encephalomyopathy (?)

Complex III (Coenzyme Q:Cytochrome c Reductase)

- Cardiomyopathy
- Kearns-Sayre syndrome (see Chapter 15)
- Myopathy and exercise intolerance with or without progressive external ophthalmoplegia

Complex IV (Cytochrome c Oxidase)

- Fatal neonatal hypotonia (see Chapter 6)
- Menkes syndrome (see Chapter 5)
- Myoclonus epilepsy and ragged-red fibers
- Progressive infantile poliodystrophy (see Chapter 5)
- Subacute necrotizing encephalomyelopathy (see Chapter 5)
- Transitory neonatal hypotonia (see Chapter 6)

Complex V (Adenosine Triphosphate Synthase)

- Congenital myopathy
- Neuropathy, retinopathy, ataxia, and dementia
- Retinitis pigmentosa, ataxia, neuropathy, and dementia

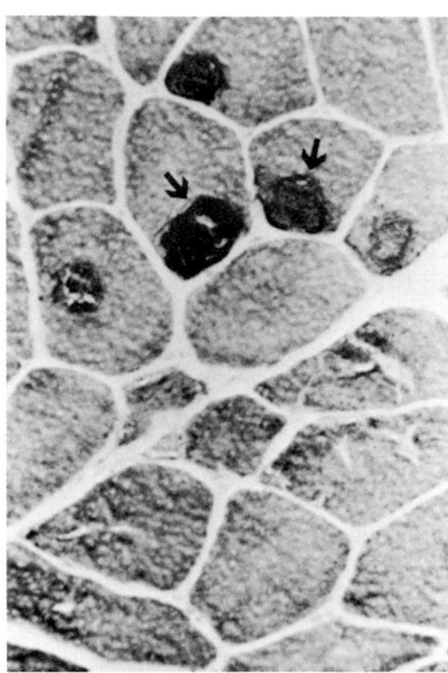

FIGURE 8-4 ■ Tubular aggregates (ATPase reaction). Dark material is present beneath the sarcolemma in type I and type II fibers (arrows).

Diagnosis. Muscle histology reveals type II atrophy. Establishing the diagnosis requires showing the biochemical defect.

Management. Dantrolene, which reduces the myofibrillar Ca^{2+} concentration by blocking Ca^{2+} release from the sarcoplasmic reticulum, provides symptomatic relief. Verapamil may also be useful.

Cramps and Tubular Aggregates

Tubular aggregates are abnormal double-walled structures that originate from the sarcoplasmic reticulum and are located in a subsarcolemmal position (Figure 8-4). Aggregates appear in the muscle biopsy specimens from patients with several neuromuscular disorders. In some families, patients have a progressive myopathy, while others only experience cramps or myalgia.

Sporadic Cases

Clinical Features. Onset is usually in the second or third decade. Cramps may occur at rest or be induced by exercise. The thigh and calf muscles become swollen, stiff, and tender. Cramping occurs more often in cold weather and at night, interfering with sleep. Myalgia is present between cramps. Episodic stiffness of the mouth and tongue interferes with speech. Cramps are not associated with myoglobinuria. Muscle mass, strength, and tendon reflexes are normal.

Diagnosis. The serum concentration of CK is normal. EMG results are normal except that in some patients the cramps are electrically silent. Muscle histology results are the basis for a diagnosis. Light and electron microscopic examinations show tubular aggregates in type II fibers. Evidence of glycogen or lipid storage is not present.

Management. The cramps do not respond to medication.

Autosomal Dominant Cases

Clinical Features. Muscle aches, cramps, and proximal weakness begin in the second decade. The cramps are exercise induced but also may occur at rest and during sleep. Usually, the legs cramp more than the arms, but the pattern varies from family to family. Weakness, when it occurs, is mild and progresses slowly.

Diagnosis. The serum concentration of CK is moderately elevated. EMG results suggest a myopathic process in some families and a neuropathic process in others. Muscle biopsy may show tubular aggregates in type I and type II fibers. Type I fiber predominance and type II hypotrophy are present in some patients.

Treatment. No treatment is available for either the myopathy or the cramps.

Familial X-Linked Myalgia and Cramps

Familial X-linked myalgia and cramps is another phenotype associated with a decreased amount of skeletal muscle dystrophin, which is usually associated with Becker muscular dystrophy (see Chapter 7). Almost all cases are male (Samaha & Quinlan, 1996), except for one female who also had hypertrophy of the calves (Malapart et al, 1995). Half of the males and the one female showed a deletion in the dystrophin gene.

Clinical Features. Symptoms begin in early childhood, frequently between 4 and 6 years of age. The boys first have cramps with exercise and then cramps at rest. Usually the limb muscles are affected, but chest pain may occur as well. The cramping continues throughout life but is not associated with atrophy or weakness. Tendon reflexes are normal.

Diagnosis. Affected family members have elevated concentrations of serum CK, especially after exercise. The EMG and muscle biopsy are usually normal or show only mild, nonspecific changes. This disorder and the McLeod phenotype (acanthocytosis, elevated serum concentration of CK, and absence of the Kell antigen) are allelic conditions. EMG and muscle specimens show nonspecific myopathic changes. DNA analysis may be normal or may show a deletion in the first third of the dystrophin gene or in exons 45–52.

Management. Pharmaceutical agents do not relieve the cramps. Exercise avoidance is the only way to avoid cramping.

Malignant Hyperthermia

Malignant hyperthermia (MH) is a disorder of calcium regulation in skeletal muscle (Rosenberg & Dirksen, 2010). Transmission is as an autosomal dominant trait. Genetic localization was first to chromosome 19q13.1 and the skeletal muscle ryanodine receptor. However, MH proved to be genetically heterogeneous, with additional loci on chromosomes 17q, 7q, 3q, and 5p (Robinson et al, 1997). Several neuromuscular disorders, such as CPT-2, muscular dystrophy, and central core disease, predispose to the syndrome. The administration of several inhalation anesthetics or succinylcholine triggers attacks of muscular rigidity and necrosis associated with a rapid rise in body temperature. Nonanesthetic triggers of rhabdomyolysis in susceptible persons include severe exercise in hot conditions, neuroleptic drugs, alcohol, and infections.

Clinical Features. The first symptoms are tachycardia, tachypnea, muscle fasciculations, and increasing muscle tone. Body temperature rises dramatically, as much as 2°C per hour. All muscles become rigid, and a progressive and severe metabolic acidosis develops. Seizures and death may occur without prompt treatment.

Diagnosis. The basis for diagnosis is the response to anesthesia or succinylcholine. The serum concentration of CK rises to 10 times the upper limit of normal. Molecular diagnosis is available in Europe for detection of three responsible genes, and in the United States for detection of ryanodine receptor (RYR1) mutations. No reliable test for identifying all susceptible individuals is available.

Management. Treatment includes termination of anesthesia, body cooling, treatment of metabolic acidosis, and intravenous injection of dantrolene, 1–2 mg/kg, and repeated every 5 to 10 minutes up to a total dose of 10 mg/kg. Pretreat individual with known or suspected malignant hyperthermia with dantrolene before using an anesthetic.

Neuroleptic Malignant Syndrome

Neuroleptic malignant syndrome, like malignant hyperthermia, is a disorder of the skeletal muscle calcium channels.

Clinical Features. Several neuroleptic agents may induce an idiosyncratic response characterized by muscle rigidity, hyperthermia, altered states of consciousness, and autonomic dysfunction in susceptible individuals. Implicated agents include phenothiazines, butyrophenones, and thioxanthenes. Persons of all ages are affected, but young men predominate. Symptoms develop over 1 to 3 days. The first symptoms are rigidity and akinesia, followed by fever, excessive sweating, urinary incontinence, and hypertension. Consciousness fluctuates, and the 20% mortality rate is due to respiratory failure.

Diagnosis. The clinical findings are the basis of diagnosis. The only helpful laboratory test results are an increased serum concentration of CK and a leukocytosis.

Management. The offending neuroleptic agent must be promptly withdrawn and general supportive care provided. Bromocriptine reverses the syndrome completely.

Rigid Spine Syndrome

Rigid spine syndrome is now recognized as the severe classic form of multi-minicore myopathy (Beggs & Agrawal, 2008), and has been linked to mutations in the *SEPN1* gene (Moghadaszadeh et al, 2001). Multi-minicore myopathy is divisible into four groups: the classic form comprises 75% of the total and the other three (moderate form with hand involvement, antenatal form with arthrogyposis, and the ophthalmoplegic form) each comprise less than 10%. The classic form is usually perinatal and characterized by neonatal hypotonia, delayed motor development, axial muscle weakness, scoliosis, and significant respiratory depression. Spinal rigidity of varying severity is present.

Clinical Features. Marked limitation in flexion of the dorsolumbar and cervical spine begin in infancy or early childhood secondary to contractures in the spinal extensors. Movement of the spine and the thoracic cage is lost. Extension of the elbow and ankles may be limited. The condition is not progressive, but scoliosis often leads to respiratory failure.

Diagnosis. The presence of multiple "minicores" visible on muscle biopsy using oxidative stains is the basis for diagnosis.

Management. Management is symptomatic.

Rippling Muscle Disease (Caveolinopathies)

Caveolin is a muscle-specific membrane protein (Bruno et al, 2007). Disorders of caveolin produce several different phenotypes within the same family. One is *rippling muscle disease* in which mechanical stimulation of muscle produces electrically silent contractions. Transmission of the disorder is by autosomal dominant inheritance. Autosomal dominant limb-girdle muscular dystrophy type 1C, as well as some cases of isolated hyperCKemia and isolated hypertrophic cardiomyopathy, are allelic disorders (Bruno et al, 2007)

Clinical Features. Frequent falls was the initial feature in children with the caveolin-3 gene mutation (Schara et al, 2002). Other features include muscle pain and cramps following exercise that persists for several hours. Stiffness occurs during rest after the child exercises or maintains posture for long periods. Percussion of muscles causes local swelling and a peculiar rippling movement that lasts for 10 to 20 seconds. Muscle hypertrophy develops. Muscle strength, tone, and coordination, as well as tendon reflexes, are normal.

Diagnosis. The serum CK concentration is mildly elevated, and muscle biopsy findings are normal. EMG of the muscle swelling after percussion shows no electrical activity. Molecular genetic diagnosis confirms the diagnosis.

Management. Management is symptomatic.

REFERENCES

Abu-Arafeh I, Russell G. Recurrent limb pain in schoolchildren. Archives of disease in Childhood 1996;74:336–9.

Beggs AH, Agrawal PB. Multiminicore disease. In: Pagon RA, Bird TD, Dolan CR, et al., eds. GeneReviews™. Seattle: University of Washington. Available at http://www.genetests.org. Last updated April 10, 2008.

Bruno C, Sotgia F, Gazzerro E, et al. Caveolinopathies. In: Pagon RA, Bird TD, Dolan CR, et al., eds. GeneReviews™. Seattle: University of Washington. Available at http://www.genetests.org. Posted May 14, 2007.

Colding-Jorgensen E, Dunø M, Vissing J. Autosomal dominant monosymptomatic myotonia permanens. Neurology 2006;67:153–5.

Deschauer M, Wieser T, Zierz S. Muscle carnitine palmitoyltransferase II deficiency: clinical and molecular genetic features and diagnostic aspects. Archives of Neurology 2005;62:37–41.

Dunø M, Colding-Jørgensen E. Myotonia congenita. In: Pagon RA, Bird TD, Dolan CR, et al., eds. GeneReviews™. Seattle: University of Washington. Available at http://www.genetests.org. PMID: 20301529. Last updated April 12, 2011.

Gregersen N, Andresen BS, Corydon MJ, et al. Mutation analysis in mitochondrial fatty acid oxidation defects: Exemplified by acyl-CoA dehydrogenase deficiencies, with special focus on genotype-phenotype relationship. Human Mutations 2001;18:169–89.

Haller RG, Wyrick P, Taivassalo T, et al. Aerobic conditioning: An effective therapy in McArdle's disease. Annals of Neurology 2006;59:922–8.

Logigian EL, et al. Mexiletine is an effective antimyotonia treatment in myotonic dystrophy type 1. Neurology 2010;74:1441–8.

Malapart D, Recan D, Leturcq F, et al. Sporadic lower limb hypertrophy and exercise induced myalgia in a woman with dystrophin gene deletion. Journal of Neurology, Neurosurgery and Psychiatry 1995;59:552–4.

Meola G, Hanna MG, Fontaine B. Diagnosis and new treatment in muscle channelopathies. Journal of Neurology, Neurosurgery and Psychiatry 2009;80:360–5.

Moghadaszadeh B, Petit N, Jaillard C. Mutations in SEPN1 cause congenital muscular dystrophy with spinal rigidity and restrictive respiratory syndrome. Nature Genetics 2001;29:17–8.

Novelli A, Valente EM, Bernardini L, et al. Autosomal dominant Brody disease cosegregates with a chromosomal (2;7)(p11.2;p12.1) translocation in an Italian family. European Journal of Human Genetics 2004;12:579–83.

Odermatt A, Taschner PEM, Scherer SW, et al. Characterization of the gene encoding human sarcolipin (SLN), a proteolipid associated with SERCA1: Absence of structural mutations in five patients with Brody disease. Genomics 1997;45:541–53.

Robinson RL, Monnier N, Wolz W, et al. A genome wide search for susceptibility loci in three European malignant hyperthermia pedigrees. Human Molecular Genetics 1997;6:953–61.

Rosenberg H, Dirksen RT. Malignant hyperthermia susceptibility. In: GeneClinics: Medical Genetics Knowledge Base [database online]. Seattle: University of Washington. Available at http://www.genetests.org. PMID: 20301325. Last updated January 19, 2010.

Samaha FJ, Quinlan JG. Myalgia and cramps: Dystrophinopathy with wide-ranging laboratory findings. Journal of Child Neurology 1996;11:21–4.

Schara U, Vorgerd M, Popovic N, et al. Rippling muscle disease in children. Journal of Child Neurology 2002;17:483–90.

Van den Berg JSP, et al. Acquired neuromyotonia: superiority of plasma exchange over high-dose intravenous human immunoglobulin. Journal of Neurology 1999;246(7):623–5.

Vissing J, Haller R. The effect of oral sucrose on exercise tolerance in patients with McArdle's disease. New England Journal of Medicine 2003;349:2503–9.

Vorgerd M, Zange J, Kley R, et al. Effect of high-dose creatine therapy on symptoms of exercise intolerance in McArdle disease. Archives of Neurology 2002;59:97–101.

CHAPTER 9

SENSORY AND AUTONOMIC DISTURBANCES

This chapter deals primarily with sensory disturbances of the limbs and trunk. Autonomic dysfunction is often associated with sensory loss but sometimes occurs alone. Chapter 17 considers sensory disturbances of the face.

SENSORY SYMPTOMS

Pain, dysesthesias, and loss of sensibility are the important symptoms of disturbed sensation. Peripheral neuropathy is the most common cause of disturbed sensation at any age. As a rule, hereditary neuropathies are more likely to cause loss of sensibility without discomfort, whereas acquired neuropathies are more likely to be painful. Discomfort is more likely than numbness to bring a patient to medical attention.

Nerve root pain generally follows a dermatomal distribution. Ordinarily, it is descripted as deep and aching. The pain is more proximal than distal and may be constant or intermittent. When intermittent, the pain may radiate in a dermatomal distribution. The most common cause of root pain in adults is sciatica associated with lumbar disk disease. Disk disease also occurs in adolescents, usually because of trauma. In children, radiculitis is a more common cause of root pain. Examples of radiculitis are the migratory aching of a limb preceding paralysis in the acute inflammatory demyelinating polyradiculoneuropathy/Guillain-Barré syndrome (see Chapter 7) and the radiating pain in a C5 distribution that heralds an idiopathic brachial neuritis (see Chapter 13).

Polyneuropathy involving small nerve fibers causes dysesthetic pain. This pain differs from previously experienced discomfort and the description is as pins and needles, tingling, or burning. It compares with the abnormal sensation felt when dental anesthesia is wearing off. The discomfort is superficial, distal, and usually symmetric. Dysesthetic pain is never a feature of hereditary neuropathies in children.

Loss of sensibility is the sole initial feature in children with sensory neuropathy. Because of the associated clumsiness, delay in establishing a correct diagnosis is common. Strength and tests of cerebellar function are normal and tendon reflexes are absent. The combination of areflexia and clumsiness should suggest a sensory neuropathy.

Table 9-1 summarizes the pattern of sensory loss as a guide to the anatomical site of abnormality and Box 9-1 a differential diagnosis of conditions with sensory deficits.

PAINFUL LIMB SYNDROMES

Three painful arm syndromes are acute idiopathic brachial neuritis (also called neuralgic amyotrophy or brachial plexitis), familial recurrent brachial neuritis, and complex regional pain syndrome (reflex sympathetic dystrophy). In the first two syndromes, muscle atrophy follows a transitory pain in the shoulder or arm. Monoplegia is the prominent feature (see Chapter 13). Although muscle atrophy also occurs in complex regional pain syndrome, pain is the prominent feature. Discussion of complex regional pain syndrome follows.

Complex Regional Pain Syndrome I

The presence of regional pain and sensory changes following a noxious event defines *complex regional pain syndrome* (CRPS). A working group of the International Association for the Study of Pain developed a new terminology that separates reflex sympathetic dystrophy (RSD) from causalgia (Rowbotham, 1998). CRPS I

TABLE 9-1 Patterns of Sensory Loss

Pattern	Site
All limbs	Spinal cord or peripheral nerve
Bothlegs	Spinal cord or peripheral nerve
Glove-and-stocking	Peripheral nerve
Legs and trunk	Spinal cord
One arm	Plexus
One leg	Plexus or spinal cord
Unilateral arm and leg	Brain or spinal cord

BOX 9-1 Disturbances of Sensation

BRACHIAL NEURITIS
- Neuralgic amyotrophy (see Chapter 13)
- Recurrent familial brachial neuropathy (see Chapter 13)

COMPLEX REGIONAL PAIN SYNDROME I (REFLEX SYMPATHETIC DYSTROPHY)

CONGENITAL INSENSITIVITY (INDIFFERENCE) TO PAIN
- Lesch-Nyhan syndrome
- Mental retardation
- With normal nervous system

FORAMEN MAGNUM TUMORS

HEREDITARY METABOLIC NEUROPATHIES
- Acute intermittent porphyria
- Hereditary tyrosinemia

HEREDITARY SENSORY AND AUTONOMIC NEUROPATHY (HSAN)
- HSAN I (autosomal dominant)
- HSAN II (autosomal recessive)
- HSAN III (familial dysautonomia)
- HSAN IV (with anhydrosis)

LUMBAR DISK HERNIATION

SYRINGOMYELIA

THALAMIC SYNDROMES

replaces the term RSD. The definition of CRPS I is defined as "a pain syndrome that develops after an injury, is not limited to the distribution of a single peripheral nerve, and is disproportional to the inciting event." CRPS II requires demonstrable peripheral nerve injury and replaces the term causalgia.

Clinical Features. The essential feature of CRPS I is sustained burning pain in a limb combined with vasomotor and pseudomotor dysfunction, leading to atrophic changes in skin, muscle, and bone following trauma. The pain is of greater severity than that expected from the inciting injury. The mechanism remains a debated issue. Catecholamine hypersensitivity may account for the decreased sympathetic outflow and autonomic features in the affected limb (Wasner et al, 2001).

The mean age at onset in children is 11 years, and girls are more often affected than are boys. CRPS I frequently follows trauma to one limb, with or without fracture. The trauma may be relatively minor, and the clinical syndrome is so unusual that a diagnosis of "hysterical" or "malingering" is common. Time until onset after injury is usually within 1 or 2 months, but the average interval from injury to diagnosis is 1 year.

The first symptom is pain at the site of injury, which progresses either proximally or distally without regard for dermatomal distribution or anatomical landmarks. Generalized swelling and vasomotor disturbances of the limb occur in 80% of children. Pain is intense, described as burning or aching, and is out of proportion to the injury. It may be maximally severe at onset or may become progressively worse for 3 to 6 months. Movement or dependence exacerbates the pain, causing the patient to hold the arm in a position of abduction and internal rotation, as if swaddled to the body. The hand becomes swollen and hyperesthetic and feels warmer than normal.

Children with CRPS I do better than do adults. Reported outcomes vary widely, probably based on the standard of diagnosis. In my own experience, most begin recovering within 6 to 12 months. Long-term pain is unusual, as are the trophic changes of the skin and bones that often occur in adults. Recovery is usually complete, and recurrence is unusual.

Diagnosis. The basis for diagnosis is the clinical features; laboratory tests are not confirmatory. Because the syndrome follows accidental or surgical trauma, litigation is commonplace, and requires careful documentation of the clinical features examination. In recent years, CRPS I has become popular on the Internet and is often self-diagnosed incorrectly. Websites caution the patient that doctors misdiagnose the condition as hysterical. The result is increasing numbers of hysterical patients seeking consultation for an incorrect, self-diagnosis of CRPS I.

One simple test is to immerse the affected limb in warm water. Wrinkling of the skin of the fingers or toes requires intact sympathetic innervation. The absence of wrinkling is evidence of a lesion in either the central or the peripheral sympathetic pathway. The other, unaffected, limb serves as a control.

Management. Management for most children is range of motion exercise and over-the-counter analgesics. Treatment of more severe syndromes includes the oral administration of guanethidine, gabapentin (Wheeler et al, 2000), prednisone with or without stellate ganglion blockade, and sympathectomy. Pregabalin at doses of 2–10 mg/kg/day divided into two doses often helps.

Erythromelalgia

Familial erythromelalgia is an autosomal dominant disorder (2q24) caused by a mutation in a gene encoding a voltage-gated sodium channel (Waxman & Dib-Hajj, 2005).

Clinical Features. Burning pain occurs in one or more limbs exposed to warm stimuli or exercise. Onset is often in the second decade. Moderate exercise, such as walking, induces burning pain, redness, and warmth of the feet and lower legs.

Diagnosis. The clinical features establish the diagnosis, especially when other family members are affected.

Management. Stopping the exercise provides relief. Sodium channel blockers (carbamazepine, phenytoin, lamotrigine, oxcarbazepine, and possibly lacosamide) are useful to prevent attacks in some families.

CENTRAL CONGENITAL INSENSITIVITY (INDIFFERENCE) TO PAIN

Most children with congenital insensitivity to pain have an hereditary sensory neuropathy. In many early reports, sensory neuropathy was not a consideration and appropriate tests not performed. This section is restricted to those children and families with a central defect. Sensory neuropathy testing is normal and mild mental retardation often associated. Several affected children are siblings with consanguineous parents. Autosomal recessive inheritance is therefore suspect. The Lesch-Nyhan syndrome is a specific metabolic disorder characterized by self-mutilation (presumably because of indifference to pain) and mental retardation without evidence of sensory neuropathy (see Chapter 5).

Clinical Features. Children with congenital insensitivity to pain come to medical attention when they begin to crawl or walk. Their parents recognize that injuries do not cause crying and that the children fail to learn the potential of injury from experience. The result is repeated bruising, fractures, ulcerations of the fingers and toes, and mutilation of the tongue. Sunburn and frostbite are common.

Examination shows absence of the corneal reflex and insensitivity to pain and temperature, but relative preservation of touch and vibration sensations. Tendon reflexes are present, an important differential point from sensory neuropathy.

Diagnosis. The results of electromyography (EMG), nerve conduction studies, and examination of the cerebrospinal fluid are normal.

Management. No treatment is available for the underlying insensitivity, but the repeated injuries require supportive care. Injuries and recurrent infections reduce longevity.

FORAMEN MAGNUM TUMORS

Extramedullary tumors in and around the foramen magnum are known for false localizing signs and for mimicking other disorders, especially syringomyelia and multiple sclerosis. In children, neurofibroma caused by neurofibromatosis is the only tumor found in this location.

Clinical Features. The most common initial symptom is unilateral or bilateral dysesthesias of the fingers. Suboccipital or neck pain occurs as well. Ignoring such symptoms is common early in the course. Numbness and tingling usually begin in one hand and then migrate to the other. Dysesthesias in the feet are a late occurrence. Gait disturbances, incoordination of the hands, and bladder disturbances generally follow the sensory symptoms and are so alarming that they prompt medical consultation.

Many patients have café au lait spots, but few have evidence of subcutaneous neuromas. The distribution of weakness may be one arm, one side, or both legs; 25 % of patients have weakness in all limbs. Atrophy of the hands is uncommon. Sensory loss may involve only one segment or may have a “cape” distribution. Diminished pain and temperature sensations are usual and other sensory disturbances may be present. Tendon reflexes are brisk in the arms and legs. Patients with neurofibromatosis may have multiple neurofibromas causing segmental abnormalities in several levels of the spinal cord.

Diagnosis. Magnetic resonance imaging (MRI) is the best method for showing abnormalities at the foramen magnum.

Management. Surgical excision of a C2 root neurofibroma relieves symptoms completely.

HEREDITARY NEUROPATHIES

Hereditary Sensory and Autonomic Neuropathies

The classification of hereditary sensory and autonomic neuropathy (HSAN) attempts to synthesize information based on natural history, mode of inheritance, and electrophysiological characteristics.

Hereditary Sensory and Autonomic Neuropathy Type I

Hereditary sensory and autonomic neuropathy type I (HSAN I) is the only HSAN transmitted as an autosomal dominant inheritance. As with other dominantly inherited neuropathies, variable expression is the rule (Nicholson, 2012). Therefore, the history alone is insufficient to determine whether the parents are affected; physical examination and electrophysiological studies are required. HSAN type I maps to chromosome 9q22.1-22.3. This disorder is caused by a mutation in the serine palmitoyl transferase long-chain base subunit 1 (*SPTLC1*) gene [3,4], although cases without SPTLC1 mutations have been described (de Andrade et al, 2009).

Clinical Features. Symptoms begin during the second decade or later. The major clinical features are lancinating pains in the legs and ulcerations of the feet. However, initial symptoms are usually insidious, and the precise onset is often difficult to date. A callus develops on the sole of the foot, usually in the skin overlying a weight-bearing bony prominence. The callus blackens, becomes necrotic, and breaks down into an ulcer that is difficult to heal. Sensory loss precedes the ulcer, but often it is the ulcer, and not the sensory loss, that first brings the patient to medical attention. Although plantar ulcers are an important feature, they are not essential for diagnosis. When the proband has typical features of plantar ulcers and lancinating pain, other family members may have sensory loss in the feet, mild pes cavus, or peroneal atrophy, and loss of the ankle tendon reflex.

Sensory loss in the hands is variable and never as severe as in the feet. Finger ulcers do not occur. Distal muscle weakness and wasting are present in all advanced cases.

Diagnosis. Autosomal dominant inheritance and sensory loss in the feet are essential for the diagnosis. The presence of plantar ulcers and lancinating pain is helpful but not essential. Clinical grounds differentiate HSAN I from familial amyloid polyneuropathy. Urinary incontinence, impotence, and postural hypotension are frequent features of amyloidosis but do not occur in HSAN I. Molecular genetic testing is available.

Electrophysiological studies show slowing of sensory nerve conduction velocity and the absence of sensory nerve action potentials. Sural nerve biopsy reveals a marked decrease or absence of myelinated fibers and a mild to moderate reduction of small myelinated fibers.

Management. No treatment is available for the neuropathy, but good foot care prevents plantar ulcers. Patients must avoid tight-fitting shoes and activities that traumatize the feet. Discontinue weight-bearing at the first sign of a plantar ulcer. Much of the foot mutilation reported in previous years was due to secondary infection of the ulcers. Warm soaks, elevation, and antibiotics prevent infection from mutilating the foot.

Hereditary Sensory and Autonomic Neuropathy Type II

Hereditary sensory and autonomic neuropathy type II (HSAN II) probably includes several disorders transmitted by autosomal recessive inheritance. A mutation in the *HSN2* gene on chromosome 12p13.3 is present in this disorder (de Andrade et al, 2009). Some cases are relatively static, and others have a progressive course. Many of the cases are sporadic; instances of parental consanguinity and affected siblings occur in some families.

Clinical Features. Symptoms probably begin during infancy and possibly at the time of birth. Infantile hypotonia is common (see Chapter 6). Unlike HSAN I, which affects primarily the feet, HSAN II involves all limbs equally, as well as the trunk and forehead. The result is a diffuse loss of all sensation; diminished touch and pressure is probably earlier and greater in extent than are temperature and pain. Affected infants and children are constantly hurting themselves without a painful response. The absence of the protection that pain provides against injury results in ulcerations and infections of the fingers and toes, stress fractures, and injuries to long bones. Loss of deep sensibility causes injury and swelling of joints, and loss of touch makes simple tasks, such as tying shoes, manipulating small objects, and buttoning buttons, difficult if not impossible. Tendon reflexes are absent throughout. Sweating diminishes in all areas of decreased sensibility, but no other features of autonomic dysfunction are present.

HSAN II may be associated with impaired hearing, taste, and smell, with retinitis pigmentosa, or with the early onset of cataracts. It is not clear whether such cases represent separate genetic disorders or are part of the phenotypic spectrum of a single genetic disorder.

Diagnosis. The diagnosis relies primarily on the history and examination. Absence of sensory nerve action potentials confirms that the congenital absence of pain is due to peripheral neuropathy and not to a cerebral abnormality. Motor nerve conduction velocities are normal, as are the morphological characteristics of motor unit potentials. Fibrillations are sometimes present. Sural nerve biopsy reveals an almost complete absence of myelinated fibers.

The boundary between HSAN II and HSAN IV (discussed later) is difficult to delineate clinically. Mental retardation and anhydrosis are more prominent in HSAN IV than in HSAN II.

Management. No treatment is available for the neuropathy. However, parents must be vigilant for painless injuries. Discoloration of the skin and swelling of joints or limbs should raise the possibility of fracture. Children must learn to avoid activities that might cause injury and to examine themselves for signs of superficial infection.

Hereditary Sensory and Autonomic Neuropathy Type III

The usual name for hereditary sensory and autonomic neuropathy type III (HSAN III) is *familial dysautonomia* or *the Riley-Day syndrome*. This disorder is present at birth. Cardinal features are hypotonia, feeding difficulties, and poor control of autonomic function. It occurs almost exclusively in patients of Jewish Ashkenazi ancestry and is associated with an absence of fungiform papillae on the tongue. A mutation in the gene encoding an IjB kinase complex-associated protein is present in this condition. Because neonatal hypotonia is prominent, the discussion is in Chapter 6.

Hereditary Sensory and Autonomic Neuropathy Type IV (Congenital Insensitivity to Pain with Anhidrosis)

Genetic transmission of hereditary sensory and autonomic neuropathy type IV (HSAN IV) is by autosomal recessive inheritance. The abnormal gene site is 1q21-22 (Bonkowski et al, 2003). Several point mutations in the nerve growth factor 1 receptor gene (*TRKA1*) have been associated with the clinical phenotype of HSAN IV. The major features are congenital insensitivity to pain, anhydrosis, and mental retardation. All the clinical abnormalities are present at birth, and while complications of the pain-free state are a continuous problem, the underlying disease may not be progressive.

Clinical Features. Anhydrosis, rather than insensitivity to pain, causes the initial symptoms. HSAN type IV patients frequently have bowel problems, recurrent syncope, and crises of hyperthermia. Affected infants have repeated episodes of fever, sometimes associated with seizures. These episodes usually occur during the summer; the cause is an inability to sweat in response to exogenous heat. Sweat glands are present in the skin but lack sympathetic innervation. Most infants are hypotonic and areflexic. Attainment of developmental milestones is slow, and, by 2 or 3 years of age, the child has had several self-inflicted injuries caused by pain insensitivity. Injuries may include ulcers of the fingers and toes, stress fractures, self-mutilation of the tongue, and Charcot joints.

Sensory examination shows widespread absence of pain and temperature sensation. Touch, vibration, and stereognosis are intact in some patients. Tendon reflexes are absent or hypoactive. The cranial nerves are intact and the corneal reflex and lacrimation are normal. Mild to moderate retardation is present in almost every case. Other features, present in some children, are blond hair and fair skin, Horner syndrome, and aplasia of dental enamel.

Diagnosis. Familial dysautonomia (HSAN III) and HSAN IV have many features in common and are easily confused. However, insensitivity to pain is not prominent in HSAN III, and fungiform papillae of the tongue are present in HSAN IV. Molecular genetic testing is now available for both disorders.

Management. No treatment is available for the underlying disease. However, constant vigilance is required to prevent injuries to the skin and bones with secondary infection.

Hereditary Sensory and Autonomic Neuropathy Type V

This is a rare disorder characterized by decreased numbers of small diameter neurons in peripheral nerves and manifested by the absence of thermal and mechanical pain perception. Genetic studies show the role of nerve growth factor beta, which is also involved in the development of the autonomic nervous system and cholinergic pathways in the brain. HSAN type V is usually reported not to cause mental retardation or cognitive decline.

Clinical Features. HSAN type V is the least frequent of all the HSANs. It is characterized by a loss of thermal and mechanical pain perception and various milder autonomic dysfunctions, with anhidrosis less marked than in patients with HSAN IV and an absence of the sympathetic skin response in nerve studies.

Both recessive and dominant modes of inheritance are possible for this condition. It was found to be associated with a mutation in the nerve growth factor beta gene (*NGFB*) in a Swedish family (Einarsdottir, 2004) and with a mutation in the neurotrophic tyrosine kinase receptor type 1 (NTRK1) in another report (Houlden et al, 2001).

Diagnosis. The diagnosis relies on the history and the absence of sympathetic skin responses. Molecular genetic testing is available.

Management. No treatment is available for the underlying disease. However, constant vigilance is required to prevent injuries to the skin and bones with secondary infection.

Metabolic Neuropathies

Acute Intermittent Porphyria

Acute intermittent porphyria is an autosomal dominant disorder that results from an error in pyrrole metabolism due to deficiency of porphobilinogen (PBG) deaminase. The gene location is 11q23.3. Individuals with similar degrees of enzyme deficiency may have considerable variation in phenotypic expression (Anderson et al, 2005).

Clinical Features. Approximately 90 % of individuals with acute intermittent porphyria never have clinical symptoms. Onset is rarely before puberty. Symptoms are periodic and occur at irregular intervals. Alterations in hormonal levels during a normal menstrual cycle or pregnancy and exposure to certain drugs, especially barbiturates, trigger attacks. The most common clinical feature of acute intermittent porphyria is an attack of severe abdominal pain, often associated with vomiting, constipation, or diarrhea. Tachycardia, hypertension, and fever may be associated. Limb pain is common, and muscle weakness often develops. The weakness is a result of a motor neuropathy that causes greater weakness in proximal than distal muscles and in the arms more than the legs. Tendon reflexes are usually decreased and may be absent in weak muscles. Approximately half of the patients have cerebral dysfunction; mental changes are particularly common, and seizures sometimes occur. Chronic mental symptoms, such as depression and anxiety, sometimes continue even between attacks.

Diagnosis. Suspect acute intermittent porphyria in people with acute or episodic neurological or psychiatric disturbances. Increased excretion of aminolevulinic acid and PBG occurs during attacks, but levels may be normal between attacks. The risk of attacks correlates with the excretion of PBG in the urine when the patient is free of symptoms. Molecular genetic diagnosis is definitive.

Management. The most important aspect of managing symptomatic disease is to prevent acute attacks by avoiding known precipitating factors. During an attack, patients frequently require hospitalization because of severe pain. Carbohydrates are believed to reduce porphyrin synthesis and should be administered intravenously daily at a dose of 300–500 g as a 10 % dextrose solution. Reports of benefit from hematin infusions, a specific feedback inhibitor of heme synthesis, are in the literature. However, hematin is neither readily available nor very soluble, and may carry a risk of renal damage.

Hereditary Tyrosinemia

Hereditary tyrosinemia type I is caused by deficiency of the enzyme fumarylacetoacetate hydrolase. Transmission of the genetic trait is by autosomal recessive inheritance and the gene map locus is 15q23-q25.

Clinical Features. The major features are acute and chronic liver failure and a renal Fanconi syndrome. However, recurrent attacks of painful dysesthesias or paralysis are a prominent feature of the disease in half of children. The attacks usually begin at 1 year of age and infection precedes the attack in half of the cases. Perhaps because of the child's age, pain localization is poor and referred to the legs and lower abdomen. Associated with the pain is axial hypertonicity that ranges in severity from mild neck stiffness to opisthotonos. Generalized weakness occurs in 30 % of attacks and may necessitate respiratory support. Less common features of attacks are seizures and self-mutilation. Between attacks, the child appears normal.

Diagnosis. The basis for diagnosis is an increased blood concentration of tyrosine and a deficiency of fumarylacetoacetate hydrolase. The cause of crises is in part by an acute axonal neuropathy. The neuropathy is demonstrable by EMG studies. Succinylacetone, a metabolite of tyrosine, accumulates and inhibits porphyrin metabolism. Definitive diagnosis is by molecular genetic testing.

Management. Nitisinone (Orfadin®), 2-(2-nitro-4-trifluoro-methylbenzyol)-1,3-cyclohexanedione, which blocks p-hydroxyphenylpyruvic acid dioxygenase, the second step in the tyrosine degradation pathway, prevents the accumulation of fumarylacetoacetate and its conversion to succinylacetone (Holme & Lindstedt, 2000). Liver transplantation is the definitive treatment.

SPINAL DISORDERS

Lumbar Disk Herniation

Trauma is the usual cause of lumbar disk herniation in children. Almost all cases occur after age 10 years. They are more common in boys than in girls and are frequently sports related. Delays in diagnosis are commonplace because lumbar disk herniation is so unusual in children.

Clinical Features. The initial features are pain and inability to function normally because of pain and inability to move the back. Straight leg raising and bending forward from the waist are impaired. Frequently the pain has been present for a long time because most children will accommodate to their disability. Examination reveals diminished sensation to pinprick in the distribution of the L5 and S1 dermatome, and diminished or absent ankle tendon reflexes in more than half of patients.

Diagnosis. Radiographs of the lumbosacral spine reveal minor congenital anomalies (hemivertebrae, sacralization of the lumbar spine) in an unusually large number of cases. MRI of the spine or myelography confirms the diagnosis.

Management. Bed rest provides immediate relief in most patients. The indication for surgical treatment is pain that persists and limits function in spite of adequate medical measures.

Syringomyelia

Syringomyelia is a generic term for a fluid-filled cavity within the substance of the spinal cord. The cavity varies in length and may extend into the brainstem. A brainstem extension is termed syringobulbia. The cavity, or syrinx, is central in the gray matter and may enlarge in all directions. The cervicothoracic region is a favorite site, but thoracolumbar syrinx also occurs, and occasionally a syrinx extends from the brainstem to the conus medullaris.

The mechanism of syrinx formation is uncertain. Cavitation of the spinal cord sometimes follows trauma and infarction, but these are not important mechanisms of syringomyelia in children. In childhood, the cause of primary syringomyelia is either a congenital malformation or a cystic astrocytoma. In the past, the two were distinguishable only by postmortem examination. Astrocytomas of the spinal cord, like those of the cerebellum, may have large cysts with only a nubbin of solid tumor. MRI has greatly enhanced antemortem diagnosis of cystic astrocytoma by showing small areas of increased signal intensity in one or more portions of the cyst. Cystic astrocytoma is more likely to produce symptoms during the first decade, whereas congenital syringomyelia becomes symptomatic in the second decade or later and is usually associated with the Chiari anomaly. Chapters 12 and 13 consider cystic astrocytoma of the spinal cord; this section deals primarily with congenital syringomyelia.

Clinical Features. The initial symptoms of syringomyelia depend on the cyst's location. Because the cavity is near the central canal, it first affects crossing fibers subserving pain and temperature. When the syrinx is in the cervical area, pain and temperature are typically lost in a "cape" or "vest" distribution. However, early involvement is often unilateral or at least asymmetric and sometimes involves the fingers before the shoulders. Preservation of touch and pressure persists until the cyst enlarges into the posterior columns or the dorsal root entry zone. Loss of pain sensibility in the hands often leads to injury, ulceration, and infection, as seen in hereditary sensory and autonomic neuropathies. Pain is prominent. Complaints include neck ache, headache, back pain, and radicular pain.

Scoliosis is common, and torticollis may be an initial sign in children with cervical cavities. As the cavity enlarges into the ventral horn, weakness and atrophy develop in the hands and may be associated with fasciculations; pressure on the lateral columns causes hyperreflexia and spasticity in the legs. Very long cavities may produce lower motor neuron signs in all limbs. Sphincter control is sometimes impaired. The posterior columns are generally the last to be affected, so that vibration sense and touch are preserved until relatively late in the course. The progress of symptoms is extremely slow and insidious. The spinal cord accommodates well to the slowly developing pressure within. Thus, at the time of consultation, a long history of minor neurological handicaps such as clumsiness or difficulty running is common.

Bulbar signs are relatively uncommon and usually asymmetric. They include hemiatrophy of the tongue with deviation on protrusion, facial weakness, dysphasia, and dysarthria. Disturbances of the descending pathway of the trigeminal nerve cause loss of pain and temperature sensations on the same side of the face as the facial weakness and tongue hemiatrophy.

Diagnosis. MRI is the diagnostic study of choice (Figure 9-1).

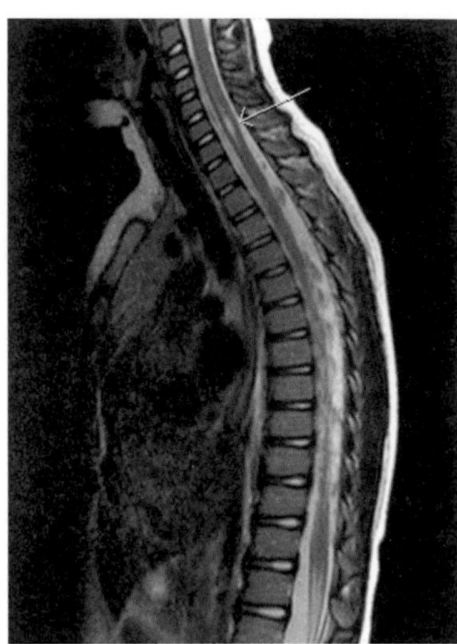

FIGURE 9-1 ■ Syrinx. T_2 sagittal MRI of spine shows a dilated central canal/cervical syrinx (arrow).

Management. Syrinxes occurring with hydrocephalus and communicating with the fourth ventricle do well following ventriculoperitoneal shunt. Syrinxes associated with Chiari I malformations collapse after shunting from the syrinx to the cerebellopontine angle, and noncommunicating syrinxes often collapse after excision of an extramedullary obstruction.

THALAMIC PAIN

The thalamic pain syndrome occurs almost exclusively in adults following infarction of the thalamus. Similar symptoms sometimes occur in patients with thalamic glioma. The location of the lesion is usually the ventroposterolateral nucleus of the thalamus. Thalamic-type pain also occurs with lesions of the parietal lobe, medial lemniscus, and dorsolateral medulla (MacGowan et al, 1997).

Clinical Features. Touching the affected limb or part of the body produces intense discomfort described as "sharp," "crushing," or "burning." Suffering is considerable, and the quality of the pain is unfamiliar to the patient. Several different modes of stimulation, such as changes in ambient temperature, auditory stimulation, and even changes in emotional state, can accentuate the pain. Despite the severity of these dysesthesias, the affected limb is otherwise anesthetic to ordinary sensory testing.

Diagnosis. The presence of thalamic pain should prompt imaging studies to determine the presence of tumor, infarction, or demyelinating disease.

Management. The combination of levodopa and a peripheral decarboxylase inhibitor may be helpful for relieving pain. If this does not prove satisfactory, administer some combination of analgesic and tranquilizing medication.

REFERENCES

Anderson KE, Bloomer JR, Bonkovsky HL, et al. Recommendations for the diagnosis and treatment of the acute porphyrias. Annals of Internal Medicine 2005;142:439–50.

Bonkowski JL, Johnson J, Carey JC, et al. An infant with primary tooth loss and palmar hyperkeratosis: A novel mutation in the NTRK1 gene causing congenital insensitivity to pain with anhydrosis. Pediatrics 2003;112:e237–41.

de Andrade DC, Baudic S, Attal N, et al. Beyond neuropathy in hereditary sensory and autonomic neuropathy type V: Cognitive evaluation. European Journal of Neurology 2008;15:712–9.

Einarsdottir E, Carlsson A, Minde J, et al. A mutation in nerve growth factor beta gene (NGFB) causes loss of pain perception. Human Molecular Genetics 2004;13:799–805.

Holme E, Lindstedt S. Nontransplant treatment of tyrosinemia. Clinical Liver Disease 2000;4:805–14.

Houlden H, King RH, Hashemi-Nejad A, et al. A novel TRK A (NTRK1) mutation associated with hereditary sensory and autonomic neuropathy type V. Annals of Neurology 2001;49:521–5.

MacGowan DGL, Janal MN, Clark WC, et al. Central poststroke pain and Wallenberg's lateral medullary infarction. Frequency, character, and determinants in 63 patients. Neurology 1997;49:120–5.

Nicholson GA. Hereditary sensory neuropathy, type 1. GeneReviews at GeneTests: Medical Genetics Information Resource [database online]. Seattle: University of Washington. Available at http://www.genetests.org. PMID: 20301564. Last updated May 3, 2012.

Rowbotham MC. Complex regional pain syndrome type I (reflex sympathetic dystrophy). More than a myth. Neurology 1998;51:4–5.

Wasner G, Schattschneider J, Heckmann K, et al. Vascular abnormalities in reflex sympathetic dystrophy (CRPS I): Mechanisms and diagnostic value. Brain 2001;124:587–99.

Waxman SG, Dib-Hajj SD. Erythromelalgia: A hereditary pain syndrome enters the molecular era. Annals of Neurology 2005;57:785–8.

Wheeler DS, Vaux KK, Tam DA. Use of gabapentine in the treatment of childhood reflex sympathetic dystrophy. Pediatric Neurology 2000;22:220–31.

CHAPTER 10

ATAXIA

The term ataxia denotes disturbances in the fine control of posture and movement. The cerebellum and its major input systems from the frontal lobes and the posterior columns of the spinal cord provide this control. The initial and most prominent feature is usually an abnormal gait. The ataxic gait is wide-based, lurching, and staggering, and it provokes disquiet in an observer for fear that the patient is in danger of falling. One observes a similar gait in people who are attempting to walk in a vehicle that has several directions of motion at once, such as a railroad train.

When an abnormality occurs in the vermis of the cerebellum, the child cannot sit still but constantly moves the body to-and-fro and bobs the head (titubation). In contrast, disturbances of the cerebellar hemispheres cause a tendency to veer in the direction of the affected hemisphere, with dysmetria and hypotonia in the ipsilateral limbs. Bifrontal lobe disease may produce symptoms and signs that are indistinguishable from those of cerebellar disease.

Loss of sensory input to the cerebellum, because of peripheral nerve or posterior column disease, necessitates constant looking at the feet to know their location in space (due to loss of proprioception). The gait is also wide-based, but is not so much lurching as careful. The foot raises high with each step and slaps down heavily on the ground. Station and gait are considerably worse with the eyes closed, and the patient may actually fall to the floor (Romberg sign). Sensory ataxia is more likely to cause difficulty with fine finger movements than with reaching for objects.

Other features of cerebellar disease are a characteristic speech that varies in volume and has an increased separation of syllables (scanning speech), hypotonia, limb and ocular dysmetria, and tremor. The differential diagnosis of a child with acute ataxia or recurrent attacks of ataxia (Box 10-1) are quite different from that of a child with chronic static or progressive ataxia (Box 10-2). Therefore, the discussion of these two presentations is separate in the text. However, one may "suddenly" become aware of what had been a slowly progressive ataxia, and children with recurrent ataxia may never recover to baseline function after each attack. Progressive ataxia superimposes on the acute attacks.

ACUTE AND RECURRENT ATAXIAS

The two most common causes of ataxia among children who were previously healthy and then suddenly have an ataxic gait are drug ingestion and acute postinfectious cerebellitis. Migraine, brainstem encephalitis, and an underlying neuroblastoma are the next considerations.

Brain Tumor

Primary brain tumors ordinarily cause chronic progressive ataxia and their discussion is later in this chapter. However, ataxia may be acute if the brain tumor bleeds or causes hydrocephalus. In addition, early clumsiness may not become apparent until it becomes severe enough to cause

BOX 10-1 Acute or Recurrent Ataxia

- Brain tumor
- Conversion reaction*
- Drug ingestion
- Encephalitis (brainstem)
- Genetic disorders
  - Dominant recurrent ataxia
  - Episodic ataxia type 1
  - Episodic ataxia type 2
  - Hartnup disease
  - Maple syrup urine disease
  - Pyruvate dehydrogenase deficiency
- Migraine
  - Basilar
  - Benign paroxysmal vertigo*
- Postinfectious/immune
  - Acute postinfectious cerebellitis
  - Miller Fisher syndrome*
  - Multiple sclerosis*
  - Myoclonic encephalopathy and neuroblastoma*
- Progressive cavitating leukoencephalopathy
- Pseudoataxia (epileptic)
- Trauma
  - Hematoma* (see Chapter 2)
  - Postconcussion*
  - Vertebrobasilar occlusion*
- Vascular disorders
  - Cerebellar hemorrhage*
  - Kawasaki disease*

*Denotes the most common conditions and the ones with disease modifying treatments

BOX 10-2 Chronic or Progressive Ataxia

BRAIN TUMORS

- Cerebellar astrocytoma*
- Cerebellar hemangioblastoma* (Von Hippel-Lindau disease)
- Ependymoma*
- Medulloblastoma*
- Supratentorial tumors* (see Chapter 4)

CONGENITAL MALFORMATIONS

- Basilar impression
- Cerebellar aplasias
- Cerebellar hemisphere aplasia
- Chiari malformation*
- Dandy-Walker malformation (see Chapter 18)
- Vermal aplasia

HEREDITARY ATAXIAS

- Autosomal dominant inheritance (see Table 10-1)
- Autosomal recessive inheritance
  - Abetalipoproteinemia
  - Ataxia-telangiectasia
  - Ataxia without oculomor apraxia
  - Ataxia with episodic dystonia
  - Friedreich ataxia
  - Hartnup disease
  - Juvenile GM_2 gangliosidosis
  - Juvenile sulfatide lipidoses
  - Maple syrup urine disease
  - Marinesco-Sjögren syndrome
  - Pyruvate dehydrogenase deficiency
  - Ramsay Hunt syndrome
  - Refsum disease (HSMN IV) (see Chapter 7)
  - Respiratory chain disorders (see Chapter 8)

X-LINKED INHERITANCE

- Adrenoleukodystrophy (see Chapter 5)
- Leber optic neuropathy (see Chapter 16)
  - With adult-onset dementia
  - With deafness
  - With deafness and loss of vision

*Denotes the most common conditions and the ones with disease modifying treatments

an obvious gait disturbance. Brain imaging is therefore a recommendation for most children with acute cerebellar ataxia.

Conversion Reaction

Clinical Features. Psychogenic gait disturbances are relatively common in children, especially girls between 10 and 15 years of age. Psychogenic symptoms are involuntary and usually protective against an overwhelming stressor. In contrast, malingering is a voluntary act. Psychogenic gait disturbances are often extreme. The child appears to sit without difficulty but when brought to standing immediately begins to sway from the waist. Stance is not wide to improve stability as it would occur in an organic ataxia. Instead, the child lurches, staggers, and otherwise travels across the room from object to object. The lurching maneuvers are often complex and require extraordinary balance. Strength, tone, sensation, and tendon reflexes are normal.

Diagnosis. The diagnosis of psychogenic gait disturbances is by observation; laboratory tests or imaging studies are not ordinarily required to exclude other possibilities.

Management. Determination of the precipitating stress is important. Conversion may represent a true call for help in a desperate situation such as sexual or physical abuse. Such cases require referral to a multispecialty team able to deal with the whole family. Fortunately, most children with psychogenic gait disturbances are responding to an immediate and less serious life stress. Identifying possible stressors, modifying surrounding circumstances and activities, and improving copying mechanisms are necessary for improvement and prevention of further psychogenic symptoms.

Dominant Recurrent Ataxias

At least two distinct genetic defects are recognized that cause episodic ataxia: episodic ataxia type 1 (EA-1) and episodic ataxia type 2 (EA-2). Both are the result of ion channel mutations. Mutations in a potassium channel gene underlie EA-1 and mutations in a voltage-dependent calcium channel underlie EA-2 (Subramony et al, 2003).

Episodic Ataxia Type 1 (Paroxysmal Ataxia and Myokymia)

EA-1 results from a mutation of the potassium channel gene *KCNA1* on chromosome 12p. The additional feature of continuous motor unit activity (see Chapter 8) suggests a defect in membrane stability affecting the central and peripheral nervous systems.

Clinical Features. The onset of attacks is usually between 5 and 7 years of age. Abrupt postural change, startle, exercise, and stress may provoke an attack. The child becomes aware of attack onset by the sensation of spreading limpness or stiffness lasting for a few seconds.

Incoordination, trembling of the head or limbs, and blurry vision often follow. Some children feel warm and perspire. Some can continue standing or walking, but most sit down. Attacks usually last for less than 10 minutes but can be as long as 6 hours. Myokymia of the face and limbs begins at about age 12 years. Physical findings include large calves, normal muscle strength, and widespread myokymia of face, hands, arms, and legs, with a hand posture resembling carpopedal spasm. Electromyography (EMG) at rest shows continuous spontaneous activity (De Vries et al, 2009)

Diagnosis. The basis for clinical diagnosis is the history of typical attacks and the family history. EMG confirms the diagnosis by showing continuous motor unit activity, most often in the hands but also in the proximal arm muscles and sometimes in the face.

Management. Some patients respond to daily antiepileptic drugs. When these fail, a trial of daily acetazolamide is reasonable.

Episodic Ataxia Type 2 (Acetazolamide-Responsive Ataxia)

EA-2, one form of spinocerebellar ataxia (SCA6), and one type of familial hemiplegic migraine all represent allelic mutations in the same calcium channel gene *CACNA1A* on chromosome 19p. About half of patients have migraine headaches; some episodes may be typical of basilar migraine (Spacey, 2011; De Vries et al, 2009).

Clinical Features. Clinical heterogeneity is considerable despite genetic localization to the 19p site. The onset is generally during school age or adolescence. The child first becomes unsteady and is then unable to maintain posture because of vertigo and ataxia. Vomiting is frequent and severe. Jerk nystagmus, sometimes with a rotary component, occurs during attacks. One to three attacks may occur each month, with symptoms lasting from 1 hour to 1 day. Attacks become milder and less frequent with age. Slowly progressive truncal ataxia and nystagmus may persist between attacks. In some patients ataxia is the only symptom, others have only vertigo, and still others have only nystagmus. Most affected individuals are normal between attacks, but some are phenotypically indistinguishable from those with SCA6 (see discussion on Progressive Hereditary Ataxias later in this chapter).

Diagnosis. The clinical features and the family history are the basis for diagnosis. Molecular diagnosis is available on a research basis. Magnetic resonance imaging (MRI) may show selective atrophy of the cerebellar vermis. Basilar artery migraine and benign paroxysmal vertigo can be distinguished from dominant recurrent ataxia because in these conditions, older family members have migraine but do not have recurrent ataxia. Further, attacks of benign paroxysmal vertigo rarely last more than a few minutes.

Management. Daily oral acetazolamide prevents recurrence of attacks in almost every case. The mechanism of action is unknown. The dose is generally 125 mg twice a day in young children and 250 mg twice a day in older children. Flunarizine, 5–10 mg/day, may serve as an alternative therapy for children with acetazolamide intolerance. Antiepileptic and antimigraine medications are without value.

Other Episodic Ataxias

Episodic ataxia type 3 (EA-3), EA-4, EA-5 and EA-6 are described. These ataxias are even less frequent and well described. EA-6 was identified as a more severe phenotype of episodic and progressive ataxia, seizures, alternating hemiplegia, and migraine headache associated with a mutation of the *SLC1A3* gene, which encodes the glial excitatory amino acid transporter EAAT1 involved in glutamate removal from the synaptic cleft (De Vries et al, 2009).

Drug Ingestion

The incidence of accidental drug ingestion is greatest between ages 1 and 4 years.

Clinical Features. An overdose of most psychoactive drugs causes ataxia, disturbances in personality or sensorium, and sometimes seizures. Toxic doses of antiepileptic drugs, especially phenytoin, may cause marked nystagmus and ataxia without an equivalent alteration in sensorium. Excessive use of antihistamines in the treatment of an infant or young child with allergy or an upper respiratory tract infection may cause ataxia. This is especially true in children with otitis media, who may have underlying unsteadiness because of middle-ear infection and possible inner ear dysfunction.

Diagnosis. Carefully question the parents or care providers of every child with acute ataxia concerning drugs intentionally administered to the child and other drugs accessible in the home. Specific inquiry concerning the use of anticonvulsant or psychoactive drugs by family members is mandatory. Screen urine for drug metabolites, and send blood for analysis when suspecting intoxication with a specific drug.

Management. Treatment depends on the specific drug ingested and its blood concentration. In most cases of ataxia caused by drug ingestion, the drug can be safely eliminated spontaneously if vital function is not compromised, if acid–base balance is not disturbed, and if liver and kidney function is normal. In life-threatening situations, dialysis may be necessary while supporting vital function in an intensive care unit. Gastric emptying has limited value when ataxia is already present.

Encephalitis (Brainstem)

Ataxia may be the initial feature of viral encephalitis affecting primarily the structures of the posterior fossa. Potential etiological agents include echoviruses, coxsackieviruses, adenoviruses, and *Coxiella burnetti* (Sawaishi et al, 1999).

Clinical Features. Cranial nerve dysfunction is often associated with the ataxia. Generalized encephalitis characterized by declining consciousness and seizures may develop later. Meningismus is sometimes present. The course is variable, and, although most children recover completely, some suffer considerable neurological impairment. Those who have only ataxia and cranial nerve palsies, with no disturbance of neocortical function, tend to recover best. Such cases are indistinguishable from the Miller Fisher syndrome on clinical grounds alone.

Diagnosis. Diagnosis requires showing a cellular response, primarily mononuclear leukocytes, in the cerebrospinal fluid, with or without some elevation of the protein content. Prolonged interpeak latencies of the brainstem auditory evoked response are evidence of an abnormality within the brainstem parenchyma and not the peripheral sensory input system. The electroencephalogram (EEG) is usually normal in children with brainstem encephalitis who have a normal sensorium.

Management. No specific treatment is available for the viral infection.

Inborn Errors of Metabolism

Hartnup Disease

Hartnup disease is a rare disorder transmitted by autosomal recessive inheritance. The abnormal gene localizes to chromosome 5p15 (Nozaki et al, 2001). The basic error is a defect of amino acid transport in kidney and small intestine. The result is aminoaciduria and the retention of amino acids in the small intestine. Tryptophan conversion is to nonessential indole products instead of nicotinamide.

Clinical Features. Affected children are normal at birth but may be slow in attaining developmental milestones. Most achieve only borderline intelligence; others are normal. Affected individuals are photosensitive and have a severe pellagra-like skin rash after exposure to sunlight. Nicotinamide deficiency causes the rash. Many patients have episodes of limb ataxia, sometimes associated with nystagmus. Mental changes, ranging from emotional instability to delirium or states of decreased consciousness, may occur. Examination reveals hypotonia and normal or exaggerated tendon reflexes. Stress or intercurrent infection triggers the neurological disturbances, which may be due to the intestinal absorption of toxic amino acid breakdown products. Most patients have both rash and neurological disturbances, but each can occur without the other. Symptoms progress over several days and last for a week to a month before recovery occurs.

Diagnosis. The constant feature of Hartnup disease is aminoaciduria involving neutral monoaminomonocarboxylic amino acids. These include alanine, serine, threonine, asparagine, glutamine, valine, leucine, isoleucine, phenylalanine, tyrosine, tryptophan, histidine, and citrulline.

Management. Daily oral administration of nicotinamide, 50–300 mg, may reverse the skin and neurological complications. A high-protein diet helps make up for the amino acid loss and the disease is rare in populations with a super-adequate diet.

Maple Syrup Urine Disease (Intermittent)

Maple syrup urine disease is a disorder of branched-chain amino acid metabolism caused by deficiency of the enzyme branched-chain keto acid dehydrogenase. The result of the deficiency is a neonatal organic acidemia. Transmission of the defect is by autosomal recessive inheritance. Three phenotypes are associated, depending on the percentage of enzyme deficiency. The classic form begins as seizures in the newborn (see Chapter 1), the intermediate form causes progressive mental retardation (see Chapter 5), and the intermittent form causes recurrent attacks of ataxia, and encephalopathy.

Clinical Features. Affected individuals are normal at birth. Between 5 months and 2 years, minor infections, surgery, or a diet rich in protein provokes episodes of ataxia, irritability, and progressive lethargy. The length of an attack is variable; most children recover spontaneously, but some die of severe metabolic acidosis. Psychomotor development remains normal in survivors.

Diagnosis. The urine has a maple syrup odor during the attack, and the blood and urine have elevated concentrations of branched-chain amino acids and ketoacids. Between attacks, the concentrations of branched-chain amino acids and ketoacids are normal in both blood and urine. Establishing the diagnosis requires showing the enzyme deficiency in cultured fibroblasts.

Management. Children with intermittent maple syrup disease need a protein-restricted diet. Some have a thiamine-responsive enzyme defect, and 1 g of thiamine a day treats the acute attacks. If this is successful, a recommended maintenance dose is 100 mg/day. The main objective during an acute attack is to reverse ketoacidosis. Allow no protein ingestion and peritoneal dialysis may be helpful in life-threatening situations.

Pyruvate Dehydrogenase Deficiency

The pyruvate dehydrogenase (PDH) complex is responsible for the oxidative decarboxylation of pyruvate to carbon dioxide and acetyl-coenzyme A (acetyl-CoA). Disorders of the complex are associated with several neurological conditions, including subacute necrotizing encephalomyelopathy (Leigh syndrome), mitochondrial myopathies, and lactic acidosis. The complex contains three main components that are termed E1, E2, and E3. E1 consists of two alpha subunits encoded on the X chromosome and two beta subunits. Episodes of intermittent ataxia and lactic acidosis characterize the X-linked form of PDH-E1 deficiency (Head et al, 2005). E1 deficiency is the most common form of PDH deficiency.

Clinical Features. The clinical features range from severe neonatal lactic acidosis and death to episodic ataxia with lactic and pyruvic acidosis and spinocerebellar degeneration. Most patients show mild developmental delay during early childhood. Episodes of ataxia, dysarthria, and sometimes lethargy usually begin after 3 years of age. In more severely affected patients, episodes may begin during infancy and are associated with generalized weakness and states of decreased consciousness. Some attacks are spontaneous, but intercurrent infection, stress, or a meal high in carbohydrate provokes others. Attacks recur at irregular intervals and may last for periods ranging from 1 day to several weeks.

The severity of neurological dysfunction in any individual probably reflects the level of residual enzyme activity. Those with generalized weakness are also areflexic and have nystagmus or other disturbances in ocular motility. Ataxia is the predominant symptom. Intention tremor and dysarthria may be present. Hyperventilation is common and metabolic acidosis may be the cause. Patients with almost complete PDH deficiency die of lactic acidosis and central hypoventilation during infancy.

Diagnosis. PDH deficiency should be suspected in children with lactic acidosis, hypotonia, progressive or episodic ataxia, the Leigh disease phenotype, and recurrent polyneuropathy. The pyruvic acid concentration is elevated, and the lactate-to-pyruvate ratio is low. The blood concentration of lactate may be elevated between attacks; lactate and pyruvate concentrations are always elevated during attacks. Some children have hyperalaninemia as well. Analysis of enzyme activity in cultured fibroblasts, leukocytes, or muscle establishes the diagnosis.

Management. The ketogenic diet is a rational treatment for PDH complex deficiency (Klepper et al, 2002). Patients are usually treated with thiamine (100–600 mg/day) and a high-fat (>55 %), low-carbohydrate diet. Unfortunately, current treatments do not prevent disease progression in most patients. In addition, daily oral acetazolamide, 125 mg twice a day in small children and 250 mg twice a day in older children, may significantly abort the attacks. The treatment of several patients with biotin, carnitine, coenzyme Q10, and thiamine supplements has not established efficacy.

Migraine

Basilar Migraine

The term basilar (artery) migraine characterizes recurrent attacks of brainstem or cerebellar dysfunction that occur as symptoms of a migraine attack. Children who experience basilar artery migraine have typical migraine with aura at other times (Kirchmann et al, 2006). Girls are more often affected than are boys. The peak incidence is during adolescence, but attacks may occur at any age. Infant-onset cases are more likely to present as benign paroxysmal vertigo.

Clinical Features. Gait ataxia occurs in approximately 50 % of patients. Other symptoms include visual loss, vertigo, tinnitus, alternating hemiparesis, and paresthesias of the fingers, toes, and corners of the mouth. An abrupt loss of consciousness may occur, usually lasting for only a few minutes. Cardiac arrhythmia and brainstem stroke are rare life-threatening complications. A severe, throbbing, occipital headache usually follows the neurological disturbances. Nausea and vomiting occur in less than one-third of cases.

Children may have repeated basilar migraine attacks, but, with time, the episodes evolve into a pattern of classic migraine. Even during attacks of classic migraine, the patient may continue to complain of vertigo and even ataxia.

Diagnosis. EEG distinguishes basilar migraine from benign occipital epilepsy. The EEG shows occipital intermittent delta activity during and just after an attack in basilar migraine and occipital sharp and spike and wave discharges in epilepsy.

Management. Treatment of basilar artery migraine is the same as for other forms of migraine (see Chapter 3). Frequent attacks require a prophylactic agent.

Benign Paroxysmal Vertigo

Benign paroxysmal vertigo is primarily a disorder of infants and preschool children but may occur in older children.

Clinical Features. Recurrent attacks of vertigo are characteristic. Vertigo is maximal at onset. True cerebellar ataxia is not present, but vertigo is so profound that standing is impossible. The child either lies motionless on the floor or wants holding. Consciousness maintains throughout the event and headache is not associated. The predominant symptoms are pallor, nystagmus, and fright. Episodes last only for minutes and may recur at irregular intervals. With time, attacks decrease in frequency and stop completely or evolve into more typical migraines. Migraine develops in 21 % (Lindskog et al, 1999).

Diagnosis. The diagnosis is primarily clinical, and laboratory tests are useful only to exclude other possibilities. A family history of migraine, though not necessarily paroxysmal vertigo, is positive in 40 % of cases. Some parents indicate that they experience vertigo with their attacks of migraine. Only in rare cases does a parent have a history of benign paroxysmal vertigo.

Management. The attacks are so brief and harmless that treatment is not required. Migraine prophylaxis may be considered when the attacks are frequent.

Postinfectious/Immune-Mediated Disorders

In many conditions discussed in this section, the underlying cause of cerebellar dysfunction and some other neurological deficits is an altered immune state. Preceding viral infections are usually incriminated but documentation is limited to only half of cases. Natural varicella infections and the varicella vaccine are definite preceding causes. No other vaccine links to acute cerebellar ataxia.

Acute Cerebellar Ataxia

Acute cerebellar ataxia usually affects children between 2 and 7 years of age, but it may occur as late as 16 years. The disorder affects both genders equally, and the incidence among family members is not increased. In the past, acute cerebellar ataxia occurred most often following varicella infection. The widespread use of varicella vaccine has made the syndrome uncommon. However, it is a complication of live-inactivated vaccine administration.

Clinical Features. The onset is explosive. A previously healthy child awakens from a nap and cannot stand. Ataxia is maximal at onset. Some worsening may occur during the first hours, but a longer progression, or a waxing and waning course, negates the diagnosis. Ataxia varies from mild unsteadiness while walking to complete inability to stand or walk. Even when ataxia is severe, sensorium is clear and the child is otherwise normal. Tendon reflexes may be present or absent; their absence suggests the *Miller Fisher syndrome*. Nystagmus, when present, is usually mild. Chaotic movements of the eyes (opsoclonus) should suggest the myoclonic encephalopathy-neuroblastoma syndrome.

Symptoms begin to remit after a few days, but recovery of normal gait takes 3 weeks to 5 months. Patients with pure ataxia of the trunk or limbs and only mild nystagmus are likely to recover completely. Marked nystagmus or opsoclonus (see the section on Myoclonic Encephalopathy/Neuroblastoma Syndrome later in this chapter), tremors of the head and trunk, or moderate irritability are usually followed by persistent neurological sequelae.

Diagnosis. The diagnosis of acute postinfectious cerebellitis is one of exclusion. Every child should have drug screening, and most will have a brain imaging study. The necessity of imaging the brain in typical cases, especially those with varicella infection, is debatable. Lumbar puncture is indicated when encephalitis is suspected.

Management. Acute postinfectious cerebellitis is a self-limited disease. Treatment is not required. Occupational therapy may facilitate activities during the recovery phase.

Miller Fisher Syndrome

Ataxia, ophthalmoplegia, and areflexia characterize the Miller Fisher syndrome. A similar disorder with ataxia and areflexia but without ophthalmoplegia is *acute ataxic neuropathy*. Some believe that Miller Fisher syndrome is a variant of Guillain-Barré syndrome; others believe that it is a form of brainstem encephalitis. In support of the hypothesis of a Guillain-Barré-like, immune-mediated hypothesis is the finding that *Campylobacter jejuni* serotype O:19 is a causative agent in both Miller Fisher syndrome and Guillain-Barré syndromes (Jacobs et al, 1995).

Clinical Features. A viral illness precedes the neurological symptoms by 5 to 10 days in 50% of cases. Either ophthalmoparesis or ataxia may be the initial feature. Both are present early in the course. The initial ocular motor disturbance is paralysis of upgaze, followed by loss of lateral gaze and then downgaze. Recovery takes place in the reverse order. Preservation of the Bell phenomenon sometimes occurs despite paralysis of voluntary upward gaze, suggesting the possibility of supranuclear palsy. Ptosis occurs but is less severe than the vertical gaze palsy.

Decreased peripheral sensory input probably causes areflexia and more prominent limb than trunk ataxia. Weakness of the limbs may be noted. Unilateral or bilateral facial weakness occurs in a significant minority of children. Recovery generally begins within 2 to 4 weeks after symptoms become maximal and is complete within 6 months.

Diagnosis. The clinical distinction between the Miller Fisher syndrome and brainstem encephalitis can be difficult. Disturbances of sensorium, multiple cranial nerve palsies, an abnormal EEG, or prolongation of the interpeak latencies of the brainstem auditory evoked response should suggest brainstem encephalitis. The cerebrospinal fluid profile in Miller Fisher syndrome parallels that of Guillain-Barré syndrome. A cellular response occurs early in the course, and protein elevation occurs later.

Management. Intravenous immunoglobulin to block antibodies and plasmapheresis to remove antibodies may be beneficial. The dose of immunoglobilin is 2 g/kg over 2 to 5 days. The outcome in untreated children is usually good.

Multiple Sclerosis

Multiple sclerosis is usually a disease of young adults, but 3–5% of cases occur in children less than 6 years of age (Ruggieri et al, 1999). The childhood forms of multiple sclerosis are similar to the adult forms. This section could just as well appear in several other chapters of the text. The advent of neuroimaging, especially magnetic resonance imaging (MRI), has heightened diagnostic accuracy (Tenembaun et al, 2007).

In a prospective study of 296 children with acute demyelination, 81 presented with focal involvement, 119 with acute disseminated encephalomyelitis (ADEM), and 96 with symptoms that suggest already established multiple sclerosis. Long-tract (motor, sensory, or sphincter) dysfunction was the commonest finding in 226 children (76%), followed by symptoms localized to the brainstem in 121 children (41%), optic neuritis in 67 children (22%), and transverse myelitis in 42 children (14%) (Mikaeloff, 2006). Monofocal presentation was more common in adolescents. Recovery from acute demyelination is variable: 85% of children with optic neuritis recover full visual acuity (Kriss et al, 1988; Visudhiphan, 1995; Wilejto et al, 2006). In published reports of 250 children with transverse myelitis, 80% were paraplegic or tetraplegic and had incontinence or severe urinary symptoms at onset, and 5% died (Banwell et al, 2007). More than 30% of survivors remain wheelchair dependent, and 70% have residual bladder control problems (Wingerchuk et al, 2006).

Clinical Features. The female-to-male ratio varies from 1.5:1 to 3:1. Ataxia, concurrent with a febrile episode, is the most common initial feature in children, followed by encephalopathy, hemiparesis, or seizures. Intranuclear ophthalmoplegia, unilateral or bilateral, develops in one-third of patients (see Chapter 15).

The clinical features that occur in multiple sclerosis are sufficiently variable that no single prototype is valid. The essential feature is repeated episodes of demyelination in noncontiguous areas of the central nervous system. Focal neurological deficits that develop rapidly and persist for weeks or months characterize an episode. Afterward the child has partial or complete recovery. Months or years separate recurrences, which are often concurrent with fever, but not with a specific febrile illness. Lethargy, nausea, and vomiting sometimes accompany the attacks in children but rarely in adults. The child is usually irritable and shows truncal and limb ataxia. Tendon reflexes are generally brisk throughout. The long-term outcome is poor.

Diagnosis. Multiple sclerosis may be the suspected diagnosis at the time of the first attack, but definitive diagnosis requires recurrence to establish a polyphasic course. Examination of the cerebrospinal fluid at the time of exacerbation reveals fewer than 25 lymphocytes/mm^3, a normal or mildly elevated protein content, and sometimes the presence of oligoclonal bands.

MRI is the technique of choice for the diagnosis of multiple sclerosis and shows occult disease in up to 80% of affected individuals at the time of first presentation (Figure 10-1). The finding of three or more white matter lesions on a T_2-weighted image MRI scan, especially if one of these lesions is in the perpendicular plane to the corpus callosum, is a sensitive predictor of definite multiple sclerosis (Frohman et al, 2003). However, the extent and severity of lesions may not correlate with the clinical syndrome. After repeated attacks, the MRI reveals thalamic grey matter loss (Mesarus et al, 2008).

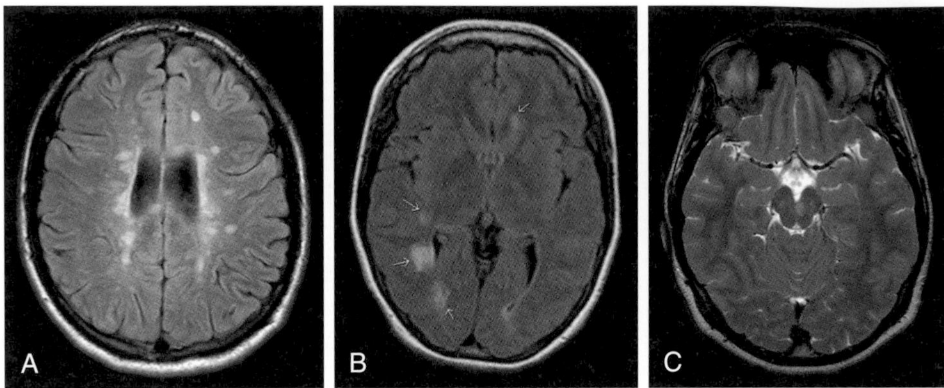

FIGURE 10-1 ■ Multiple sclerosis. (A) T_2 flair axial MRI shows multiple demyelinating lesions. (B) Axial flair showing multiple demyelinating lesions (arrows). (C) T_2 axial MRI showing midbrain central demyelination.

Management. The treatment of multiple sclerosis in children is similar to that in adults, and the outcome is no more favorable. Acute exacerbations require a short course of corticosteroids. Following an initial administration of methylprednisolone, 500–1000 mg, depending on the age, a tapering dose schedule is used. Experience is not available in children with the drugs used to prevent relapses in adults.

Myoclonic Encephalopathy/ Neuroblastoma Syndrome

Myoclonic encephalopathy is a syndrome characterized by opsoclonus (chaotic irregular eye movements), myoclonic ataxia (irregular shock-like muscle contractions), and encephalopathy. The pathophysiological mechanism is an altered immune state. Initially, the syndrome was attributed either to the presence of occult neuroblastoma or to an unknown cause. With improved imaging techniques, almost all cases appear to be neuroblastoma related. A single patient report associated the opsoclonus-myoclonus syndrome with a benign ovarian teratoma (Fitzpatrick et al, 2008). Two to three percent of children with neuroblastoma develop a myoclonic encephalopathy. A specific causal antibody is not established but a neuronal surface antibody is a suspect (Blaes et al, 2005).

Clinical Features. The mean age at onset is 18 months, with a range from 1 month to 4 years (Russo et al, 1997). Unlike acute postinfectious cerebellitis and Miller Fisher syndrome, in which neurological symptoms are fully expressed within 1 to 2 days, the evolution of symptoms in myoclonic encephalopathy may take a week or longer.

Either ataxia or chaotic eye movements may bring the child to medical attention. Almost half of affected children show personality change or irritability, suggesting the presence of a more diffuse encephalopathy. Some look ataxic, but the imbalance is actually myoclonus, constant rapid muscular contractions that have an irregular occurrence and a widespread distribution (see Chapter 14). Opsoclonus is a disorder of ocular muscles that is similar to myoclonus. Spontaneous, conjugate, irregular jerking of the eyes in all directions is characteristic. The movements are most prominent with attempts to change fixation and are then associated with blinking or eyelid flutter. Opsoclonus persists even in sleep and becomes more severe with agitation.

Diagnosis. The clinical features are the basis for diagnosis of myoclonic encephalopathy. Laboratory investigation is required to determine the underlying cause. An occult neuroblastoma is the expected cause in all children with recurrent ataxia or the myoclonic encephalopathy syndrome. Neuroblastoma is also the likely cause when an acute ataxia progresses over several days or waxes and wanes.

The occult neuroblastoma is equally likely to be in the chest or the abdomen. In contrast, only 10–15 % of neuroblastomas are in the chest when myoclonic encephalopathy is absent. The usual studies to detect neuroblastoma are MRI of the chest and abdomen (Figure 10-2), and measurement of the urinary excretion of homovanillic acid and vanillylmandelic acid.

Management. Long-term neurological outcome does not depend on finding and removing the tumor. Partial or complete remission of the neurological symptoms may occur regardless of whether neuroblastoma is present. In most children, a prolonged course follows, with waxing and waning of neurological dysfunction. Either adrenocorticotropic hormone or oral corticosteroids provide partial or complete relief of symptoms in 80 % of patients. Marked improvement usually

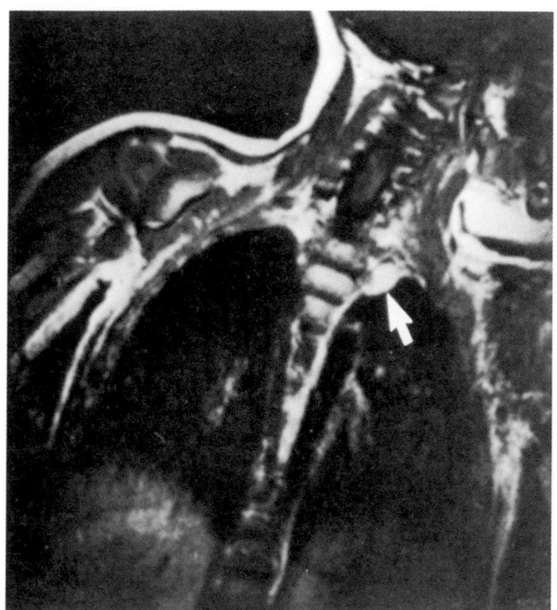

FIGURE 10-2 ■ MRI demonstrates an apical neuroblastoma (arrow) in a child with normal radiographs and CT of the chest.

occurs 1 to 4 weeks after initiation of therapy. Relapses occur after discontinuing therapy but may also occur while treatment is in progress. On long-term follow-up, two-thirds showed mild neurological deficits, and the remainder showed little or none (Hayward et al, 2001).

Childhood Ataxia with Central Nervous System Hypomyelination/ Vanishing White Matter

Vanishing white matter disease is one of the most prevalent inherited childhood leukoencephalopathies. Characteristic of this disorder are recurrent attacks of demyelination similar to acute disseminated encephalomyelitis triggered by febrile illnesses, minor head injury or acute fright often leading to severe neurological deterioration and coma. The classical phenotype is characterized by early childhood onset of chronic neurological deterioration, dominated by cerebellar ataxia. Most patients die a few years after onset. The defect resides in one of the five subunits of eukaryotic translation initiation factor eIF2B, which is an essential factor in all cells of the body for protein synthesis and its regulation under different stress conditions. Some familial cases suggest a genetic basis (Van der Knaap, 2006).

Clinical Features. Age of onset is from infancy to early childhood (Naidu et al, 2005). Most children are developmentally normal prior to the first attack but some show mild delay. Gait disturbances are usually the initial feature, usually ataxia but sometimes dystonia or spasticity. Repeated attacks cause neurological deterioration and death occurs during childhood.

Diagnosis. This disorder is readily confused with ADEM at onset. However, the cranial MRI, which shows a patchy leukoencephalopathy with cavitation in affected areas, is not a feature of ADEM. With time, the cavities coalesce to form large white matter cysts that spare gray matter until late in the course. Chemical abnormalities such as elevated lactate in brain, blood, and cerebrospinal fluid are inconsistent.

Management. Management is symptomatic. Corticosteroids have no value.

Pseudoataxia (Epileptic Ataxia)

Clinical Features. Ataxia and other gait disturbances can be the only clinical features of seizure activity. Both limb and gait ataxia may be present, and the child's epilepsy may be undiagnosed. If the child is already taking antiepileptic drugs, a toxic drug effect is often the initial diagnosis. During the ataxic episode, the child may appear inattentive or confused. Like other seizure manifestations, ataxia is sudden in onset and episodic.

Diagnosis. The absence of nystagmus suggests that ataxia is a seizure manifestation and not caused by drug toxicity. The usual EEG findings concurrent with ataxia are prolonged, generalized, 2–3 Hz spike-wave complexes that have a frontal predominance. This is the typical EEG finding in the Lennox-Gastaut syndrome (see Chapter 1). Such discharges are ordinarily associated with myoclonic jerks or akinetic seizures. Either one occurring briefly, but repeatedly, could interrupt smooth movement and produce ataxia.

Management. Pseudoataxia usually responds to anticonvulsant drugs.

Trauma

Mild head injuries are common in children and are an almost daily occurrence in toddlers. Recovery is always complete despite considerable parental concern. More serious head injuries, associated with loss of consciousness, seizures, and cerebral contusion, are less common but still account for several thousand deaths in children annually. Ataxia may follow even mild head injuries. In most cases, ataxia is part of the so-called postconcussion syndrome, in which imaging studies do not show any structural derangement of the nervous system. In others, a cerebellar contusion or posterior fossa hematoma may be present (see Chapter 2). Ataxia may also follow cervical injuries, especially during sports.

Postconcussion Syndrome

Clinical Features. Many adults complain of headache, dizziness, and mental changes following even a mild head injury. Some of these symptoms also occur after head injury in children and probably represent a transitory derangement of cerebral function caused by the trauma. Even mild head trauma can cause a cerebral axonopathy, which may explain the persistence of symptoms.

In infants and small children, the most prominent postconcussive symptom is ataxia. This is not necessarily a typical cerebellar ataxia but may be only an unsteady gait. No limb dysmetria is present, and other neurological functions are normal.

In older children with postconcussive syndromes, headache and dizziness are as common as ataxia. The headache is usually low grade and transient. When the headache worsens and becomes chronic it is usually an *analgesic-induced headache* (see Chapter 3). Gait is less disturbed, possibly because an older child better compensates for dizziness, but still the sensation of unsteadiness is present.

Diagnosis. The clinical syndrome is the basis for diagnosis. Cranial computed tomography (CT) at the time of injury to exclude intracranial hemorrhage is normal but MRI may show foci of high signal intensity on T_2-weighted images, indicating axonal injury.

Management. Ataxia usually clears completely within 1 month and always within 6 months. Decreased activity and caution to prevent falls during the time of ataxia is the only treatment need.

Vascular Disorders

Cerebellar Hemorrhage

Spontaneous cerebellar hemorrhage in children, in the absence of a coagulopathy, is due to arteriovenous malformation, even though less than 10 % of intracranial arteriovenous malformations in children are in the cerebellum. The two major features of cerebellar hemorrhage are ataxia and headache. Even small bleedings may lead to hydrocephalus due to the location in the posterior fossa. Neurosurgery consultation is indicated as shunting, evacuation of blood or posterior fossa decompression may be acutely needed.

Kawasaki Disease

Kawasaki disease is a systemic vasculitis that occurs predominantly in infants and children.

Clinical Features. Five of the following six criteria are required for diagnosis: fever, conjunctival injection, reddening of the oropharynx and lips, indurative edema of the limbs, polymorphic exanthems, and lymphadenopathy. Arthralgia, carditis, and aseptic meningitis may be associated features. Kawasaki disease is identical with childhood polyarteritis nodosa.

Multiple infarcts may occur in the brain. Acute ataxia, facial palsy, ocular motor palsies, and hemiplegia may occur. The neurological and coronary artery complications make Kawasaki a serious illness with guarded prognosis.

Diagnosis. Clinical features of multisystem disease are essential for diagnosis. Abnormal laboratory findings include an increased sedimentation rate, a positive test for C-reactive protein, and increased serum complement and globulin levels. Skin biopsy shows the typical histopathological changes of arteritis.

Management. Intravenous immune globulin, 2 g/kg over 2 to 5 days, and high-dose aspirin in the acute phase is an effective method of treatment.

Vertebrobasilar Occlusion

Trauma to the vertebrobasilar arteries may occur with childhood injuries including sports and chiropractic manipulation. Bony canals encase the vertebral arteries from C2 to the foramen magnum. Sudden stretching of the arteries by hyperextension or hyperflexion of the neck causes endothelial injury and thrombosis.

Clinical Features. The onset of symptoms is within minutes or hours of injury. Vertigo, nausea, and vomiting are the initial symptoms of brainstem ischemia. Occipital headache may be present as well. Ataxia is due to incoordination of the limbs on one side. It may be maximal at onset or progress over several days. Examination shows some combination of unilateral brainstem disturbances (diplopia, facial weakness) and ipsilateral cerebellar dysfunction.

Diagnosis. CT or MRI shows a unilateral infarction in the cerebellar hemisphere. Infarction of the lateral medulla may occur as well. Arteriography localizes the arterial thrombosis.

Management. Many children recover completely in the months that follow injury. The benefit of antiplatelet versus anticoagulation is not established.

CHRONIC OR PROGRESSIVE ATAXIA

Brain tumor is always an initial concern when progressive ataxia develops in previously normal children, especially if headache is present as well (see Box 10-2). Congenital abnormalities that cause ataxia are often associated with some degree of cognitive impairment. The onset of symptoms may occur during infancy or be delayed until adult life. Friedreich ataxia is the most common hereditary form of progressive ataxia. The causes of chronic or progressive ataxia are usually easy to diagnose, and many are treatable. Failure to establish a diagnosis can have unfortunate consequences for the child.

Brain Tumors

Approximately 85 % of primary brain tumors in children 2 years to 12 years of age are located in the posterior fossa. Supratentorial tumors predominate in children less than 2 years and older than 12 years. Seventy percent of primary brain tumors are gliomas; only 5 % of central nervous system tumors arise from the spinal cord. Neuroectodermal tumors are the second most common malignancy of childhood and the most common solid tumors. The four major tumors of the posterior fossa are cerebellar astrocytoma, brainstem glioma, ependymoma, and primitive neuroectodermal tumors (medulloblastoma). The initial feature of brainstem glioma is cranial nerve dysfunction and not ataxia (see Chapter 15). Although this discussion is limited to tumors of the posterior fossa, it is important to remember that supratentorial brain tumors may also cause ataxia. Approximately one-quarter of children with supratentorial brain tumors have gait disturbances at the time of their first hospitalization, and many show signs of cerebellar dysfunction. Gait disturbances occur with equal frequency whether supratentorial tumors are in the midline or the hemispheres, whereas cerebellar signs are more common with midline tumors.

Cerebellar Astrocytoma

Cerebellar astrocytomas comprise 12 % of brain tumors in children. The tumor usually grows slowly in the cerebellar hemisphere and consists of a large cyst with a mural nodule. It may be in the hemisphere, in the vermis, in both the hemisphere and vermis, or may occupy the fourth ventricle. Midline tumors are likely to be solid.

Clinical Features. Occurrence is equal in both genders. The peak incidence is at 5 to 9 years of age but may be as early as infancy. Headache is the most common initial complaint in school-age children, whereas unsteadiness of gait and vomiting are the initial symptoms in preschool children. Headache can be insidious and intermittent; typical morning headache and vomiting are rare. The first complaints of headache and nausea are nonspecific and often attributed to a flu-like illness. Only when symptoms persist is the possibility of increased intracranial pressure considered. In infants and small children, separation of cranial sutures often relieves the symptoms of increased intracranial pressure. For this reason, gait disturbances without headache or vomiting are the common initial sign of cerebellar astrocytoma in infants.

Papilledema is present in most affected children at initial examination but is often absent in infants with separation of cranial sutures. Ataxia is present in three-quarters, dysmetria in half, and nystagmus in only a quarter. Ataxia varies in severity from a wide-based, lurching gait to a subtle alteration of gait observed only with tandem walking or quick turning. Its cause is partly the cerebellar location of the tumor and partly hydrocephalus. When the tumor is in the cerebellar hemisphere, ipsilateral or bilateral dysmetria may be present. Other neurological signs sometimes present in children with cerebellar astrocytoma are abducens palsy, multiple cranial nerve palsies, stiff neck, and head tilt.

Diagnosis. MRI is the best imaging study for diagnosis.

Management. Children with life-threatening hydrocephalus should undergo a shunting procedure as the first step in treatment. The shunt relieves many of the symptoms and signs, including ataxia. Corticosteroids are sufficient to relieve pressure in many children with less severe hydrocephalus.

The 5-year survival rate after surgical removal approaches 95 %. The mural nodule must be located and removed at surgery or the tumor may recur. The amount of tumor resected is difficult to determine at the time of resection, and postoperative imaging studies improve upon the surgeon's estimate. The need for adjuvant radiotherapy is not established.

The total removal of deeper tumors that involve the floor of the fourth ventricle is rare. Local recurrence is common after partial resection. Repeat surgery may be curative in some cases, but postoperative radiation therapy appears to offer a better prognosis following partial resection. The overall disease-free survival rates following either surgery alone or surgery and radiotherapy are 92 % at 5 years and 88 % at 25 years. Low-grade cerebellar astrocytomas never require chemotherapy, regardless of the degree of surgical resection.

High-grade cerebellar astrocytoma (glioblastoma) is rare in children. More than 30 % of childhood patients have dissemination of tumor through the neuraxis (spinal cord drop metastases). Examination of cerebrospinal fluid for cytological features and complete myelography always follow surgical resection in patients with glioblastoma. An abnormal result in either indicates whole-axis radiation therapy.

Cerebellar Hemangioblastoma (Von Hippel-Lindau Disease)

Von Hippel-Lindau (VHL) disease is a multisystem disorder transmitted by autosomal dominant inheritance (Schimke et al, 2009). The most prominent features are hemangioblastomas of the cerebellum and retina, and pancreatic cysts. All children with cerebellar hemangioblastomas have VHL disease. Among adults, 60 % have isolated tumors and do not have the genetic defect. The expression of VHL disease is variable even within the same kindred. The most common features are cerebellar and retinal hemangioblastoma (59 %), renal carcinoma (28 %), and pheochromocytoma (7 %).

Clinical Features. Mean age at onset of cerebellar hemangioblastoma in VHL disease is 32 years; onset before 15 is unusual. The initial features are headache and ataxia. Retinal hemangioblastomas occur at a younger age and may cause visual impairment from hemorrhage as early as the first decade. They may be multiple and bilateral and appear on ophthalmoscopic examination as a dilated artery leading from the disk to a peripheral tumor with an engorged vein. Spinal hemangioblastomas are intramedullary in location and lead to syringomyelia. Pheochromocytomas occur in 7–19 % of patients and may be the only clinical manifestation.

Diagnosis. Suspect the diagnosis in individuals with any of the following: more than one hemangioblastoma of the central nervous system, an isolated hemangioblastoma associated with a visceral cyst or renal carcinoma, or any known manifestation with a family history of disease. Molecular genetic testing of the VHL gene detects mutations in nearly 100 % of patients. The gene for VHL disease is a tumor-suppressor gene that maps to chromosome 3p25. Clinical testing allows the identification of asymptomatic, affected family members who need annual examinations to look for treatable abnormalities. Such examinations should include indirect ophthalmoscopy and renal ultrasound, as well as gadolinium-enhanced MRI of the brain every 3 years.

Management. Cryotherapy or photocoagulation of smaller retinal lesions can lead to complete tumor regression without visual loss. The treatment of cerebellar hemangioblastoma is surgically and total extirpation is the rule.

Ependymoma

The derivation of posterior fossa ependymoma is the cells that line the roof and floor of the fourth ventricle. These tumors can extend into both lateral recesses and grow out to the cerebellopontine angle. They account for 10 % of primary brain tumors in children.

Clinical Features. Eight percent of all childhood brain tumors are ependymomas. The peak incidence in children is from birth to 4 years. The incidence in both genders is equal. The clinical features evolve slowly and are often present for several months before initial consultation. Symptoms of increased intracranial pressure are the first feature in 90 % of children. Disturbances of gait and coordination, neck pain, or cranial nerve dysfunction are the initial features in the remainder. Half of affected children have ataxia, usually of the vermal type, and one-third has nystagmus. Head tilt or neck stiffness is present in one-third of children and indicates extension of tumor into the cervical canal.

Although steady deterioration is expected, some children have an intermittent course. Episodes of headache and vomiting, ataxia, and even nuchal rigidity last for days or weeks and are then followed by periods of well-being. The cause of the intermittent symptoms is transitory obstruction of the fourth ventricle or aqueduct by the tumor acting in a ball-valve fashion.

Diagnosis. Only two grades of ependymoma are recognized: classic (benign) and anaplastic (malignant). Because ependymomas typically arise in the ependymal linings of ventricles, tumors may spread through the entire neuraxis. A typical MRI appearance of a fourth ventricular ependymoma is a homogeneously enhancing solid mass that extends out of the foramina of Luschka or Magendie with associated obstructive hydrocephalus. Marked dilation of the ventricular system is usual. Evaluation includes contrast-enhanced MRI scans of the brain and entire spinal cord as well as cytological evaluation of the CSF.

Management. The single most important factor determining prognosis is the degree of resection (Perilongo et al, 1998). The goals of surgery are to relieve hydrocephalus and to remove as much tumor as possible without damaging the fourth ventricle. Irradiation to the posterior fossa usually follows surgery, but not neuraxis radiation, unless the diagnosis of leptomeningeal spread is established. Poor prognostic features include an age of less than 2 to 5 years at diagnosis, brainstem invasion, and a radiation dose of less than 4500 cGy (Paulino et al, 2002).

Medulloblastoma

Medulloblastoma is a primitive neuroectodermal tumor (PNET) of the posterior fossa with the capacity to differentiate into neuronal and glial tissue. Most tumors are in the vermis or fourth ventricle, with or without extension into the cerebellar hemispheres. Approximately 10% are in the hemisphere alone. Medulloblastomas represent approximately 85% of intracranial PNETs and 15% of all pediatric brain tumors. Data from the National Cancer Institute's Surveillance, Epidemiology, and End Results (SEER) registry indicates an increasing incidence of medulloblastoma (McNeil et al, 2002).

Clinical Features. Ninety percent of cases have their onset during the first decade and the remainder during the second decade. Medulloblastoma is the most common primary brain tumor with onset during infancy.

The tumor grows rapidly, and the interval between onset of symptoms and medical consultation is generally brief: 2 weeks in 25% of cases and less than a month in 50%. Vomiting is an initial symptom in 58% of children, headache in 40%, an unsteady gait in 20%, and torticollis or stiff neck in 10%. The probable cause of prominent vomiting, with or without headache, as an early symptom is tumor irritation of the floor of the fourth ventricle. Gait disturbances are more common in young children and refusal to stand or walk is characteristic rather than by ataxia.

Two-thirds of children have papilledema at the time of initial examination. Truncal ataxia and limb ataxia are equally common, and both may be present. Only 22% of children have nystagmus. Tendon reflexes are hyperactive when hydrocephalus is present and hypoactive when the tumor is causing primarily cerebellar dysfunction.

Diagnosis. CT or MRI easily identifies medulloblastoma (Figure 10-3). The tumors are vascular and become enhanced when contrast medium is used.

Management. The combined use of surgical extirpation, radiation therapy, and chemotherapy greatly improves the prognosis for children with medulloblastoma. The role of surgery is to provide histological identification, debulk the tumor, and relieve obstruction of the fourth ventricle. Ventriculoperitoneal shunting reduces intracranial pressure even before decompressive resection. The treatment of children less than 3 years of age at diagnosis is with chemotherapy alone or chemotherapy with field radiotherapy.

The overall 5-year survival rate is approximately 40%. Survival is better (60–70%) in children who have gross total tumor resection compared with partial resection or biopsy. Craniospinal radiation increases survival better than local field radiation. The use of adjuvant chemotherapy significantly improves survival. Most initial recurrences occur at the primary site. One histological variant, anaplastic large cell medulloblastoma, carries a poorer prognosis because of a higher risk for early metastatic involvement and recurrence (Eberhart et al, 2002). The presence of dissemination is the single most important factor that correlates with outcome (Helton et al, 2002).

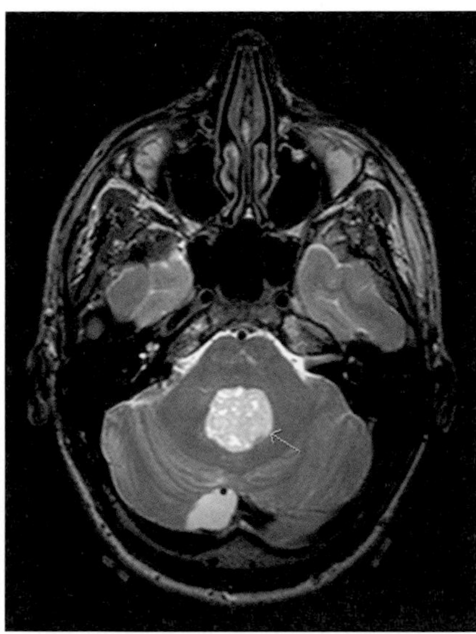

FIGURE 10-3 ■ Medulloblastoma. T_2 axial MRI shows (arrow) a heterogeneous cystic mass in the vermis of cerebellum and an incidental subarachnoid cyst.

Congenital Malformations

Basilar Impression

Basilar impression is a disorder of the craniovertebral junction. Posterior displacement of the odontoid process compresses the spinal cord or brainstem.

Clinical Features. The first symptoms are often head tilt, neck stiffness, and headache. Minor trauma to the head or neck frequently precipitates the onset of symptoms. Examination shows ataxia, nystagmus, and hyperreflexia.

Diagnosis. MRI is the best method to visualize both the cervicomedullary junction and an associated Chiari malformation or syringobulbia.

Management. Surgical decompression of the foramen magnum usually relieves symptoms.

Cerebellar Malformations

Congenital Hemisphere Hypoplasia. Congenital hypoplasia of the cerebellum can be unilateral or bilateral. More than half of patients with bilateral disease have an identifiable genetic disorder transmitted by autosomal recessive inheritance. The common histological feature is the absence of granular cells, with relative preservation of Purkinje cells. Unilateral cerebellar hypoplasia is not associated with genetic disorders. In some hereditary forms, granular cell degeneration may continue postnatally and cause progressive cerebellar dysfunction during infancy.

Clinical Features. Developmental delay and hypotonia are the first features suggesting a cerebral abnormality in the infant. Titubation of the head is a constant feature, and some combination of ataxia, dysmetria, and intention tremor is noted. A jerky, coarse nystagmus is usually present. Tendon reflexes may be increased or diminished. Those with hyperactive reflexes probably have congenital abnormalities of the corticospinal tract in addition to cerebellar hypoplasia. Seizures occur in some hereditary and some sporadic cases. Other neurological signs and symptoms may be present, depending on associated malformations. Cognitive impairment is a constant feature but varies from mild to severe.

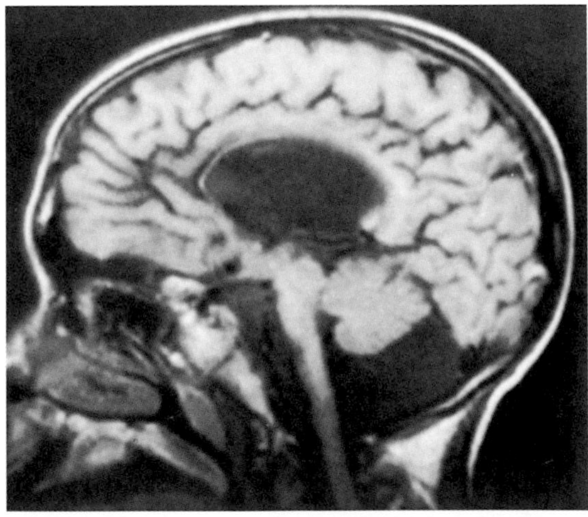

FIGURE 10-4 ■ Aplasia of the cerebellum associated with thinning of the corpus callosum.

Diagnosis. MRI is diagnostic (Figure 10-4). It shows not only the extent of cerebellar hypoplasia but also associated anomalies. The folial pattern of the cerebellum is prominent, and there is compensatory enlargement of the fourth ventricle, cisterna magna, and vallecula.

Management. No treatment is available.

Vermal Aplasia. Aplasia of the vermis is relatively common and often associated with other midline cerebral malformations. All or part of the vermis may be missing, and, when the vermis is incomplete, the caudal portion is usually lacking. Dominantly inherited aplasia of the anterior vermis is a rare condition.

Clinical Features. Partial agenesis of the cerebellar vermis may be asymptomatic. Symptoms are nonprogressive and vary from only mild gait ataxia and upbeating nystagmus to severe ataxia.

Complete agenesis causes titubation of the head and truncal ataxia. Vermal agenesis is frequently associated with other cerebral malformations, producing a constellation of symptoms and signs referable to neurological dysfunction. Two such examples are the *Dandy-Walker malformation* (see Chapter 18) and the *Joubert syndrome* (Figure 10-5).

The Joubert syndrome consists of four recessively inherited syndromes characterized by a characteristic facies, oculomotor apraxia, and hyperpnea intermixed with central apnea in the neonatal period (Valente et al, 2005). One of the phenotypes includes malformations in several viscera. Cerebellar vermal agenesis is a constant feature of the Joubert syndrome, but several other cerebral malformations are usually present as well. All patients are cognitively impaired, and some are microcephalic. Several affected children have died unexpectedly, possibly from respiratory failure.

Diagnosis. MRI shows agenesis of the vermis of the cerebellum with enlargement of the cisterna magna. Other cerebral malformations, such as agenesis of the corpus callosum, are also associated.

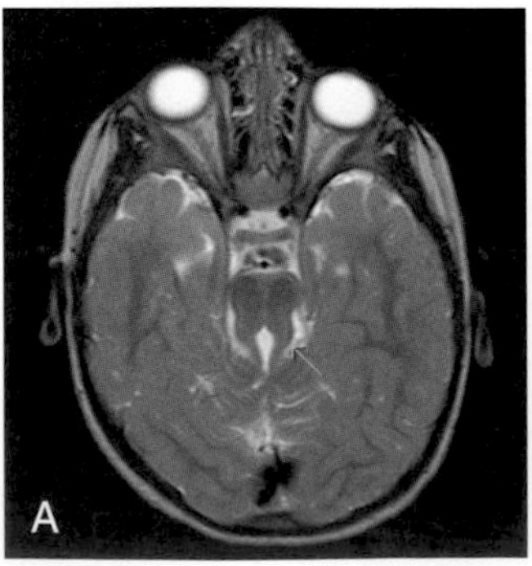

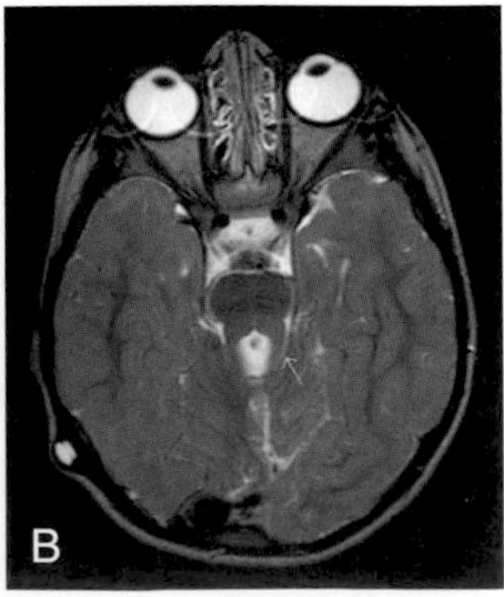

FIGURE 10-5 ■ Joubert syndrome. T_2 axial MRIs of siblings with the molar tooth sign.

Management. No treatment is available.

X-Linked Cerebellar Hypoplasia. Some families with cerebellar hemispheric and vermal hypoplasia have a genetic defect that maps to the short arm of the X chromosome (Bertorini, 2000).

Clinical Features. Hypotonia, mild dysphagia, and delayed motor development are present from birth. By age of 4 years, action tremor of the upper limbs and slow eye movements are noted. In adult life, neurological symptoms include moderate dysarthria, unsteady gait with truncal and locomotor ataxia, intention tremor, and limitation of vertical gaze with slow conjugate eye movements. Male family members showing delayed developmental milestones also show some combination of nonprogressive ataxia, dysarthria, and external ophthalmoplegia. Intelligence is normal.

Diagnosis. Brain MRI shows severe global atrophy of the cerebellar vermis and hemispheres.

Management. Treatment is supportive.

Chiari Malformations

The *type I Chiari malformation* is a displacement of the cerebellar tonsils and posterior vermis of the cerebellum through the foramen magnum, compressing the spinomedullary junction. The *type II Chiari malformation* has an additional downward displacement of a dysplastic lower medulla and a lumbosacral meningomyelocele (see Chapter 12). A molecular genetic hypothesis of ectopic expression of a segmentation gene in the rhombomeres explains the several cerebellar and brainstem anomalies, as well as the defective basioccipital and supraoccipital bone formation (Sarnat et al, 2002).

Clinical Features. The widespread use of MRI has shown that Chiari I malformations are often an incidental finding on neuroimaging studies in children with epilepsy or migraines. When symptomatic, the onset is frequently during adolescence or adult life. Major clinical features are headache, head tilt, pain in the neck and shoulders, ataxia, and lower cranial nerve dysfunction. Physical signs vary among patients and may include weakness of the arms, hyperactive tendon reflexes in the legs, nystagmus, and ataxia. Children with chronic headaches and Chiari I often suffer from migraines and analgesic induced headaches. The physical finding should be considered an incidental finding in children with normal neurological exam and lack of symptoms other than headaches.

Diagnosis. MRI provides the best visualization of posterior fossa structures. The distortion of the cerebellum and the hindbrain is precisely identified (Figure 10-6).

Management. Surgical decompression of the foramen magnum to at least the C3 vertebra is the recommended treatment. Significant improvement occurs in more than half of patients.

Progressive Hereditary Ataxias

Autosomal Dominant Inheritance

Spinocerebellar Degenerations. A genotypic classification of the dominantly inherited ataxias has replaced the phenotypic classification that included *Marie's ataxia*, *olivopontocerebellar atrophy*, and *spinocerebellar atrophies* (SCA) (Bird, 2012). Table 10-1 lists the progressive autosomal dominant ataxias with onset in childhood. The genetic abnormality is usually a trinucleotide repeat. The original description of SCA3 was in Portuguese families from the Azores and named *Machado-Joseph disease*.

Clinical Features. The clinical features overlap, and genetic testing is the best method for diagnosis. Table 10-1 indicates a few distinguishing clinical features.

Diagnosis. DNA-based genetic tests are available for the diagnosis of SCA1, SCA2, SCA3, SCA6, SCA7, and DRPLA.

Management. Treatment is symptomatic and, depending on the disease, may include anticonvulsants, muscle relaxants, and assistive devices.

Hypobetalipoproteinemia

Clinical Features. Several different disorders are associated with hypocholesterolemia, and reduced, but not absent, concentrations of

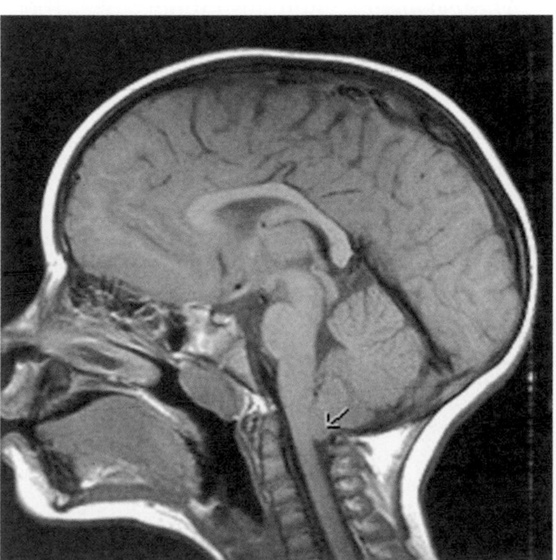

FIGURE 10-6 ■ Chiari type I malformation. T_1 sagittal MRI shows downward displacement of the cerebellar tonsils (arrow).

TABLE 10-1 **Autosomal Dominant Cerebellar Ataxias: Clinical Characteristics**

Disease	Average onset (range in years)	Clinical features (all include ataxia)
SCA1	4th decade (<10 to >60)	Pyramidal signs, peripheral neuropathy
SCA2	3rd–4th decade (<10 to >60)	Slow saccadic eye movement, peripheral neuropathy, decreased DTRs, dementia
SCA3	4th decade (10–70)	Pyramidal and extrapyramidal signs; lid retraction, nystagmus, decreased saccade velocity; amyotrophic fasciculations, sensory loss
SCA4	4th–5th decade (19–59)	Sensory axonal neuropathy
SCA5	3rd–4th decade (10–68)	Early onset, slow course
SCA7	3rd–4th decade (1/2–60)	Visual loss with retinopathy
SCA12	3rd (8–55)	Early tremor, late dementia
DRPLA	Rare (USA) (8–20) 20% (Japan) (40–60s)	Early onset correlates with shorter duration; chorea, seizures, dementia, myoclonus

ADCA, autosomal dominant cerebellar ataxias; DRPLA, dentatorubral-pallidoluysian atrophy; DTRs, deep tendon reflexes; EA, episodic ataxia; SCA, spinocerebellar ataxia.

(Adapted from Bird TD. Ataxia overview. In: GeneClinics: Medical Genetics Knowledge Base [database online]. Seattle: University of Washington. Available at http://www.geneclinics.org. PMID 20301317. Last updated April 26, 2012.)

apolipoprotein B and apolipoprotein A. Some patients with this lipid profile have no neurological symptoms; others have severe ataxia beginning in infancy. Malabsorption does not occur, but the infant fails to thrive and has progressive fatty cirrhosis of the liver. Severe hypotonia and absence of tendon reflexes are present in the first months.

Diagnosis. The diagnosis is a consideration in children with unexplained progressive ataxia. The total serum lipid content is normal, but the concentration of triglycerides is increased. Reduced concentrations of total high- and low-density lipoprotein cholesterol concentrations and apolipoproteins are characteristic.

Management. Administration of 1000–10 000 mg/day of DL-α-tocopherol prevents many of the complications of hypobetalipoproteinemia. Vitamins A and K supplements are also required.

Autosomal Recessive Inheritance

Ataxia is a feature of many degenerative disorders but is a presenting or cardinal feature in the disorders discussed in this section.

Abetalipoproteinemia. Molecular defect(s) in the gene for the microsomal triglyceride transfer protein (MTTP) at chromosome 4q22-q24 causes abetalipoproteinemia. Transmission is by autosomal recessive inheritance. Other terms for the disorder are *acanthocytosis* and the *Bassen-Kornzweig syndrome*. MTTP catalyzes the transport of triglyceride, cholesteryl ester, and phospholipid from phospholipid surfaces. The results are fat malabsorption and a progressive deficiency of vitamins A, E, and K.

Clinical Features. Fat malabsorption is present from birth, and most newborns come to medical attention because of failure to thrive, vomiting, and large volumes of loose stool. A correct diagnosis is possible at that time.

Delayed psychomotor development occurs during infancy. A cerebellar ataxia develops in one-third of children during the first decade and in almost every child by the end of the second decade. Tendon reflexes are usually lost by 5 years of age. Progressive gait disturbances, dysmetria, and difficulty performing rapid alternating movements characterize the limb ataxia, which progresses until the third decade and then becomes stationary. Proprioceptive sensation in the hands and feet is lost, while pinprick and temperature sensations are less severely affected. Sensory loss results from demyelination in the posterior columns of the spinal cord and the peripheral nerves.

Retinitis pigmentosa is an almost constant feature. The age at onset is variable but is usually during the first decade. The initial symptom is night blindness. Nystagmus is common and its cause may be either the cerebellar disturbance or the loss of central vision.

Diagnosis. Severe anemia, with hemoglobin levels less than 8 g/dL (5 mmol/L), is common in young children but not in adults. The anemia, which may result from malabsorption, corrects with parenteral supplementation of iron or folate. Plasma cholesterol levels are less than 100 mg/dL (2.5 mmol/L), and triglyceride levels are less than 30 mg/dL (0.3 mmol/L). The absence of apolipoprotein B in plasma confirms the diagnosis. Measure the parents' plasma apolipoprotein B concentrations as well as the child's.

In abetalipoproteinemia, the heterozygote is normal; if partial deficiency of apolipoprotein B is present, the diagnosis of familial hypobetalipoproteinemia is more likely.

Management. The cause of the neurological complications of abetalipoproteinemia is chronic vitamin E deficiency. Dietary fat restriction and large oral doses of vitamin E (100 mg/kg/day) prevent the onset of symptoms or arrest their progression.

Ataxia-Telangiectasia. Ataxia-telangiectasia (AT) primarily affects the nervous and immune systems (Gatti, 2010). The gene associated with AT is a large gene located at chromosome 11q22-23, and more than 100 mutations have been discovered. The gene product is involved in cell-cycle progression and the checkpoint response to DNA damage. Transmission is by autosomal recessive inheritance.

Clinical Features. The principal feature is a progressive truncal ataxia that begins during the first year. In infants, choreoathetosis develops instead of, or in addition to, ataxia. The ataxia begins as clumsiness and progresses so slowly that cerebral palsy is often the erroneous diagnosis. Oculomotor apraxia is present in 90% of patients but may be mild at first and overlooked (see Chapter 15). Many children have a dull or expressionless face. Intellectual development is normal at first but often lags with time. One-third of children ultimately function in the mildly retarded range.

Telangiectasia usually develops after 2 years of age and sometimes as late as age 10. It first appears on the bulbar conjunctivae, giving the eyes a bloodshot appearance. Similar telangiectasia appears on the upper half of the ears, on the flexor surfaces of the limbs, and in a butterfly distribution on the face. Sun exposure or irritation exacerbates the telangiectasia.

Recurrent sinopulmonary infection is one of the more serious features of the disease and reflects an underlying immunodeficiency. The synthesis of antibodies and certain immunoglobulin subclasses is disturbed because of disorders of B-cell and helper T-cell function. Serum and salivary IgA is absent in 70–80% of children, and IgE is absent or diminished in 80–90%. The IgM concentration may be elevated in compensation for the IgA deficiency. The thymus has an embryonic appearance, and the α-fetoprotein concentration is elevated in most patients.

Taken together, the many features of this disease suggest a generalized disorder of tissue differentiation and cellular repair. The result is a malignancy risk of 38%. Most are lymphoma and lymphocytic leukemia. Two-thirds of patients are dead by 20 years of age. Infection is the most common cause of death, and neoplasia is second.

Diagnosis. Suspect the diagnosis in infants with some combination of ataxia, chronic sinopulmonary infections, and oculomotor apraxia. As the child gets older, the addition of telangiectasia to the other clinical features makes the diagnosis a certainty. Complete studies of immunocompetence are required. Ninety percent of patients with AT have an elevated α-fetoprotein concentration and approximately 80% have decreased serum IgA, IgE, or IgG. Especially characteristic is a selective deficiency of the IgG_2 subclass. Molecular genetic testing is available in children with a compatible clinical syndrome and normal serum concentrations of α-fetoprotein and immunoglobulin.

The acanthocyte is an abnormal erythrocyte characterized by thorny projections from the cell surface that prevent normal rouleau formation and cause a very low erythrocyte sedimentation rate. Between 50% and 70% of peripheral erythrocytes undergo transformation to acanthocytes. Acanthocytes also occur in association with other neurological disorders in which lipoproteins are normal (see Chapter 14).

Management. Treat all infections vigorously. Intravenous antibiotics are sometimes required for what would otherwise be a trivial sinusitis in a normal child. Patients with AT are exquisitely sensitive to radiation, which produces cellular and chromosomal damage. Radiation may be a precipitant in the development of neoplasia. Therefore, despite the frequency of sinopulmonary infections minimize radiation exposure.

Ataxia with Oculomotor Apraxia Type 1. This disorder may be mistaken for AT but is a different genetic disorder (Coutinho et al, 2010).

Clinical Features. Development is normal during the first year, but a slowly progressive ataxia develops during childhood. The onset of progressive gait imbalance is usually 7 years, but ranges from 2–16 years. Dysarthria, dysmetria, and mild intention tremor follow. Oculomotor apraxia is a late feature and progresses to external ophthalmoplegia. A severe, progressive neuropathy results in generalized areflexia, quadriplegia, and atrophy of the hands and feet. Chorea and arm dystonia are common. Intellect is normal in some and impaired in others.

Diagnosis. Molecular genetic testing is clinically available.

Management. Treatment is supportive.

Ataxia with Oculomotor Apraxia Type 2. This disorder may be mistaken for AT but is a different genetic disorder (Moreira & Koenig, 2011).

Clinical Features. The onset of symptoms is between age 3 and 30 years. The features include ataxia caused by cerebellar atrophy, an axonal sensorimotor neuropathy, and oculomotor apraxia.

Diagnosis. The serum concentration of α-fetoprotein is elevated. Molecular genetic testing is clinically available.

Management. Treatment is supportive.

Friedreich Ataxia. Friedreich ataxia is the most common recessively inherited ataxia. The cause is an unstable triplet repeat of the frataxin gene on chromosome 9q13 (Bidichandani et al, 2012). The size at which the expansion causes disease is not established.

Clinical Features. The onset is usually between 2 and 16 years of age, but symptoms may begin later. The initial feature is ataxia or clumsiness of gait in 95 % of cases and scoliosis in 5 %. The ataxia is slowly progressive and associated with dysarthria, depressed tendon reflexes, extensor plantar responses, foreshortening of the foot creating a high arch, and loss of position and vibration senses. Two-thirds of patients have a hypertrophic cardiomyopathy and 10 % have diabetes mellitus. An atypical presentation occurs in 25 %. These atypical syndromes include any of the following features: (1) onset after age 25 years; (2) present tendon reflexes; and (3) spastic paraparesis without ataxia.

Diagnosis. The clinical features suggest the diagnosis and molecular genetic testing provides confirmation. Motor nerve conduction velocities in the arms and legs are slightly slower than normal. In contrast, sensory action potentials are absent or markedly reduced in amplitude. Spinal somatosensory evoked responses are usually absent. Common changes on the electrocardiogram (ECG) are reduced amplitude of T waves and left or right ventricular hypertrophy. Arrhythmias and conduction defects are uncommon.

Management. The underlying disturbance is not curable, but symptomatic treatment is available. Surgical stabilization prevents severe scoliosis. Regular ECG and chest radiographs to determine heart size are useful to monitor the development of cardiomyopathy. Chest pain on exertion responds to propranolol, and congestive heart failure responds to digitalis. Patients with diabetes require insulin treatment.

Juvenile GM_2 Gangliosidosis. The transmission of all juvenile forms of both α- and β-hexosaminidase-A deficiency are by autosomal recessive inheritance. Some, like *Tay-Sachs disease*, are restricted to Ashkenazi Jews, whereas others occur in individuals of non-Jewish descent (see Chapter 5). In all of these conditions, GM_2 gangliosides are stored within the central nervous system.

Clinical Features. A progressive ataxic syndrome occurs in patients with late-onset hexosaminidase-A deficiency. Age at onset is usually before 15 years. Family members may believe that affected children are only clumsy, before neurological deterioration becomes evident. Intention tremor, dysarthria, and limb and gait ataxia are prominent.

Diagnosis. Any child with an apparent "spinocerebellar degeneration" may have juvenile GM_2 gangliosidosis. Diagnosis requires the measurement of α- and β-hexosaminidase activity in fibroblasts. Molecular genetic diagnosis is used for genetic counseling.

Management. Specific treatment is not available.

Juvenile Sulfatide Lipidosis. Sulfatide lipidosis (*metachromatic leukodystrophy*) is a disorder of central and peripheral myelin metabolism usually caused by deficient activity of the enzyme arylsulfatase A. The defective gene is on chromosome 22q. Discussion of the late infantile form is in Chapters 5 and 7. The usual cause of the juvenile form is arylsulfatase deficiency, but a secondary cause is saposin B deficiency.

Clinical Features. Juvenile sulfatide lipidosis begins later and has a slower course than the late infantile disease. Onset is usually between 4 and 12 years. Initial symptoms are poor school performance, behavioral change, and a gait disturbance. Spasticity, progressive gait and limb ataxia, seizures, and mental deterioration follow. Peripheral neuropathy is not a prominent clinical feature, but prolonged motor conduction velocities are usual late in the course. Protein concentration in the cerebrospinal fluid may be normal or only slightly elevated.

Progression is relatively rapid. Most children deteriorate into a vegetative state and die within 10 years. The time from onset to death ranges from 3 to 17 years and the age at onset does not predict the course.

Diagnosis. MRI shows widespread demyelination of the cerebral hemispheres. Late-onset disease may resemble multiple sclerosis. Diagnosis requires the demonstration of reduced or absent arylsulfatase A in peripheral leukocytes. Those with reduced amounts require testing for saposin B deficiency. Molecular genetic testing is available.

Management. Allogenic bone marrow transplantation, when used early in the course, slows the rate of progression.

Marinesco-Sjögren Syndrome. Cerebellar ataxia, congenital cataracts, and mental retardation are the characteristic features of the Marinesco-Sjögren syndrome. This complex has many causes. Some families have a mitochondrial disorder. Other families have congenital cataracts, delayed motor development, ataxia, demyelinating peripheral neuropathy, and dysmorphic facial features (Merlini et al, 2002)

Clinical Features. A constant feature is cataracts, which may be congenital or develop during infancy. The type of cataract varies and is not specific. Dysarthria, nystagmus, and ataxia of the trunk and limbs characterize the cerebellar dysfunction during infancy. Strabismus and hypotonia are frequently present in childhood. Developmental delay is a constant feature but varies from mild to severe. Other features include short stature, delayed sexual development, pes valgus, and scoliosis.

Although the onset of symptoms is in infancy, progression is slow or stationary. Ataxia leads to wheelchair confinement by the third or fourth decade, and shortening of life span is significant.

Diagnosis. The basis of diagnosis is the clinical and neuroimaging studies. *SIL1* is the only gene associated with Marinesco-Sjögren syndrome. Molecular genetic testing is available on a research basis only.

Management. Treatment is supportive.

Other Metabolic Disorders. Descriptions of *Hartnup disease* and *maple syrup urine disease* are in the section on acute or recurrent ataxia. After an acute attack of these diseases, some patients never return to baseline but instead have chronic progressive ataxia. Such patients require screening for metabolic disorders (Table 10-2). Refsum disease is an inborn error of phytanic acid metabolism and transmission is by autosomal recessive inheritance. The cardinal features are retinitis pigmentosa, chronic or recurrent polyneuropathy, and cerebellar ataxia. Affected individuals usually have either night blindness or neuropathy (see Chapter 7).

Disorders of pyruvate metabolism and of the respiratory chain enzymes cause widespread disturbances in the nervous system and are described in Chapters 5, 7, and 8. The common features among the several disorders of mitochondrial metabolism include lactic acidosis, ataxia, hypotonia, ophthalmoplegia, mental retardation, and peripheral neuropathy. A raised concentration of blood lactate or the production of lactic acidosis by administration of a standard glucose tolerance test suggests a mitochondrial disorder. Deficiency of pyruvate dehydrogenase may produce acute, recurrent, or chronic ataxias and is discussed in the section on acute or recurrent ataxia. Respiratory chain disorders produce a combination of ataxia, dementia, myoclonus, and seizures.

TABLE 10-2 Metabolic Screening in Progressive Ataxias

Disease	Abnormality
Blood	
Abetalipoproteinemia	Lipoproteins, cholesterol
Adrenoleukodystrophy	Very-long-chain fatty acids
Ataxia-telangiectasia	IgA, IgE, α-fetoprotein
Hypobetalipoproteinemia	Lipoproteins, cholesterol
Mitochondrial disorders	Lactate, glucose-lactate tolerance
Sulfatide lipidoses	Arylsulfatase A
Urine	
Hartnup disease	Amino acids
Maple syrup urine disease*	Amino acids
Fibroblasts	
Carnitine acetyltransferase deficiency*	Carnitine acetyltransferase
GM_2 gangliosidosis	Hexosaminidase
Refsum disease	Phytanic acid
Bone Marrow	
Neurovisceral storage	Sea-blue histiocytes

*Denotes the most common conditions and the ones with disease modifying treatments

X-Linked Inheritance

Ataxia may be the initial feature of the infantile form of *adrenoleukodystrophy* (see Chapter 5). The clinical features of adrenoleukodystrophy can mimic a spinocerebellar degeneration and requires consideration in any family with only males affected. An X-linked ataxia associated with hypotonia, deafness, and loss of vision in early childhood occurs in some families. Other families have only ataxia and deafness. The abnormal gene site and gene product are not established, and it is not possible to know if these are allelic or different disorders.

REFERENCES

Banwell B, Ghezzi A, Bar-Or A, et al. Multiple sclerosis in children: clinical diagnosis, therapeutic strategies, and future directions. Lancet Neurology 2007;6:887–902.

Bertorini E, des Portes V, Zanni G, et al. X-linked congenital ataxia: a clinical and genetic study. American Journal of Medical Genetics 2000:53–6.

Bidichandani SI, Delatycki MB, Ashizawa A. Freidreich ataxia. In: GeneClinics: Medical Genetics Knowledge Base [database online]. Seattle: University of Washington. Available at http://www.geneclinics.org. PMID: 20301458. Last updated February 2, 2012.

Bird TD. Ataxia overview. In: GeneClinics: Medical Genetics Knowledge Base [database online]. Seattle: University of Washington. Available at http://www.geneclinics.org. PMID: 20301317. Last updated April 26, 2012.

Blaes F, Fuhlhuber V, Korfei M, et al. Surface-binding autoantibodies to cerebellar neurons in opsoclonus syndrome. Annals of Neurology 2005;58:313–7.

Coutinho P, Barbot C, Céu Moreira M, et al. Ataxia with oculomotor apraxia type 1 [AOA1]. GeneClinics: Medical Genetics Knowledge Base [database online]. Seattle: University of Washington. Available at http://www.geneclinics.org. PMID: 20301629. Last updated June 22, 2010.

De Vries B, Mamsa H, Stam AH, et al. Episodic ataxia associated with EAAT1 mutation C186S affecting glutamate reuptake. Archives of Neurology 2009;66(1):97–101.

Eberhart CG, Kepner JL, Goldthwaite PT, et al. Histopathologic grading of medulloblastomas: A Pediatric Oncology Group study. Cancer 2002;94:552–60.

Fitzpatrick AS, Gray OM, McConville J, et al. Opsoclonus-myoclonus syndrome associated with benign ovarian teratoma. Neurology 2008;70:1292–3.

Frohman EM, Goodin DS, Calabresi PA, et al. The utility of MRI in suspected MS. Report of the Therapeutics and Technology Assessment Subcommittee of the American Academy of Neurology. Neurology 2003;61:602–11.

Gatti RA. Ataxia-telangiectasia. In: GeneClinics: Medical Genetics Knowledge Base [database online]. Seattle: University of Washington. Available at http://www.geneclinics.org. PMID: 20301790. Last updated March 11, 2010.

Hayward K, Jeremy RJ, Jenkins S, et al. Long-term neurobehavioral outcomes in children with neuroblastoma and opsoclonus-myoclonus-ataxia syndrome: relationship to MRI findings and anti-neuronal antibodies. Journal of Pediatrics 2001;139:552–9.

Head RA, Brown RM, Zolkipli Z, et al. Clinical and genetic spectrum of pyruvate dehydrogenase deficiency: Dihydrolipoamide acetyltransferase (E2) deficiency. Annals of Neurology 2005;58:234–41.

Helton KJ, Gajjar A, Hill DA, et al. Medulloblastoma metastatic to the suprasellar region at diagnosis: a report of six cases with clinicopathologic correlation. Pediatric Neurosurgery 2002;38:111–7.

Jacobs BC, Endtz H, van der Meche FG, et al. Serum anti-GQ1b IgG antibodies recognize surface epitopes on Campylobacter jejuni from patients with Miller Fisher syndrome. Annals of Neurology 1995;37:260–4.

Kirchmann M, Thomsen LL, Oleson J. Basilar type migraine: Clinical, epidemiologic, and genetic features. Neurology 2006;66:880–6.

Klepper J, Leiendecker B, Bredahl R, et al. Introduction of a ketogenic diet in young infants. Journal of Inherited Metabolic Diseases 2002;25:449–60.

Kriss A, Francis DA, Cuendet F, et al. Recovery after optic neuritis in childhood. Journal of Neurology, Neurosurgery and Psychiatry 1988;51:1253–8.

Lindskog U, Ödkvist L, Noaksson L, et al. Benign paroxysmal vertigo in childhood: A long-term follow-up. Headache 1999;39:33–7.

McNeil DE, Cote TR, Clegg L, et al. Incidence and trends in pediatric malignancies medulloblastoma/primitive neuroectodermal tumor: a SEER update. Medical Pediatric Oncology 2003;39:190–4.

Merlini L, Gooding R, Lochmuller H, et al. Genetic identity of Marinesco-Sjogren/myoglobinuria and CCFDN syndromes. Neurology 2002;58:231–6.

Mesarus S, Rocco MA, Absinto A, et al. Evidence of thalamic grey matter loss in pediatric multiple sclerosis. Neurology 2008;70:1107–13.

Mikaeloff Y, Suissa S, Vallée L, et al. First episode of acute CNS inflammatory demyelination in childhood: prognostic factors for multiple sclerosis and disability. Journal of Pediatrics 2004;144:246–52.

Moreira M-C, Koenig M. Ataxia with oculomotor apraxia type 2 (AOA2). In: GeneClinics: Medical Genetics Knowledge Base [database online]. Seattle: University of Washington. Available at http://www.geneclinics.org. PMID: 20301333. Last updated December 8, 2011.

Naidu S, Bibat G, Lin D, et al. Progressive cavitating leukoencephalopathy: A novel childhood disease. Annals of Neurology 2005;58:929–38.

Nozaki J, Dakeishi M, Ohura T, et al. Homozygosity mapping to chromosome 5p15 of a gene responsible for Hartnup disorder. Biochemical and Biophysical Research Communications 2001;284:255–60.

Paulino AC, Wen BC, Buatti JM, et al. Intracranial ependymomas: an analysis of prognostic factors and patterns of failure. American Journal of Clinical Oncology 2002;25:117–22.

Perilongo G, Massimino M, Sotti G, et al. 1998 Analyses of prognostic factors in a retrospective review of 92 children with ependymoma: Italian Pediatric Neuro-Oncology Group. Medical Pediatric Oncology 1998;29:79–85.

Ruggieri M, Polizzi A, Pavone L, et al. Multiple sclerosis in children less under 6 years of age. Neurology 1999;53:478–84.

Russo C, Cohen SL, Petruzzi J, et al. Long-term neurological outcome in children with opsoclonus-myoclonus associated with neuroblastoma: A report of the Pediatric Oncology Group. Medical Pediatric Oncology 1997;29:284–8.

Sarnat HB, Benjamin DR, Siebert JR, et al. Agenesis of the mesencephalon and metencephalon with cerebellar hypoplasia: Putative mutation in the EN2 gene. Report of 2 cases in early infancy. Pediatric and Developmental Pathology 2002;5:54–68.

Sawaishi Y, Takahashi I, Hirayama Y, et al. Acute cerebellitis caused by Coxiella burnetti. Annals of Neurology 1999;45:124–7.

Schimke RN, Collins DL, Stolle CA. Von Hippel-Lindau syndrome. In: GeneClinics: Medical Genetics Knowledge Base [database online]. Seattle: University of Washington. Available at http://www.geneclinics.org. PMID: 20301636. Last updated December 22, 2009.

Spacey S. Episodic ataxia type 2. In: GeneClinics: Medical Genetics Knowledge Base [database online]. Seattle: University of Washington. Available at http://www.geneclinics.org. PMID 20301674. Last updated December 8, 2011.

Subramony SH, Schott K, Raike RS, et al. Novel CACNAiA mutation causes febrile episodic ataxia with interictal cerebellar deficits. Annals of Neurology 2003;54:725–31.

Tenembaum S, Chitnis T, Ness J, et al. Acute disseminated encephalomyelitis. Neurology 2007;68(16 Suppl 2):S23–36.

Valente EM, Marsh SE, Castori M, et al. Distinguishing the four genetic causes of Joberts syndrome-related disorders. Annals of Neurology 2005;57:513–9.

Van der Knaap MS, Pronk JC, Scheper GC. Vanishing white matter disease. Lancet Neurology 2006; May 5:413–42.

Visudhiphan P, Chiemchanya S, Santadusit S. Optic neuritis in children: recurrence and subsequent development of multiple sclerosis. Pediatric Neurology 1995;13:293–5.

Wilejto M, Shroff M, Buncic JR, et al. The clinical features, MRI findings, and outcome of optic neuritis in children. Neurology 2006;67:258–62.

Wingerchuk DM, Pittock SJ, Lucchinetti CF, et al. Revised diagnostic criteria for neuromyelitis optica. Neurology 2006;66:1485–9.

CHAPTER 11

HEMIPLEGIA

The approach to children with hemiplegia must distinguish between acute hemiplegia, in which weakness develops within a few hours, and chronic progressive hemiplegia, in which weakness evolves over days, weeks, or months. The distinction between an acute and an insidious onset should be easy but can be problematic. In children with a slowly evolving hemiplegia, missing early weakness is possible until an obvious level of functional disability is attained, by which time the hemiplegia seems new and acute.

An additional presentation of hemiplegia found in infants who come to medical attention because of developmental delay is slowness in meeting motor milestones and early establishment of hand preference. Children should not establish a hand preference until the second year. Such children may have a static structural problem from birth (*hemiplegic cerebral palsy*), but the clinical features are not apparent until the child is old enough to use the affected limbs.

Magnetic resonance imaging (MRI) is the diagnostic modality of choice for investigating all forms of hemiplegia. It is especially informative to show migrational defects in hemiplegic cerebral palsy associated with seizures. Magnetic resonance arteriography (MRA) is sufficiently informative in visualizing the vascular structures to obviate the need for arteriography in most children.

HEMIPLEGIC CEREBRAL PALSY

The term hemiplegic cerebral palsy comprises several pathological entities that result in limb weakness on one side of the body. In premature infants, the most common cause is periventricular hemorrhagic infarction (see Chapter 4). In term infants, the underlying causes are often cerebral malformations, cerebral infarction, and intracerebral hemorrhage. Imaging studies of the brain are useful to provide the family with a definitive diagnosis.

The usual concern that brings infants with hemiplegia from birth for a neurological evaluation is delayed crawling or walking. Abnormalities of the legs are the focus of attention. Unilateral facial weakness is never associated, probably because bilateral corticobulbar innervation of the lower face persists until birth. Epilepsy occurs in half of children with hemiplegic cerebral palsy.

Infants with injury to the dominant hemisphere can develop normal speech in the nondominant hemisphere, but it is at the expense of visuoperceptual and spatial skills. Infants with hemiplegia and early-onset seizures are an exception; they show cognitive disturbances of verbal and nonverbal skills.

Congenital Malformations

Migrational defects comprise the majority of congenital malformations causing infantile hemiplegia (Figure 11-1). The affected hemisphere is often small and may show a unilateral perisylvian syndrome in which the sylvian fossa is widened (Sébire et al, 1996). Chapter 17 describes a bilateral perisylvian syndrome with speech disturbances. Seizures and mental retardation are often associated. As a rule, epilepsy is more common when congenital malformations cause infantile hemiplegia than when the cause is stroke.

Neonatal Infarction

Cerebral infarction from arterial occlusion occurs more often in full-term newborns than in premature newborns. MRI shows three patterns of infarction: (1) *arterial border zone infarction* is associated with resuscitation and caused by hypotension; (2) *multiartery infarction* is not often associated with perinatal distress and may be caused by congenital heart disease, disseminated intravascular coagulation, and polycythemia; and (3) *single-artery infarction* can result from injury to the cervical portion of the carotid artery during a difficult delivery owing to either misapplication of obstetric forceps or hyperextension and rotation of the neck with stretching of the artery over the lateral portion of the upper cervical vertebrae. *However, trauma is a rare associated event, and the cause of most single-artery infarctions, especially large infarctions in the frontal or parietal lobes, is unexplained.*

Clinical Features. Some newborns with large single-artery infarcts appear normal at birth but develop repetitive focal seizures during the first 4 days postpartum. Ten percent of neonatal seizures are caused by stroke. Most of these will later show a hemiparesis that spares the face. When neonatal seizures do not occur, hemiparesis including early handedness during infancy

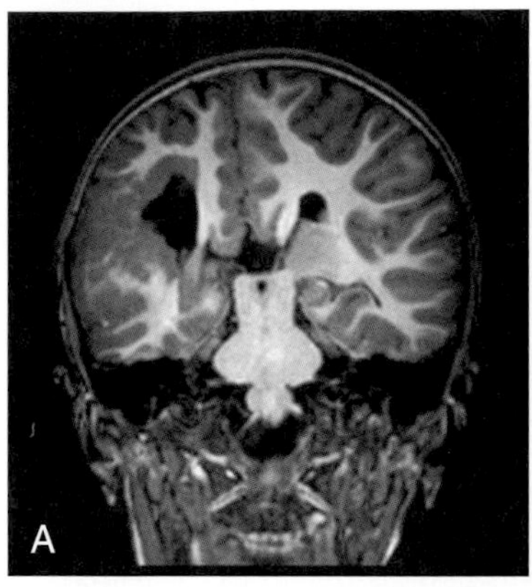

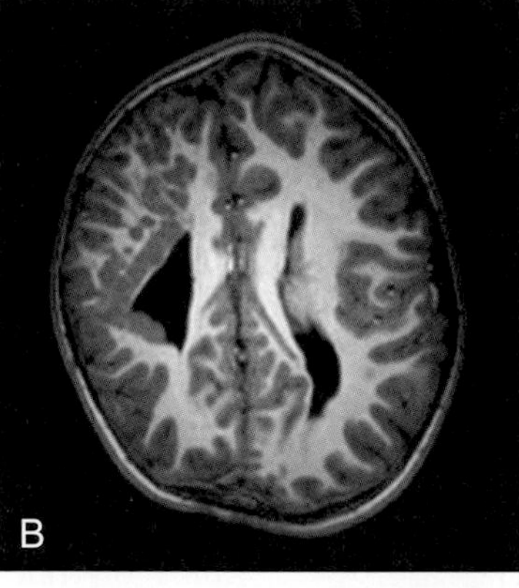

FIGURE 11-1 ■ Closed lip schizencephaly with periventricular heterotopias. (A) T_1 coronal MRI; (B) axial MRI.

brings the child to neurological attention (Lee et al, 2005; Roach et al, 2008). Many such children develop epilepsy during childhood and some have cognitive impairment.

Diagnosis. MRI with or without MRA and MRV (magnetic resonance venography) is the preferred modality for diagnosis of stroke. Diffusion-weighted images are the best sequence for visualization of ischemic areas. Ultrasound is satisfactory to detect large infarcts in the complete distribution of the middle cerebral artery. The size of the defect on MRI correlates directly with the probability of later hemiplegia (Mercuri et al, 1999). Follow-up imaging studies may show either unilateral enlargement of the lateral ventricle or porencephaly in the distribution of the middle cerebral artery contralateral to the hemiparesis. Hemiatrophy of the pons contralateral to the abnormal hemisphere may be an associated feature.

Maternal use of cocaine during pregnancy can cause cerebral infarction and hemorrhage in the fetus. Cocaine is detectable in the newborn's urine during the first week postpartum.

Management. Provide supportive care for all type of strokes. Correct dehydration and anemia when present. Neonates with prothrombotic states or tendency for cardiogenic emboli may benefit from the use of unfractionated heparin (UFH) or low-molecular-weight heparin (LMWH). Give vitamin B and folate to neonates with methylenetetrahydrofolate reductase (MTHFR) mutation in an effort to normalize homocysteine levels. The use of LMWH may have a place in cerebral venous sinus thrombosis when the clot is expanding or multiple sinuses are involved. Thrombolytic agents are not recommended as the safety and efficacy in newborns is unknown (Roach et al, 2008). Antiepileptic drugs are often needed for seizure control (see Chapter 1). Rehabilitative measures may help improve the level of function when sequelae occur.

Neonatal Hemorrhage

Intracranial hemorrhage affects 1 % of full-term neonates (Gradnitzer et al, 2002). Small unilateral parietal or temporal hemorrhages occur almost exclusively in term newborns and are not associated with either trauma or asphyxia. Larger hemorrhages into the temporal lobe sometimes result when obstetric forceps apply excessive force to the lateral skull, but more often they are idiopathic. Intraventricular hemorrhage may be an associated feature.

Clinical Features. Newborns with small hemorrhages are normal at birth and seem well until seizures begin any time during the first week. The symptoms of larger hemorrhages may be apnea, seizures, or both. Seizures are usually focal, and hemiplegia or hypotonia is present on examination. Some infants recover completely, whereas others show residual hemiplegia and cognitive deficits.

Diagnosis. Seizures and apnea usually prompt lumbar puncture to exclude the possibility of sepsis. The cerebrospinal fluid is grossly bloody. Computed tomography (CT) shows hemorrhage, and follow-up studies show focal encephalomalacia.

Management. Correction of significant thrombocytopenia, replacement of coagulation factors when applicable, vitamin K for all neonates and higher doses for certain factor deficiencies (maternal use of warfarin, phenobarbital or phenytoin), and ventricular drain sometimes followed by ventriculoperitoneal (VP) shunt is needed for intraventricular bleeds with hydrocephalus. Correct anemia and dehydration when present, and treat seizures when they coexist (Roach et al, 2008).

ACUTE HEMIPLEGIA

The sudden onset of an acute, focal neurological deficit suggests either a vascular, epileptic or migraine mechanism (Box 11-1). Strokes

BOX 11-1 Differential Diagnosis of Acute Hemiplegia

Alternating hemiplegia
Asthmatic amyotrophy (see Chapter 13)
Cerebrovascular disease*
Diabetes mellitus
Epilepsy
Hypoglycemia (see Chapter 2)
Kawasaki disease (see Chapter 10)
Migraine*
Trauma
Tumor*

*Denotes the most common conditions and the ones with disease modifying treatments

manifest as abrupt onset of the weakness within seconds, seizures within couple of minutes; migraines tend to manifest their neurologic signs over several minutes. Infants and children who have acute hemiplegia are divisible almost equally into two groups according to whether or not epilepsia partialis continua precedes the hemiplegia. Both groups may have seizures on the paretic side after hemiplegia is established. Cerebral infarction, usually in the distribution of the middle cerebral artery, accounts for one-quarter of cases in which seizures precede the hemiplegia and more than half of cases in which hemiplegia is the initial feature. Whatever the cause, the probability of a permanent motor deficit is almost 100 % when the initial feature is epilepsia partialis continua and about 50 % when it is not.

Alternating Hemiplegia

This is a rare and poorly understood clinical syndrome with hemiplegia as a cardinal feature (Swoboda et al, 2004). Considerations of its nosological identity include migraine, epilepsy, and familial paroxysmal choreoathetosis. Most cases are sporadic, but some families show mutations in a sodium-potassium ATPase gene also implicated in familial hemiplegic migraine type 2. The clinical spectrum of both disorders, expanded by mutation analysis, now overlaps.

Clinical Features. Onset is from birth to 18 months (mean, 8 months). The initial features are mild developmental delay and abnormal eye movements. Motor attacks may be hemiplegia, dystonia, or both. As a rule, young infants have more dystonic features and older children are more likely to have flaccid hemiplegia. Brief episodes of monocular or binocular nystagmus, lasting for 1 to 3 minutes, are often associated with both dystonic and hemiplegic attacks. Because the attack-onset is abrupt, dystonia is often mistaken for a seizure and hemiplegia for a stroke. Most reports of epileptic seizures in infants with this syndrome are probably dystonic attacks.

The duration of hemiplegia varies from minutes to days, and intensity waxes and wanes during a single episode. During long attacks, hemiplegia may shift from side to side or both sides may be affected. The arm is usually weaker than the leg, and walking may not be impaired. Hemiplegia disappears during sleep and reappears on awakening but not immediately.

Dystonic episodes may primarily affect the limbs on one side, causing hemidystonia, or affect the trunk, causing opisthotonic posturing. Some children scream during attacks as if in pain. Headache may occur at the onset of an attack but not afterward. Writhing movements that suggest choreoathetosis may be associated. Mental slowing occurs early in the course and mental regression follows later. Stepwise neurological impairment occurs as well, as if recovery from individual attacks is incomplete.

Diagnosis. Results of electroencephalography (EEG), cerebral arteriography, and MRI are normal. The diagnosis relies entirely on the clinical features.

Management. Anticonvulsant and antimigraine medications have consistently failed to prevent attacks or prevent progression. However, topiramate prophylaxis prevented recurrent attacks in a single case report (Di Rosa et al, 2006). Flunarizine, a calcium channel blocking agent, reduces the frequency of attacks, but its efficacy is not established. Other calcium channel blocking agents and anticonvulsant drugs have not been useful.

Alternating hemiplegia and dopa-responsive dystonia (see Chapter 14) share the feature of episodic dystonia with diurnal variation, and infants with attacks of dystonia should receive a trial of levodopa-carbidopa.

Cerebrovascular Disease

The annual incidence of stroke in children after the newborn period is approximately 2.3 per 100 000 (Fullerton et al, 2003). This represents a significant decline over the past 20 years (Fullerton et al, 2002). Half are ischemic and half are nontraumatic intracerebral and subarachnoid hemorrhages (Lanthier et al, 2002). The incidence rate is slightly higher in black than in white children and lowest in Hispanic children. Girls have a lower incidence than boys, but the gender and racial differences are not attributable to head injuries or sickle cell disease. Approximately 25 % of ischemic strokes in children are associated with a known risk factor (Box 11-2).

BOX 11-2 Causes of Stroke

CEREBROVASCULAR MALFORMATIONS
- Arteriovenous malformation
- Fibromuscular dysplasia
- Hereditary hemorrhagic telangiectasia
- Sturge-Weber syndrome

COAGULOPATHIES/HEMOGLOBINOPATHIES
- Antiphospholipid antibodies/lupus anticoagulant
- Congenital coagulation defects*
- Disseminated intravascular coagulation
- Drug-induced thrombosis
- Malignancy
- Sickle cell anemia/disease*
- Thrombocytopenic purpura

HEART DISEASE
- Arrhythmia
- Atrial myxoma
- Bacterial endocarditis
- Cardiac catheterization
- Cardiomyopathy
- Cyanotic congenital defects*
- Mitral valve prolapse*
- Prosthetic heart valve
- Rhabdomyoma
- Rheumatic heart disease

TRAUMA
- Arterial dissection*
- Blunt trauma to neck
- Intraoral trauma
- Vertebral manipulation

VASCULITIS
- Carotid infection
- Drug abuse (amphetamines and cocaine)
- Hemolytic-uremic syndrome (see Chapter 2)
- Hypersensitivity vasculitis
- Isolated angiitis
- Kawasaki disease (see Chapter 10)
- Meningitis* (see Chapter 4)
- Mixed connective tissue disease
- Systemic lupus erythematosus
- Takayasu arteritis
- Varicella infection

VASCULOPATHIES
- Fabry disease
- Homocystinuria* (see Chapter 5)
- Mitochondrial encephalopathy, lactic acidosis, and stroke (MELAS)
- Moyamoya disease

*Denotes the most common conditions and the ones with disease modifying treatments

The coexistence of multiple risk factors predicts a poor outcome.

Stroke is always a consideration when a previously healthy child suddenly becomes hemiparetic or develops any focal neurological disturbance. MRI (diffusion-weighted images) with or without MRA and MRV is the preferred diagnostic modality. Clinical features vary with the age of the child and the location of the stroke. Hemiparesis, either immediately or as a late sequela, is one of the more common features.

CT scan may show decreased density, effacement of sulci and loss of differentiation between gray and white matter and may enhance with contrast material. These changes may be subtle or absent in the first 24 hours after stroke. Cerebral infarction is often superficial, affecting both gray and white matter, and is in the distribution of a single artery. Multiple infarcts suggest either embolism or vasculitis. Small, deep lesions of the internal capsule are rare but can occur in infants.

Box 11-3 lists inherited states promoting cerebral infarction and Table 11-1 summarizes the evaluation of a child with cerebral infarction. The usual line of investigation includes tests for coagulopathies, vaculitis, and vasculopathies, a search for cardiac sources of emboli, and cerebral arteriography. The basic evaluation for prothrombotic disorders may include prothrombin time and activated partial thromboplastin time and a complete blood cell count, including platelets, protein C, protein S and antithrombin III levels, activated protein C resistance, plasminogen, fibrinogen, homocysteine, antiphospholipid antibody screen, lipoprotein(a), and a cholesterol panel. Genetic testing may include screening for the factor V Leiden mutation, the prothrombin *20210A* gene, and the MTHFR mutation.

An area of increased density on a noncontrast-enhanced CT identifies intracerebral hemorrhage. Edema frequently surrounds the area of increased density and may produce a mass effect with shift of midline structures.

Arteriovenous Malformations

Supratentorial malformations may cause acute or chronic progressive hemiplegia. Intraparenchymal hemorrhage causes acute hemiplegia. The major clinical features of hemorrhage into a hemisphere are loss of consciousness, seizures, and hemiplegia. Large hematomas cause midline structures to shift and increase intracranial pressure. Chapter 4 contains the discussion of arteriovenous malformations. MRA, CT angiogram or direct angiogram are the best techniques to visualize the malformation.

BOX 11-3 Inherited States Promoting Cerebral Infarction

ACTIVATED PROTEIN C RESISTANCE

Factor V Leiden mutation

DEFICIENCIES

Antithrombin III
Protein C
Protein S

OTHER GENETIC FACTORS

Elevated antiphospholipid antibodies and lupus anticoagulant
Elevated factor VIII levels, and low plasminogen or high fibrinogen.
Elevated lipoprotein(a)
Plasminogen activator inhibitor promoter polymorphism (PAI 1)
Prothrombin gene *20210* mutation
MTHFR gene defect

Brain Tumors

The usual cause of acute hemiplegia from brain tumor is hemorrhage into or around the tumor. Hemorrhage may hide the underlying tumor on CT and MRI is more informative (see Chapter 4). Tumors may also cause a slowly progressive hemiparesis with or without increased intracranial pressure, disk edema or seizures.

Carotid and Vertebral Artery Disorders

Cervical Infections. Unilateral and bilateral occlusions of the cervical portion of the internal carotid arteries may occur in children with a history of chronic tonsillitis and cervical lymphadenopathy. Whether this is cause and effect or coincidence is uncertain. Tonsillitis may cause carotid arteritis.

Unilateral cerebral infarction may occur in the course of cat-scratch disease (see Chapter 2) and mycoplasma pneumonia. In both diseases, the presence of submandibular lymph node involvement is associated with arteritis of the adjacent carotid artery. Necrotizing fasciitis is a serious cause of inflammatory arteritis with subsequent occlusion of one or both carotid arteries. The source of parapharyngeal space infection is usually chronic dental infection. Mixed aerobic and anaerobic organisms are isolated on culture.

Clinical Features. The usual sequence in cervical arteritis is fever and neck tenderness followed by sudden hemiplegia. Bilateral hemiplegia may occur when both sides are infected.

Diagnosis. Culture of the throat or lymph node specimens is required to identify the offending organism or organisms. Arteriography, CT angiogram or MRA identifies the site and extent of carotid occlusion.

Management. An aggressive course of antibiotic therapy, especially for necrotizing fasciitis, is mandatory. The outcome is variable, and recovery may be partial or complete.

TABLE 11-1 Evaluation of Cerebral Infarction

Blood	
Activated protein C resistance, antiphosphospholipid antibodies, apolipoproteins, cholesterol (high and low density lipoproteins), complete blood count, culture, erythrocyte sedimentation rate, factor V, free protein S, lactic acid, Leiden mutation, lupus anticoagulant, plasminogen, protein C, serum homocystine, triglycerides	Bacterial endocarditis Homocystinuria Hypercoaguable state Hyperlipidemia Leukemia Lupus erythematosus MELAS Polycythemia Sickle cell anemia Vasculitis
Urine	
Cocaine, urinalysis	Cocaine abuse Homocystinuria Nephritis Nephrosis
Heart	
Echocardiography, electrocardiography	Bacterial endocarditis Congenital heart disease Mitral valve prolapse Rheumatic heart disease
Brain	
Arteriography, magnetic resonance imaging	Arterial dissection Arterial thrombosis Arteriovenous malformation Fibromuscular hypoplasia Moyamoya disease Vasculitis

Fibromuscular Dysplasia. Fibromuscular dysplasia is an idiopathic segmental nonatheromatous disorder of the renal arteries and the extracranial segment of the internal carotid artery within 4 cm of its bifurcation. Seven percent of patients also have intracerebral aneurysms.

Clinical Features. Transitory ischemic attacks and stroke are the only clinical features of fibromuscular dysplasia. Fibromuscular dysplasia is primarily a disease of women over 50 years of age but can occur in children.

Diagnosis. Arteriography shows an irregular contour of the internal carotid artery in the neck resembling a string of beads. Suspect concomitant fibromuscular dysplasia of the renal arteries if hypertension is present.

Management. Either operative transluminal balloon angioplasty or carotid endarterectomy are options to treat the stenosis. The long-term prognosis in children is unknown.

Trauma to the Carotid Artery. Children may experience carotid thrombosis and dissection from seemingly trivial injuries, such as during exercise and sports, and can also occur without known cause in otherwise normal children (Rafay et al, 2006). They also occur in child abuse (grabbing and shaking the neck) or from injuries to the carotid artery during a fall, when the child has a blunt object (e.g., pencil, lollipop) in the mouth. Other risk factors for carotid dissection include fibromuscular dysplasia, Ehlers-Danlos syndrome type IV, Marfan syndrome, coarctation of the aorta, cystic medial necrosis, autosomal dominant polycystic kidney disease, osteogenesis imperfecta, atherosclerosis, extreme arterial tortuosity, moyamoya syndrome, and pharyngeal infections (Roach et al, 2008).

Clinical Features. Usually, a delay of several hours and sometimes days separate the injury from the onset of symptoms. The delay probably represents the time needed for thrombus to form within the artery. Clinical features usually include hemiparesis, hemianesthesia, hemianopia, and aphasia when the dominant hemisphere is affected. Deficits may be transitory or permanent, but some recovery always occurs. Seizures are rare.

Diagnosis. MRA safely visualizes carotid dissection and occlusion.

Management. In children with cervicocephalic arterial dissection (CCAD), use either Unfractionated heparin (UFH) or Low molecular weight heparin (LMWH) as a bridge to oral anticoagulation with warfarin. It is common and reasonable to treat a child with CCAD with either subcutaneous LMWH or warfarin for 3 to 6 months. Alternatively, an antiplatelet agent may be used. Continue therapy beyond 6 months when symptoms recur or when there is radiographic evidence of a residual abnormality of the dissected artery. Surgery such as bypass or extracranial to intracranial shunts may be considered in patients who continue to have symptoms from a CCAD while on medical therapy. Do not give anticoagulation medication to children with an intracranial dissection or with subarachnoid hemorrhage from CCAD (Roach et al, 2008).

Trauma to the Vertebral Artery. Vertebral artery thrombosis or dissection may follow minor neck trauma, especially rapid neck rotation. The site of occlusion is usually at the C1–C2 level. Boys are more often affected than are girls (Ganesan et al, 2002).

Clinical Features. The usual features of vertebral artery injury are headache and brainstem dysfunction. Repeated episodes of hemiparesis associated with bitemporal throbbing headache and vomiting may occur and are readily misdiagnosed as basilar artery migraine. The outcome is relatively good, survival is the rule, and chronic neurological disability is unusual.

Diagnosis. The clue to diagnosis is the presence of one or more areas of infarction on CT or MRI. The possibility of stroke leads to an arteriographic study, which reveals the vertebral artery occlusion.

Management. Long-term aspirin prophylaxis is a common recommendation, but not proven effective.

Cocaine Use

Cocaine is a potent vasoconstrictor that causes infarction in several organs. Stroke occurs mainly in young adults and may follow any route of administration. The interval from administration to stroke is usually unknown but may be minutes to hours. Intracerebral hemorrhage and subarachnoid hemorrhage are more common than cerebral infarction and often occur in people with underlying aneurysms or arteriovenous malformations. Vasospasm or vasculitis is the probable cause of infarction.

Diabetes Mellitus

Acute but transitory attacks of hemiparesis occur in children with insulin-dependent diabetes mellitus. Complicated migraine is a suggested mechanism, but the pathophysiology remains unknown.

Clinical Features. Attacks frequently occur during sleep in a child with a respiratory illness. Hemiparesis is present on awakening; weakness is greater in the face and arm than in the leg. Sensation is intact, but aphasia is present if the dominant hemisphere is affected. Tendon reflexes may be depressed or brisk in the affected arm, and an extensor plantar response is usually present. Headache is a constant feature and may be unilateral or generalized. Some patients are nauseated. The family does not have a history of migraine. Attacks last for 3 to 24 hours, and recovery is complete. Recurrences are common.

Diagnosis. Stroke is not a complication of juvenile insulin-dependent diabetes, except during episodes of ketoacidosis (see Chapter 2). Head CT in children with transitory hemiplegia does not show infarction.

Management. Although some children have further attacks, a method for prevention of recurrences is not established.

Epilepsy

Hemiparetic Seizures

Todd paralysis is a term used to describe hemiparesis that lasts for minutes or hours and follows a focal or generalized seizure. It occurs most often following prolonged seizures, especially those caused by an underlying structural abnormality.

Hemiparesis may be a seizure manifestation as well as a postictal event. Such seizures are *hemiparetic* or *focal inhibitory* seizures. Todd paralysis may be difficult to distinguish from hemiparetic seizures because it is not always clear whether a seizure preceded the hemiparesis or whether the hemiparesis is ictal or postictal.

Clinical Features. The initial feature may be a brief focal seizure followed by flaccid hemiparesis or the abrupt onset of flaccid monoparesis or hemiparesis. Consciousness is not impaired, and the child seems well otherwise. The severity and distribution of weakness fluctuate, affecting one limb more than the other and sometimes the face. Tendon reflexes are normal in the hemiparetic limbs, but the plantar response may be extensor.

Diagnosis. EEG shows recurrent spike- and slow-wave discharges over the hemisphere contralateral to the weakness. A radioisotope scan shows increased focal uptake in the affected hemisphere during the ictal phase and decreased uptake between seizures. Results of MRI, CT, and cerebral arteriography may be normal.

Management. The treatment is with the same drugs used for the treatment of partial seizures such as levetiracetam, oxcarbazepine, and lamotrigine (see Chapter 1).

Heart Disease

Congenital Heart Disease

Cerebrovascular complications of congenital heart disease are most likely in children with cyanotic heart conditions. The usual complications are venous sinus thrombosis in infants and embolic arterial occlusion in children. Emboli may occur from valvular vegetations or bacterial endocarditis. In either case, the development of cerebral abscess is a major concern. Cerebral abscess of embolic origin is exceedingly uncommon in children younger than 2 years of age with congenital heart disease and occurs only as a complication of meningitis or surgery.

Children with complex congenital heart disease are at risk for cardioembolic stroke, thrombotic stroke, and watershed infarcts from drops in perfusion pressure. The rates of stroke in children with complex congenital heart disease vary with (1) the severity of the malformation; (2) the number of corrective surgeries required; (3) anesthetic techniques during surgery; (4) patient selection; and (5) length of follow-up. The greatest risk for children with congenital heart disease occurs at the time of surgery or cardiac catheterization (Roach, 2002). Cerebral dysgenesis is an important consideration in children with congenital heart disease. Postmortem studies show a 10–29 % prevalence of associated cerebral malformations. Children with hypoplastic left heart syndrome are especially at risk for associated dysgenetic brain lesions.

Clinical Features. Venous thrombosis occurs most often in infants with cyanotic heart disease who are dehydrated and polycythemic. One or more sinuses may occlude. Failure of venous drainage always increases intracranial pressure. Hemiparesis is a major clinical feature and may occur first on one side and then on the other with sagittal sinus obstruction. Seizures and decreased consciousness are associated features. The mortality rate is high in infants with thrombosis of major venous sinuses, and most survivors have neurological morbidity.

Children with cyanotic heart disease are at risk for arterial embolism when vegetations are present within the heart or because of the right-to-left shunt, which allows peripheral emboli to bypass the lungs and reach the brain. The potential for cerebral abscess formation increases in children with right-to-left shunt because decreased arterial oxygen saturation lowers cerebral resistance to infection.

The initial feature is sudden onset of hemiparesis associated with headache, seizures, and loss of consciousness. Seizures are at first focal and recurrent but later become generalized.

Diagnosis. MRI is the preferred procedure for the detection of venous thrombosis and emboli. A pattern of hemorrhagic infarction occurs adjacent to the site of venous thrombosis, and multiple areas of infarction are associated with embolization.

The CT appearance may be normal during the first 12 to 24 hours following embolization. By the next day, the study shows a low-density lesion. Although the sequence is consistent with a sterile embolus, the possibility of subsequent abscess formation is a consideration. Repeat enhanced CT or MRI studies within 1 week reveal ring enhancement if an abscess developed.

Management. Treatment for congestive heart failure may reduce the possibility of cardiogenic embolism and stroke. Repairing the congenital heart defect reduces the risk of subsequent stroke (this is unknown with patent foramen ovale, PFO). UFH or LMWH is given until warfarin is adjusted for children with a cardiac embolism unrelated to a PFO who are judged to have a high risk for recurrent embolism. Alternatively, it is reasonable to use LMWH initially in this situation and to continue it instead of warfarin. In children with a risk of cardiac embolism, it is reasonable to continue either LMWH or warfarin for at least 1 year or until the lesion responsible for the risk has been corrected. If the risk of recurrent embolism is judged to be high, it is reasonable to continue anticoagulation indefinitely as long as it is well tolerated. For children with a suspected cardiac embolism unrelated to a PFO with a lower or unknown risk of stroke, it is reasonable to begin aspirin and to continue it for at least 1 year. Surgical repair or transcatheter closure is reasonable in individuals with a major atrial septal defect (not for PFO) both to reduce the stroke risk and to prevent long-term cardiac complications. Anticoagulant therapy is not used for individuals with native valve endocarditis (Roach et al, 2008). Antibiotics are very important to decrease the possibility of transformation into abscess in cases of endocarditis.

Treatment for venous thrombosis is primarily supportive and directed toward correcting dehydration and controlling increased intracranial pressure. Dexamethasone is useful to decrease cerebral volume, but osmotic diuretics may cause further thrombosis. The infarction is usually hemorrhagic, and anticoagulants are contraindicated. Distinguishing a septic from a sterile thrombosis is impossible, and all infants receive antibiotic treatment.

Mitral Valve Prolapse

Mitral valve prolapse is a familial disorder present in 5 % of children. It is usually asymptomatic but estimated to cause recurrent attacks of cerebral ischemia in 1 in every 6000 cases each year. Sterile emboli from thrombus originating either from the prolapsing leaflet or at its junction with the atrial wall cause the recurrent attacks.

Clinical Features. The initial feature is usually a transitory ischemic attack in the distribution of the carotid circulation producing partial or complete hemiparesis. Weakness usually clears within 24 hours, but recurrent episodes, not necessarily in the same arterial distribution, are the rule. Basilar insufficiency is less common and usually results in visual field defects. The interval between recurrences varies from weeks to years. Permanent neurological deficits occur in less than 20 % of individuals.

Diagnosis. Only 25 % of patients have late systolic murmurs or a midsystolic click. In the remainder, a cardiac examination is normal. Two-dimensional echocardiography is required to establish the diagnosis.

Management. No treatment is needed for asymptomatic children with auscultatory or electrocardiographic (ECG) abnormalities, nor is specific treatment available for a transient ischemic attack. However, once a child has suffered a transitory attack of ischemia, administer daily aspirin to reduce the likelihood of further thrombus formation in the heart.

Rheumatic Heart Disease

The frequency and severity of rheumatic fever and rheumatic heart disease in North America have been decreasing for several decades. Unfortunately, a mini epidemic of acute rheumatic fever recurs every 5–10 years in the United States. Rheumatic heart disease involves the mitral valve in 85 % of patients, the aortic valve in 54 %, and the tricuspid and pulmonary valves in less than 5 %. The source of cerebral emboli is either valvular vegetations or septic emboli due to infective endocarditis.

Clinical Features. The main features of mitral valve disease are cardiac failure and arrhythmia. Aortic valve disease is often asymptomatic. Neurological complications are always due to bacterial endocarditis except in the immediate postoperative period, when embolization is the likely explanation. Symptoms are much the same as in congenital heart disease, except that cerebral abscess is less common.

Diagnosis. Rheumatic heart disease is an established diagnosis long before the first stroke. Multiple blood cultures identify the organism and select the best drug for intravenous antibiotic therapy.

Management. Bacterial endocarditis requires vigorous intravenous antibiotic therapy.

Hypercoagulable States

A prethrombotic condition is present in 20–50 % of children presenting with arterial ischemic stroke and 33–99 % of children with cerebral venous sinus thrombosis (Barnes & DeVeber, 2006; Bonduel et al, 1999; DeVeber et al, 1998).

Abnormalities of blood cells or blood cell concentration may place the child at risk for hemorrhagic or ischemic stroke. Low platelet count due to autoimmune thrombocytopenia or bone marrow suppression may lead to hemorrhage. Anything that increases blood viscosity, such as sickled cells, polycythemia, or chronic hypoxia, may predispose to arterial or venous infarct. Dehydration is associated with arterial strokes and cerebrovascular thrombosis (CVT), possibly because it increases viscosity. Anemia is a risk factor for arterial ischemic infarction and CVT, possibly due to alterations in hemodynamics or imbalances in thrombotic pathways.

Risk factors for a prothrombotic state include recurrent episodes of deep vein thrombosis or pulmonary emboli, especially if they occur at a young age, or a family history of thrombotic events. The likelihood of stroke from most prothrombotic states seems to be relatively low, but the stroke risk increases when other risk factors are present. Thus, it is reasonable to test for the most common prothrombotic states even when another explanation for the stroke is present. Hypercoagulable states include antithrombin III, protein C or protein S deficiencies, activated protein C resistance, factor V Leiden mutation, prothrombin gene mutation (*G20210A*), antiphospholipid antibody syndrome, elevated levels of lipoprotein A and homocysteine. Protein C deficiency and the genetic polymorphisms collectively (factor V Leiden, prothrombin gene mutation, thermolabile form of the MTHFR gene) may be independent risk factors in children for recurrent arterial stroke. Cerebral venous and, less often, cerebral arterial thromboses may occur in patients with paroxysmal nocturnal hemoglobinuria. Polycythemia rubra vera, essential thrombocythemia, and disseminated intravascular coagulation may lead to cerebral infarction or intracranial hemorrhage (Roach et al, 2008). Thrombosis also accompanies secondary to transitory hematological abnormalities associated with intercurrent illness. For example, idiopathic nephrotic syndrome is associated with decreased antithrombin and CVT (Fluss et al, 2006).

Clinical Features. The typical features of venous thrombosis are headache and obtundation caused by increased intracranial pressure, seizures, and successive hemiplegia on either side. Suspect an inherited hypercoaguable state in children with recurrent venous thromboses, a family history of venous thrombosis, or thrombosis at an unusual site (see Table 11-1). Arterial thromboses usually cause ischemic stroke in the distribution of a single cerebral artery.

Diagnosis. Suspect venous thrombosis when hemiplegia and increased intracranial pressure develop suddenly. The diagnosis of sagittal sinus thromboses is suggested when parasagittal hemorrhage or infarction is associated with absence of the normal flow void in the sagittal sinus on MRI. Cerebral arteriography is the more definitive procedure. Box 11-4 summarizes laboratory studies.

Management. Provide supportive care for all type of strokes. Correct dehydration and anemia when present. In prothrombotic states, the child may benefit from the use of UFH or LMWH. Give vitamin B6, B12 and folate to children with MTHFR mutation in an effort to normalize homocysteine levels.

Ventricular drain sometimes followed by VP shunt is needed for intraventricular bleeds with hydrocephalus. Correct anemia and dehydration when present. Remove risk factors such as smoking and oral contraception when possible. Treat seizures when they coexist (Roach et al, 2008). Symptomatic treatment includes decreasing intracranial pressure, treating seizures when present, and rehydrating the patient without increasing cerebral edema.

BOX 11-4 Progressive Hemiplegia

- Adrenoleukodystrophy (see Chapter 5)
- Arteriovenous malformation (see Chapter 4)
- Brain abscess (see Chapter 4)
- Cerebral hemisphere tumor (see Chapter 4)
- Demyelinating diseases
- Late-onset globoid leukodystrophy (see Chapter 5)
- Multiple sclerosis (see Chapter 10)
- Sturge-Weber syndrome

Hypocoagulable States

Common congenital coagulation factor deficiencies include deficiencies of coagulation factor VIII (hemophilia A), coagulation factor IX (hemophilia B), and von Willebrand factor. A deficiency of any factor that regulates coagulation places the child at risk for hemorrhage.

Management. Correction of significant thrombocytopenia, replacement of coagulation factors when applicable, vitamin K for all neonates and higher doses for certain factor deficiencies (maternal use of warfarin, phenobarbital or phenytoin), and ventricular drain sometimes followed by VP shunt is needed for intraventricular bleeds with hydrocephalus. Correct anemia and dehydration when present, and treat seizures when they coexist (Roach et al, 2008).

Ischemic Arterial Infarction

Capsular Stroke

Small, deep infarcts involving the internal capsule occur in adults with hypertensive angiopathy. They also occur, but very rarely, in infants and young children. The onset of weakness is sudden and may occur during sleep or wakefulness.

Clinical Features. The face and limbs are involved, and a typical hemiplegic posture and gait develop. Hypalgesia and decreased position sense are difficult to demonstrate in infants but are demonstrable in older children. Larger infarcts affecting the striatum and the internal capsule of the dominant hemisphere cause speech disturbances. At the onset of hemiplegia, the child is mute and lethargic. As speech returns, evidence of dysarthria and aphasia develops. Eventually speech may become normal. Hemiparesis may clear completely, but some children have residual weakness.

Diagnosis. MRI is the modality of choice to confirm the diagnosis (diffusion-weighted images) of internal capsule infarcts.

Management. Some anticoagulation or thrombolytic treatments may apply for certain etiologies as mentioned earlier in this chapter. Initiate a rehabilitative treatment program once the child's condition is stable.

Cerebral Artery Infarction

Acute infantile hemiplegia may result from infarction in the distribution of the middle cerebral artery or one of its branches, the posterior cerebral artery, or the anterior cerebral artery.

Clinical Features. Sudden hemiplegia is the typical initial feature. Hemianesthesia, hemianopia, and aphasia (with dominant hemisphere infarction) are present as well. Some children are lethargic at the onset of symptoms, but consciousness is seldom lost completely.

Epilepsia partialis continuans precedes hemiplegia in approximately one-third of cases. When this is the case, permanent hemiplegia is a constant feature and epilepsy is common. When hemiplegia occurs without seizures, half of the patients recover completely and partial paralysis persists in the remainder.

Diagnosis. Complete occlusion of the middle cerebral artery produces a large area of hypodensity on CT involving the cortex, underlying white matter, basal ganglia, and internal capsule. Occlusion of superficial branches of the middle cerebral artery produces a wedge-shaped area of hypodensity extending from the cortex into the subjacent white matter. Table 11-1 lists studies for hypercoaguable states.

Management. Very few case reports describe children with ischemic stroke treated with intra-arterial or intravenous tissue plasminogen activator (Carlson et al, 2001). Few children present within the mandated 3 hours of infarct onset, and guidelines are not available on using intravenous or intra-arterial thrombolytics in children.

Lipoprotein Disorders

Familial lipid and lipoprotein abnormalities may cause premature cerebrovascular disease in infants and children. Genetic transmission of these disorders is by autosomal dominant inheritance.

Clinical Features. Ischemic episodes cause transitory or permanent hemiplegia, sometimes associated with hemianopia, hemianesthesia, and aphasia. Affected families have a history of cerebrovascular and coronary artery disease developing at an early age.

Diagnosis. Most children have low plasma concentrations of high-density lipoprotein cholesterol, others have high plasma concentrations of triglycerides, and some have both. The mechanism of arteriosclerosis is lipoprotein mediated endothelial damage with secondary thrombus formation.

Management. Dietary treatment, lipid-lowering medications, and daily aspirin administration comprise the management program.

Mitochondrial Encephalopathy, Lactic Acidosis, and Stroke

The most common mutation in mitochondrial encephalopathy, lactic acidosis, and stroke (MELAS) is in the mitochondrial gene *MTTL1* encoding tRNA (Leu-UUR) (DiMauro & Hirano, 2010).

Clinical Features. MELAS is a multisystem disorder with onset between 2 and 10 years. Early psychomotor development is usually normal, but short stature is common. First onset of symptoms is frequently between the ages of 2 and 10 years. The most common initial symptoms are generalized tonic-clonic seizures, recurrent headaches, anorexia, and recurrent vomiting. Exercise intolerance or proximal limb weakness can be the initial feature. Seizures are often associated with stroke-like episodes of transient hemiparesis or cortical blindness. These stroke-like episodes may be associated with altered consciousness and may be recurrent. The cumulative residual effects of the stroke-like episodes gradually impair motor abilities, vision, and mentation, often by adolescence or young adulthood. Sensorineural hearing loss is common.

Affected children are usually normal at birth. Failure to thrive, growth retardation, and progressive deafness are characteristic of onset during infancy. In later-onset cases, the main neurological features are recurrent attacks of prolonged migraine-like headaches and vomiting, seizures (myoclonic, focal, generalized) that often progress to status epilepticus, the sudden onset of focal neurological defects (hemiplegia, hemianopia, aphasia), and encephalopathy. Mental deterioration, when present, occurs anytime during childhood. Neurological abnormalities are initially intermittent and then become progressive, leading to coma and death.

Diagnosis. MRI shows multifocal infarction-like areas that do not conform to definite vascular territories. The initial lesions are often in the occipital lobes; progressive disease affects the cerebral and cerebellar cortices, the basal ganglia, and the thalamus. The concentration of lactate in the blood, magnetic resonance spectroscopy and cerebrospinal fluid is elevated. Muscle biopsy specimens show *ragged-red fibers* (see Chapter 7). Molecular diagnosis is commercially available. The blood leukocyte DNA reveals the A3243G mutation in 80% of MELAS patients (Roach et al, 2008).

Management. Specific treatment is not available, but a cocktail of vitamins is often used. The administration of coenzyme Q10 (50–100 mg three times a day) and L-carnitine (1000 mg three times a day) has benefited some patients. Idebenone, a form of coenzyme Q10, which crosses the blood-brain barrier more efficiently, may also be beneficial. Anecdotal reports indicated that dichloroacetate, which reduces blood lactate by activating the pyruvate dehydrogenase complex, is useful. However, a subsequent, controlled study showed a toxic effect on peripheral nerves.

Oral administration of L-arginine attenuates the severity of exacerbations when administered in the acute phase (Koga et al, 2005). It also reduces the frequency of exacerbations when given interictally. Confirmation by a double-blind study is required.

Moyamoya Disease

Moyamoya is not a disease, but rather a chronic, progressive, noninflammatory vasculopathy secondary to several other disorders. The end-result is a slowly progressive, bilateral occlusion of the internal carotid arteries starting at the carotid siphon. Occlusion of the basilar artery may occur as well. Associated conditions include sickle cell anemia, trisomy 21, neurofibromatosis 1, ventricular septal defect, mitral valve stenosis, and tetralogy of Fallot. Because the occlusion is slowly progressive, multiple anastomoses form between the internal and external carotid arteries. The result is a new vascular network at the base of the brain composed of collaterals from the anterior or posterior choroidal arteries, the basilar artery, and the meningeal arteries. On angiography, these telangiectasias produce a hazy appearance, as if a puff of smoke, from which is derived the Japanese word moyamoya (Figure 11-2). The disorder is worldwide in distribution, with a female-to-male bias of 3:2.

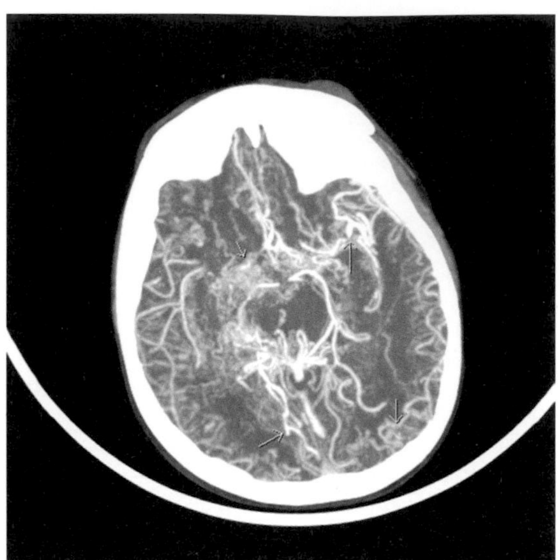

FIGURE 11-2 ■ Moyamoya disease. CT angiogram shows narrowing of vessels, leptomeningeal and basilar collaterals and tortuous vessels (arrows).

Clinical Features. The initial symptoms vary from recurrent headache to abrupt hemiparesis. Infants and young children tend to have an explosive onset characterized by the sudden development of complete hemiplegia affecting the face and limbs. The child is at least lethargic and sometimes comatose. When the child is sufficiently alert, examination may reveal hemianopia, hemianesthesia, and aphasia. Some children have chorea of the face and all limbs, which is worse on one side. Recovery follows, but before it is complete new episodes of focal neurological dysfunction occur on either the same or the opposite side. These episodes include hemiparesis, hemianesthesia, or aphasia, alone or in combination. The outcome is generally poor. Most children will have chronic weakness on one or both sides, epilepsy, and mental retardation. Some have died.

Recurrent transient ischemic attacks are an alternative manifestation. Characteristic of the attacks are episodic hemiparesis and dysesthesias lasting for minutes or hours, not associated with loss of consciousness. Frequently, hyperpnea or excitement triggers attacks, which may recur daily. After 4 or 5 years, the attacks cease but residual deficits persist.

Repeated episodes of monoparesis or symptoms of subarachnoid hemorrhage are other possible features of moyamoya disease. Monoparesis generally occurs after infancy and subarachnoid hemorrhage after 16 years of age.

Diagnosis. The typical "puff of smoke" may be seen by MRA, CT angiogram or catheter angiogram. CT or MRI may show large cerebral infarction caused by stenosis in the internal carotid artery. Definitive diagnosis requires arteriographic demonstration of bilateral stenosis in the distal internal carotid arteries and the development of collaterals in the basal ganglia and meninges. Studies should include a search for an underlying vasculopathy or coagulopathy.

Management. Treatment options depend on finding the underlying cause and severity of the disease. Indications for revascularization surgery include progressive ischemic symptoms or evidence of inadequate blood flow or cerebral perfusion reserve in an individual without a contraindication to surgery. Techniques to minimize anxiety and pain during hospitalizations may reduce the possibility of stroke caused by hyperventilation-induced vasoconstriction. Management of systemic hypotension, hypovolemia, hyperthermia, and hypocarbia during the intraoperative and perioperative periods may also reduce the risk of perioperative stroke in these children. Aspirin is a reasonable choice in asymptomatic patients or after revascularization surgery (Roach et al, 2008).

Sickle Cell Disease

Sickle cell disease (SCD) is a genetic disorder of African-American children transmitted by autosomal recessive inheritance. It is the most common hematological disorder associated with cerebrovascular accidents. The term encompasses a group of disorders associated with mutations in the *HBB* gene and defined by the presence of hemoglobin S (Hb S). Sickle cell anemia (Hb SS) accounts for 60–70 % of SCD in the United States. The other forms of SCD result from co-inheritance of Hb S with other abnormal globin β-chain variants (Bender & Hobbs, 2012).

Silent infarcts occur in the distribution of small vessels. The most common underlying lesion is an intracranial arterial stenosis or obstruction, often seen in the proximal middle cerebral and anterior cerebral arteries. Sickled erythrocytes cause chronic injury to the vessel endothelium, resulting in a narrow lumen. Subarachnoid hemorrhage and intraparenchymal hemorrhage also can occur.

Prior to modern therapy, neurological complications occurred in up to 25 % of homozygotes and also may occur at times of stress, such as surgery, in heterozygotes. The abnormal erythrocytes clog large and small vessels, decreasing total, hemispheric, or regional blood flow. Cerebral infarction usually occurs in the region of arterial border zones.

Clinical Features. The major systemic features are jaundice, pallor, weakness, and fatigability from chronic hemolytic anemia. Half of homozygotes show symptoms by 1 year, and all have symptoms by 5 years of age. The incidence of cerebral infarction varies among studies but may be as high as 46 % (Steen et al, 2003). Strokes occur at the time of a thrombotic, vaso-occlusive crisis. Dehydration or anoxia is often the cause of a crisis. Fever and pain in the abdomen and chest are characteristic. Focal or generalized seizures are the initial neurological feature in 70 % of patients. Vasculopathy and hypoperfusion cause epilepsy in children with SCD (Prengler et al, 2005). After the seizures have ended, hemiplegia and other focal neurological deficits are noted. Some recovery follows, but there is a tendency for recurrent strokes, epilepsy, and cognitive impairment. Strokes affecting both hemispheres produce a pseudobulbar palsy with brainstem dysfunction.

The worst case is a child in coma and has meningismus. Diffuse decrease in cerebral blood flow associated with subarachnoid or intracerebral hemorrhage is the usual cause. The mortality rate is high.

Diagnosis. The presence of significant quantities of Hb S establish the diagnosis. High-performance liquid chromatography, isoelectric focusing, or hemoglobin electrophoresis are used to quantify Hb S. Mutation analysis is available. Most affected children have an established diagnosis long before their first stroke. CT or MRI documents the extent of cerebral infarction and hemorrhage. After several such crises, cortical atrophy may be present. Cerebral arteriography offers little additional information and carries the risk of increasing ischemia.

Management. Acute management of ischemic stroke resulting from sickle cell disease should include optimal hydration, correction of hypoxemia, and correction of systemic hypotension

Stroke preventive treatment includes periodic transfusions to reduce the percentage of sickle hemoglobin in children 2 to 16 years of age with an abnormal tarnscranial doppler (TCD) resulting from SCD. In fact, this is the best preventive therapy for stroke when compared with other etiologies. Children with SCD and a confirmed stroke should be placed on a regular program of red cell exchange transfusion in conjunction with measures to prevent iron overload. For acute cerebral infarction, exchange transfusion designed to reduce sickle hemoglobin to less than 30% total hemoglobin is reasonable. In children with SCD, it is reasonable to repeat a TCD annually if normal and to repeat the test in 1 month, if abnormal. Borderline and mildly abnormal TCD studies may be repeated in 3 to 6 months. Hydroxyurea may be used in children and young adults with SCD and stroke who cannot continue on long-term exchange transfusion. Surgical revascularization procedures may be considered in children with SCD with moyamoya (Roach et al, 2008).

Hydroxyurea, the most prescribed therapy for SCD, benefits individuals with SCD by induction of Hb F synthesis. Hb F synthesis decreases sickling, improves red cell survival, lowers the white blood cell count, and acts as a vasodilator. Hydroxyurea treatment decreases acute painful episodes, episodes of acute chest syndrome, and the need for transfusion; survival is not improved (Steinberg et al, 2003).

Stem cell transplantation from a normal matched sibling stem cell donor or one with sickle cell trait can be curative (Walters et al, 2000).

Vasculopathies

Hypersensitivity Vasculitis. The term hypersensitivity vasculitis covers several disorders that have a known underlying cause (drugs, infection) and a characteristic purpura of the legs and a venulitis. Neurological complications occur only in Henoch-Schönlein purpura, for which an antecedent infection is the probable cause.

Clinical Features. The systemic features of Henoch-Schönlein purpura are fever, a purpuric rash on the extensor surfaces of the limbs, and abdominal pain with nausea and vomiting. Joint and renal disturbances may be present. Almost half of affected children have headache and abnormalities on EEG. Focal neurological deficits occur in one-third of patients, with hemiplegia accounting for half of these cases. A seizure may precede hemiplegia. Associated with hemiplegia are hemianesthesia, hemianopia, and aphasia. These deficits may be permanent.

Diagnosis. CT or MRI shows infarction, hemorrhage, or both.

Management. Corticosteroids treat the underlying disease.

Isolated Angiitis of the Central Nervous System. Isolated angiitis of the central nervous system (CNS) is an inflammation of small cerebral vessels. It is rare in children. The clinical features are recurrent headache, sometimes of a migrainous type, encephalopathy, and stroke. Arteriography shows multiple areas of irregular narrowing of the cerebral vessels. Corticosteroid therapy may be beneficial, but additional treatment with pulse cyclophosphamide is often required.

Systemic Lupus Erythematosus. Several collagen vascular disorders can cause neurological disturbances in adults, but systemic lupus erythematosus (SLE) is the main cause in children. SLE is an episodic multisystem, autoimmune disease, characterized by the presence of antinuclear antibodies (ANA), especially antibodies to double-stranded DNA. SLE accounts for 4.5% of patients seen in pediatric rheumatology clinics. The onset of SLE is uncommon before adolescence. In childhood, the ratio of affected girls to boys is 4.5:1. Mixed connective tissue disease is a rare cause of either large vessel occlusion or hemorrhage secondary to fibrinoid necrosis.

Clinical Features. Most children have fever, arthralgia, and skin rash at the time of diagnosis. The clinical features of lupus in children are generally similar to those in adults, except for a higher incidence of hepatosplenomegaly, chorea, nephritis, and avascular necrosis.

Neurological features are present in one-quarter of children at the time of diagnosis and in 30–60% sometime during the course. CNS involvement usually indicates a severe clinical course. Neuropsychiatric abnormalities are almost a constant feature. The prevalence of recurrent headaches is 71%, migraine 36%, cognitive disorders 55%, isolated seizures 47%, epilepsy 15%, acute confusional state 35%, dysesthesia or paresthesia 14%, transient ischemic attacks 12%, and cerebrovascular accident (CVA) 8%. Chorea and myositis are rare complications. Unlike systemic complaints, neurological disturbances are likely to progress or develop anew even after initiating treatment.

Vasculitis in SLE is rare and affects small arterioles and venules. Perivasculitis is more common. CVAs occur mainly in patients with hypertension or severe renal and cardiac disease. They are associated with positive results on serological tests for syphilis and the presence of lupus anticoagulant.

Hemiplegia usually follows a seizure and the cause may be either cerebral infarction or hemorrhage. Neurological episodes during treatment are often complications of immunosuppression, such as fungal meningitis, rather than primary complications of the underlying disease.

Diagnosis. The diagnosis of lupus requires a compatible clinical syndrome and the detection of an abnormal titer of ANA. ANA is present in almost all patients. Antibodies to double-stranded DNA are pathognomonic for SLE and present in almost all patients with active disease. Antibodies to extractable nuclear antigen (Sm, Ro/SS-A, La/SS-B, RNP), and anti-histone antibodies are strongly associated with SLE. Anti-Sm is highly specific for the disease. Rheumatoid factor is present in 10–30 % of cases. The presence of anticardiolipin antibodies is associated with hemolytic anemia and thrombotic events. CT or MRI of the head is useful to determine the presence of hemorrhage or infarction. Results of cerebral arteriography may be normal.

Management. The usual treatment of the CNS manifestations of SLE is high-dose oral or intravenous corticosteroids after excluding an infectious process. Several studies support the use of both steroids and cyclophosphamide in treating CNS lupus. In patients with antiphospholipid antibodies and platelet count greater than 70 000/mm^3, low-dose aspirin therapy is recommended. Anticoagulation with heparin followed by warfarin is required for children with stroke and antiphospholipid antibodies.

Takayasu Arteritis. Takayasu's arteritis, also known as *the pulseless disease*, is a chronic inflammatory, large-vessel vasculitis affecting the aorta and its major branches. The cause is unknown.

Clinical Features. Onset usually occurs between 15 and 20 years of age but may occur as early as infancy. Ninety percent of patients are female and most are of Japanese ethnicity. The most common features are fever, weight loss, myalgias, arthralgia, hypertension, absent pulses, and vascular bruits. The cause of neurological manifestations of the disease is cerebral hypoperfusion secondary to stenosis of the carotid and vertebral arteries, and complications of hypertension. Stroke occurs in only 5–10 % of patients. Focal seizures and sudden hemiplegia characterize the stroke. Examination reveals loss of radial pulses, and sometimes a carotid bruit.

Diagnosis. CT reveals a focal hypodense area, indicating infarction. Arteriography shows involvement of the ascending aorta and its major branches. Cardiac catheterization is necessary to define the full extent of arteritis. Some vessels have a beaded appearance; others terminate abruptly and have prestenotic dilatation.

Management. Treatment consists of corticosteroids and immunosuppressive agents such as methotrexate. Small series have shown usefulness of anti-tumor necrosis factor agents. Management of hypertension is critical, and antiplatelet agents are useful in preventing thrombosis. Surgical intervention, angioplasty, and stent placement sometimes are required.

Early diagnosis and treatment can lead to full recovery.

Infections

Hemiplegia occurs during the course of bacterial meningitis, resulting from vasculitis or venous thromboses, and during the course of viral encephalitis, especially herpes simplex, resulting from parenchymal necrosis. In both bacterial and viral infections, prolonged or repetitive focal seizures precede the hemiplegia. Brain abscess may cause hemiplegia, but its evolution is usually slowly progressive rather than acute.

Varicella

Arterial ischemic strokes may occur during the course of varicella infection, and probably after varicella immunization, 1 week to several months after the appearance of rash (Sébire et al, 1999). The infarcts are small and located in the basal ganglia and internal capsule.

Migraine

Migraine is an hereditary disorder associated with, but not caused by, paroxysmal alterations in cerebral blood flow. Transitory neurological abnormalities may accompany the attack. The cause is a primary neuronal disturbance rather than cerebral ischemia. However, cerebral infarction may occur in adolescents during a prolonged attack of classic migraine. Such instances may represent something more than ordinary migraine. Mitochondrial disorders and channelopathies are possible mechanisms. The occurrence of focal motor deficits, usually hemiplegia or ophthalmoplegia (see Chapter 15), during an occasional migraine attack is called complicated migraine. In some families, hemiplegic migraine is a familial trait.

Complicated Migraine

Clinical Features. The family has a history of migraine, but other family members have not experienced hemiplegia during an attack. The evolution of symptoms is variable but usually includes scintillating or simple scotomas, unilateral dysesthesias of the hand and mouth, and unilateral weakness of the arm and face usually sparing the leg. Occurring concurrently with hemiparesis is a throbbing frontotemporal headache contralateral to the affected hemisphere. Nausea and vomiting follow. The patient falls asleep and usually recovers function on awakening. Hemiparesis lasts for less than 24 hours.

Diagnosis. Migraine is a clinical diagnosis that relies on a positive family history of the disorder. During an attack of hemiplegic migraine, an EEG focus of polymorphic delta activity is present in the hemisphere contralateral to the weakness. Neuroimaging studies are unnecessary.

Management. See Chapter 3 for a summary of migraine management.

Familial Hemiplegic Migraine

Familial hemiplegic migraine (FHM) differs from complicated migraine because other family members with migraine have had at least one hemiplegic attack. Transmission of the trait is by autosomal dominant inheritance. Three genetic loci exist (Jen, 2009). *FHM1* on chromosome 19p is allelic with the gene for hereditary paroxysmal cerebellar ataxia and encodes a calcium channel (*CACNA1A*)). *FHM2* is allelic for alternating hemiplegia and encodes a sodium-potassium ATPase pump. Mutations in a sodium channel *(SCN1A)* cause FHM3.

Clinical Features. Hemiplegia is an essential feature. Associated features may include visual disturbance, sensory loss, such as numbness or paresthesias of the face or a limb, and difficulty with speech. Attacks are stereotyped, occur primarily in childhood or adolescence, may be precipitated by trivial head trauma, and rarely occur more often than once a year. The hemiplegia, although more severe in the face and arm, also affects the leg, and always outlasts the headache. Hemianesthesia of the hemiplegic side is a prominent feature. Aphasia occurs when the dominant hemisphere is affected. Confusion, stupor, or psychosis may be present during an attack. The psychosis includes both auditory and visual hallucinations, as well as delusions. Occasionally, patients have fever and a stiff neck.

Symptoms last for 2 or 3 days. When the attack is over, the neurological deficits usually resolve completely, but permanent sequelae are possible. A gaze-evoked nystagmus may persist between attacks. Recurrent hemiplegic attacks may occur on either the same or the opposite side. Families with linkage to chromosome 1 may experience seizures during severe attacks.

Diagnosis. The basis for diagnosis is the clinical findings and family history. The diagnostic criteria are: (1) fulfills criteria for migraine with aura; (2) the aura includes some degree of hemiparesis and the hemiparesis may be prolonged; and (3) at least one first-degree relative has identical attacks. Molecular testing for mutations in *CACNA1A* is available on a clinical basis. Mutations in *ATP1A2* cause FHM2, and mutations in *SCN1A* cause FHM3. Molecular genetic testing of *ATP1A2* and *SCN1A* is available on a research basis only.

Management. Acetazolamide is a useful prophylactic agent in several channelopathies and may be useful in children with FHM1. A trial of standard migraine prophylactic drugs (tricyclic antidepressants, beta-blockers, calcium channel blockers) for all FHM types is reasonable. In general, avoid vasoconstricting agents to minimize stroke risk. Cerebral angiography is hazardous as it may precipitate a severe attack.

Trauma

Trauma accounts for half of all deaths in children. Approximately 10% of traumatic injuries in children are not accidental. Head injury is the leading cause of death from child abuse, and half of survivors have permanent neurological handicaps.

Epidural hematoma, subdural hematoma, cerebral laceration, and intracerebral hemorrhage can produce focal signs such as hemiplegia. However, brain swelling is such a prominent feature of even trivial head injury in children that diminished consciousness and seizures are the typical clinical features (see Chapter 2).

Tumors

The initial clinical feature of primary tumors of the cerebral hemispheres is more likely to be chronic progressive hemiplegia than acute hemiplegia. However, tumors may cause acute hemiplegia when they bleed or provoke seizures and are a consideration in the evaluation of acute hemiplegia.

CHRONIC PROGRESSIVE HEMIPLEGIA

The important causes of chronic progressive hemiplegia are brain tumor, brain abscess, and arteriovenous malformations. Increased intracranial pressure is the initial feature of all three. Their discussion is in Chapter 4. Progressive hemiplegia is sometimes an initial feature of demyelinating diseases (see Chapters 5 and 10; see Table 11-1).

Sturge-Weber Syndrome

The Sturge-Weber syndrome (SWS) is a sporadic neurocutaneous disorder characterized by the association of a venous angioma of the pia mater with a port-wine stain of the face. Other findings include cognitive impairment, contralateral hemiparesis and hemiatrophy, and homonymous hemianopia. The syndrome occurs sporadically and in all races.

Clinical Features. The clinical features are highly variable, and individuals with cutaneous lesions and seizures but with normal intelligence and no focal neurological deficit are common. The cutaneous angioma is usually present at birth. It is flat and variable in size but usually involves the upper lid. The size of the cutaneous angioma does not predict the size of the intracranial angioma. It is unilateral in 70 % of children and ipsilateral to the venous angioma of the pia. Even when the facial nevus is bilateral, the pial angioma is usually unilateral. The characteristic neurological and radiographic features of SWS may be present without the cutaneous angioma. Only 10–20 % of children with a port-wine nevus of the forehead have a leptomeningeal angioma. Bilateral brain lesions occur in at least 15 % of children.

Seizures occur in 80 % of children with SWS. Onset is generally within the first year and the seizure type is usually focal motor, sometimes leading to partial or generalized status epilepticus (see Chapter 1). Eighty percent of children with SWS who have seizures in the first year will show developmental delay and cognitive impairment.

Hemiparesis, contralateral to the facial angioma, occurs in up to 50 % of children. Hemiparesis often appears after a focal-onset seizure and progresses in severity after subsequent seizures. Transitory episodes of hemiplegia, not related to clinical or EEG evidence of seizure activity, may occur. Some episodes are associated with migraine-like headache, and others occur in the absence of other symptoms and cerebral ischemia may be the cause. Glaucoma occurs in 71 % of children with SWS, usually developing in the first decade.

Diagnosis. The association of neurological abnormalities and a port-wine stain of the face should suggest SWS. The pial angioma is best visualized by a contrast-enhanced MRI and only rarely by angiography.

Management. The seizures are often difficult to control with anticonvulsant medications. Hemispherectomy sometimes improves seizure control and promotes normal intellectual development. Hemispherectomy is an option in cases of epilepsy refractory to medical treatment and progressive hemisphere dysfunction. A limited resection suffices for some children. In general, the surgical considerations in children with SWS are similar to those used with other epileptic patients. Early hemispherectomy is the recommended procedure when focal seizure onset is in infancy.

REFERENCES

Barnes C, Deveber G. Prothrombotic abnormalities in childhood ischaemic stroke. Thrombosis Research 2006;118:67–74.

Bender MA, Hobbs W. Sickle cell disease. In: Pagon RA, Bird TD, Dolan CR, et al., eds. GeneReviews™ [Internet]. Seattle: University of Washington. Available at http://www.geneclinics.org. PMID: 20301551. Last updated May 17, 2012.

Bonduel M, Sciuccata G, Hepner M, et al. Prethrombotic disorders in children with arterial ischemic stroke and sinovenous thrombosis. Archives of Neurology 1999;56:967–71.

Carlson MD, Leber S, Deveikis J, et al. Successful use of rt-PA in pediatric stroke. Neurology 2001;57:157–8.

DeVeber G, Monagle P, Chan A, et al. Prothrombotic disorders in infants and children with cerebral thromboembolism. Archives of Neurology 1998;55:1539–43.

DiMauro S, Hirano M. MELAS. In: Pagon RA, Bird TD, Dolan CR, et al., eds. GeneReviews™ [Internet]. Seattle: University of Washington. Available at http://www.geneclinics.org. PMID: 20301411. Last updated October 14, 2010.

Di Rosa G, Spano M, Pustorino G, et al. Alternating hemiplegia of childhood successfully treated with topiramate: 18 months of follow-up. Neurology 2006;66:146.

Fluss J, Geary DG, deVeber G. Cerebral sinovenous thrombosis and idiopathic nephrotic syndrome in childhood: Report of four new cases and review of the literature. European Journal of Pediatrics 2006;165:709–16.

Fullerton HJ, Chetkovitch DM, Wu YW, et al. Deaths from stroke in US children, 1979 to 1998. Neurology 2002;59:34–9.

Fullerton HJ, Wu YW, Zhao S, et al. Risk of stroke in children. Ethnic and gender disparities. Neurology 2003;61:189–94.

Ganesan V, Chong WK, Cox TC, et al. Posterior circulation stroke in childhood. Risk factors and recurrence. Neurology 2002;59:1552–6.

Gradnitzer E, Urlesberger B, Maurer U, et al. Cerebral hemorrhage in term newborn infants: An analysis of 10 years (1989-1999). Wiener Klinische Wochenschrift 2002;152:9–13.

Jen JC. Familial Hemiplegic Migraine. In: Pagon RA, Bird TD, Dolan CR, et al., eds. GeneReviews™ [Internet]. Seattle: University of Washington. Available at http://www.geneclinics.org. PMID: 20301562. Last updated September 8, 2009.

Koga Y, Akita Y, Nishioka J, et al. L-Arginine improves the symptoms of strokelike episodes in MELAS. Neurology 2005;64:710–2.

Lanthier S, Carmant L, David M, et al. Stroke in children. The coexistence of multiple risk factors predicts poor outcome. Neurology 2002;54:371–8.

Lee J, Croen LA, Lindan C, et al. Predictors of outcome in perinatal arterial stroke: A population-based study. Annals of Neurology 2005;58:303–8.

Mercuri E, Rutherford M, Cowan F, et al. Early prognostic indicators of outcome in infants with neonatal cerebral infarction: A clinical, electroencephalogram, and magnetic resonance imaging study. Pediatrics 1999;103:39–46.

Prengler M, Pavlakis SG, Boyd S, et al. Sickle cell disease: Ischemia and seizures. Annals of Neurology 2005; 58:290–302.

Rafay MF, Armstrong D, Deveber G, et al. Craniocervical arterial dissection in children: Clinical and radiographic presentation and outcome. Journal of Child Neurology 2006;21:8–16.

Roach ES. Etiology of stroke in children. Seminars in Pediatric Neurology 2002;7:244–60.

Roach ES, Golomb MR, Adams R, et al. Management of stroke in infants and children: A scientific statement from a special writing group of the American Heart Association Stroke Council and the Council on Cardiovascular Disease in the Young. Stroke 2008;39:2644–91.

Sébire G, Husson B, Dusser A, et al. Congenital unilateral perisylvian syndrome: Radiological basis and clinical correlations. Journal of Neurology, Neurosurgery and Psychiatry 1996;61:52–6.

Sébire G, Meyer L, Chabrier S. Varicella as a risk factor for cerebral infarction in childhood: A case-control study. Annals of Neurology 1999;45:679–80.

Steen RG, Xiong X, Langston JW, et al. Brain injury in children with sickle cell disease: Prevalence and etiology. Annals of Neurology 2003;54:564–72.

Steinberg MH, Barton F, Castro O, et al. Effect of hydroxyurea on mortality and morbidity in adult sickle cell anemia: risks and benefits up to 9 years of treatment. Journal of the American Medical Association 2003;289:1645–51.

Swoboda KJ, Kanavakis E, Xaidara A, et al. Alternating hemiplegia of childhood or familial hemiplegic migraine? A novel ATP1A2 mutation. Annals of Neurology 2004;55:884–7.

Walters MC, Storb R, Patience M, et al. Impact of bone marrow transplantation for symptomatic sickle cell disease: An interim report. Multicenter investigation of bone marrow transplantation for sickle cell disease. Blood 2000;95:1918–24.

CHAPTER 12

PARAPLEGIA AND QUADRIPLEGIA

In this text, the term *paraplegia* denotes partial or complete weakness of both legs, and the term *quadriplegia* denotes partial or complete weakness of all limbs, thereby obviating need for the terms paraparesis and quadriparesis. Many conditions described fully in this chapter are abnormalities of the spinal cord. The same spinal abnormality can cause paraplegia or quadriplegia, depending on the location of the injury. Therefore, the discussion of both is together in this chapter.

APPROACH TO PARAPLEGIA

Weakness of both legs, without any involvement of the arms, suggests an abnormality of either the spinal cord or the peripheral nerves. Ordinarily, a pattern of distal weakness and sensory loss, muscle atrophy, and absent tendon reflexes provides recognition of peripheral neuropathies (see Chapters 7 and 9). In contrast, spinal paraplegia causes spasticity, exaggerated tendon reflexes, and a dermatomal level of sensory loss. Disturbances in the conus medullaris and cauda equina, especially congenital malformation, may produce a complex of signs in which spinal cord or peripheral nerve localization is difficult. Indeed, both may be involved. Spinal paraplegia may be asymmetric at first, and then the initial feature is monoplegia (see Chapter 13). When anatomical localization between the spinal cord and peripheral nerves is difficult, electromyography (EMG) and nerve conduction studies are useful in making the distinction.

Cerebral abnormalities sometimes cause paraplegia. In such a case, the child's arms as well as the legs are usually weak. However, leg weakness is so much greater than arm weakness that paraplegia is the chief complaint. It is important to remember that both the brain and the spinal cord may be abnormal and that the abnormalities can be in continuity (syringomyelia) or separated (Chiari malformation and myelomeningocele).

SPINAL PARAPLEGIA AND QUADRIPLEGIA

Box 12.1 lists conditions that cause acute, chronic, or progressive spinal paraplegia. In the absence of trauma, spinal cord compression and myelitis are the main causes of an acute onset or rapidly progressive paraplegia. Spinal cord compression from any cause is a medical emergency requiring rapid diagnosis and therapy to avoid permanent paraplegia. Corticosteroids have the same anti-inflammatory effect on the spinal cord as on the brain and provide transitory decompression before surgery.

Several techniques are available to visualize the spinal cord. Each has its place, and sometimes the use of more than one technique achieves a comprehensive picture of the disease process. However, magnetic resonance imaging (MRI) is clearly the procedure of choice to visualize the spine, and should be used first. Computed tomography (CT) and radioisotope bone scanning are useful for visualizing the vertebral column, especially when osteomyelitis is a consideration. Isotope bone scans localize the process but rarely provide an etiology.

Symptoms and Signs

Clumsiness of gait, refusal to stand or walk, and loss of bladder or bowel control are the common complaints of spinal paraplegia. Clumsiness of gait is the usual feature of slowly progressive disorders. When functional decline is sufficiently insidious, the disturbance may go on for years without raising concern. Refusal to stand or walk is a symptom of an acute process. When a young child refuses to support weight, the underlying cause may be weakness, pain, or both.

Scoliosis is a feature of many spinal cord disorders. It occurs with neural tube defects, spinal cord tumors, and several degenerative disorders. It also occurs when the paraspinal muscles are weaker on one side of the spine than on the other side. The presence of scoliosis, in females before puberty and in males of all ages, should strongly suggest either a spinal cord disorder or a neuromuscular disease (see Chapters 6 and 7).

Abnormalities in the skin overlying the spine, such as an abnormal tuft of hair, pigmentation, a sinus opening, or a mass, may indicate an underlying dysraphic state. Spina bifida is usually an associated feature.

Foot deformities and especially stunted growth of a limb are malevolent signs of lower spinal cord dysfunction. The usual deformity is

BOX 12-1 Spinal Paraplegia

CONGENITAL MALFORMATIONS
- Arachnoid cyst
- Arteriovenous malformations
- Atlantoaxial dislocation
- Caudal regression syndrome
- Dysraphic states
- Chiari malformation
- Myelomeningocele
- Tethered spinal cord
- Syringomyelia (see Chapter 9)

FAMILIAL SPASTIC PARAPLEGIA
- Autosomal dominant
- Autosomal recessive
- X-linked recessive

INFECTIONS
- Asthmatic amyotrophy (see Chapter 13)
- Diskitis
- Epidural abscess
- Herpes zoster myelitis
- Polyradiculoneuropathy (see Chapter 7)
- Tuberculous osteomyelitis

LUPUS MYELOPATHY

METABOLIC DISORDERS
- Adrenomyeloneuropathy (adrenoleukodystrophy)
- Argininemia
- Krabbe disease

NEONATAL CORD INFARCTION

TRANSVERSE MYELITIS
- Devic disease
- Encephalomyelitis
- Idiopathic
- Trauma

CONCUSSION
- Epidural hematoma
- Fracture dislocation

NEONATAL CORD TRAUMA (SEE CHAPTER 6)

TUMORS
- Astrocytoma
- Ependymoma
- Ewing's sarcoma
- Neuroblastoma

foreshortening of the foot (pes cavus). In such cases, disturbances of bladder control are often an associated feature.

Brief, irregular contractions of small groups of muscles that persist during sleep characterize *spinal myoclonus*. The myoclonic contractions are often mistaken for seizure activity or fasciculations. The cause of myoclonus is irritation of pools of motor neurons and interneurons, usually by an intramedullary tumor or syrinx. The dermatomal distribution of the myoclonus localizes the site of irritation within the spinal cord. Alternatively, spinal myoclonus can present as sequelae from severe traumatic or hypoxic brain injury, due to disinhibition of anterior horn cells or multifocal cortical hyperexcitability (Werhahn et al, 1997).

Congenital Malformations

Some congenital malformations, such as caudal regression syndrome and myelomeningocele, are obvious at birth. Many others do not cause symptoms until adolescence or later. Congenital malformations are always a consideration when progressive paraplegia appears in childhood.

Arachnoid Cysts

Arachnoid cysts of the spinal cord, like those of the brain (see Chapter 4), are usually asymptomatic and discovered incidentally on imaging studies. Familial cases should suggest neurofibromatosis type 2 (see Chapter 5).

Clinical Features. Arachnoid cysts may be single or multiple and are usually thoracic. Symptomatic arachnoid cysts are unusual in childhood and encountered more often in adolescents and young adults. The features are back or radicular pain and paraplegia. Standing intensifies symptoms, and changes in position may relieve or exacerbate symptoms. The pain tends to increase in severity with time.

Diagnosis. MRI is the diagnostic modality of choice. The cyst has the same MRI characteristics as cerebrospinal fluid.

Management. Shunting of a symptomatic cyst is curative. However, it is common to blame a subarachnoid cyst for symptoms that have another cause.

Arteriovenous Malformations

Arteriovenous malformations of the spinal cord are uncommon in childhood and even rarer in infancy, although case reports do exist (Barrow et al, 1994).

Clinical Features. The progression of symptoms is usually insidious, and the time from onset to diagnosis may be several years. Subacute or chronic pain is the initial feature in one-third of patients and subarachnoid hemorrhage in one-quarter. Paraplegia is an early feature in only one-third, but monoplegia or paraplegia is present in almost all children at the time of diagnosis. Most children have a slowly progressive spastic paraplegia and loss of bladder control.

When subarachnoid hemorrhage is the initial feature, the malformation is more likely to be in the cervical portion of the spinal cord. Blunt trauma to the spine may be a precipitating factor. The onset of paraplegia or quadriplegia is then acute and associated with back pain. Back pain and episodic weakness that improve completely or in part may be initial features in some children, but impairment is progressive. This type of presentation is misleading, and the diagnosis often delayed.

Diagnosis. MRI is the first step in diagnosis. It distinguishes intramedullary from dural and extramedullary locations of the malformation and even allows recognition of thrombus formation. Arteriography is still necessary to demonstrate the intramedullary extent of the malformation and all of the feeding vessels.

Management. The potential approaches to therapy for intraspinal and intracranial malformations are similar (see Chapter 4).

Atlantoaxial Dislocation

The odontoid process is the major factor preventing dislocation of C1 onto C2. True aplasia of the odontoid process is rare and leads to severe instability. Hypoplasia of the odontoid process can occur alone or as part of Morquio syndrome, other mucopolysaccharidoses, Klippel-Feil syndrome (see Chapter 18), several types of genetic chondrodysplasia, and some chromosomal abnormalities (Crockard & Stevens, 1995). Asymptomatic atlantoaxial subluxation may occur in 20% of children with Down syndrome secondary to congenital hypoplasia of the articulation of C1 and C2; symptomatic dislocation is much less common.

Clinical Features. Congenital atlantoaxial dislocation produces an acute or slowly progressive quadriplegia that may begin any time from the neonatal period to adult life. When the onset is in a newborn, the clinical features resemble an acute infantile spinal muscular atrophy (see Chapter 6). The infant has generalized hypotonia with preservation of facial expression and extraocular movement. The tendon reflexes are absent at first but then become hyperactive.

Dislocations during childhood frequently follow a fall or head injury. In such cases, symptoms may begin suddenly and include not only those of myelopathy but also those related to vertebral artery occlusion.

Morquio syndrome is primarily a disease of the skeleton, with only secondary abnormalities of the spinal cord. Beginning in the second year or thereafter, the following features develop in affected children: prominent ribs and sternum, knock-knees, progressive shortening of the neck, and dwarfism. The odontoid process is hypoplastic or absent. Acute, subacute, or chronic cervical myelopathy develops, sometimes precipitated by a fall. Loss of endurance, fainting attacks, and a "pins and needles" sensation in the arms characterize an insidious onset of symptoms.

The essential feature of the *Klippel-Feil syndrome* is a reduced number and abnormal fusion of cervical vertebrae. As in Morquio syndrome, the head appears to rest directly on the shoulders, the posterior hairline is low, and head movement in all directions is limited. Elevation of the scapulae and deformity of the ribs (*Sprengel deformity*) are often present. Weakness and atrophy of the arm muscles and mirror movements of the hands are features of evolving paraplegia. Associated abnormalities may be present in the genitourinary, cardiac, and musculoskeletal systems.

Symptomatic atlantoaxial dislocation in children with Down syndrome may occur anytime from infancy to the twenties. Females are more often affected than are males. Symptoms include neck pain, torticollis, and an abnormal gait. Spinal cord compression is progressive and leads to quadriplegia and urinary incontinence.

Diagnosis. C1 usually moves anteriorly to C2. Flexion radiographs assess the separation between the dens and the anterior arch of C1. MRI is best to view the relationship between the cord and the subluxing bones. Flexion-extension plain films of the cervical spine are often used to make the diagnosis, but CT or MRI may be more useful to assess for associated abnormalities. The neck of children with trisomy 21 should not be flexed for lumbar puncture as this may dislocate the atlantoaxial join and cause acute spinal cord compression.

Management. Surgical stabilization of the atlantoaxial junction is a consideration in any child with evidence of spinal cord compression. The choice of surgical procedure depends on the mechanism of compression.

Caudal Regression Syndrome

The term caudal regression syndrome covers several malformations of the caudal spine that range from sacral agenesis to sirenomelia, in which the legs are fused together (also known as Mermaid syndrome). The mechanism of caudal regression is incompletely understood, but some cases are clearly genetic in origin, while approximately 20% of mothers of children with caudal dysgenesis have insulin-dependent diabetes mellitus (Lynch et al, 2000). Although the name implies regression of a normally formed cord, defects in neural tube closure and prosencephalization are often associated features. The clinical spectrum varies from absence of the lumbosacral spinal cord, resulting in small, paralyzed legs, to a single malformed leg associated with malformations of the rectum and genitourinary tract.

Chiari Malformation

The type I Chiari malformation is extension of the cerebellar tonsils through the foramen magnum, sometimes with associated hydrosyringomyelia. The type II malformation combines the cerebellar herniation with distortion and dysplasia of the medulla and occurs in more than 50 % of children with lumbar myelomeningocele. The herniated portion may become ischemic and necrotic and can cause compression of the brainstem and upper cervical spinal cord.

Ectopic expression of a segmentation gene in the rhombomeres may explain the Chiari malformation and also the brainstem anomalies, myelodysplasia, and the defective bone formation that results in a small posterior fossa (Sarnat, 2004).

Clinical Features. Most Chiari I malformations are discovered as an incidental finding on an MRI ordered because of headache. The malformation is rarely the cause of the headache. The initial features of a symptomatic Chiari malformation are usually insidious. Oropharyngeal dysfunction is a presenting feature in 35 % of children less than 6 years of age, followed by scoliosis (23 %) and head and neck pain (23 %) (Greenlee et al, 2002). Among older children, headache and neck pain are the first features in 38 % and weakness in 56 %. Eighty percent show motor deficits on examination, usually atrophy and hyporeflexia in the arms and spasticity and hyperreflexia in the legs. Sensory loss and scoliosis are each present in half of cases.

Type II malformation should be suspected in every child with myelomeningocele. The child may have hydrocephalus secondary to aqueductal stenosis or by an obstruction of the outflow of cerebrospinal fluid from the fourth ventricle due to herniation. Respiratory distress is the most important feature of the Chiari II malformation. Rapid respirations, episodes of apnea, and Cheyne-Stokes respirations may occur. Other evidence of brainstem compression includes poor feeding, vomiting, dysphagia, and paralysis of the tongue. Sudden cardiorespiratory failure is the usual cause of death.

Diagnosis. MRI is the best method to visualize the posterior fossa and cervical cord. CT is useful to further delineate bony abnormalities.

Management. Posterior fossa decompression is the usual technique to manage newborns with myelomeningocele and respiratory distress caused by the Chiari malformation. Unfortunately, the results are not encouraging. Posterior fossa decompression is usually successful in relieving symptoms of cord compression in older children without myelomeningocele. Ventriculoperitoneal shunt may be required as well.

Myelomeningocele

Dysraphia comprises all defects in the closure of the neural tube and its coverings. Closure occurs during the third and fourth weeks of gestation. The mesoderm surrounding the neural tube gives rise to the dura, skull, and vertebrae but not to the skin. Therefore, defects in the final closure of the neural tube and its mesodermal case do not preclude the presence of a dermal covering.

Despite extensive epidemiological studies, the causes of myelomeningocele remain unknown. Causes are likely to be multifactorial, including both genetic and environmental factors. Because women who have previously had a child with dysraphia have an approximate 2 % risk of recurrence, prenatal diagnosis is available to prevent repetition.

α-Fetoprotein, the principal plasma protein of the fetus, is present in amniotic fluid. The concentration of α-fetoprotein in the amniotic fluid increases when plasma proteins exude through a skin defect. Prenatal diagnosis is possible by the combination of measuring the maternal serum concentration of α-fetoprotein and ultrasound examination of the fetus.

The incidence of dysraphic defects has been declining in the United States and the United Kingdom. Antenatal screening alone does not explain the decline; changes in critical environmental factors may be important. Because the ingestion of folic acid supplements during early pregnancy reduces the incidence of neural tube defects, the consumption of 0.4 mg of folic acid daily is advisable for all women of childbearing age. Women with a prior history of delivering a child with a neural tube defect should take 4 mg/day of folic acid from at least 4 weeks before conception through the first 3 months of pregnancy.

Clinical Features. Spina bifida cystica, the protrusion of a cystic mass through the defect, is an obvious deformity of the newborn's spine. More than 90 % are thoracolumbar. Among newborns with spina bifida cystica, the protruding sac is a meningocele without neural elements in 10–20 % and is a myelomeningocele in the rest. Meningoceles tend to have a partial dermal covering and are often pedunculated, with a narrow base connecting the sac to the underlying spinal cord. Myelomeningoceles usually have a broad base, lack epithelial covering, and ooze a combination of cerebrospinal fluid and serum. Portions of the dome contain exposed remnants of the spinal cord.

In newborns with spina bifida cystica, it is important to determine the extent of neurological dysfunction caused by the myelopathy, the potential for the development of hydrocephalus, and the presence of other malformations in the nervous system and in other organs. When myelomeningocele is the only deformity, the newborn is alert and responsive and has no difficulty in feeding. Diminished consciousness or responsiveness and difficulty in feeding should suggest perinatal asphyxia or cerebral malformations such as hydrocephalus. Cyanosis, pallor, or dyspnea suggests associated malformations in the cardiovascular system. Multiple major defects are present in approximately 30% of cases.

The spinal segments involved can be determined by locating the myelomeningocele with reference to the ribs and iliac crest. Several patterns of motor dysfunction are observable depending on the cyst's location. Motor dysfunction results from interruption of the corticospinal tracts and from dysgenesis of the segmental innervation. At birth, the legs are flaccid, the hips are dislocated, and arthrogryposis of the lower extremities is present. Spastic paraplegia, a spastic bladder, and a level of sensory loss develop in infants with a thoracic lesion. Segmental withdrawal reflexes below the level of the lesion, which indicate the presence of an intact but isolated spinal cord segment below the cyst, are present in half of patients. Infants with deformities of the conus medullaris maintain a flaccid paraplegia, have lumbosacral sensory loss, lack a withdrawal response in the legs, and have a distended bladder with overflow incontinence.

Only 15% of newborns with myelomeningocele have clinical evidence of hydrocephalus at birth, but ultrasound detects hydrocephalus in 60% of affected newborns. Hydrocephalus eventually develops in 80%. The first clinical features of hydrocephalus often follow the repair of the myelomeningocele, but the two are not related. Aqueductal stenosis and the Chiari malformation are the cause of hydrocephalus in the majority of infants with myelomeningocele.

Diagnosis. Examination alone establishes the diagnosis of spina bifida cystica. EMG may be useful to clarify the distribution of segmental dysfunction. Cranial ultrasound to look for hydrocephalus is required for every newborn. MRI is useful to define malformations of the brain, especially the Chiari malformation (see Figure 10-6). Therapeutic decisions may require such information. Even in the absence of hydrocephalus at birth, repeat ultrasound examinations in 2 to 4 weeks are required to evaluate ventricular size.

Management. The chance of surviving the first year is poor without back closure shortly postpartum. However, closure is not a surgical emergency and delays of a week or longer do not influence the survival rate. Other factors associated with increased mortality are a high spinal location of the defect and clinical hydrocephalus at birth. The long-term outcome depends on the degree of neurological deficit from the spinal defect and any associated brain abnormalities.

Tethered Spinal Cord

A thickened filum terminale, a lipoma, a dermal sinus, or diastematomyelia may anchor the conus medullaris to the base of the vertebrae. Spina bifida occulta is usually an associated feature. As the child grows, the tether causes the spinal cord to stretch and the lumbosacral segments to become ischemic. The mitochondrial oxidative metabolism of neurons is impaired, and neurological dysfunction follows.

Dermal sinus is a midline opening of the skin usually marked by a tuft of hair or port-wine stain. An abnormal invagination of ectoderm into the posterior closure site of the neural tube causes the problem. Most sinuses terminate subcutaneously as a blind pouch or dermoid cyst. Others extend through a spina bifida to the developing neuraxis, at which point they attach to the dura or the spinal cord as a fibrous band or dermoid cyst. Such sinuses tether the spinal cord and serve as a route for bacteria from the skin to reach the subarachnoid space and cause meningitis.

Diastematomyelia consists of a bifid spinal cord (also called diplomyelia) that is normal in the cervical and upper thoracic regions and then divides into lateral halves (Figure 12-1). Two types of diastematomyelia occur with equal frequency. In one type, a dural sheath surrounds each half of the cord and a fibrous or bony septum separates the two halves. Once the cord separates, it never rejoins. In the other type, a single dural sheath surrounds both halves and a septum is not present. The two halves rejoin after one or two segments. Therefore, the cause of spinal cord splitting is not the presence of a septum, but rather a primary disturbance in the formation of luminal borders caused by faulty

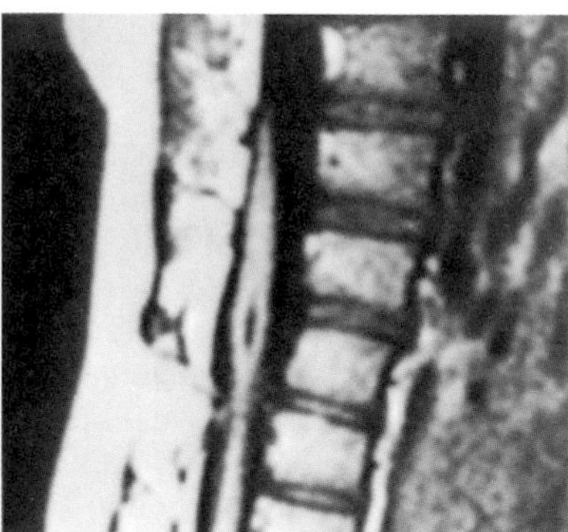
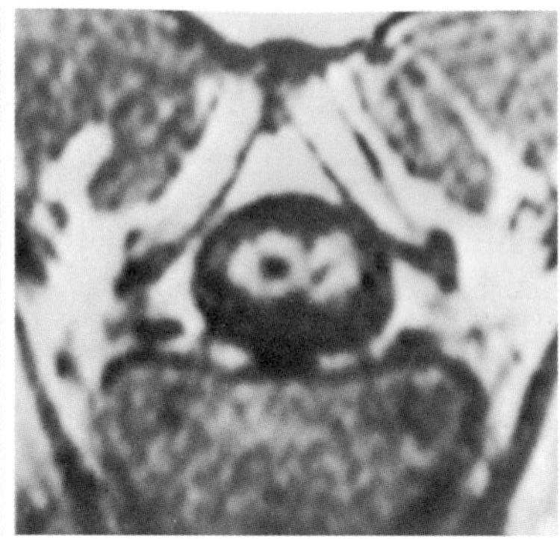

FIGURE 12-1 ■ Diplomyelia. MRI shows two cords with two central canals. Longitudinal section shows an enlarged segment with a cystic center.

closure of the neural tube. It is usually associated with other dysraphic disturbances such as spina bifida occulta or cystica.

Clinical Features. The initial features of a tethered spinal cord occur at any age from infancy to young adulthood. The clinical features vary with age. External signs of spinal dysraphism (tuft of hair, subcutaneous lipoma, and dermal sinus) are present in more than half of patients, and spina bifida occulta or sacral deformity is present in almost 90 %.

Infants and young children are most likely to show clumsiness of gait, stunted growth, or deformity of one foot or leg, and disturbances in bladder or bowel function. These may occur alone or in combination. Consequently, the first specialist consulted may be an orthopedic surgeon, urologist, neurologist, or neurosurgeon. The progression of symptoms and signs is insidious, and a static problem is the first diagnosis in most children. Children with only a clumsy gait or disturbances in urinary control tend to have normal or exaggerated tendon reflexes and an extensor plantar response. In some children, diminished or absent ankle tendon reflexes are noted on one or both sides. Children with foot deformity usually have pes cavus and stunted growth of the entire leg. The other leg may appear normal or have a milder deformity without a growth disturbance. Diminished tendon reflexes in the deformed foot are more likely than increased reflexes.

The initial feature of tethered spinal cord in older children and adolescents is either clumsiness of gait or scoliosis. Bilateral, but mild, foot deformities are sometimes present and urinary incontinence and constipation reported. Exaggerated knee and ankle tendon reflexes are usual, and the plantar response is usually extensor.

Diagnosis. EMG is not a useful screening procedure, as the results are usually abnormal. Radiographs of the spine may show a spina bifida, but MRI is the appropriate diagnostic test and is particularly useful in the detection of lumbosacral lipoma. The essential feature of a tethered spinal cord is a low-lying conus medullaris. At 28 weeks' gestation, the tip of the conus is at the L3 vertebral level. It generally raises one level by 40 weeks' gestation. A conus that extends below the L2 to L3 interspace in children 5 years and older is always abnormal.

Management. Surgical relief of the tethering prevents further deterioration of neurological function and improves preexisting deficits in up to 50 % of children (Cornette et al, 1998).

Hereditary Spastic Paraplegia

Hereditary spastic paraplegia (HSP) is a heterogeneous group of genetic disorders in which the prominent clinical feature is progressive spastic paraplegia. Some families have *pure* or *uncomplicated* HSP, in which neurological impairment is limited to progressive spastic paraplegia, a hypertonic urinary bladder disturbance, and mild diminution of vibration and position sense. Others have *complicated* or *complex* HSP in which the spastic paraplegia is associated with other neurological findings such as seizures, dementia, amyotrophy, extrapyramidal disturbance, or peripheral neuropathy (Fink, 2009). Genetic transmission of HSP is by autosomal dominant inheritance in 70 % of cases and by autosomal recessive inheritance in 25 %. Genetic heterogeneity exists even within the dominant and recessive forms. The X-linked form is uncommon, usually congenital, and almost always *complicated*.

Autosomal Dominant Inheritance

Children with autosomal dominant spastic paraplegia may have pure or complicated spastic paraplegia.

Clinical Features. The age at onset ranges from infancy to late adulthood, with the mean at 29 years. Early and late onset cases may occur among members of the same family. Motor milestones are normal in affected infants except for toe walking. Frequently, the diagnosis in such children is cerebral palsy, especially if the affected parent is asymptomatic or has only a mildly stiff gait. Increased tone is more prominent than weakness. Tone increases slowly for several years and then stabilizes. At this point, the child may have minimal stiffness of gait or be unable to stand or walk.

Usually, tendon reflexes are brisk in the legs and arms, and ankle clonus may be present. Occasional children with absent or diminished ankle tendon reflex have an associated axonal neuropathy. Increased reflexes are usually the only sign of involvement of the arms. Vibratory and position sense are diminished in half of patients. Urinary symptoms, usually in the form of frequency and urgency, and pes cavus deformities each occur in one-third of affected children.

Diagnosis. Familial spastic paraplegia is difficult to diagnose in the absence of a family history, and then becomes a diagnosis of exclusion. This is especially true in childhood in whom dominant transmission is usual. MRI of the brain and spinal cord is usually normal. The differential diagnosis includes multiple sclerosis, structural abnormalities involving the spinal cord, B12 deficiency, adrenomyeloneuropathy and other leukodystrophies, and dopa-responsive dystonia. The diagnosis of HSP is suspect in any child with very slowly progressive spastic paraplegia. Laboratory studies are not helpful except to exclude other conditions such as adrenoleukodystrophy and argininemia. DNA based diagnosis is now available for almost all subtypes.

Management. Several centers use botox injections to relieve spasticity. Many children require ankle-foot orthoses to improve gait. Treatment is not available for the underlying condition.

Autosomal Recessive Inheritance

Autosomal recessive inheritance of hereditary spastic paraplegia may be pure or complicated. Both forms are genetically heterogeneous. Autosomal recessive cases account for 15–20 % of the total (Hedera & Bandmann, 2008).

Clinical Features. Spastic paraplegia may begin during infancy or be delayed until adolescence. Involvement of other neurological systems follows. The common associated features, alone or in combination, include cerebellar dysfunction, pseudobulbar palsy, sensory neuropathy, and pes cavus.

Children with sensory neuropathy lose the once hyperactive tendon reflexes in the legs. Some show developmental delay and never achieve bladder control. When sensory loss is progressive, the symptoms resemble those of familial sensory neuropathies described in Chapter 9. The outcome varies from mild disability to wheelchair dependence.

Diagnosis. In the absence of a family history, the course of disease may suggest cerebral palsy until the progressive nature of the spasticity is recognized. Sensory neuropathy with mutilation of digits may lead to the erroneous diagnosis of syringomyelia. Laboratory tests are useful only to exclude other diagnoses. Argininemia, a treatable cause of autosomal recessive progressive spastic paraplegia, is a consideration (Cederbaum & Crombez, 2012).

Management. No treatment is available for the underlying defect, but the sensory neuropathy requires supportive care (see Chapter 9).

Infections

Primary myelitis from acquired immune deficiency syndrome is uncommon in children and not discussed in this section.

Diskitis (Disk Space Infection)

Disk space infection is a relatively uncommon disorder of childhood in which one disk space is infected secondary to subacute osteomyelitis of the adjacent vertebral bodies. The cause is bacterial infection. *Staphylococcus aureus* is the organism most often grown on culture of disk material removed by needle biopsy and is probably the major cause. Blood cultures are often negative, likely because the infection is subacute. Biopsy is typically unnecessary.

Clinical Features. The initial feature is either difficulty walking or back pain. Difficulty walking occurs almost exclusively in children less than 3 years of age. The typical child has a low-grade or no fever, is observed to be limping, and may refuse to stand or walk. This symptom complex evolves over 24 to 48 hours. Affected children prefer to lie on their sides rather than to rest supine, resist standing, and then seem uncomfortable and walk with a shuffling gait. Examination shows loss of lumbar lordosis and absolute resistance to flexion of the spine. The hips or back are sometimes tender.

Pain as an initial feature occurs more often after 3 years of age. The pain may be vertebral or rarely abdominal. When abdominal, the pain gradually increases in intensity and may radiate from the epigastrium to the umbilicus or pelvis. Abdominal pain in association with low-grade fever and an elevated peripheral white blood cell count invariably suggests the possibility of appendicitis or other intra-abdominal disease. Fortunately, abdominal pain is the least common presenting feature.

Back pain is the most common complaint. Older children may indicate a specific area of pain and tenderness. Younger children may have only an abnormal posture intended to splint the painful area. Back pain usually leads to prompt diagnosis because attention immediately directs to the spine. Examination reveals loss of lumbar lordosis and decreased movement of the spine, especially flexion.

Diagnosis. Disk space infection is a consideration in all children who have sudden back pain or refuse to walk, and in whom there are no specific neurological abnormalities. Strength, tone, and tendon reflexes in the legs are normal. Radiographs of the spine reveal narrowing of the affected intervertebral space, most often in the lumbar region but sometimes as high as the C5 to C6 positions. MRI is the best method to demonstrate inflammation within the disk. It shows osteomyelitis of the surrounding vertebrae as well as of the disk space (Figure 12-2).

Management. Antibiotics are effective in treating the infection. Initiate intravenous antibiotics as soon as diagnostic confirmation is complete. Immobilization is not necessary because the children are nearly asymptomatic when discharged from hospital.

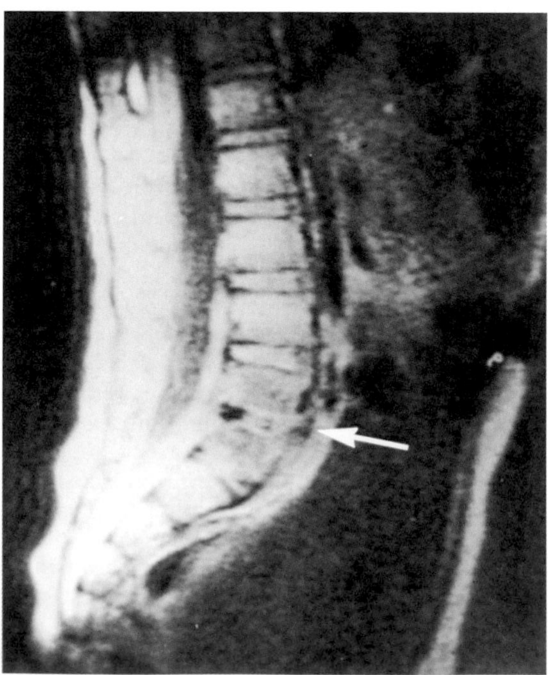

FIGURE 12-2 ■ Diskitis. MRI reveals collapse of the disk space (arrow) and demineralization of the adjoining vertebral bodies.

Herpes Zoster Myelitis

Immunosuppressed individuals may experience reactivation of the varicella-zoster virus that had been latent in sensory ganglia following primary chickenpox infection.

Clinical Features. The spinal cord becomes involved within 3 weeks after a truncal rash appears. The myelopathy usually progresses for 3 weeks, but progression may last as long as 6 months in immunocompromised patients. Cord involvement is bilateral in 80 % of cases.

Diagnosis. Diagnosis depends on recognition of the characteristic herpetic rash at the dermatomal level of the myelitis. Unfortunately, the myelitis sometimes precedes the onset of rash. Images of the spine are required to exclude other causes. The cerebrospinal fluid shows a pleocytosis and protein elevation that is greatest at the time of maximal neurological deficit.

Management. Treatment with corticosteroids and acyclovir is a standard practice, although their benefit is uncertain.

Tuberculous Osteomyelitis

Tuberculosis causes vertebral infection by hematogenous dissemination. Any level of the vertebral column may be affected. The infection usually begins in one vertebral body and then spreads to adjacent vertebrae and the surrounding soft tissue. Fewer than 20 % of patients with tuberculous osteomyelitis have symptoms of spinal cord dysfunction. The pathophysiological mechanisms include epidural abscess, arteritis, and vertebral collapse. In addition, tuberculous granuloma of the spine may occur in the absence of vertebral disease.

Clinical Features. Tuberculosis of the vertebrae and spine, also known at Pott disease or tuberculous spondylitis, is primarily a disease of children and young adults in countries with high rates of tuberculosis infection, although in the United States it is more typically seen in immunocompromised adults. Young children with vertebral osteomyelitis not extending to the spinal cord may refuse to walk because of pain, and their symptoms may mimic paraplegia. The prominent features are fever, anorexia, and back pain. In children less than 10 years of age, infection is generally diffuse, affecting several vertebrae and adjacent tissues. Older children tend to have localized infection, but with a higher incidence of spinal cord compression. The symptoms and signs of spinal cord compression from tuberculosis are similar to those described for epidural abscess, except that progression is slower.

Diagnosis. The cerebrospinal fluid is usually under pressure and shows a pleocytosis with polymorphonuclear leukocytes predominating early in the course and lymphocytes predominating in the later stages. The total cell count rarely exceeds 500 cells/mm^3. Protein concentrations are elevated, and glucose concentrations are depressed. Stained smears show acid-fast organisms and the organism can be isolated on cultures of the cerebrospinal fluid.

Early stages of vertebral osteomyelitis can be shown by a technetium bone scan or plain radiographs. The search for contiguous abscess requires MRI. As the disease progresses, radiographs reveal collapse of adjacent vertebrae and gibbus formation (structural kyphosis).

Management. Treatment of tuberculous osteomyelitis and meningitis are similar, although the length of treatment differs. For tuberculous osteomyelitis in children, the Centers for Disease Control and Prevention recommends isoniazid, rifampin, and pyrazinamide for 8 weeks, followed by 4 to 7 months of isoniazid and rifampin. In situations where isoniazid resistance is suspected, the addition of ethambutol should be considered, although this is not routinely used in children. In cases of tuberculous meningitis and disseminated tuberculosis, treatment needs to be continued for 9 to 12 months. Direct observed therapy should be used in all children with tuberculosis.

Lupus Myelopathy

Transverse myelopathy is a rare complication of systemic lupus erythematosus. The usual features are back pain, rapidly progressive paraplegia, and bowel and bladder dysfunction. Sensory loss is not a constant feature. The protein concentration of the cerebrospinal fluid is elevated. Recovery is poor and mortality is high.

Metabolic Disorders

Adrenomyeloneuropathy

Adrenomyeloneuropathy (AMN) is the most common phenotype of adrenoleukodystrophy accounting for 40–50% of cases (Moser et al, 2012). The etiology is impaired ability to oxidize very-long-chain fatty acids (see Chapter 5). Genetic transmission is by X-linked inheritance.

Clinical Features. Paraplegia begins after age 20 years and is slowly progressive throughout adult life. Intellectual impairment is usual and prolonged survival is the rule (van Geel et al, 1997). Most patients develop Addison's disease, which predates the paraplegia almost half of the time. A sensory neuropathy may be associated. Approximately 20% of female heterozygotes develop clinical disease.

Diagnosis. Multiple sclerosis is a common misdiagnosis among female heterozygotes. The demonstration of increased plasma concentrations of very-long-chain fatty acids is essential for diagnosis.

Management. Symptomatic males require regular assessment of adrenal function and corticosteroid replacement therapy for adrenal insufficiency. Unfortunately, corticosteroid replacement therapy has no effect on nervous system involvement. Bone marrow transplantation is an option for boys and adolescents who are in early stages of symptom development with evidence of brain involvement on MRI. Bone marrow transplantation carries the risk of morbidity and mortality and is not recommended for patients without MRI evidence of brain involvement (Shapiro et al, 2000). Dietary therapy and other pharmacological agents have not proven to be useful.

Arginase Deficiency

Arginase catalyzes the metabolism of arginine to ornithine and urea in the urea cycle. Arginase deficiency is the least common of all urea cycle disturbances. Genetic transmission is as an autosomal recessive trait (Cederbaum & Crombez, 2012).

Clinical Features. Motor and cognitive development slows in early childhood and then regresses. Most children develop a progressive spastic paraplegia or quadriplegia. Other features may include recurrent vomiting and seizures.

Diagnosis. The serum concentration of arginine is elevated, and 90% of children have elevated blood concentrations of ammonia. There is typically no detectable arginase activity in red blood cells. In the United States, most infants are diagnosed based on the expanded newborn screen. Molecular genetic testing is available.

Management. Dietary protein restriction may slow the progression of the disorder and sometimes cause improvement.

Krabbe Disease

The early infantile form of Krabbe disease (globoid leukodystrophy) causes psychomotor regression (see Chapter 5) and a peripheral neuropathy (see Chapter 7). The disorder is due to mutations of the gene encoding glycosylceramidase *(GALC)* at chromosome site 14q31 (Wenger, 2011).

A late-onset form of the disease, with onset from childhood to adolescence, may show only a pure spastic paraplegia or more often spastic paraplegia and visual loss. Many patients with late-onset disease are compound heterozygotes, having one copy of two different mutations associated with enzyme deficiency. Hematopoietic stem cell transplantation in presymptomatic infants and older individuals with mild symptoms may improve and preserve cognitive function, but peripheral nervous system function may deteriorate. Allogeneic hematopoietic stem cell transplantation slows the progress of late-onset disease.

Neonatal Cord Infarction

Infarction of the spinal cord is a hazard in newborns undergoing umbilical artery catheterization. The artery of Adamkiewicz arises from the aorta at the level of T10 to T12 and is the major segmental artery to the thoracolumbar spinal cord. Placing the catheter tip between levels T10 and T11 may cause embolization of the artery resulting in acute and sometimes irreversible paraplegia. A similar syndrome occurs among premature or small-for-date newborns in the absence of catheterization. The mechanism in such cases is unknown but hypotension may be causal.

Transverse Myelitis

Transverse myelitis is an acute demyelinating disorder of the spinal cord that evolves in hours or days. The incidence is 1–4 new cases per million people per year (Transverse Myelitis Consortium Working Group, 2002). The age distribution shows peaks in the second and fourth decades. It may occur alone or in combination with demyelination in other portions of the nervous system. The association of transverse myelitis and optic neuritis is *Devic disease*, also known as neuromyelitis optica; acute demyelination throughout the neuraxis is *acute disseminated encephalomyelitis*.

Multiple sclerosis is usually suspect in adults with transverse myelitis, although only 20 % ultimately develop other demyelinating lesions. The symptoms of multiple sclerosis in childhood are as diverse as they are in adults (see Chapter 10).

The exact cause of transverse myelitis is unknown, and may include infectious or autoimmune processes. Several viral agents have been theorized to cause transverse myelitis, including hepatitis A, mumps, varicella, herpes simplex, cytomegalovirus, Epstein-Barr virus, and echovirus. However, definitively proving causation is difficult due to the fact that school-age children average four to six "viral" episodes annually. Therefore, approximately half of children with any illness report a history of a viral infection within the preceding 30 days. Similarly, despite several case reports, no established cause-and-effect relationship exists between any licensed vaccines and demyelinating disorders of the central nervous system.

Clinical Features. Mean age at onset is 9 years. Symptoms progress rapidly, attaining maximal deficit within 2 days. The level of myelitis is usually thoracic and demarcated by the sensory loss. Asymmetric leg weakness is common. The bladder fills and does not empty voluntarily. Tendon reflexes may be increased or reduced. Recovery typically begins after 6 days but is often incomplete. Visual acuity should be carefully checked to rule out Devic disease; in children with unreliable or inconsistent visual acuity tests, a formal ophthalmologic examination may be needed. Transverse myelitis has a spectrum of severity; a significant minority are unable to walk 30 feet at 3 years after the illness. Age less than 3 years at onset has, surprisingly, been associated with worse long-term outcomes, contradicting previous assumptions that the plasticity of the young central nervous system would allow more robust recovery. In rare instances, the disease can be fatal. Approximately 75 % of patients have permanent sensory disturbances, and impaired bladder control is the most common long-term sequelae, occurring in 80 % of children (Pidcock et al, 2007).

Several children have a relapsing myelitis in which attacks of acute myelitis recur over months or years. A percentage of these children will ultimately develop multiple sclerosis or neuromyelitis optica, and therefore require close monitoring by a neurologist familiar with demyelinating disease.

Diagnosis. MRI of the spine excludes acute cord compression and sometimes shows signal change and edema at the level of myelitis. Cranial MRI excludes disease that is more widespread. CSF studies often demonstrate increased white blood cells and protein, but are rarely positive for oligoclonal bands or elevated IgG index.

Management. The recommended treatment protocol is high-dose intravenous methylprednisolone (20 mg/kg/day, maximum 1 g/day) for 3 to 5 days, followed by tapering doses of oral prednisone over 4 to 6 weeks. Intravenous immunoglobulin and plasmapheresis are second-line interventions. Physical and occupational therapy may be needed.

Devic Disease (Neuromyelitis Optica/ NMO)

Devic disease is a distinct disorder and is not a subset of multiple sclerosis. The cause seems to be an autoimmune mechanism that targets the aquaporin 4 protein in the astrocytic cell membrane.

Clinical Features. A history of anorexia or a flu-like syndrome a few days or a week before the first neurological symptoms is common. The anorexia and fever may be part of the acute demyelinating illness rather than a viral infection. Myelitis precedes optic neuritis in 13% of patients and follows it in 76%; myelitis and neuritis occur simultaneously in 10%. The child remains irritable while the neurological symptoms are evolving.

Bilateral optic neuritis occurs in 80% of patients (see Chapter 16). Diminished visual acuity in both eyes may be present at onset, or one eye may become affected before the other. Loss of vision is acute and accompanied by pain. The initial ophthalmoscopic examination may have normal results but more often shows bilateral papilledema. The pupils dilate and the light response is sluggish.

Back pain and leg discomfort herald myelitis. The legs become weak, and the patient has difficulty standing and walking. Paraplegia becomes complete; it is first flaccid and then becomes spastic. Tendon reflexes first diminish and later become brisk and are associated with extensor plantar responses. The bladder is spastic, and the patient has overflow incontinence. In some patients, one detects a sensory level, but more often the sensory deficit is patchy and difficult to delineate in an irritable child. The course is variable. Some patients develop an encephalomyelitis (see following section on Diffuse Encephalomyelitis), some have permanent paraplegia, and some have a relapsing course with repeated episodes of myelitis (Wingerchuk & Weinshenker, 2003). Most children recover, but not always completely.

Diagnosis. MRI of the spine excludes spinal cord compression syndrome, and MRI of the head excludes other demyelinating lesions (Figure 12-3). The cerebrospinal fluid in children with Devic disease is usually abnormal. The protein content is mildly to moderately increased, and a mixed pleocytosis of neutrophils and mononuclear cells is present. The presence of anti-NMO (neuromyelitis optica) antibodies clinches the diagnosis.

Management. A course of corticosteroids is usual for children with Devic disease. The regimen is the same as for diffuse encephalomyelitis. Bladder care with intermittent catheterization is imperative, as are measures to prevent bedsores and infection. The child often requires physical and occupational therapy.

Diffuse Encephalomyelitis

Discussion of diffuse encephalomyelitis is in the section on Devic syndrome and in Chapter 2. The major clinical difference from Devic disease is that both the cerebral hemispheres and spinal cord are affected. Cerebral demyelination may precede, follow, or occur concurrently with the myelitis.

Clinical Features. In addition to the myelitis, an encephalopathy characterized by decreased consciousness, irritability, and spastic quadriplegia occurs. If the brainstem is affected, dysphagia, fever, cranial nerve palsies, and irregular respiration are present.

Diagnosis. MRI is required in order to appreciate the full extent of demyelination. The cerebral hemispheres contain multiple white matter lesions that become confluent (see Figure 2-2), and may have lesions in the cerebellum and brainstem. Measures of very-long-chain fatty acids exclude adrenoleukodystrophy.

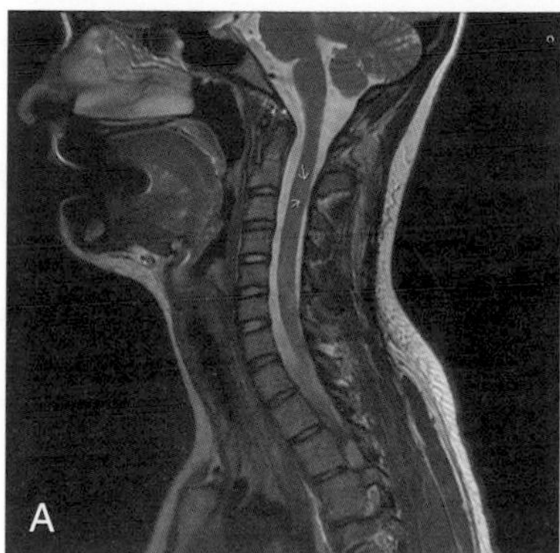

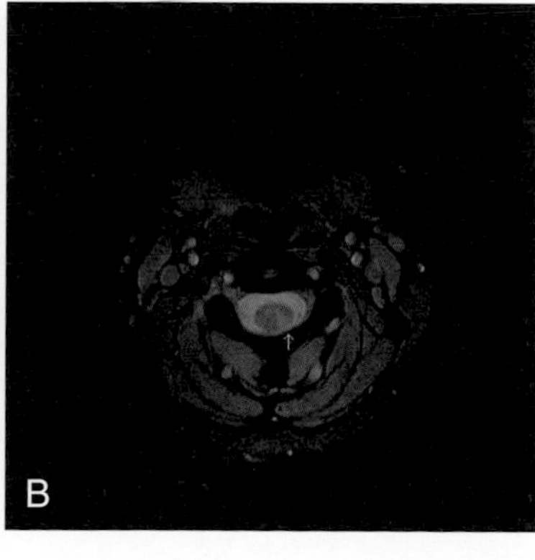

FIGURE 12-3 ■ Multiple sclerosis. C2 to C3 segment demyelinating lesion in (A) sagittal and (B) transverse T_2 MRI.

Management. Most authorities agree with the use of corticosteroid treatment. Methylprednisolone 20 mg/kg/day (up to 1 g daily) for 3 to 5 days is the typical initial treatment, which is then tapered over a 4-week period, depending on the response. The benefit of such a course of therapy is not established, and some patients become corticosteroid dependent and relapse after stopping prednisone. There may be an overlap with other demyelinating diseases such as multiple sclerosis, and the child may require long-term immunosuppression.

Trauma

Spinal cord injuries are relatively rare, especially before adolescence. The major cause is motor vehicle accidents, followed by sports-related injuries. The injuries affect the cervical spinal cord in 65 % of cases before 15 years of age and in 71 % of cases before 9 years of age. Fifteen percent of patients have injuries at multiple levels. Neurological function that is intact immediately after the injury remains intact afterward, and even those with incomplete function are likely to recover. Evidence of complete transection on initial examination indicates that paralysis is permanent.

Compressed Vertebral Body Fractures

Clinical Features. Compression fractures of the thoracolumbar region occur when a child jumps or falls from a height greater than 10 feet and lands in a standing or sitting position. Transection of the spinal cord has not occurred, but spinal cord concussion may cause paraplegia. Back pain at the fracture site is immediate and intense. Nerve root compression causes pain that radiates into the groin and legs.

Diagnosis. Thoracolumbar radiographs reveal the fracture and MRI of the spinal cord is normal.

Management. Immobilization relieves the back pain and promotes healing of the fracture.

Fracture Dislocation and Spinal Cord Transection

Motor vehicle accidents are the usual cause of spinal cord transection from fracture dislocation of the vertebral column. A forceful flexion of the spine fractures the articular facets and allows the vertebral body to move forward or laterally, with consequent contusion or transection of the spinal cord. The common sites of traumatic transection are the levels C1 to C2, C5 to C7, and T12 to L2.

Clinical Features. Neurological deficits at and below the level of spinal cord contusion or transection are immediate and profound. Many children with fracture dislocations sustained head injuries at the time of trauma and are unconscious.

Immediately after the injury, the child has flaccid weakness of the limbs below the level of the lesion associated with loss of tendon and cutaneous reflexes (spinal shock). In high cervical spinal cord lesions, eliciting the knee and ankle tendon reflexes, anal reflex, and plantar response may be possible during the initial period of spinal shock. Spinal shock lasts for approximately 1 week in infants and young children and up to 6 weeks in adolescents.

First, the superficial reflexes return, then the plantar response becomes one of extension, and finally massive withdrawal reflexes (mass reflex) appear. Trivial stimulation of the foot or leg triggers the mass reflex, usually in a specific zone unique to the patient. The response at first is dorsiflexion of the foot, flexion at the knees, and flexion and adduction at the thighs. Later, contractions of the abdomen, sweating, piloerection, and emptying of the bladder and bowel occur. During this time of heightened reflex activity the tendon reflexes return and become exaggerated.

Below the level of injury, sensation is lost to a variable degree, depending on the completeness of the transection. When the injury is incomplete, sensation begins to return within weeks and may continue to improve for up to 2 years. Patients with partial or complete transections may complain of pain and tingling below the level of injury.

In addition to the development of a small, spastic bladder, autonomic dysfunction includes constipation, lack of sweating, orthostatic hypotension, and disturbed temperature regulation.

Diagnosis. Radiographs of the vertebrae readily identify fracture dislocations. Imaging of the spinal cord produces further information on the presence of compressive hematomas and the structural integrity of the spinal cord (Figure 12-4). The presence of a complete block on myelography indicates a poor prognosis for return of function.

Management. The immediate treatment of fracture dislocation is to reduce the dislocation and prevent further damage to the cord by the use of corticosteroids, surgery, and immobilization. An intravenous infusion of methylprednisolone, 30 mg/kg within the first 8 hours after injury followed by 4 mg/kg/hour for 23 hours, significantly reduces neurological morbidity. A discussion of the long-term management of

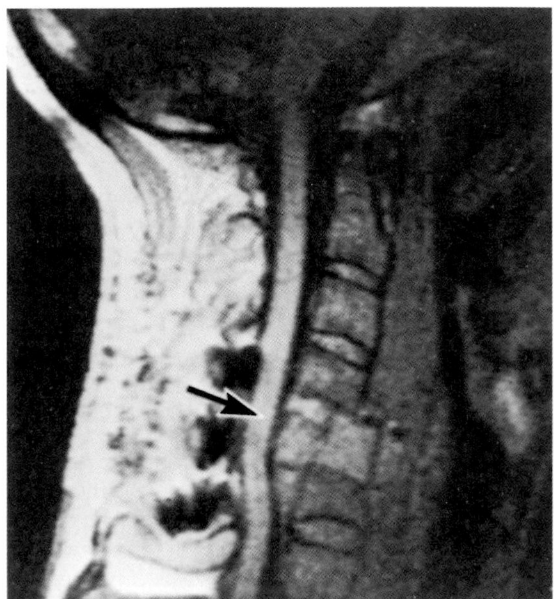

FIGURE 12-4 ■ Fracture dislocation. C4 is dislocated on C5, causing compression (arrow) of the cord.

spinal cord injuries is beyond the scope of this text. Specialized centers provide the best results.

Spinal Cord Concussion

A direct blow on the back may produce a transitory disturbance in spinal cord function. The cause of dysfunction is edema (spinal shock); the spinal cord is intact.

Clinical Features. Most injuries occur at the level of the cervical cord or the thoracolumbar juncture. The major clinical features are flaccid paraplegia or quadriplegia, a sensory level at the site of injury, loss of tendon reflexes, and urinary retention. Recovery begins within a few hours and is complete within a week.

Diagnosis. At the onset of weakness, a spinal cord compression syndrome, such as epidural hematomas, is a consideration, and an imaging study of the spine is necessary.

Management. The indications for methylprednisolone treatment are in the section on fracture dislocation and spinal cord transection.

Spinal Epidural Hematoma

Spinal epidural hematoma usually results from direct vertebral trauma and is especially common in children with an underlying bleeding tendency. The hematoma causes symptoms by progressive compression of the cord, and the clinical features are like any other extradural mass lesion. MRI is usually the basis for diagnosis. Treatment is surgical evacuation.

Tumors of the Spinal Cord

Ewing's sarcoma accounts for nearly 20% of cases of spinal cord compression in children over 5 years of age, while neuroblastoma is the most common cause in younger children. Astrocytoma and ependymoma are the main primary tumors. Motor deficits, usually paraplegia, are an early feature in 86% of spinal cord tumors and back pain in 63%.

Astrocytoma

Chapter 9 discusses the problems of differentiating cystic astrocytoma of the spinal cord from syringomyelia (see section on Syringomyelia).

Clinical Features. Astrocytomas are usually long and may extend from the lower brainstem to the conus medullaris. The initial features of multiple-segment spinal astrocytomas may occur in the arms or legs. Weakness of one arm is characteristic of one syndrome. Pain in the neck may be associated, but bowel and bladder function are normal. Examination shows mild spastic weakness of the legs. The solid portion of the tumor is in the neck, and its caudal extension is cystic.

Progressive spastic paraplegia, sometimes associated with thoracic pain, characterizes a second syndrome. Scoliosis may be associated. In these patients, the solid portion of the tumor is in the thoracic or lumbar region. When solid tumor extends into the conus medullaris, tendon reflexes in the legs may be diminished or absent and bowel and bladder function are impaired.

Intra-axial tumors of the cervicomedullary junction are often low-grade and have an indolent course. They may cause cranial nerve dysfunction or spinal cord compression. Difficulty swallowing and nasal speech are the main features of cranial nerve dysfunction (see Chapter 17).

Diagnosis. MRI is the definitive diagnostic procedure. It allows visualization of both the solid and cystic portions of the tumor (Figure 12-5).

Management. Evaluating proposed treatment options is difficult because the natural history of the tumor is one of slow progression. The 5-year survival rate with low-grade astrocytoma is greater than 90%. Complete resection should be attempted using microsurgical technique. Remove the solid portion and aspirate the cystic portion. MRI is repeated 1, 6, and 12 months after surgery. The benefits of radiation and chemotherapy are still under investigation.

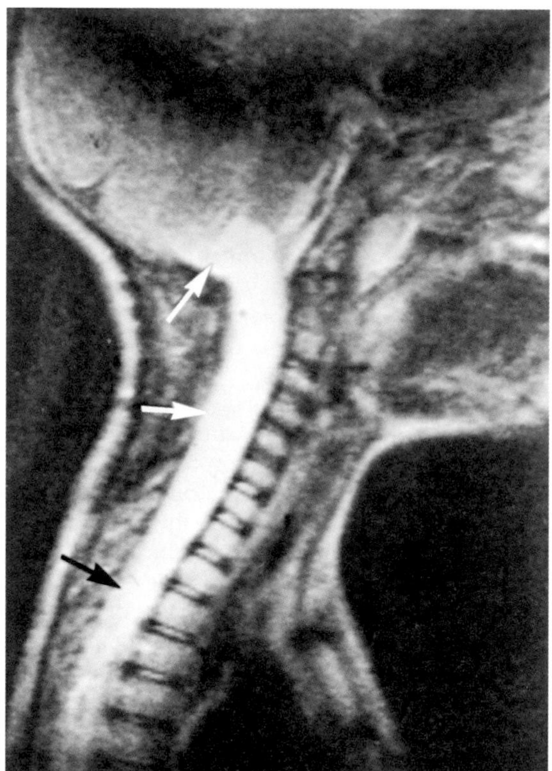

FIGURE 12-5 ■ Astrocytoma of the cervical cord. The tumor demonstrates an intense signal (arrows) on T_2-weighted images.

Ependymoma

Ependymomas are composed primarily of ependymal cells and arise from the lining of the ventricular system or central canal. They are more often intracranial than intraspinal in children. When intraspinal, they tend to be located in the lumbar region or in the cauda equina but may occur anywhere along the neuraxis.

Clinical Features. Clinical features vary with the location of the tumor. The initial feature may be scoliosis, pain in the legs or back, paresthesia, or weakness in one or both legs. Delay in diagnosis is frequent when scoliosis is the only sign. Eventually, all children have difficulty walking, and this feature usually leads to appropriate diagnostic testing.

Stiff neck and cervical pain that is worse at night are the early features of cervical ependymomas. Tumors of the cauda equina may sometimes rupture and produce meningismus, fever, and pleocytosis mimicking bacterial meningitis. Spastic paraplegia is the usual finding on examination. Cervical tumors cause weakness of one arm as well. Tumors of the cauda equina produce flaccid weakness and atrophy of leg muscles associated with loss of tendon reflexes.

Diagnosis. MRI is the primary modality for imaging tumors of the spinal cord. Lumbar puncture, when indicated, shows an elevated protein content in the cerebrospinal fluid.

Management. Microsurgical techniques make possible the complete removal of intramedullary ependymomas. The role of postoperative local radiation therapy in treating benign tumors is uncertain. Malignant ependymomas of the spinal cord are unusual in children but require total neuraxis irradiation when present.

Neuroblastoma

Neuroblastoma is the most common extracranial solid tumor of infancy and childhood. Neurological dysfunction results from direct invasion, metastasis, and by distant "humoral" effects (see Chapter 10). Half of cases occur before 2 years of age and 60% occur before 1 year. The derivation of neuroblastoma is cells of the sympathetic chain and cranial ganglia. Tumors in a paraspinal location may extend through a neural foramen and compress the spinal cord.

Clinical Features. Paraplegia is the initial manifestation of neuroblastoma extending into the epidural space from a paravertebral origin. Because most affected children are infants, the first symptom is usually refusal to stand or walk. Mild weakness may progress to complete paraplegia within hours or days. Examination generally reveals a flaccid paraplegia, a distended bladder, and exaggerated tendon reflexes in the legs. Sensation may be difficult to test.

Diagnosis. Radiographs of the chest usually show the extravertebral portion of the tumor, and MRI delineates the extent of spinal compression.

Management. In children with acute spinal cord compression, high-dose corticosteroids, before surgical extirpation and radiation therapy, provide some symptomatic relief. The survival rate in infants with neuroblastoma confined to a single organ is greater than 60%.

Cerebral Paraplegia and Quadriplegia

Almost all progressive disorders of the brain that result in quadriplegia also have dementia as an initial or prominent feature (see Chapter 5). Pure paraplegia of cerebral origin is unusual. At the very least, the patient has impairment of fine finger movements and increased tendon reflex activity in the arms. Pure paraplegia should always direct attention to the spinal cord.

Cerebral Palsy

Cerebral palsy (CP) is a nonprogressive disorder of posture or movement caused by a lesion of the developing brain (Ashwal et al, 2004). The prevalence of moderately severe cases is approximately 2 per 1000 live births; the prevalence of CP has increased among very small premature infants, as more have survived. Reduced life expectancy is the norm in children with CP who are immobile, with profound cognitive impairment, or require special feeding (Strauss et al, 1998). Otherwise, children with CP may live well into adult life. CP is often a misdiagnosis for several slowly progressive disorders (Table 12-1). Perinatal asphyxia is a known cause of CP but accounts for only a minority of cases. Prenatal factors are a more important cause but are difficult to identify with precision in an individual patient.

In general, head MRI is appropriate in every child with CP in order to identify the brain abnormality. In contrast, only selected patients require metabolic and genetic evaluations.

CP is not always a permanent condition. Many infants with only mild motor impairments improve and achieve normal motor function in childhood. Unfortunately, up to 25 % of such children are cognitively impaired or have some behavioral disturbance. Traditionally, the classification of CPs is by the pattern of motor impairment. The spastic types are paraplegia or diplegia, quadriplegia, and hemiplegia (see Chapter 11). The hypotonic types are ataxic (see Chapter 10) and athetoid (see Chapter 14).

TABLE 12-1 **Slowly Progressive Disorders Sometimes Misdiagnosed as Cerebral Palsy**

Condition	Chapter
Polyneuropathy	
GM_1 gangliosidosis type II	5
Hereditary motor and sensory neuropathies	7
Infantile neuroaxonal dystrophy	5
Metachromatic leukodystrophy	5
Ataxia	
Abetalipoproteinemia	10
Ataxia-telangiectasia	10
Friedreich ataxia	10
Spasticity-Chorea	
Familial spastic paraplegia	12
Glutaric aciduria type I	14
Lesch-Nyhan syndrome	5
Niemann-Pick disease type C	5
Pelizaeus-Merzbacher disease	5
Rett syndrome	5

Spastic Diplegia (Paraplegia). Diplegia means weakness of all four limbs, but that the legs are weaker than the arms. The motor impairment in the arms may be limited to increased responses of tendon reflexes; the classification of such children is *paraplegia*. Periventricular leukomalacia is the usual cause of spastic diplegia in children born prematurely. In neonates and especially in premature infants, the periventricular white matter represents a watershed area and is vulnerable to hypoxic insults. Cystic lesions in the white matter are often unilateral or at least asymmetric, causing a hemiplegia superimposed on spastic diplegia.

Clinical Features. Many children with spastic diplegia have normal tone, or even hypotonia, during the first 4 months. The onset of spasticity in the legs is insidious and slowly progressive during the first year. Four-point creeping is impossible because of leg extension. Either rolling or crawling on the floor with the belly on the ground achieves movement. The milestone of sitting up alone develops late or is never achieved. From the supine position, the infant pulls to a standing rather than a sitting position. Later, bending forward at the waist, to compensate for the lack of flexion at the hip and knee, and placing one hand on the floor for balance accomplishes sitting posture. Most children with spastic diplegia stand on their toes, with flexion at the knees and an increased lumbar lordosis. Leg spasticity makes walking difficult but is achievable by throwing the body forward or from side to side to transfer weight.

Examination shows spasticity of the legs and less spasticity of the arms. All limbs show exaggerated tendon reflexes. Reflex sensitivity and responsiveness are increased; percussion at the knee causes a crossed adductor response. Ankle clonus and an extensor plantar response are usually present. When vertically suspended, the legs cross at the thigh because of strong adductor muscle contractions (*scissoring*).

Subluxation or dislocation of the hips is relatively common in children with severe spasticity; the cause, in part, is from the constant adduction of the thighs and by insufficient development of the hip joint resulting from delayed standing or inability to stand.

Diagnosis. Spastic diplegia is a clinical diagnosis. MRI easily identifies abnormalities in the deep white matter secondary to periventricular leukomalacia, but children with a known history of perinatal distress secondary to prematurity do not require follow-up imaging studies. It is important not to mistake CP for a progressive disease of the brain or cervical portion of the spine. Features that suggest a progressive disease are a family history of CP, deterioration of mental function, loss of motor skills previously obtained, atrophy of muscles, and sensory loss.

Management. There are probably as many methods to manage spastic diplegia and quadriplegia as there are children with CP. In general, a multidisciplinary approach, including infant stimulation, physical therapy, and occupational therapy, helps the child achieve an adequate functional status. Controlled clinical trials are rarely accomplished, and one such trial concluded that physical therapy offered no short-term advantage. It is possible that the main benefit from physical therapy is to maintain range of motion over the long term. Most drugs to relieve spasticity have marginal benefit and often cause unacceptable sedation. Levodopa improves motor function without sedation (Brunstrom et al, 2000).

Injections of botulinum toxin and placement of a baclofen pump are useful procedures for the treatment of spasticity. Pump placement is just below the skin at the waistline. The pump is 3 inches in diameter and 1 inch thick and connects to a small catheter through which the baclofen releases. The pump releases medication at prescribed intervals, which adjusts through an external programmer. Refills, needed every 2 to 3 months, require a return visit to the doctor. The refill is injected by syringe through the skin and into the pump. After 5 to 7 years, the battery life ends and the pump is surgically removed to replace the battery. Initiate a program of physical therapy that maintains the desired range of motion postoperatively.

Spastic Quadriplegia. All limbs are affected, the legs often more severely than the arms. The term *double hemiplegia* is applied if the arms are worse than the legs. Intrauterine disease, usually malformations, is the cause of most spastic quadriplegia. Hypoxic-ischemic encephalopathy of the term newborn accounts for a minority of cases.

Clinical Features. Developmental delay is profound, and identification of the infant as neurologically abnormal occurs early. Failure to meet motor milestones, abnormal posturing of the head and limbs, and seizures are the common reasons for neurological evaluation. In severely affected children, the characteristic supine posture is retraction of the head and neck, flexion of the arms at the elbows with the hands clenched, and extension of the legs. Infantile reflexes (Moro and tonic neck) are obligatory and stereotyped and persist after 6 months of age. Microcephaly is frequently an associated feature.

Because of damage to both hemispheres, supranuclear bulbar palsy (dysphagia and dysarthria) is common. Disturbances in vision and ocular motility are frequently associated features, and seizures occur in 50% of affected children.

Diagnosis. The clinical findings are the basis for diagnosis. Laboratory studies are useful when the underlying cause is not obvious or the possibility of a genetically transmitted defect exists. MRI of the brain is especially useful to show malformations.

Management. Treatment is the same as described in the section on spastic diplegia (paraplegia).

REFERENCES

Ashwal S, Russman BS, Blasco PA, et al. Practice parameter: Diagnostic assessment of the child with cerebral palsy. Report of the Quality Standards Subcommittee of the American Academy of Neurology and the Practice Subcommittee of the Child Neurology Society. Neurology 2004;62:851–63.

Barrow DL, et al. Intradural premedullary arteriovenous fistulas (type IV spinal cord arteriovenous malformations). Journal of Neurosurgery 1994;81(2):221–9.

Brunstrom JE, Bastian AJ, Wong M, et al. Motor benefit from levodopa in spastic quadriplegic cerebral palsy. Annals of Neurology 2000;47:662–5.

Cederbaum S, Crombez MA. Arginase deficiency. In: GeneClinics: Medical Genetics Knowledge Base [database online]. Seattle: University of Washington. Available at http://www.geneclinics.org. PMID: 20301338. Last updated February 9, 2012.

Cornette L, Verpoorten C, Lagae L, et al. Tethered cord syndrome in occult spinal dysraphism. Timing and outcome of surgical release. Neurology 1998;50:1761–5.

Crockard HA, Stevens JM. Craniovertebral junction anomalies in inherited disorders: Part of the syndrome or caused by the disorder? European Journal of Pediatrics 1995;154:504–12.

Fink JK. Hereditary spastic paraplegia overview. In: GeneClinics: Medical Genetics Knowledge Base [database online]. Seattle: University of Washington. Available at http://www.geneclinics.org. PMID: 20301682. Last updated February 3, 2009.

Greenlee JDW, Donovan KA, Hasan DM, et al. Chiari I malformation in the very young child: The spectrum of presentations and experience in 31 children under age 6 years. Pediatrics 2002;110:1212–9.

Hedera P, Bandmann O. Complicated autosomal recessive spastic paraplegia. Neurology 2008;70:1375–6.

Lynch SA, Wang Y, Strachan T, et al. Autosomal dominant sacral agenesis: Currarino syndrome. Journal of Medical Genetics 2000;37:561–6.

Moser HW, Moser AB, Steinberg SJ, et al. X-Linked adrenoleukodystrophy. In: GeneClinics: Medical Genetics Knowledge Base [database online]. Seattle: University of Washington. Available at http://www.geneclinics.org. PMID: 20301491. Last updated April 19, 2012.

Pidcock FS, Krishnan C, Crawford TO, et al. Acute transverse myelitis in childhood. Center-based analysis of 47 cases. Neurology 2007;68(18):1474–80.

Sarnat HB. Regional ependymal upregulation of vimentin in Chiari II malformation, aqueductal stenosis, and hydromyelia. Pediatric Developmental Pathology 2004;7(1):48–60.

Shapiro E, Krivit W, Lockman L, et al. Long-term effect of bone-marrow transplantation for childhood-onset cerebral X-linked adrenoleukodystrophy. Lancet 2000;356:713–8.

Strauss DJ, Shavelle RM, Anderson TW. Life expectancy of children with cerebral palsy. Pediatric Neurology 1998;18:143–9.

Transverse Myelitis Consortium Working Group. Proposed diagnostic criteria and nosology of acute transverse myelitis. Neurology 2002;59:499–505.

van Geel BM, Assies J, Wanders RJA, et al. X linked adrenoleukodystrophy: Clinical presentation, diagnosis, and therapy. Journal of Neurology, Neurosurgery and Psychiatry 1997;63:4–14.

Wenger DA. Krabbe disease. In: GeneClinics: Medical Genetics Knowledge Base [database online]. Seattle: University of Washington. Available at http://www.geneclinics.org. PMID: 20301416. Last updated March 31, 2011.

Werhahn KJ, et al. The clinical features and prognosis of chronic posthypoxic myoclonus. Movement Disorders 1997;12(2):216–20.

Wingerchuk DM, Weinshenker BG. Neuromyelitis optica. Clinical predictors of a relapsing course and survival. Neurology 2003;60:848–53.

CHAPTER 13

MONOPLEGIA

Weakness or paralysis of a limb is usually due to pathology of the spine and the proximal portion of nerves. Monoplegia may also be the initial presentation of a hemiplegia, paraplegia, or quadriplegia. Therefore, one must also consult the differential diagnosis of spinal paraplegia provided in Box 12-1 and the table and boxes in Chapter 11 referring to the differential diagnosis of cerebral hemiplegia.

APPROACH TO MONOPLEGIA

Either pain or weakness may cause refusal to use a limb. The cause of most painful limbs is orthopedic or rheumatologic (arthritis, infection, and tumor). A trivial pull on an infant's arm may dislocate the radial head and cause an apparent monoplegia. Pain followed by weakness is a feature of plexitis.

Box 13-1 summarizes the differential diagnosis of acute monoplegia. Plexopathies and neuropathies are the leading causes of pure monoplegia. Stroke often affects one limb more others, usually the arm more than the leg. The presentation may suggest monoplegia, but careful examination often reveals increased tendon reflexes and an extensor plantar response in the seemingly unaffected limb. Any suggestion of hemiplegia rather than monoplegia, or increased tendon reflexes in the paretic limb, should focus attention on the brain and cervical cord as the pathological site.

Chronic progressive brachial monoplegia is uncommon. When it occurs, one should suspect syringomyelia and tumors of the cervical cord or brachial plexus. Chronic progressive weakness of one leg suggests a tumor of the spinal cord or a neurofibroma of the lumbar plexus. A monomelic form of spinal muscular atrophy, affecting only one leg or one arm, should be considered when progressive weakness is unaccompanied by sensory loss.

BOX 13-1 Differential Diagnosis of Acute Monoplegia

COMPLICATED MIGRAINE* (SEE CHAPTER 11)

DISLOCATION OF THE RADIAL HEAD

HEMIPARETIC SEIZURES* (SEE CHAPTER 11)

MONOMELIC SPINAL MUSCULAR ATROPHY

PLEXOPATHY AND NEUROPATHY

- Acute neuritis
  - Asthmatic plexitis
  - Idiopathic plexitis*
  - Osteomyelitis plexitis
  - Poliomyelitis (see Chapter 7)
  - Tetanus toxoid plexitis
- Hereditary
  - Hereditary brachial neuritis
  - Hereditary neuropathy with liability to pressure palsy
- Injury
  - Lacerations
  - Pressure injuries
  - Traction injuries*

STROKE (SEE BOX 11-2)

*Denotes the most common conditions and the ones with disease modifying treatments

SPINAL MUSCULAR ATROPHIES

The first report of a monomelic form of spinal muscular atrophy was from Asia but the condition is probably equally common among Europeans. The terms used to describe the entity are *benign focal amyotrophy* and *monomelic amyotrophy*. While trauma and immobilization of the limb may precede the onset of atrophy by several months, a cause-and-effect relationship is not established.

The transmission of the familial form is by autosomal recessive inheritance. Two affected brothers had a mutation in the superoxide dismutase 1 gene. In one set of male identical twins, both developed atrophy of first one hand and then the other.

Clinical Features. Onset is usually in the second or third decade and has a male preponderance. The initial features are usually weakness and atrophy in one limb, the arm in 75% and the leg in 25% of cases. Tendon reflexes in the involved limb are hypoactive or absent. Sensation is normal. The weakness and atrophy affect only one limb in half of cases and spread to the contralateral limb in the remainder. Tremor of one or both hands is often associated with wasting. The appearance of fasciculations heralds weakness and atrophy. Progression is slow, and spontaneous arrest within 5 years is the rule. However, another limb may become weak after a gap of 15 years.

Diagnosis. Needle electromyography (EMG) studies of all limbs are essential to show the extent of involvement. The studies are often normal at onset and show a denervation pattern 3 to 4 weeks later. Motor conduction is normal. Magnetic resonance imaging (MRI) of the spine and plexus is required to exclude a tumor.

Management. Physical therapy, occupational therapy, splinting, and bracing are the main supportive treatment options.

PLEXOPATHIES

Acute Idiopathic Plexitis

Acute plexitis is a demyelinating disorder of the brachial or lumbar plexus thought to be immune mediated. Brachial plexitis is far more common than lumbar plexitis.

Brachial Plexitis

Brachial plexitis (*brachial neuritis, neuralgic amyotrophy*) occurs from infancy to adult life. Prior tetanus toxoid immunization has occurred in 10–20% of childhood and adult cases and in almost all infants. The site of immunization does not correlate with the limb involved.

Clinical Features. The onset of symptoms is usually explosive. Pain is the initial feature in 95% of patients. Pain localization is to the shoulder but may be more diffuse or limited to the lower arm, and tends to be severe. It may awaken the patient, and the description is "sharp, stabbing, throbbing, or aching." The duration of pain, which is frequently constant, varies from several hours to 3 weeks. As the pain subsides, weakness appears. Weakness is in the distribution of the upper plexus alone in half of patients and the entire plexus in most of the rest. Lower plexitis alone is unusual. Although the initial pain abates, paresthesias may accompany the weakness. Two-thirds of people report improved strength during the month after onset. Upper plexus palsies improve faster than do lower plexus palsies. Among all patients, one-third recovers within 1 year, three-quarters by 2 years, and 90% by 3 years. After 3 years, further improvement may occur but permanent residua are expected. Recurrences are unusual and less severe than the initial episode.

Diagnosis. Pain and weakness in one arm are also symptoms of spinal cord compression, indicating the need for spinal cord imaging studies. However, when the onset is characteristic of brachial plexus neuritis, the clinical features alone establish the diagnosis. Diagnostic tests are not essential. The cerebrospinal fluid is usually normal. A slight lymphocytosis and mild elevation in protein content are sometimes noted. EMG and nerve conduction studies are helpful in showing the extent of plexopathy. Electrical evidence of bilateral involvement may be present in patients with unilateral symptoms.

Management. Gabapentin between 20 and 60 mg/kg/day divided into three or four doses, and pregabalin, a more effective choice, at 3–10 mg/kg/day divided into two doses, are helpful in controlling neuropathic pain but not the paresthesias or weakness associated with the plexopathy. Corticosteroids do not affect the outcome. Recommend range of motion exercises until strength recovers and occupational therapy to deal with any possible deficit.

Lumbar Plexitis

Lumbar plexitis occurs at all ages and is similar to brachial plexitis, except that it affects the leg instead of the arm. The mechanism is probably the same as in brachial plexitis.

Clinical Features. Fever is often the first symptom and pain in one or both legs. The pain has an abrupt onset and may occur in a femoral or sciatic distribution. Sciatica, when present, suggests disk disease. Young children refuse to stand or walk, and older children limp. Weakness may develop concurrently with pain or be delayed for as long as 3 weeks. The onset of weakness is insidious and often difficult to date, but usually it begins 8 days after the onset of pain. Weakness progresses for a week and then stabilizes. Tendon reflexes are absent in the affected leg but are present in other limbs.

Recovery is characterized first by abatement of pain and then by increasing strength. The average time from onset of pain to maximal recovery is 18 weeks, with a range of 8 weeks to several years. Functional recovery is almost universal, but mild weakness may persist.

Diagnosis. The sudden onset of pain and weakness in one leg suggests spinal cord or disk disease. MRI of the spine is a means of excluding other disorders; the results are invariably normal in lumbar plexitis. The cerebrospinal fluid is normal except for a mild elevation of the protein concentration. EMG performed 3 weeks after onset shows patchy denervation.

Management. Gabapentin between 20 and 60 mg/kg/day divided into three or four doses, and pregabalin, a more effective choice, 3–10 mg/kg/day divided into two doses, are helpful in controlling the neuropathic pain but not the paresthesias or weakness associated with the plexopathy. Corticosteroids do not affect the outcome. Recommend range of motion exercises until strength recovers and occupational therapy to deal with any possible deficit.

Acute Symptomatic Plexitis

Asthmatic Amyotrophy (Hopkins Syndrome)

Sudden flaccid paralysis of one or more limbs, resembling poliomyelitis, may occur during recovery from an asthmatic attack. All affected children had previously received poliomyelitis vaccine. The etiologic mechanism for this syndrome is unknown. Infection by a neurotropic virus other than poliovirus is a possibility. Adenovirus, echovirus, and coxsackievirus have been isolated from stool, throat, or cerebrospinal fluid in some cases. A recent case report suggests a possible atopic myelitis (Pavone et al, 2010).

Clinical Features. Age at onset is from 1 to 11 years, and the male-to-female ratio is 7:4. The interval between the asthmatic attack and the paralysis is 1 to 11 days, with an average of 5 days. Monoplegia occurs in 90%, with the arm involved twice as often as the leg. The other 10% have hemiplegia or diplegia. Meningeal irritation is not present. Sensation is intact, but the paralyzed limb is painful in half of cases. Recovery is incomplete, and all affected children have some degree of permanent paralysis.

Diagnosis. Asthmatic amyotrophy is primarily a clinical diagnosis based on the sequence of events. The diagnosis requires distinction from paralytic poliomyelitis and idiopathic brachial neuritis. The basis for excluding paralytic poliomyelitis is normal cerebrospinal fluid in asthmatic amyotrophy. A few white blood cells may be present in the cerebrospinal fluid but never to the extent encountered in poliomyelitis, and the protein concentration is normal. EMG during the acute phase shows active denervation of the paralyzed limb, but the pattern of denervation does not follow the radicular distribution expected in a brachial neuritis.

Management. Gabapentin and pregabalin may be helpful in controlling neuropathic pain. Other analgesia may be needed. As with plexitis, physical and occupational therapy are often required.

Hereditary Brachial Plexopathy

The two major phenotypes of *focal familial recurrent neuropathy* are hereditary brachial plexopathy (also called *hereditary neuralgic amyotrophy*) and hereditary neuropathy with liability to pressure palsies (see section on Mononeuropathies later in this chapter). The phenotypes can be confused because isolated nerve palsies may occur in hereditary brachial plexopathy, and brachial plexopathy occurs in patients with hereditary neuropathy with a liability to pressure palsies. Transmission of both disorders is by autosomal dominant inheritance, but the underlying mutations are at different sites on chromosome 17. The mutation responsible for hereditary brachial plexopathy is *SEPT9* located in chromosome 17q25 (Hoque et al, 2008; Stögbauer et al, 2000).

Clinical Features. Hereditary brachial plexopathy may be difficult to distinguish from idiopathic brachial plexitis in the absence of a family history or a patient's history of similar episodes. Events that may trigger an attack in genetically predisposed individuals include infection, emotional stress, strenuous use of the affected limb, and childbirth. Immunization, which may precipitate sporadic brachial plexopathies, is not a factor in the genetic form.

Two different courses exist with only one type per family suggesting the possibility of genetic heterogeneity (van Alfen et al, 2000). Characteristic of the *classic course* is severe attacks with relatively symptom free intervals. Patients with the *chronic course* experience interictal persistence of pain and weakness. The initial attack usually occurs during the second or third decade but may appear at birth. Attributing palsies at birth to trauma is common despite the positive family history. Weakness resolves completely, only to recur later.

Severe arm pain exacerbated by movement characterizes the attack. Weakness follows in days to weeks, which is usually maximal within a few days and always by 1 month. The entire plexus may be involved, but more often only the upper trunk is affected. Even with total plexus involvement, the upper plexus is weaker than other parts. Examination shows proximal arm weakness. Distal weakness may be present as well. Tendon reflexes are absent from affected muscles. Weakness persists for weeks to months and is associated with atrophy and fasciculations. Pain, which is frequently the only sensory finding, subsides after the first week.

Recovery begins weeks to months after attaining maximal weakness. Return of function is usually complete, although some residual weakness may persist after repeated attacks. The frequency of attacks is variable; several attacks may occur within a single year, but the usual pattern is two or three attacks per decade.

Occasionally children have an episode of lumbar plexopathy. Pain in the thigh and proximal weakness are characteristic. Brachial and lumbar plexopathies are never concurrent, although bilateral brachial plexopathy is a relatively common event. Isolated cranial nerve palsies may occur in families with hereditary brachial plexopathy. The vagus nerve is the one most often affected and causes hoarseness and dysphagia.

Other cranial neuropathies result in transitory facial palsy and unilateral hearing loss.

Diagnosis. The family history, early age at onset, unique triggering events, recurrences, and involvement of other nerves differentiate hereditary brachial plexopathy from idiopathic brachial neuritis. EMG shows a diffuse axonopathy in the affected arm and some evidence of denervation in the asymptomatic arm. Asymptomatic legs are electrically normal.

Management. Symptomatic treatment with gabapentin at doses between 20 and 60 mg/kg/day divided into three or four doses and pregabalin, a more effective choice, at doses of 3–10 mg/kg/day divided into two doses are helpful in controlling the neuropathic pain. Corticosteroids do not affect the outcome. Recommend range of motion exercises until strength recovers and occupational therapy to deal with any possible deficit.

Neonatal Traumatic Brachial Neuropathy

The incidence of neonatal brachial plexus birth injuries is estimated at 1:1000 live births. The cause of obstetric brachial plexus palsies is excessive traction on the plexus. Upper plexus injuries occur when pulling the head and arm away from each other. This occurs in the vertex position when the head is pulled forcefully to deliver the aftercoming shoulder or when normal contractions force the head and neck downward with the shoulder trapped by the pelvis. Injuries in the breech position occur when pulling the arm downward to free the aftercoming head or when rotating the head to occipitoanterior when the shoulder is fixed. Complete (upper and lower) plexus injuries occur during vertex deliveries when traction is exerted on a prolapsed arm and in breech deliveries when the trunk is pulled downward but an aftercoming arm is fixed.

Clinical Features. Most neonatal brachial plexus injuries occur in large full-term newborns of primiparous mothers, especially when the fetus is malpositioned and the delivery is long and difficult. The traditional division of brachial plexus injuries is into those involving the upper roots (named for *Erb* and *Duchenne*) and those involving the lower roots (named for *Klumpke*). However, solitary lower root injuries are unusual. In 88 %, the palsy affects only the C5 through C7 cervical roots and 12 % have a complete plexus palsy. Bilateral, but not necessarily symmetrical, involvement occurs in 8 % of cases.

Because the upper plexus (C5 to C7) is always involved, the posture of the arm is typical and reflects weakness of the proximal muscles. The arm is adducted and internally rotated at the shoulder and is extended and pronated at the elbow, so that the partially flexed fingers face backward. Extension of the wrist is lost and the fingers fisted. The biceps and triceps reflexes are absent. Injuries that extend higher than the C4 segment result in ipsilateral diaphragmatic paralysis.

Newborns with complete brachial plexus palsies have flaccid, dry limbs with neither proximal nor distal movement. A Horner syndrome (ptosis, miosis, anhydrosis) is sometimes associated. Sensory loss to pinprick is present with partial or complete palsies but may not conform to the segmental pattern of weakness.

Diagnosis. Recognition of brachial plexus palsy is by the typical posture of the arm and by failure of movement when the Moro reflex is tested. Because the injury often takes place during a long and difficult delivery, asphyxia may be present as well. In such cases, generalized hypotonia may mask the focal arm weakness. Approximately 10 % of newborns with brachial plexus injuries have facial nerve palsy and fractures of the clavicle or humerus.

Management. The spontaneous recovery rate is approximately 70 %. One goal of therapy is to prevent the development of contractures. Range of motion exercises prevents contractures while splinting, or other forms of immobilization, causes them. Significant recovery occurs throughout the first year, but infants who show no improvement in strength at the end of 6 months are unlikely to show functional improvement later. Surgical reconstruction of the plexus (nerve grafts, nerve reattachment, neuroma excision, etc.) is a consideration in infants with no evidence of some spontaneous recovery at 3 to 6 months. However, the benefit of reconstructive surgery is not well established.

Osteomyelitis-Neuritis

Apparent limb weakness caused by pain is a well-recognized phenomenon. However, a true brachial neuritis may occur in response to osteomyelitis of the shoulder. Ischemic nerve damage caused by vasculitis is the assumed mechanism.

Clinical Features. Osteomyelitis-neuritis occurs predominantly during infancy. The initial feature is a flaccid arm without pain or tenderness. Body temperature may be normal at first but soon becomes elevated. Pain develops on movement of the shoulder, and tenderness to palpation follows. No swelling is present. The biceps and triceps reflexes may be depressed or absent.

Diagnosis. Suspect osteomyelitis of the proximal humerus when brachial plexitis develops during infancy. Radiographs of the humerus become abnormal at the end of the first week, when they show destruction of the lateral margin of the humerus, but radioisotope bone scan shows a focal area of uptake in the proximal humerus, the scapula, or both shortly after onset. After 3 weeks, EMG shows patchy denervation in the muscles innervated by the upper plexus. These results support the idea that this is a true plexitis and not just a painful limb.

Aspirates from the shoulder joint or blood culture identify the organism. Group B *Streptococcus* is often isolated in specimens from young infants. Older children have other bacterial species.

Management. Three to 4 weeks of intravenous antibiotics is the recommended treatment. Recovery of arm strength may be incomplete.

Postnatal Injuries

Brachial Plexus. Traction and pressure injuries of the brachial plexus are relatively common because of its superficial position. Motor vehicle and sports accidents account for the majority of severe injuries. However, mild injuries also occur in the following situations: (1) when an adult suddenly yanks a child's arm, either protectively or to force movement; (2) by a blow to the shoulder, such as in a football scrimmage or from the recoil of a rifle; (3) because of prolonged wearing of a heavy backpack; (4) when the arm is kept hyperextended during surgery; and (5) by pressure in the axilla from poorly positioned crutches.

Clinical Features. Mild injuries do not affect all portions of the plexus equally. Diffuse weakness is uncommon. Pain may be an important initial feature, and sensory loss is uncommon. Recovery begins within days or weeks and is complete. Atrophy does not occur.

More severe injuries are usually associated with fractures of the clavicle and scapula, and dislocation of the humerus. The upper plexus is generally affected more severely than is the lower plexus, but complete paralysis may be present at the onset. Sensory loss is less marked than weakness, and the two may not correspond in distribution. Pain is common, not only from the plexopathy but also from the bone and soft tissue injuries. The most painful injuries are those associated with root avulsion.

Tendon reflexes are absent, and atrophy develops in denervated muscle. Recovery progresses from proximal to distal and Tinel sign plots the recovery: tingling in the distal part of a limb caused by tapping over the regenerating segment of a nerve. Complete reinnervation, when it occurs, may take several months or years. The completeness of recovery depends on the severity and nature of the injury. Pressure and traction injuries in which anatomical integrity is not disturbed recover best, whereas injuries that tear the nerve or avulse the root do not recover at all.

Diagnosis. EMG is useful in identifying the pattern of nerve injury and in providing information on the prognosis. Even with mild traction injuries, the amplitude of motor and sensory action potentials attenuates and motor and sensory conduction slows.

Management. Mild injuries do not require treatment other than range of motion exercises. For more severe traction injuries, resting the limb for the first month is usually necessary. During that time, provide analgesia as needed for pain and electrically stimulate muscles away from the site of injury, to maintain tone. Initiate range of motion exercises once pain subsides.

Prompt correction is required of fractures and dislocations that cause pressure on the brachial plexus. Lacerated nerves require surgical restoration of anatomical integrity.

Lumbar Plexus. Injuries of the lumbar plexus are much less common than are injuries of the brachial plexus. The pelvis and the heavy muscles of the hip provide considerable protection from direct trauma.

Clinical Features. Lumbar plexus injuries are usually associated with fracture dislocation of the pelvis. Motor vehicle accidents or falls from a considerable height are required to produce sufficient force to fracture the pelvis. Therefore, the patient usually has multiple injuries, and the lumbar plexus injury may be the last identified. Lumbar plexus injuries produce a patchy weakness that is difficult to differentiate from mononeuritis multiplex.

Diagnosis. EMG helps distinguish plexus injuries and nerve injuries.

Management. Fracture-dislocations require treatment to relieve pressure on the plexus. As with brachial plexus injuries, the completeness of recovery depends on the anatomical integrity of the nerves.

Plexus Tumors

Plexus tumors in childhood are rare. The most common primary tumor is the plexiform neurofibroma (Figure 13-1). These can affect either the brachial or the lumbar plexus. They grow very slowly and cause progressive but selected weakness

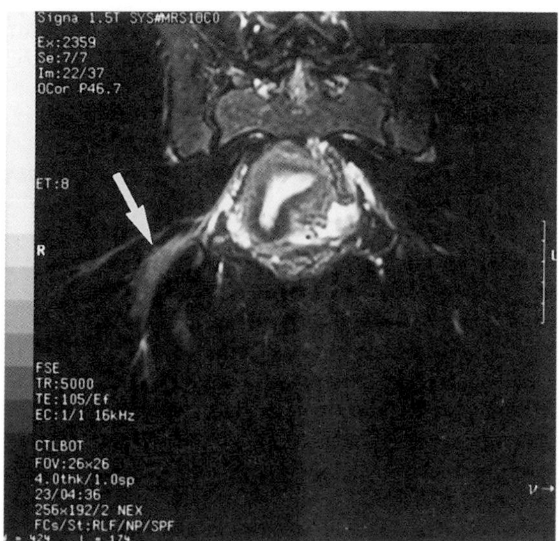

FIGURE 13-1 ■ Neurofibroma of the lumbar plexus. MRI of the plexus using a subtraction technique shows enlargement of the sciatic nerve (arrow).

over several years. Secondary tumors of the brachial plexus are the neuroblastoma and primitive neuroectodermal tumors arising in the chest.

MRI visualizes plexus tumors when fat subtraction techniques are used.

Mononeuropathies

Radial Neuropathy

Radial nerve injuries usually occur in the spinal groove of the humerus, just below the takeoff of the motor branch to the triceps muscle. Injury may occur with fractures of the humerus or by external pressure. Such pressure usually results when a sleeping or sedated patient is in a position that compresses the nerve between the humerus and a hard surface, such as an operating room table or chair.

Isolated radial nerve injuries may occur in newborns with a history of failure of progression of labor. These may result from prolonged radial nerve compression (Hayman et al, 1999).

Clinical Features. Wrist drop and finger drop are characteristic of injuries to the radial nerve within the spiral groove. The brachioradialis muscle may be weak and its tendon reflex lost. Sensory disturbances are restricted to the back of the hand near the base of the thumb. With the wrist dropped, a fist is mechanically difficult to make but the finger flexors are not weak.

Diagnosis. Electrophysiological studies are useful for locating the site of injury and assessing the anatomical integrity of the nerve and the prognosis for recovery.

Management. Pressure injuries recover completely in 6 to 8 weeks. During that time, a splint is useful for placing the wrist in extension so that the patient can flex the fingers.

Ulnar Neuropathy

The most common site of ulnar injury is the elbow. This injury may result from external pressure, recurrent dislocation of the nerve from its groove, and fracture of the distal humerus.

Clinical Features. Paresthesias on the ulnar side of the hand, the little finger, and the ring finger are experienced. Tapping the ulnar groove increases the discomfort. Hand strength is lost, and the intrinsic muscles become wasted. The little finger and the adjacent side of the ring finger have diminished or absent sensation.

Diagnosis. Electrophysiological techniques localize the injury along the course of the nerve.

Management. Minor pressure injuries do not require treatment, and recovery is complete within a few weeks. Injuries to the elbow that cause fracture or nerve dislocation require surgical repair.

Median Neuropathy

The cause of nontraumatic median neuropathies is compression of the nerve in the carpal tunnel and traumatic injuries at the elbow. In children, a storage disease such as mucolipidosis may cause nerve compression in the carpal tunnel, but idiopathic cases occur as well. Fracture at the elbow is the usual cause of traumatic median neuropathy.

Clinical Features. The most common features are numbness and pain in the hand. Nontraumatic median neuropathy is often bilateral. Weakness and atrophy are more likely to occur in traumatic injuries of the nerve than in carpal tunnel entrapment.

Diagnosis. EMG is useful to localize the lesion, especially when surgical decompression is an option.

Management. Surgical decompression may be beneficial for both nontraumatic and traumatic injuries. Immobilization is helpful in cases of repetitive injury.

Peroneal Neuropathy

The peroneal nerve lies in a superficial position adjacent to the fibula. External pressure readily compresses the nerve against the bone. This most often occurs in children who have undergone significant weight loss or trauma to the nerve. EMG documented a prenatal peroneal palsy, presumably caused by pressure, in one newborn (Jones et al, 1996).

Clinical Features. The prominent feature is an acute, painless foot drop. Both dorsiflexion and eversion of the foot are weak. Sensation is usually intact, but sometimes there is numbness over the lower lateral leg and dorsum of the foot. When only the deep branch of the peroneal nerve is involved, sensory loss is restricted to a small triangle between the first two toes. Complete or significant spontaneous recovery is the rule except after considerable trauma.

Diagnosis. Electrodiagnosis is useful to discriminate peroneal nerve lesions from disturbances of the fifth lumbar root.

Management. A foot drop brace is a useful aid to walking until recovery is complete.

Hereditary Neuropathy with Liability to Pressure Palsy

The characteristic feature of hereditary neuropathy with liability to pressure palsy (also called *tomaculous neuropathy*) is the development of a mononeuropathy following trivial trauma. In some cases, the brachial plexus is affected. Transmission of the disorder is as an autosomal dominant trait, caused by deletion of the gene encoding peripheral myelin protein-22 caused by a deletion in chromosome 17p11.2 (Bird, 2010; Li et al, 2002).

Clinical Features. The first episode usually occurs during the second or third decade. Typical precipitating factors include sleeping on a limb, body contact in sports, constrictive clothing, or positioning during surgery. Individuals quickly learn to avoid activities that provoke episodes. Superficial nerves (radial, ulnar, median, peroneal) are the ones most commonly affected. The resulting mononeuropathy is painless and affects both motor and sensory fibers. Tendon reflexes are lost. Recovery is complete within days to weeks.

Diagnosis. Except for the family history, the first episode might suggest ordinary pressure palsy, although the trivial nature of the trauma should alert the physician to the underlying neuropathy. Consider the diagnosis in children with repeated neuropathies or multifocal neuropathies even in the absence of a family history.

Molecular genetic testing establishes the diagnosis. Electrophysiological studies show slow conduction time, not only in the affected limb but also in all limbs. Other family members may show generalized slowing of conduction between attacks.

Management. No treatment is available for the underlying neuropathy. Alterations in lifestyle may be needed to avoid pressure palsies. A wrist splint is useful for carpal tunnel syndrome and an ankle-foot orthotic for foot drop. Protective pads at elbows or knees may prevent pressure and trauma to local nerves. Advise patients against sitting with legs crossed, leaning on elbows, and activities requiring repetitive movements. Despite the best effort, some patients eventually develop a generalized motor and sensory neuropathy.

REFERENCES

Bird T. Hereditary neuropathy with liability to pressure palsy In: GeneClinics: Medical Genetics Knowledge Base [database online]. Seattle: University of Washington. Available at http://www.geneclinic.org. PMID: 20301566. Last updated May 11, 2010.

Hayman M, Roland EH, Hill A. Newborn radial nerve palsy: Report of four cases and review of published reports. Pediatric Neurology 1999;21:648–51.

Hoque R, Schwendimann RN, Kelley RE, et al. Painful brachial plexopathies in SEPT9 mutations: Adverse outcome related to comorbid states. Journal of Clinical Neuromuscular Disease 2008;9:379–84.

Jones Jr HR, Herbison GJ, Jacobs SR, et al. Intrauterine onset of a mononeuropathy: Peroneal neuropathy in a newborn with electromyographic findings at age one day compatible with prenatal onset. Muscle and Nerve 1996;19:88–91.

Li J, Krajewski K, Shy ME, Lewis RA. Hereditary neuropathy with liability to pressure palsy. The electrophysiology fits the name. Neurology 2002;58:1769–73.

Pavone P, Longo MR, Scalia F, et al. Recurrent Hopkin's syndrome: A case report and review of the literature. Journal of the Neurological Sciences 2010;297:89–91.

Stögbauer F, Young P, Kuhlenbaumer G, et al. Hereditary recurrent focal neuropathies. Clinical and molecular features. Neurology 2000;54:546–51.

van Alfen N, van Engelen BGM, Reinders JWC, et al. The natural history of hereditary neuralgic amyotrophy in the Dutch population. Two distinct types? Brain 2000;123:718–23.

CHAPTER 14

Movement Disorders

Involuntary movements are usually associated with abnormalities of the basal ganglia and their connections and occur in several different neurological disorders. Abnormal movements can be the main or initial features of disease, or they can occur as a late manifestation. Discussion of the former type is in this chapter, and the latter in other chapters.

APPROACH TO THE PATIENT

Movement disorders are difficult to describe; they require visualization. If abnormal movements are not present at the time of examination, instruct the parents to videotape the movements at home. Some relatively common movements are recognizable by description, but the rich variety of abnormal movements and postures that may occur defies classification. The most experienced observer will mistake, at times, one movement for another or will have difficulty conceptualizing the nature of an abnormal movement.

Many abnormal movements are paroxysmal or at least intermittent. Motion, excitement, startle, emotional upset, or sleep induces some movements. The physician should ask what makes the movement worse and if it is action-induced. Ask children to perform the action during the examination. Paroxysmal movements raise the question of epilepsy. Indeed, the concurrent presence of seizures and involuntary movements characterize many neurological disorders of childhood. *Nocturnal paroxysmal dystonia*, once thought a movement disorder, is actually frontal lobe epilepsy (see Chapter 1). The clinical and conceptual distinction between spinal myoclonus and myoclonic seizures can be difficult. The following guidelines are useful to distinguish involuntary movements from seizures: (1) involuntary movements, with the exception of spinal myoclonus and periodic movements of sleep, abate or disappear during sleep and seizures persist or may worsen; (2) involuntary movements usually have a more stereotyped appearance and, with the exception of acute drug reactions, are more persistent than seizures; (3) loss of consciousness or awareness is characteristic of seizures but not involuntary movements; and (4) epileptiform activity on electroencephalography (EEG) accompanies seizures, but not involuntary movements.

Involuntary contractions of a muscle that do not move a joint may be fasciculations, focal seizures, or myoclonus. Low-amplitude jerking movements that move a joint or muscles may be focal seizures, chorea, myoclonus, tics, or hemifacial spasm. High-amplitude jerking movements that move a limb or limbs may be seizures, ballismus, or myoclonus. Slow, writhing movements and abnormal posturing may be due to athetosis, dystonia, continuous motor unit activity (see Chapter 8), or seizures. The possible causes of rhythmic movements may be tremor, seizures, or myoclonus.

CHOREA AND ATHETOSIS

Chorea is a rapid movement affecting any part of the body that the patient often incorporates into a voluntary movement in an attempt to hide it. The movements are random but neither rhythmic nor stereotyped, and they migrate from side-to-side and limb-to-limb. Because the involuntary movement flows into a voluntary movement, it gives the appearance of constant movement (restlessness). *Akathisia*, an inward compulsion to move (discussed later) also causes the appearance of restlessness. Depending on the condition, chorea may be unilateral or bilateral and may affect the face and trunk as well as the limbs. An observer cannot precisely describe chorea because it has no fixed form.

Chorea is more readily observed when separated from the superimposed voluntary movement that follows. Ask the child to raise both hands upward beside the head with the palms facing each other. Low-amplitude jerking movements occur, which turns the arm into pronation. When the child lightly grips the examiner's fingers, the grip alternately tightens and loosens, as if the patient is "milking" the examiner's hands. Hypotonia is common in many conditions causing chorea. Tendon reflexes may be normoreactive, but, at times, a choreic movement occurs during the patellar response, producing an extra kick. Children move their tongue constantly, in and out, when asked to maintain it protruded (motor impersistence).

Athetosis is a low-amplitude chorea. It is low-amplitude, writhing movements of the limbs that may occur alone but is often associated with chorea (choreoathetosis). The usual cause of athetosis without chorea is perinatal brain injury. Kernicterus was once a major cause of choreathetosis but is now a rare event. Perinatal asphyxia is now the predominant etiology. Many children with athetosis have atonic cerebral palsy, and others have spastic diplegia.

Ballismus is a high-amplitude chorea. It is a high-amplitude, violent flinging of a limb from the shoulder or pelvis. In adults, it may occur in limbs contralateral to a vascular lesion in the subthalamic nucleus; in children, it is usually associated with chorea and seen in cerebral palsy, kernicterus, Sydenham chorea and lupus erythematosus.

Tardive dyskinesia is a complex syndrome usually characterized by buccolingual masticatory movements that include tongue protrusion, lip smacking, puckering, and chewing. It is decidedly uncommon in children. Dopamine antagonist drugs (neuroleptics and antiemetics) are the usual cause of tardive dyskinesia. It may be a subtype of chorea, or at least a related disorder, and is sometimes associated with choreiform movements of the limbs. Most children thought to have developed tardive dyskinesia usually turn out to have motor tics. The incidence of tardive dyskinesia with both first and second generation neuroleptic drugs (0.3–0.4 % and 0.77 %, respectively) in children is significantly less than the rates reported in adults (0.6–0.8 % and 5%, respectively) (Correll & Kane, 2007).

Boxes 14-1 and 14-2 summarize the differential diagnosis of chorea and choreoathetosis. Chorea is a cardinal feature of the conditions listed in Box 14-1. The details of many such conditions are elsewhere in the text because concurrent features are more prominent. Although abnormal movements are the only manifestation, the description of familial paroxysmal choreoathetosis is in Chapter 1 because it is more likely to be confused with epilepsy than with other causes of chorea.

Box 14-2 contains a partial list of conditions in which chorea and choreoathetosis may occur, but in which they are either late features or at least not prominent early in the course. Movement disorders are a relatively common feature of several cerebral degenerative disorders. In contrast, chorea and seizures may be confused when chorea develops during an acute illness such as bacterial meningitis, metabolic encephalopathies, or encephalitis. At times, the movement disorder is due to the underlying brain disorder and at times to drugs used in treatment.

BOX 14-1 Differential Diagnosis of Chorea as an Initial or Prominent Symptom

CARDIOPULMONARY BYPASS SURGERY

GENETIC DISORDERS

- Abetalipoproteinemia (see Chapter 10)
- Ataxia-telangiectasia (see Chapter 10)
- Benign familial chorea
- Fahr disease
- Familial paroxysmal choreoathetosis (see Chapter 1)
- Glutaric aciduria
- Hepatolenticular degeneration (Wilson disease)
- Huntington disease (see Chapter 5)
- Lesch-Nyhan syndrome (see Chapter 5)
- Machado-Joseph disease (see Chapter 5)
- Neuroacanthocytosis

DRUG-INDUCED MOVEMENT DISORDERS

- Anticonvulsants
- Antiemetics*
- Oral contraceptives
- Psychotropic agents*
- Stimulants*
- Theophylline

SYSTEMIC CONDITIONS

- Hyperthyroidism*
- Lupus erythematosus*
- Pregnancy* (chorea gravidarum)
- Sydenham* (rheumatic) chorea

TUMORS OF CEREBRAL HEMISPHERE (SEE CHAPTER 4)

*Denotes the most common conditions and the ones with disease modifying treatments

Cardiopulmonary Bypass Surgery

Severe choreoathetosis is a complication of up to 10 % of children with congenital heart disease following cardiopulmonary bypass surgery and profound hypothermia. Deep hypothermia and circulatory arrest are not essential factors in the pathophysiology but are often associated. The mechanism of basal ganglia injury is unknown.

Clinical Features. Most affected children are more than 1 year of age and have cyanotic heart disease with systemic to pulmonary collaterals. Choreoathetosis begins within 2 weeks postoperatively and may be associated with oral-facial dyskinesias, hypotonia, affective changes, and pseudobulbar signs. Some children have only mild chorea that resolves spontaneously within 2 months. Others may have severe exhausting chorea, unresponsive

BOX 14-2 Conditions That May Include Chorea

ALTERNATING HEMIPLEGIA (SEE CHAPTER 11)

BILATERAL STRIATAL NECROSIS (SEE DYSTONIA)

CEREBRAL PALSY*

- Congenital malformations (see Chapters 5 and 18)
- Intrauterine disease (see Chapter 1)
- Perinatal asphyxia (see Chapter 1)
- Unknown causes

GENETIC DISORDERS

- Ceroid lipofuscinosis (see Chapter 5)
- Guanidinoacetate methyltransferase deficiency (see Chapter 1)
- Idiopathic torsion dystonia
- Incontinentia pigmenti (see Chapter 1)
- Pantothenate kinase-associated neurodegeneration
- Pelizaeus-Merzbacher disease (see Chapter 5)
- Phenylketonuria* (see Chapter 5)
- Porphyria (see Chapter 7)

INFECTIOUS DISEASES

- Bacterial meningoencephalitis (see Chapter 4)
- Viral encephalitis (see Chapter 2)

METABOLIC ENCEPHALOPATHIES (SEE CHAPTER 2)

- Addison disease
- Burn encephalopathy
- Hypernatremia*
- Hypocalcemia*
- Hypoparathyroidism*
- Vitamin B12 deficiency

RETT SYNDROME (SEE CHAPTER 5)

VASCULAR

- Moyamoya disease (see Chapter 11)
- Poststroke (see Chapter 11)

*Denotes the most common conditions and the ones with disease modifying treatments

to treatment, which results in either death or severe neurological morbidity. Expect cognitive disturbance in half of survivors (du Plessis et al, 2002).

Diagnosis. The clinical features are the only basis for diagnosis. Magnetic resonance imaging (MRI) results are often normal during the acute illness.

Management. Sedation prevents exhaustion in severely affected children. The choreoathetosis is often refractory to drug therapy. Clonazepam, gabapentin, and pregabalin may prove useful to reduce the movement.

Drug-Induced Chorea

Choreiform movements and akathisia or dystonic posturing may occur as effects of drugs, especially dopamine antagonists. Chorea is more often a consequence of the abrupt discontinuation of dopamine antagonist. Akathisia is more likely to be a dose-related effect, whereas dystonia is usually an idiosyncratic reaction (see the section on Dystonia later in this chapter). Phenytoin and ethosuximide may induce chorea as a toxic or idiosyncratic manifestation. Oral contraceptives may induce chorea. The mechanism is unknown. Neuroleptics are associated with idiosyncratic dystonic reactions and tardive dyskinesia, and stimulant drugs (dextroamphetamine and methylphenidate) are associated with chorea, akathisia, and tics (see the section on Tic and Tourette Syndrome later in this chapter).

Tardive Dyskinesia

The term tardive dyskinesia denotes drug-induced choreiform movements that occur late in the course of drug therapy. These movements are often limited to the lingual, facial, and buccal muscles. Drug-induced buccolingual dyskinesia is unusual in children.

Tardive dyskinesias are most often associated with drugs used to modify behavior (neuroleptics), such as phenothiazines, haloperidol, risperdone, quetiapine or olanzapine, and antiemetics such as metoclopramide and prochlorperazine; they also occur in children with asthma treated with theophylline. The estimated annual incidence of tardive dyskinesia in children taking neuroleptic drugs is less than 1% (Correll & Kane, 2007). The incidence after long-term exposure in children is reported as high as 9.8%, still less than the 23.4% reported in adults (Jankovic & Mejia, 2010).

Clinical Features. Tardive dyskinesia is a complex of stereotyped movements. It usually affects the mouth and face, resembles chewing, and includes tongue protrusion and lip smacking; the trunk may be involved in rocking movements and the fingers in alternating flexion and extension resembling piano playing. Limb chorea, dystonia, myoclonus, tics, and facial grimacing may be associated features. Stress exacerbates the movements and sleep relieves them.

Symptoms appear months to years after the start of therapy and are not related to changes in dosage. In children, discontinuing the drug usually stops the movement, but the movements may remain unchanged in adults.

Diagnosis. Drug-induced dyskinesia is suspected in any child who shows abnormal movements of the face or limbs while taking neuroleptic drugs. The distinction of tardive dyskinesia from facial tics is important in children with Tourette syndrome and the distinction of facial mannerisms from tics in children with schizophrenia.

Management. Discontinue all neuroleptic drugs as quickly as possible when symptoms of dyskinesia develop. This may not be practical when psychosis requires drug therapy. In such circumstances, the movements sometimes respond to diazepam.

Emergent Withdrawal Syndrome

Chorea and myoclonus may appear for the first time after abruptly discontinuing or reducing the dosage of neuroleptic drugs. Lingual-facial-buccal dyskinesia may be present as well. The symptoms are self-limited and cease in weeks to months. Slow tapering of neuroleptics reduces the possibility of this syndrome. Reintroduction of the medication with slower withdrawal may be helpful in cases triggered by abrupt removal of a dopamine blocking agent (Jankovic & Mejia, 2010).

Genetic Disorders

Cerebellar ataxia is often the initial feature of abetalipoproteinemia and ataxia-telangiectasia. Chorea may occur in both conditions, but only in ataxia-telangiectasia does chorea occur without ataxia. Huntington disease is an important cause of chorea and dystonia, but in children the initial feature is declining school performance. The discussion of Huntington disease in children is in Chapter 5.

Benign Familial (Hereditary) Chorea

Benign familial chorea is a rare disorder transmitted by autosomal dominant inheritance (Kleiner-Fisman et al, 2003). The gene locus is on chromosome 14q. Benign familial chorea and familial paroxysmal choreoathetosis (see Chapter 1) may be genetically related disorders.

Clinical Features. The onset of chorea is usually in early childhood, often when the child is beginning to walk. Delayed motor development may be associated. Other possible features are intention tremor, dysarthria, hypotonia, and athetosis. Intelligence is normal. Most children have only chorea, which declines in intensity by adolescence. Adults may be asymptomatic or may have mild hypotonia and ataxia.

Diagnosis. Benign familial chorea may be difficult to distinguish from other causes of chorea in children, especially familial paroxysmal chorea. A family history of the disorder is critical to diagnosis, but difficult to obtain when parents show incomplete expression. Chorea is continuous and not episodic or paroxysmal. Neuroimaging studies and EEG results are normal.

Management. Chlorpromazine or haloperidol is beneficial in some individuals.

Fahr Disease

Fahr disease is the combination of encephalopathy and progressive calcification of the basal ganglia. *Idiopathic basal ganglia calcification* (IBGC) is another term applied to the same condition (Sobrido et al 2007). Calcification of the basal ganglia occurs with infectious, metabolic, and genetic disorders. Inheritance of IBGC disease is as an autosomal dominant trait (chromosome 14q). Most affected people are asymptomatic (Bodaty et al, 2002). The pathogenesis is unclear.

Clinical Features. Onset may be in childhood, but the usual age is in the third to fifth decades. The core clinical features of IBGC are neuropsychiatric and movement disorders. The expression of IBGC varies within a family.

Diagnosis. Diagnosis requires bilateral calcification of the basal ganglia associated with neurological deterioration and the absence of an underlying metabolic disorder. The most common area of calcification is the globus pallidus. However, additional areas of involvement include the putamen, caudate, dentate, thalamus, and cerebral white matter. Every child with basal ganglia calcification requires assessment of parathyroid function to exclude the possibility of either hyperparathyroidism or pseudohypoparathyroidism.

Management. Specific treatment is not available. Symptoms may respond to drug therapy.

Neuroacanthocytosis (Choreoacanthocytosis)

The term neuroacanthocytosis encompasses several disorders including autosomal recessive chorea-acanthocytosis and X-linked McLeod syndrome (Walker et al, 2007). Familial and nonfamilial cases of a progressive neurological disorder exist in which the main features are chorea and acanthocytosis with normal lipoprotein levels. The acanthocyte is an abnormal erythrocyte that has thorny projections from the cell surface. Acanthocytosis occurs in at least three neurological syndromes: McLeod syndrome (see Chapter 8), neuroacanthocytosis, and abetalipoproteinemia (see Chapter 10). The clinical features in severe cases of McLeod syndrome may be similar to those of neuroacanthocytosis.

Clinical Features. Onset is usually in adult life but may occur as early as the first decade. The most consistent neurological findings are impairment of frontal lobe function and psychiatric symptoms. Tics, oromandibular dyskinesia and dystonia, and self-mutilation of the lips may be associated features. Phenotypic variability is considerable and may include axonal neuropathy, loss of tendon reflexes, dementia, seizures, and neurosis.

Diagnosis. The association of acanthocytes or echinocytes (cells with rounded projections) and neurological disease in the absence of lipoprotein abnormality is required for diagnosis. Exclusion of McLeod syndrome is by testing for the Kell antigen.

Management. Only symptomatic treatment is available. Death occurs 10 to 20 years after onset.

Paroxysmal Choreoathetosis

Paroxysmal choreoathetosis occurs in children who are otherwise normal and in children with an obvious underlying static encephalopathy. The normal children have a genetic disease, familial paroxysmal choreoathetosis (see Chapter 1), and the abnormal children may have one of several nongenetic disorders. Acquired paroxysmal choreoathetosis occurs most often in children with cerebral palsy. Either hemiplegia or diplegia may be present, and the involuntary movements affect only the paretic limbs. The onset of the movement disorder often begins 10 or more years after the acute encephalopathy.

Systemic Disorders

Hyperthyroidism

Chapter 15 discusses the ocular manifestations of thyrotoxicosis. Tremor is the most common associated movement disorder. Chorea is unusual, but, when present, may affect the face, limbs, and trunk. The movements cease when the child becomes euthyroid.

Lupus Erythematosus

Clinical Features. Lupus-associated chorea is uncommon but may be the initial feature of the disease. Onset of symptoms is 7 years before to 3 years after the appearance of systemic features. It is indistinguishable from Sydenham chorea in appearance. The average duration is 12 weeks, but one-quarter of patients have recurrences. Additional neurological features of lupus (ataxia, psychosis, and seizures) are common in children who have chorea but occur only after the appearance of systemic symptoms. Therefore, chorea may be a solitary manifestation of disease.

Diagnosis. The diagnosis is clear in children with known lupus erythematosus. When chorea is the initial feature of lupus, the diagnosis is more problematic. The erythrocyte sedimentation rate may be elevated in both lupus and Sydenham chorea and is not a distinguishing feature. The presence of elevated concentrations of antinuclear antibodies and anti-DNA lupus antibodies is critical to diagnosis.

Management. The treatment of children with neurological manifestations of lupus erythematosus requires high doses of corticosteroids. The overall outcome is poor.

Pregnancy (Chorea Gravidarum)

Chorea of any cause beginning in pregnancy is chorea gravidarum. Rheumatic fever was once the most frequent cause but it is now the antiphospholipid antibody syndrome, with or without systemic lupus erythematosus.

Clinical Features. The onset of chorea is usually during the second to fifth month of pregnancy but may begin postpartum. Cognitive change may accompany the chorea. Symptoms usually resolve spontaneously within weeks to months.

Diagnosis. Women who develop chorea during pregnancy require studies for the rheumatic fever, antiphospholipid antibody syndrome, and systemic lupus erythematosus.

Management. This is a self-limited condition, and drugs should be used cautiously so as not to harm the fetus. Pimozide, risperidone and haloperidol may be useful.

Sydenham (Rheumatic) Chorea

Sydenham chorea is the most common cause of acquired chorea in children. It is a cardinal feature of rheumatic fever and is sufficient alone to make the diagnosis. Rheumatic chorea occurs primarily in populations with untreated streptococcal infections. One hypothesis is that a mistaken antibody attack against cells in the basal ganglia occurs after exposure of genetically predisposed children to group A, β-hemolytic streptococcus infection.

Clinical Features. The onset is frequently insidious and diagnosis often delayed. Chorea, hypotonia, dysarthria, and emotional lability are cardinal features. Difficulty in school may bring the child to medical attention. Chorea causes the child to be restless, and discipline by the teacher results in emotional stress. Obsessive-compulsive behavior may be present and the behavioral change considered a sign of mental illness.

Examination reveals a fidgeting child with migratory chorea of limbs and face. Initially, the chorea may be unilateral, but eventually becomes generalized in most patients. Efforts to conceal chorea with voluntary movement only add to the appearance of restlessness. Gradual improvement occurs over several months. Most recover completely. Rheumatic valvular heart disease develops in one-third of untreated patients.

Diagnosis. The clinical features establish the diagnosis. Laboratory tests are not confirmatory. The differential diagnosis includes lupus-associated chorea and drug-induced chorea. Examine the blood for lupus antinuclear antibodies and thyroid function. The onset of Sydenham chorea is usually 4 months after the provocative streptococcal infection, and the antistreptolysin O titer may be then back to normal or only slightly increased. During the time of illness, T_2-weighted MRI images may show increased signal intensity in the putamen and globus pallidus that resolves when the child has recovered.

Management. Most importantly, evaluate the heart by echocardiogram as subclinical valvular involvement is common and changes the management with addition of aspirin and close monitoring. Dopamine blocking agents such as pimozide usually control acute neurological symptoms without producing sedation. If pimozide does not relieve the symptoms, benzodiazepines, phenothiazines, or haloperidol are therapeutic options. The treatment of all children with Sydenham chorea is the same as for acute rheumatic fever: penicillin in high doses for 10 days to eradicate active streptococcal infection and prophylactic penicillin therapy until age 21.

DYSTONIA

Repetitive muscle contractions that are sustained at the peak and result in torsional postures characterize dystonia. The appearance is one of an abnormal posture rather than an involuntary movement. The muscle contractions can affect the limbs, trunk, or face (*grimacing*). Involvement may be of a single body part (*focal dystonia*), two or more contiguous body parts (*segmental dystonia*), the arm and leg on one side of the body (*hemidystonia*), or one or both legs and the contiguous trunk and any other body part (*generalized dystonia*).

Box 14-3 summarizes the differential diagnosis of abnormal posturing. Continuous motor unit activity (see Chapter 8) may be difficult to distinguish from dystonia by clinical inspection alone, especially when only one or two limbs are affected. Electromyography distinguishes the two disorders in many cases.

BOX 14-3 Differential Diagnosis of Abnormal Posturing

- Dystonia*
- Hysteria
- Muscular dystrophy
- Myotonia
- Neuromyotonia
- Rigidity
- Spasticity*
- Stiff man syndrome

*Denotes the most common conditions and the ones with disease modifying treatments

Persistent focal dystonias are relatively common in adults but are unusual in children except when drug induced. Most dystonias in children begin focally and eventually become generalized. Children with focal, stereotyped movements of the eyelids, face, or neck are much more likely to have a tic than focal dystonia. Box 14-4 lists childhood forms of focal dystonia.

Generalized dystonia usually begins in one limb. The patient has difficulty performing an act rather than a movement, so that the foot becomes dystonic when walking forward but may not be dystonic when sitting, standing, or running. Sensory tricks are maneuvers such as the patient touching his or her chin, which result in transient control of the dystonia.

Drug-Induced Dystonia

Acute Reactions

Focal or generalized dystonia may occur as an acute idiosyncratic reaction following a first dose of dopamine antagonist (antiemetics and antipsychotics). Possible reactions include trismus, opisthotonos, torticollis, and oculogyric crisis. Difficulty with swallowing and speaking may occur. Metoclopramide, a nonphenothiazine antiemetic that blocks postsynaptic dopamine receptors, may produce acute and delayed (tardive) dystonia. The acute reactions are usually self-limited or respond to treatment with anticholinergics such as benztropine, but they may be prolonged and resistant to therapy. A dose of diphenhydramine may resolve the acute reaction. I always instruct my patients to have some diphenoydramine available when starting dopamine-blocking agents.

BOX 14-4 Differential Diagnosis of Dystonia in Childhood

Focal Dystonia

- Blepharospasm
- Dopa-responsive dystonia*
- Drug-induced dystonia
- Generalized dystonia beginning as focal dystonia
- Torticollis
- Writer's cramp

Generalized Genetic Dystonias

- Ataxia with episodic dystonia (see Chapter 10)
- Ceroid lipofuscinosis (see Chapter 5)
- Dopa-responsive dystonia*
- Familial paroxysmal choreoathetosis (see Chapter 1)
- Glutaric acidemia type I
- Hallervorden-Spatz disease
- Hepatolenticular degeneration (Wilson disease)
- Huntington disease (see Chapter 5)
- Idiopathic torsion dystonia
- Infantile bilateral striatal necrosis
- Leber disease (see Chapter 16)
- Machado-Joseph disease (see Chapter 10)
- Mitochondrial disorders (see Chapters 5, 8, and 11)
- Transient paroxysmal dystonia of infancy (see Chapter 1)

Generalized Symptomatic Dystonias

- Perinatal cerebral injury (see Chapter 1)
- Postinfectious
- Poststroke
- Posttraumatic
- Toxin-induced
- Tumor-induced

Hemidystonia

- Alternating hemiplegia (see Chapter 11)
- Antiphospholipid syndrome (see Chapter 11)
- Basal ganglia tumors
- Neuronal storage disorders

*Denotes the most common conditions and the ones with disease modifying treatments

BOX 14-5 Differential Diagnosis of Blepharospasm in Childhood

- Continuous motor unit activity
- Drug-induced
- Encephalitis
- Hemifacial spasm
- Hepatolenticular degeneration (Wilson disease)
- Huntington disease
- Hysteria
- Myokymia
- Myotonia
- Schwartz-Jampel syndrome
- Seizures

Tardive Dystonia

Usually, tardive dystonia has a generalized distribution in children, but occurs as a focal disturbance in adults. Tetrabenazine is helpful in most patients, and anticholinergic drugs offer relief in others.

Focal Dystonias

Blepharospasm

Blepharospasm is an involuntary spasmodic closure of the eyes. Box 14-5 summarizes the differential diagnosis for children. Essential blepharospasm, an incapacitating condition, is a disorder of middle or late adult life and never begins in childhood. Tics account for almost all cases of involuntary eye closure in children.

BOX 14-6 Differential Diagnosis of Torticollis and Head Tilt

- Benign paroxysmal torticollis*
- Cervical cord syringomyelia (see Chapter 12)
- Cervical cord tumors (see Chapter 12)
- Cervicomedullary malformations* (see Chapters 10 and 18)
- Diplopia* (see Chapter 15)
- Dystonia
- Familial paroxysmal choreoathetosis (see Chapter 1)
- Juvenile rheumatoid arthritis
- Posterior fossa tumors (see Chapter 10)
- Sandifer syndrome
- Spasmus nutans* (see Chapter 15)
- Sternocleidomastoid injuries
- Tics and Tourette syndrome*

*Denotes the most common conditions and the ones with disease modifying treatments

Eye fluttering occurs during absence seizures (see Chapter 1) but is not confused with dystonia. Focal dystonia involving eye closure in children is usually drug induced.

Baclofen, clonazepam, trihexyphenidyl, and injections of botulinum A toxin are often successful in treating blepharospasm and orofacial dystonia in adults.

Torticollis

Box 14-6 summarizes the differential diagnoses of torticollis and head tilt. The first step in diagnosis is to distinguish fixed from nonfixed torticollis. In fixed torticollis, the neck is not moveable to the neutral position. The causation may be a structural disturbance of the cervical vertebrae or may occur when pain prevents movement.

Evidence of concurrent dystonia in the face or limbs indicates the need for further evaluation directed at underlying causes of dystonia. When torticollis and corticospinal tract signs (hyperactive tendon reflexes, ankle clonus, or extensor plantar responses) are associated, suspect a cervical spinal cord disturbance, and order a cervical MRI. Symptoms of increased intracranial pressure indicate a posterior fossa tumor with early herniation. When torticollis is the only abnormal feature, the underlying causes are focal dystonia, injury to the neck muscles, and juvenile rheumatoid arthritis.

Nonfixed torticollis that occurs in attacks suggests benign paroxysmal torticollis, familial paroxysmal choreoathetosis, or familial dopa-responsive dystonia (Schneider et al, 2006). The combination of head tilt and nystagmus in infants is termed *spasmus nutans* (see Chapter 15).

Benign Paroxysmal Torticollis. The underlying cause of benign paroxysmal torticollis is unknown. A migraine variant, closely related to benign paroxysmal vertigo (see Chapter 10), is the apparent cause in some infants but not in others.

Clinical Features. Onset is usually in the first year. Head tilting to one side (not always the same side) and slight head rotation characterize the episodes. The child may resist efforts to return the head to a neutral position, but overcoming the resistance is possible. Some children have no other symptoms, whereas others have pallor, irritability, malaise, and vomiting. Most attacks last for 1 to 3 days, end spontaneously, and tend to recur three to six times a year. Children who are old enough to stand and walk become ataxic during attacks.

With time, the attacks may evolve into episodes characteristic of benign paroxysmal vertigo or classic migraine, or may simply cease without further symptoms. The disorder may occur in siblings indicating a genetic factor, but usually the family history only reveals migraine.

Diagnosis. Suspect the disorder in any infant with attacks of torticollis that remit spontaneously and pursue a family history of migraine. Familial paroxysmal choreoathetosis and familial paroxysmal dystonia do not begin during early infancy. Sandifer syndrome, intermittent retrocollis associated with reflux, is an alternative consideration.

Management. No treatment is available or needed for the acute attacks.

Writer's Cramp

Writer's cramp is a focal, task-specific dystonia. It may occur only when writing, or when performing other specific manual tasks such as typing or playing the piano (occupational cramp). The cramp is more often isolated but may be associated with other focal dystonias, such as torticollis, or with generalized dystonia.

Clinical Features. Onset is usually after 20 years of age but may be in the second decade. In writer's cramp or other task-specific dystonias, the dystonic postures occur when the patient attempts to write or perform the task. The initial features are any of the following: aching in the hand when writing, loss of handwriting neatness or speed, and difficulty in holding writing implements. All three symptoms are eventually present. Dystonic postures occur when the patient attempts to write. During writing, the hand and arm lift from the paper, and the fingers may flex or extend. Writing with the affected hand becomes impossible and the patient learns to write with the nondominant hand, which may also become dystonic.

Symptoms are at first intermittent and are especially severe when others observe the writing. Later the movement occurs with each attempt at writing. Some patients have life-long difficulty with using the dominant hand for writing and may have difficulty with other manual tasks as well. Others experience remissions and exacerbations. Progression to generalized dystonia is rare.

Diagnosis. Unfortunately, people often attribute the cause of writers or other task specific dystonias to psychological factors despite the lack of associated psychopathological features. Early diagnosis can save considerable expense and concern. Distinguish isolated focal dystonia and generalized dystonia with focal onset. Thoroughly explore the family history and repeat the examination to determine the presence of dystonia in other body parts.

Management. Botulinum toxin type A is used to treat focal dystonias. Oral medications are the same as those used to treat generalized dystonia used in patients with focal dystonia (see section on Idiopathic Torsion Dystonia later in this chapter).

Generalized Genetic Dystonias

The classification of autosomal dominant dystonias (DYT) uses a numeric system. Three DYTs are important entities in childhood.

Dopa-Responsive Dystonia

Other names for dopa-responsive dystonia include dystonia-parkinsonism syndrome, dystonia with diurnal variation, and Segawa disease. The cause of the syndrome is either of two different genetic abnormalities. The inheritance of one type is as an autosomal dominant trait and the other as an autosomal recessive trait. The dominant type is due to mutations in the gene for GTP cyclohydrolase 1, the cofactor for tyrosine hydroxylase (Furukawa, 2012); the recessive form is due to mutations in the tyrosine hydroxylase gene (Swoboda & Furukawa, 2008). Most reported cases of "juvenile parkinsonism" are probably variants of dopa-responsive dystonia.

Clinical Features. The onset of GTP cyclohydrolase 1-deficient dopa-responsive dystonia is approximately 6 years of age. The initial feature is usually foot dystonia, which causes a gait disturbance. Parkinsonian-like symptoms follow. Diurnal fluctuation in the severity of symptoms is common. Symptoms improve considerably on awakening, and worsen later in the day. Arm dystonia with abnormal hand posturing and postural tremor sometimes appears first. Examination reveals brisk deep-tendon reflexes in the legs and ankle clonus. A gradual progression to generalized dystonia follows. Intellectual, cerebellar, sensory, or autonomic disturbances do not occur.

Tyrosine hydroxylase deficiency has a broader phenotype. Onset is often in infancy. Some have mild dystonia and others have a parkinsonian-like syndrome and encephalopathy. Marked variation in expressivity occurs between affected members of the same kindred. Age at onset is usually between 4 and 8 years but may be as early as infancy and as late as age 12 years. Incorrect diagnosis of early-onset cases is common; cerebral palsy is the common misdiagnosis. The initial feature is nearly always a gait disturbance caused by leg dystonia. Flexion at the hip and knee and plantar flexion of the foot cause toe walking. Both flexor and extensor posturing of the arms develop, finally parkinsonian features such as cogwheel rigidity, mask-like facies, and bradykinesia appears. The disease reaches a plateau in adolescence. Postural or intention tremor occurs in almost half of patients, but typical parkinsonian tremor is unusual.

In some families, dystonia is predominantly cervical in location. Additional symptoms may include a postural tremor and laryngeal dystonia. The genetic defect in such cases is not the same as for dopa-responsive dystonia (Schneider et al, 2006).

Diagnosis. Every child with dystonia should be treated with a trial dose of *sinemet*, the original brand of carbidopa-levodopa. The response in affected children is dramatic. Some generic preparations are less effective; therefore I prefer the brand name Sinemet® for a diagnostic trial. Molecular genetic testing is available on a clinical basis for both forms of dopa-responsive dystonia.

Management. A small dose of carbidopa-levodopa usually provides immediate and complete relief in most patients, even when initiating treatment long after symptoms begin. No other dystonia responds so well. Initiate carbidopa-levodopa therapy at the lowest possible dose and slowly increase it until a response is established. Long-term therapy is beneficial and required. Symptoms return after discontinuing the drug. Trihexyphenidyl, in doses lower than ordinarily needed to treat idiopathic torsion dystonia, and bromocriptine are also partially effective.

Glutaric Acidemia Type I

Glutaric acidemia type I is a rare inborn error in the catabolism of lysine, hydroxylysine, and tryptophan. Genetic transmission is by autosomal recessive inheritance. Deficiency of glutaryl-coenzyme-A dehydrogenase causes the disorder.

Clinical Features. Megalencephaly is usually present at birth. Neurological findings may be otherwise normal. Two patterns of illness occur in affected infants (Bjugstad et al, 2000). In two-thirds of infants, the initial feature is an acute encephalopathy characterized by somnolence, irritability, and excessive sweating. Seizures sometimes occur. The prognosis in such cases is poor. Afterward, development regresses and progressive choreoathetosis and dystonia occur.

The other pattern is more insidious and the prognosis better. Affected infants are at first hypotonic and later have mild developmental delay and dyskinesias. Cerebral palsy is a common misdiagnosis (see Chapter 12).

Diagnosis. Metabolic acidosis may be present. Abnormal urinary concentration of glutaric, 3-hydroxyglutaric, 3-hydroxybutyric, and acetoacetic acids are detectable. Showing the enzyme deficiency in cultured fibroblasts establishes the diagnosis. Molecular genetic testing and prenatal diagnosis are available. Computed tomography often shows diffuse attenuation of cerebral white matter and cerebral atrophy, most marked in the frontal and temporal lobes.

Management. Disease progression slows in patients with little or no neurological disease by oral carnitine supplementation together with the immediate administration of fluids, glucose, electrolytes, and antipyretics during febrile illnesses (Strauss et al, 2007).

Hepatolenticular Degeneration (Wilson Disease)

Genetic transmission of hepatolenticular degeneration is by autosomal recessive inheritance. The defective gene site is chromosome 13q14-q21, and the abnormal gene product is the main copper transporter moving copper from the hepatocytes into the bile. Mutations that completely prevent function of the gene produce a more severe phenotype than certain types of missense mutations. Tissue damage occurs after excessive copper accumulation in the liver, brain, and cornea.

Clinical Features. Wilson disease can present with hepatic, neurological, or psychiatric disturbances, alone or in combination. The age at onset ranges from 3 to over 50 years (Cox & Roberts, 2006). *Hepatic failure is the prominent clinical feature in children less than 10 years of age, usually without neurological symptoms or signs.* Neurological manifestations with only minimal symptoms of liver disease are more likely when the onset of symptoms is in the second decade. A single symptom, such as a disturbance of gait or speech, is often the initial feature and may remain unchanged for years. Eventually the initial symptoms worsen and new features develop (dysarthria, dystonia, dysdiadochokinesia, rigidity, gait and postural abnormalities, tremor, and drooling). Dystonia of bulbar muscles is responsible for three prominent features of the disease: dysarthria, a fixed pseudosmile (risus sardonicus), and a high-pitched whining noise on inspiration.

Psychiatric disturbances precede the neurological abnormalities in 20% of cases. They range from behavioral disturbances to paranoid psychoses. Dementia is not an early feature of the disease.

The Kayser-Fleischer ring, a yellow-brown granular deposit at the limbus of the cornea, is a certain indicator of the disease. The cause is copper deposition in the Descemet membrane. It is present in almost all patients with neurological manifestations, although it may be absent in children with liver disease alone.

Diagnosis. Hepatolenticular degeneration is a consideration in any child with acquired and progressive dysarthria and dystonia. The association of chronic liver disease with the neurological disturbances increases the probability of hepatolenticular degeneration. The detection of low serum copper and ceruloplasmin concentrations and increased urinary copper excretion or the demonstration of a Kayser-Fleischer ring by slit-lamp examination establishes the diagnosis. Ninety-six percent of patients will have a serum ceruloplasmin concentration of less than 20 mg/dL, corresponding to less than 56 g/dL of ceruloplasmin copper. Molecular genetic testing of the *ATP7B* gene (chromosomal locus 13q14.3-q21.1) is clinically available.

Management. Treatment is life-long. Copper chelating agents (e.g., penicillamine or trientine) that increase urinary excretion of copper are the primary treatment for Wilson disease. The dose of D-penicillamine is 250 mg four times a day for children more than 10 years of age and half as much for younger children. Ingestion of penicillamine is always on an empty stomach together with a daily dose of 25 mg pyridoxine. Measures of 24-hour urine copper excretion confirm chelation. Urinary copper values should run 5–10 times normal. Improvement is slow, and neurological improvement frequently takes several months. Worsening may occur during the first months of therapy, but this should not be a cause for alarm. Early treatment provides satisfactory results, without excess morbidity and mortality.

Oral administration of zinc interferes with absorption of copper and is useful after initial decoppering with a chelating agent. Antioxidants, such as vitamin E, help to prevent tissue damage, particularly to the liver. Liver transplantation is required for patients who fail to respond or cannot tolerate medical therapy. All siblings of patients with Wilson disease require careful screening for disease and early treatment.

Idiopathic Torsion Dystonia

Early-onset idiopathic torsion dystonia (DYT1) (dystonia musculorum deformans) is transmitted by autosomal dominant inheritance with reduced penetrance (30–40%) and variable expression. The gene locus is chromosome 9q34 (de Leon & Bressman, 2010). The frequency of idiopathic torsion dystonia in Ashkenazi Jews is five to ten times greater than in other groups. Nonfamilial cases probably represent autosomal dominant inheritance with incomplete penetrance.

Clinical Features. Age at onset has a bimodal distribution; for early onset the median is 9 years, and for late onset the median is 45 years. The early onset cases are more genetically homogeneous.

The limbs usually become dystonic before the trunk. The initial features may be in the arms, legs, or larynx. Early leg involvement is more common in children than in adults. Despite the focal features at onset, dystonia always generalizes in children, affecting the limbs and trunk.

Spontaneous stabilization is the rule, but remission is unusual. The eventual outcome varies from complete disability to functional independence.

Other clinical features include dysarthria, orofacial movements, dysphagia, postural tremor, and blepharospasm. Mental deterioration does not occur, but, as a group, patients with familial disease have a lower IQ than those with sporadic cases.

Diagnosis. The clinical features of dystonic movements and postures and the family history suggest the diagnosis. Normal perinatal history, no exposure to drugs, no evidence of intellectual or corticospinal deterioration, and no demonstrable biochemical disorder exclude other possibilities. Molecular genetic testing confirms the diagnosis.

Management. Medical management is often ineffective. Deep brain stimulation of the bilateral globus pallidum is useful in many patients (Volkmann & Benecke, 2002). High-dose anticholinergic therapy (trihexyphenidyl, 30 mg/day) provides the best medical results. While children tend to tolerate higher doses than adults, confusion and memory impairment may limit usefulness. Other drugs that may be of value include baclofen, carbamazepine, and benzodiazepines. All juvenile-onset dystonic patients deserve a trial of L-dopa to exclude dopa-responsive dystonia. Botulinum toxin is useful for selected focal problems.

Infantile Bilateral Striatal Necrosis

Bilateral striatal necrosis (BSN) occurs in several genetic disorders that share pathological features of bilateral, symmetric, spongy degeneration of the corpus striatum and degeneration of the globus pallidus (Straussberg et al, 2002). *Familial infantile striatal degeneration* is rare, and inheritance can be autosomal recessive or mitochondrial. The familial form has an insidious onset and a slowly progressive course; the sporadic form is associated with acute systemic illness. Many features of BSN overlap with Leigh syndrome and metabolic disorders, such as glutaric acidemia I and methylmalonic aciduria. Onset is in infancy or early childhood.

Clinical Features. Three clinical syndromes are associated with infantile BSN. One type has an insidious onset during infancy or childhood and a long clinical course that includes dystonia, cognitive impairment, seizures, and death. Most of these cases are probably mitochondrial disorders; one affected child had a point mutation in the mitochondrial ATPase 6 gene. A clinical and pathological overlap exists between progressive infantile BSN, subacute necrotizing encephalomyelopathy (see Chapter 5), and Leber hereditary optic neuropathy (see Chapter 16).

A second syndrome begins as an acute encephalopathy, usually following a febrile illness with nausea and vomiting. The major features are dystonia and tremor. The severity of symptoms may fluctuate at the time of intercurrent illness. Some children recover spontaneously; others are permanently impaired.

The third syndrome, described in Arab kinships, may have a wider distribution. The etiology may be defective transport of biotin across the blood-brain barrier. Transmission is probably by autosomal recessive inheritance. Onset is usually between age 3 and 5 years. The first symptoms are confusion, dysarthria, and dysphagia. Cranial nerve palsies, cogwheel rigidity, dystonia, and quadriparesis follow the initial features.

Diagnosis. The observation of static or progressive striatal necrosis on serial MRI examinations suggests the diagnosis.

Management. All features of biotin-responsive BSN respond to administration of biotin, 5–10 mg/kg/day, but reappear within 1 month after biotin is discontinued. All children with evidence of BSN deserve a trial of biotin.

Pantothenate Kinase-Associated Neurodegeneration

Pantothenate kinase-associated neurodegeneration (PKAN), previously called *Hallervorden-Spatz syndrome*, is a neurodegeneration with brain iron accumulation (Gregory & Hayflick, 2010). It is a genetic disorder transmitted as an autosomal recessive trait. The abnormality is in the *pank2* gene located on chromosome locus 20p13. Two other genetic disorders causing iron deposition in the globus pallidus are *aceruloplasminemia* and *neuroferritinopathy*. Both have adult onset and are not discussed in this text.

Clinical Features. The characteristic features of PKAN are progressive dystonia and basal ganglia iron deposition. The disorder becomes symptomatic between 2 and 10 years of age in more than half of patients but may appear as late as the third decade. The initial feature is progressive rigidity, first in the foot, causing an equinovarus deformity, and then in the hand. Other features are choreoathetosis, rigidity, and dysarthria. Two-thirds of patients have a pigmentary retinopathy (Hayflick et al, 2003). Mental deterioration and spasticity follow, with progression to spastic immobility and death within 5 to 10 years.

Diagnosis. The MRI features and molecular genetic testing are the basis for antemortem diagnosis. T_2-weighted MRI shows low-intensity signal images from the globus pallidus with a central area of increased signal intensity, *the eye-of-the-tiger sign* (Figure 14-1). Postmortem examination shows degeneration of the pallidum and substantia nigra with deposition of iron-containing material.

Management. Agents that chelate iron have not proved effective. Symptomatic treatment for dystonia includes intramuscular botulinum toxin, baclofen pump placement, oral trihexyphenidyl, and deep brain stimulation.

Rapid-Onset Dystonia-Parkinsonism

Rapid-onset dystonia-parkinsonism (DYT12) is a separate autosomal dominant form of dystonia characterized by an unusually rapid evolution of signs and symptoms (Brashear & Ozelius, 2011).

Clinical Features. The disorder is characterized by the acute (hours) or subacute (days to weeks) development of generalized dystonia and parkinsonism that involves the face and arms more than the legs. Symptoms respond poorly to treatment with levodopa. Age at onset is 4 to 55 years. Severe bulbar symptoms such as dysarthria, drooling, and orofacial dystonia are associated. Some show hypertonicity and hyperreflexia.

Diagnosis. Diagnosis depends on the clinical features. Molecular genetic testing is available on a research basis.

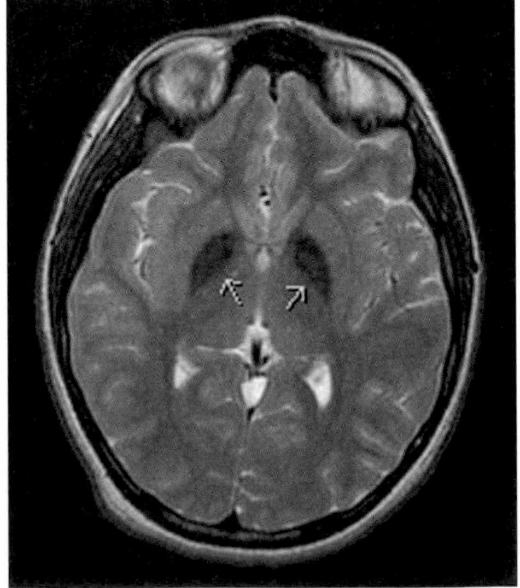

FIGURE 14-1 ■ Pantothenate kinase-associated neurodegeneration (Hallervorden-Spatz syndrome). T_2 axial MRI shows the characteristic iron deposition in the globus pallidus, the eye-of-the-tiger sign (arrows).

Management. A trial of levodopa is reasonable in any child with new-onset dystonia even though it is not effective in this disorder. When dopa fails, then high dosages of benzodiazepines or trihexyphenidyl may provide symptomatic relief. Children tolerate high dosages when the dose is slowly increased; adults rarely tolerate such high dosages.

Symptomatic Generalized Dystonia

An underlying tumor, active encephalopathy, or prior brain damage can cause dystonia.

Clinical Features. The onset of dystonia may be at the time of an acute encephalopathy, after the acute phase is over, or several years later, when the encephalopathy is static. Delayed-onset chorea and dystonia in children with perinatal disturbances such as asphyxia or kernicterus usually begin by 2 to 3 years of age but may begin in adolescence. After involuntary movements appear, they tend to become progressively more severe, but intellectual decline is not an associated feature. Delayed-onset dystonia may have a generalized distribution.

Hemidystonia most often occurs after stroke or head injury but may be a symptom of neuronal storage diseases or tumors of the basal ganglia, alternating hemiplegia, and the antiphospholipid antibody syndrome (see Chapter 11). The dystonic limbs are contralateral to the damaged basal ganglia.

Diagnosis. Children with a known cause for the development of dystonia or chorea do not require extensive studies. The new symptoms are discouraging for patients and families who have adjusted to a fixed neurological deficit. Provide assurance that the new symptoms are not evidence of new brain degeneration, but only the appearance of new symptoms from old lesions. This sequence is most likely when injury is perinatal and brain maturation is required to manifest involuntary movements.

The appearance of hemidystonia, even with a known predisposing event, necessitates MRI to look for localized changes that may require treatment, such as an expanding cyst. Consider the possibility of tumor in children who had been neurologically intact before hemidystonia appeared.

Management. The drugs used to treat symptomatic dystonia are no different from those used for genetic dystonia, but the results may not be as favorable. Botulinum toxin may be useful when specific muscle contractions are causing severe disability.

Hemifacial Spasm

Involuntary, irregular contractions of the muscles innervated by one facial nerve characterize hemifacial spasm. This is a very rare condition in children. The spasms may develop because of aberrant regeneration following facial nerve injury, secondary to posterior fossa tumor, or without apparent cause.

Clinical Features. Spasms are embarrassing and disturbing but not painful. The orbicularis oculi muscles are the muscles affected first and most commonly, causing forced closure of the eye. As facial muscles on one side become affected, they pull the mouth to one side. Spasms may occur several times a minute, especially during times of stress. The subsequent course depends on the underlying cause.

Diagnosis. Hemifacial spasm in children may be mistaken for a focal seizure. The stereotyped appearance of the spasm and a concurrent normal EEG are distinguishing features. Suspect posterior fossa tumor in every child with hemifacial spasm. Brain MRI is required in every instance unless symptoms are explained by a history of prior facial nerve injury.

Management. Some patients respond to treatment with carbamazepine at anticonvulsant doses (see Chapter 1), but most do not respond to medical therapy. Injection of botulinum toxin into the muscles in spasm is the treatment of choice. Surgical procedures to relieve pressure on the facial nerve from adjacent vessels are of questionable value.

MIRROR MOVEMENTS

Mirror movements are involuntary movements of one side of the body, usually the hands, which occur as mirror reversals of an intended movement on the other side of the body. They are normal during infancy and tend to disappear before 10 years of age, coincident with myelination of the corpus callosum. Persistence of mirror movements may be a familial trait caused by ipsilateral and contralateral organization of the corticospinal pathways. Obligatory mirror movements are abnormal even in infants and suggest a congenital abnormality at the cervicomedullary junction.

MYOCLONUS

The term myoclonus encompasses several involuntary movements characterized by rapid muscle jerks. They are less frequent and severe during sleep, but may not disappear. Myoclonus may be rhythmic or nonrhythmic; focal, multifocal, or generalized; or spontaneous or activated by movement (action myoclonus) or sensory stimulation (reflex myoclonus).

The distinction of nonepileptic myoclonus from tic, chorea, tremor, and seizures is easily accomplished. Tics are usually more complex and stereotyped movements than myoclonus and briefly suppressed by voluntary effort; myoclonus is not voluntarily suppressible. Chorea is more random than myoclonus and often incorporated into voluntary movement; myoclonus is never part of a larger movement. Rhythmic myoclonus and tremor look alike and are difficult to distinguish clinically. Tremor is a continuous to-and-fro movement, whereas rhythmic myoclonus has a pause between movements.

Box 14-7 summarizes the etiological classification of myoclonus. Physiological myoclonus

BOX 14-7 Etiological Classification of Myoclonus

Physiological
- Anxiety-induced
- Exercise-induced
- Sleep jerks and nocturnal myoclonus

Essential

Epileptic (see Chapter 1)

Symptomatic
- Post-central nervous system injury
  - Hypoxia (see Chapter 2)
  - Trauma (see Chapter 2)
  - Stroke (see Chapter 11)
- Basal ganglia degenerations
  - Idiopathic torsion dystonia
  - Hallervorden-Spatz disease
  - Hepatolenticular degeneration (Wilson disease)
  - Huntington disease (see Chapter 5)
- Drug-induced
  - Carbamazepine
  - Levodopa
  - Tricyclic antidepressants
- Lysosomal storage diseases (see Chapter 5)
- Metabolic encephalopathies (see Chapter 2)
  - Dialysis syndromes
  - Disorders of osmolality
  - Hepatic failure
  - Renal failure
- Myoclonic encephalopathy (see Chapter 10)
  - Idiopathic
  - Neuroblastoma
- Spinal cord tumor (see Chapter 12)
- Spinocerebellar degenerations (see Chapter 10)
- Toxic encephalopathies (see Chapter 2)
- Viral encephalitis

occurs in normal people when falling asleep, during sleep (nocturnal myoclonus), when waking up, and during times of anxiety. Nocturnal myoclonus is a rhythmic jerking of the legs during sleep that is common in children. It requires distinction from the restless legs syndrome, a genetic disorder transmitted by autosomal dominant inheritance (Earley, 2003). Leg discomfort at rest, relieved by movement, characterizes the syndrome. Misdiagnosis of such symptoms as "growing pains" is common. Periodic limb movements mainly occur during sleep but also during wakefulness.

Epileptic myoclonus is associated with epileptiform activity on the EEG (see Chapter 1). The causes of symptomatic myoclonus include drugs, electrolyte abnormalities, a cerebral injury, or part of a generalized progressive encephalopathy.

Essential Myoclonus

Essential myoclonus is a chronic condition of focal, segmental, or generalized jerking aggravated by action or stress. Affected people are otherwise normal. Occurrence is usually sporadic, but, when familial, transmission is by autosomal dominant inheritance.

Clinical Features. Onset is in the first or second decade. Both genders are equally affected. The movements are predominantly in the face, trunk, and proximal muscles. While usually generalized, they may be restricted to one side of the body. No other neurological disturbances develop, and life expectancy is not affected. Essential tremor may be present in the same family.

Diagnosis. The clinical features and family history establish the diagnosis. Careful neurological examination, EEG, and brain imaging exclude symptomatic and epileptic myoclonus. Even then, a period of observation and repeat laboratory investigations may be necessary to eliminate other causes.

Management. Mild essential myoclonus does not require treatment. Botulinum toxin type A injection into the affected muscles often reduces the movement. Levetiracetam and clonazepam are the drugs of choice in those requiring therapeutic intervention. Carbamazepine, tetrabenazine, and valproate are useful in symptomatic myoclonus and may be beneficial in generalized myoclonus as well.

Symptomatic Myoclonus

Myoclonus is often a symptom of an underlying neurological disease. Generalized myoclonus is the rule when the cause is a diffuse, progressive encephalopathy (such as lysosomal storage diseases) and segmental when the lesion is focal in the brainstem or spinal cord. Multifocal myoclonus may occur as a nondose-dependent side effect of carbamazepine therapy in children.

Posthypoxic Myoclonus (Lance-Adams Syndrome)

Posthypoxic myoclonus is a form of action myoclonus in patients who have suffered an episode of hypoxia. It does not follow hypoxic-ischemic encephalopathy of the newborn. Single or repetitive myoclonic jerks occur when voluntary movement is attempted. Facial and pharyngeal muscle myoclonus interferes with speech and swallowing. Cerebellar disturbances are usually associated findings.

Myoclonus usually begins during recovery from anoxic encephalopathy and once started never remits. It may respond to levetiracetam, valproate, 5-hydroxytryptophan, or clonazepam.

Segmental (Focal) Myoclonus

Segmental myoclonus is an involuntary contraction of contiguous muscles innervated by the brainstem or spinal cord. It may be rhythmic or nonrhythmic. Rhythmic segmental myoclonus looks like a focal seizure. The underlying causes in children are limited mainly to demyelinating diseases and intrinsic tumors. Cystic astrocytoma of the spinal cord is the major cause of spinal myoclonus and may be the initial feature (see Chapter 12).

Palatal myoclonus is the most common segmental myoclonus of brainstem origin. Unilateral or bilateral rhythmic contractions of the palate (80–180 per minute) that usually persist during sleep are characteristic. It may be associated with rhythmic contractions of the eyes, larynx, neck, diaphragm, trunk, and limbs. Lesions in the central tegmental tract or the dentato-olivary pathways cause palatal myoclonus. The median interval between the precipitating cause and the onset of palatal myoclonus is 10 to 11 months. Clonazepam and tetrabenazine are the most useful drugs in the treatment of segmental myoclonus.

RESTLESS LEGS SYNDROME

Once thought exclusively a disorder of adults, the increased laboratory investigation of sleep disorders in children reveals a small percentage with restless legs syndrome (Kotagal & Silber,

2004). At least four different genetic disorders are associated with the restless legs syndrome.

Clinical Features. The essential elements of the syndrome are an urge to move the legs, usually accompanied by uncomfortable or unpleasant sensations in the legs. These elements begin or worsen during periods of rest or inactivity such as lying or sitting; they are partially or totally relieved by movement and worse in the evening or at night (Allen et al, 2003). Sleep disturbances are associated. Almost two-thirds have a positive family history with mothers affected three times more often than fathers.

Diagnosis. Diagnosis is established on the basis of the clinical features. A sleep laboratory study is useful to diagnose this disorder and associated sleep disorders. Eighty percent of affected children have deficient serum ferritin blood concentrations.

Treatment. Oral iron is the initial intervention in those with low serum ferritin blood concentrations. Pharmacotherapy includes pramipexole, clonazepam, or gabapentin.

STEREOTYPIES

Stereotypies in children are commonly not associated with underlying pathology. In these cases they tend to be transient and outgrown when the child detects they are not socially well seen. Stereotypies are repeated, purposeless movements that may be simple or complex. Simple stereotypies are foot or finger tapping and hair curling. Complex stereotypies range from shuddering attacks to sequential movements of the head, arms, and body. They appear intentional. Occasionally, a history of similar movements is present in other family members.

The main differential diagnosis is with seizures and complex tics. Seizures are never as stereotyped. Complex tics are more difficult to differentiate. Stereotypies differ from tics in that suppression of the movement does not cause tension, and other features of the Tourette syndrome are not present. Stereotypies tend to disappear as the child ages. Treatment is neither needed nor effective. The best management is to ignore the movements.

TIC AND TOURETTE SYNDROME

Tics are stereotyped movements (motor tic) or utterances (verbal tic) that are sudden, brief, and purposeless. A tic can be accurately described and reproduced by an observer (e.g., "he blinks his eyes," "she clears her throat"). Tics are suppressible, but this requires significant effort and is not recommended. Stress exacerbates tics, relaxation reduces tics and sleep makes them stop.

Tourette syndrome is any combination of verbal and motor tics. It is not a separate disease, but rather part of a phenotypic spectrum that includes simple motor tic, attention deficit disorder, and obsessive-compulsive behavior (Jankovic, 2001). Transmission of the syndrome is as a highly penetrant, autosomal dominant trait in which males more commonly express tics and attention deficit disorder and females express obsessive-compulsive behavior. Bilineal transmission is common and may correlate with the severity of disease. Two abnormal gene loci are identified (13q31 and 11q23) (OMIM, 2007).

In addition to the strong evidence for a genetic basis for Tourette syndrome, environmental factors also play a role. Stimulants provoke tics in predisposed children, and streptococcal infection may cause the sudden onset of severe tic or obsessive-compulsive disorder. The term PANDAS (*pediatric autoimmune neuropsychiatric disorders associated with streptococcal infection*) acknowledges the association between streptococcal infection and the acute exacerbation of chorea or tics (Dale et al, 2001).

Clinical Features. Most affected children have normal intelligence; however, their school performance often is affected by inattentiveness from attention deficit disorder or overfixation on a single thought from their obsessive-compulsive traits. There is a higher incidence of behavioral disturbances in children with Tourette syndrome. Consider the movement disorder and the behavioral disturbances to each be an expression of the same underlying genetic defect; one does not cause the other.

Onset is any time from 2 to 15 years of age, with the mean between 6 and 7 years. The most severe period of tic severity is between 8 and 12 years of age, and half of children are tic-free by age 18 years. Often, neck muscles are the first affected, causing a head movement in which the child appears to be tossing hair back from the face. New motor tics develop either in place of, or in addition to, existing tics. They usually affect the head, eyes, or face. Common tics include blinking, grimacing, lip smacking, and shrugging of one or both shoulders.

The initial verbal tics are usually clearing of the throat, a snorting or sniffing noise, and coughing. Many children who make sniffing or coughing noises will undergo an extensive evaluation for allergies and undergo treatment that does not result in improvement in the noises. Grunting and hissing are other verbal tics. Uttering profanities (coprolalia) is rare in children. The patient is able to suppress profane language, when it occurs, and replace profanities with barking or coughing noises.

Symptoms wax-and-wane spontaneously and in response to stress and excitement. Tics usually become less frequent when children are out of school. While some children outgrow their tics, some have life-long difficulty and others have prolonged remissions with recurrence in middle age or later.

A large percentage of children with tics have an attention deficit disorder (ADD) and obsessive-compulsive disorder. The characteristics of attention deficit disorder are hyperactivity (ADHD), short attention span, restlessness, poor concentration, and impaired impulse control. Stimulants treat ADHD, but, unfortunately, all stimulants, including caffeine, have the potential to accentuate tics in genetically predisposed children.

Characteristics of obsessive-compulsive behavior include ritualistic actions and thoughts, which may include touching things repeatedly, placing objects in a certain place, washing and rewashing hands, obsessive thoughts about sex or violence, and counting objects. The following questions elicit a history of obsessive-compulsive behavior in family members: Do you routinely go back and check the door and lights after you leave the house? Do you have routines in the way that you clean the house or fold clothes? Eliciting a history in family members may further support the diagnosis.

Diagnosis. The clinical features establish the diagnosis. Laboratory tests are not helpful and are unnecessary in obvious cases. EEG, MRI, and psychological test results are normal. The serum concentration of neuronal autoantibodies does not differentiate PANDAS and Tourette syndrome from controls (Singer et al, 2005). Tics do not ordinarily occur in degenerative diseases of the nervous system or as an adverse reaction to drugs. Drug-induced tics are the potentiation of Tourette syndrome in a genetically predisposed child. Carbamazepine and lamotrigine, as well as amphetamine and methylphenidate, may trigger the symptoms. Withdrawal of the potentiating drug does not always stop the tics.

Management. Most children with tics and Tourette syndrome do not require drug treatment. The decision to prescribe medication depends on whether the tics bother the child. Drug therapy is not required if the tics bother the parents but do not disturb the child's life. Tell the parents that the tics are not a sign of progressive neurological or mental illness, that they may worsen with stress, and will diminish in frequency if ignored. Caffeine ingestion may exacerbate tics and should be reduced or removed from the diet.

Drug treatment is difficult to evaluate because the disorder's natural history is one of exacerbation and remission. The most useful drugs to control tics are pimozide, fluphenazine, ziprasidone, and haloperidol. The incidence of adverse effects is very low when small doses are used. The dosage of pimozide is initially 1 mg/day and is increased 1 mg each week as needed. The maintenance dosage is usually 2–4 mg/day and never exceeds 10 mg/day. The initial dose of fluphenazine is 1 mg/day and increased 1 mg each week. The usual maintenance dosage is 2–6 mg/day; never exceed 10 mg/day. Start haloperidol as a single dose of 0.5 mg at night and slowly increase 0.5 mg each week until tics are reasonably controlled or adverse reactions are noted. The usual maintenance dosage is 1–3 mg/day in two divided doses.

The major toxic effects of all three drugs are sedation, irritability, and depression of appetite. Dystonia and akathisia are idiosyncratic reactions. Clonidine and guanfacine are less effective in suppressing tics but safer and with better side effect profiles. In addition they often help with ADD symptoms. Dosing starts with clonidine 0.05 mg qd and may be increased up to 0.2 mg bid if tolerated, with sedation being the main side effect. Guanfacine is less sedating and just as effective. Begin with 0.5 mg qd and increase up to 2 mg bid as needed. A long-acting guanfacine is also available with doses ranging from 1 to 4 mg qd.

The majority of children with tics also suffer from anxiety and obsessive-compulsive disorder traits, which may interfere with social skills and learning. Treating this component often results in a more relaxed child, with secondary reduction in the frequency of tics. Citalopram or escitalopram are often my first choice in treating children with Tourette's syndrome. Start titration from 2 to 20 mg in the case of citalopram, or 1 to 10 mg in the case of escitalopram over 4 weeks. Some children may need higher doses. A few children develop anhedonia as a side effect of selective serotonin reuptake inhibitors. In those cases sertraline 25–100 mg qd may be a better choice.

The long-term outcome for children with tics is difficult to ascertain. Many reports indicate that tics improve and may cease during adult life, but a recent report indicates that tics were still present in 90 % of adults with childhood-onset tics (Pappert et al, 2003).

TREMOR

Tremor is an involuntary oscillating movement with a fixed frequency. The product of tremor frequency and amplitude is constant; because frequency decreases with age, amplitude increases. Shuddering, cerebellar ataxia or dysmetria, and asterixis are not tremors because they lack rhythm. Myoclonus may be rhythmic but the movement interrupts between oscillations.

All normal people have a low-amplitude physiological tremor, inherent in maintaining a posture, which is easily observed when holding a laser pointer steady. Physiological tremor enhances to a clinically detectable level in some situations (anxiety, excitement, exercise, fatigue, stress) and by drugs (adrenergic agonists, nicotine, prednisone, thyroid hormone, and xanthines). Hyperthyroidism is routinely associated with enhanced physiological tremor.

Parkinsonism is a common cause of pathological tremors in adults, but it does not occur in children except when drug induced or as part of a complex degenerative disorder. Typical parkinsonian tremor is seldom present in these situations. Essential (physiological) tremor is the major cause of tremor in children.

Essential Tremor

Essential (familial) tremor, which is an enhanced physiological tremor, is a monosymptomatic condition transmitted as an autosomal dominant trait. Two different gene loci are responsible. One maps to chromosome 3q13 (Louis et al, 2001) and the other to chromosome 2p25-p22 (Higgins et al, 2003).

Clinical Features. Childhood- and adult-onset cases are similar. The tremor usually appears in the second decade but can begin as early as 2 years of age. Only limbs in use show the tremor. The head, face, and neck are sometimes affected. The head tremor is usually mild and has a "no-no" appearance. The tremor frequency in the limbs is typically between 4 and 8 Hz. Essential tremor may impair function, especially schoolwork, and therefore disturbs the patient. In young children, the tremor has the appearance of restlessness or clumsiness. Only later does the tremor display an *action tremor* quality.

Greater precision of movement enhances the tremor. Therefore, tremor appears first and most prominently in the hands. It is further enhanced by anxiety, concentrated effort to stop the tremor, and fatigue. Essential tremor is generally life-long.

Diagnosis. Essential tremor in children is often mistaken for cerebellar dysfunction because it occurs with action (intention). The two are easily differentiated because essential tremor is rhythmic and not dysmetric (does not become worse at the endpoint) and because it is not associated with other signs of cerebellar dysfunction.

Management. Not all children with essential tremor require treatment. Medication should be reserved for situations in which tremor impairs function. Propranolol, 1–2 mg/kg/day, or primidone, 2–10 mg/kg/day, are effective to control tremor in 70% of cases. Other options include topiramate (Ondo et al, 2006). A surgical option for individuals with incapacitating essential tremor is deep brain stimulation of the ventral intermediate nucleus of the thalamus (Vaillencourt et al, 2003). Alcohol ingestion relieves essential tremor, but this treatment should be discouraged.

Paroxysmal Dystonic Head Tremor

Clinical Features. Paroxysmal dystonic head tremor is an uncommon nonfamilial syndrome of unknown cause. The major feature is attacks of horizontal head tremor (frequency 5–8 Hz), as if the person were saying "no." Onset occurs in adolescence, and all patients in the literature as well as three adolescents in our own practice were male. The attacks vary from 1 to 30 minutes, are not provoked by any single stimulus, and cannot be suppressed. A head tilt predates the onset of tremor by 5 to 10 years. The attacks are life-long but do not progress to other neurological symptoms. Results of the examination are otherwise normal.

Diagnosis. Imaging studies of the brain show no abnormalities. In an infant, the combination of head nodding and head tilt would be diagnosed as spasmus nutans even in the absence of nystagmus (see Chapter 15), and perhaps the underlying mechanism is similar.

Management. Daily use of clonazepam reduces the frequency and severity of attacks, but the head tilt may persist.

REFERENCES

Allen RP, Picchietti D, Hening WA, et al. Restless legs syndrome diagnosis and epidemiology workshop at the National Institutes of Health: International Restless Legs Syndrome Study Group. Sleep Medicine 2003;4:101–19.

Bjugstad KB, Goodman SI, Freed CR. Age at symptom onset predicts severity of motor impairment and clinical outcome of glutaric acidemia type 1. Journal of Pediatrics 2000;137:681–6.

Bodaty H, Mitchell P, Luscombe G, et al. Familial idiopathic basal ganglia calcification (Fahr's disease) without neurological, cognitive and psychiatric symptoms is not linked to the IBGC1 locus on chromosome 14. Human Genetics 2002;110:8–14.

Brashear A and Ozelius L. Rapid onset dystonia-parkinsonism. In: GeneClinics: Medical Genetics Knowledge Base [database online]. Seattle: University of Washington. Available at http://www.geneclinics.org. PMID: 20301294. Last updated August 25, 2011.

Correll C, Kane JM. One-year incidence rates of tardive dyskinesia in children and adolescents treated with second generation antipsychotics: A systematic review. Journal of Child and Adolescent Psychopharmacology 2007;17(5):647–55.

Cox DW, Roberts EA. Wilson Disease. In: GeneClinics: Medical Genetics Knowledge Base [database online]. Seattle: University of Washington. Available at http://www.geneclinics.org. Last updated 24 January 2006.

Dale RC, Church AJ, Cardoso F, et al. Poststreptococcal acute disseminated encephalomyelitis with basal ganglia involvement and auto-reactive antibasal ganglia antibodies. Annals of Neurology 2001;50:588–95.

de Leon, DMS, Bressman SB. Early-onset primary dystonia (DYT1). In: GeneClinics: Medical Genetics Knowledge Base [database online]. Seattle: University of Washington. Available at http://www.geneclinics.org. PMID: 20301665. Last updated November 23, 2010.

du Plessis AJ, Bellinger DC, Gauvreau K, et al. Neurologic outcome of choreoathetoid encephalopathy after cardiac surgery. Pediatric Neurology 2002;27:9–17.

Earley CJ. Restless legs syndrome. New England Journal of Medicine 2003;348:2103–9.

Furukawa Y. GTP Cyclohydrolase 1-deficient dopa-responsive dystonia In: GeneClinics: Medical Genetics Knowledge Base [database online]. Seattle: University of Washington; Available at http://www.geneclinics.org. PMID: 20301681 Last updated May 3, 2012.

Gregory A, Hayflick S. Pantothenate kinase-associated neurodegeneration. In: GeneClinics: Medical Genetics Knowledge Base [database online]. Seattle: University of Washington. Available at http://www.geneclinics.org. PMID: 20301663. Last updated March 23, 2010.

Hayflick SJ, Westaway SK, Levinson B, et al. Genetic, clinical, and radiographic delineation of Hallervorden-Spatz syndrome. New England Journal of Medicine 2003;348:33–40.

Higgins JJ, Jankovic J, Lombardi RQ, et al. Haplotype analysis of the ETM2 locus in essential tremor. Neurogenetics 2003;4:185–9.

Jankovic J, Mejia NI. Tardive dyskinesia and withdrawal emergent syndrome in children. Expert Review of Neurotherapeutics 2010;10(6):893–901.

Jankovic J. Tourette's syndrome. New England Journal of Medicine 2001;345:1184–92.

Kleiner-Fisman G, Rogaeva W, Houle S, et al. Benign hereditary chorea: Clinical, genetic, and pathological findings. Annals of Neurology 2003;54:244–7.

Kotagal S, Silber MH. Childhood-onset restless leg syndrome. Annals of Neurology 2004;56:803–7.

Louis ED. Essental tremor. New England Journal of Medicine 2001;345:887–91.

Ondo WG, Jankovic J, Connor GS, et al. Topiramate in essential tremor, placebo-controlled trial. Neurology 2006;66:672–7.

Online Mendelian Inheritance in Man, OMIM (TM). Gilles de la Tourette syndrome. Baltimore, MD: Johns Hopkins University. MIM Number:137580. Available at http://omim.org/entry/137580. Date last edited 6/21/2010.

Pappert EJ, Goetz CG, Louis ED, et al. Objective assessments of longitudinal outcome in Gilles de la Tourete syndrome. Neurology 2003;61:936–40.

Schneider SA, Mohire MD, Trender-Gerhardt I, et al. Familial dopa-responsive cervical dystonia. Neurology 2006;66:599–601.

Singer HS, Hong JA, Yoon BA, et al. Serum autoantibodies do not differentiate PANDA and Tourette syndrome from controls. Neurology 2005;65:1701–7.

Sobrido MJ, Hopfer S, Geschwind DH. Familial idiopathic basal ganglia calcification. In: GeneClinics: Medical Genetics Knowledge Base [database online]. Seattle: University of Washington. Available at http://www.geneclinics.org. Last updated September 20, 2007.

Strauss KA, Lazovic J, Wintermark M, et al. Multimodal imaging of striatal degeneration in Amish patients with glutaryl-CoA dehydrogenase deficiency. Brain 2007;130:1905–20.

Straussberg R, Shorer Z, Weitz R, et al. Familial infantile bilateral striatal necrosis. Clinical features and response to biotin treatment. Neurology 2002;59:983–9.

Swoboda K, Furukawa Y. Tyrosine hydroxylase deficiency. In: GeneClinics: Medical Genetics Knowledge Base [database online]. Seattle: University of Washington. Available at http://www.geneclinics.org. PMID: 20301610. Last updated February 8, 2008.

Vaillencourt DE, Sturman MM, Metmann LV, et al. Deep brain stimulation of the VIM thalamic nucleus modifies several features of essential tremor. Neurology 2003;61:919.

Volkmann J, Benecke R. Deep brain stimulation for dystonia: Patient selection and evaluation. Movement Disorders 2002;17(Suppl 3):S112–5.

Walker RH, Jung HH, Dobson-Stone C, et al. Nerologic phenotypes associated with acanthocytosis. Neurology 2007;68:92–8.

CHAPTER 15

Disorders of Ocular Motility

The maintenance of binocular vision requires harmonious function of the visual sensory system, gaze centers, ocular motor nerves, neuromuscular junction, and ocular muscles. This chapter deals with nonparalytic strabismus, paralytic strabismus (ophthalmoplegia), gaze palsies, ptosis, and nystagmus. The discussion of visual and pupillary disorders is in Chapter 16.

NONPARALYTIC STRABISMUS

Strabismus (squint), or abnormal ocular alignment, affects 3–4% of preschool children. Many individuals have a latent tendency for ocular misalignment, *heterophoria*, which becomes apparent only under stress or fatigue. During periods of misalignment, the child may have diplopia or headache. Constant ocular misalignment is *heterotropia.* Children with heterotropia suppress the image from one eye to avoid diplopia. If only one eye fixates continuously, visual acuity may be lost permanently in the other (developmental amblyopia).

In nonparalytic strabismus, the amount of deviation in different directions of gaze is relatively constant (comitant). Each eye moves through a normal range when tested separately (*ductions*), but the eyes are disconjugate when used together (*versions*). Many children with chronic brain damage syndromes, such as malformations or perinatal asphyxia, have faulty fusion or faulty control of conjugate gaze mechanisms (nonparalytic strabismus). In neurologically normal children, the most common cause of nonparalytic strabismus is either a genetic influence or an intraocular disorder. Ocular alignment in the newborn is usually poor, with transitory shifts of alignment from convergence to divergence. Ocular alignment usually establishes by 3 to 4 weeks of age but may not occur until 5 months. Approximately 2% of newborns exhibit tonic downward deviation of the eyes during the waking state. Constant ocular alignment usually begins after 3 months of age. The eyes assume a normal position during sleep and are able to move upward reflexively.

Esotropia

Esotropia is a constant inward deviation (convergence) of the eyes. It is called alternating esotropia when fixation occurs with both eyes. Unilateral esotropia is when fixation occurs continuously with the opposite eye. Early onset esotropia presents before 6 months of age. The observation of accommodative esotropia is usually between 2 and 3 years of age, and may be undetected until adolescence.

Clinical Features. Children with infantile esotropia often alternate fixation between eyes and may cross-fixate, i.e., look to the left with the right eye and to the right with the left eye. The misalignment is sufficient that family members see that a problem exists. Some children fixate almost entirely with one eye and are at risk for permanent loss of visual acuity, *developmental amblyopia*, in the other.

Accommodative esotropia occurs when accommodation compensates for hyperopia. Accommodation more sharply focuses the blurred image. Because convergence accompanies accommodation, one eye turns inward. Some children with accommodative esotropia cross-fixate and use each eye alternatively, while the other maintains fixation. However, if one eye is more hyperopic than the other eye, only the better eye fixates and the unused eye has a considerable potential for amblyopia.

Diagnosis. An ophthalmologist should examine the eyes to determine whether hyperopia is present.

Management. Eyeglasses correct hyperopic errors. The treatment of early onset esotropia, in which only one eye fixates, consists of alternate eye patching to prevent ambliopia. Early corrective surgery is required for persistent esotropia. Esotropia presenting after 6 years of age raises concern for a posterior fossa disorder such as a Chiari malformation.

Exotropia

Exotropia is an outward divergence of the eyes. It may be intermittent (exophoria) or constant (exotropia).

Clinical Features. Exophoria is a relatively common condition that begins before 4 years of age. It is most often evident when the child is fatigued and fixating on a far object or in bright sunlight. The natural history of the condition is unknown. Exotropia may be congenital but poor vision in the outward-turning eye is also a cause.

Diagnosis. Exotropia is an indication to examine the eye for intraocular disease.

Management. In children with intermittent exotropia, the decision to perform corrective surgery depends on the frequency and degree of the abnormality. When exotropia is constant, treatment depends on the underlying cause of visual loss.

OPHTHALMOPLEGIA

The causes of paralytic strabismus include disorders of the ocular motor nerves, the ocular muscles, or neuromuscular junction. Table 15-1 summarizes the muscles, the nerves, and their functions. The eyes no longer move together and diplopia is experienced. Strabismus and diplopia worsen when the child looks in the direction of action of the paralyzed muscle.

Congenital Ophthalmoplegia

Testing of eye movements is uncommon in newborns and ophthalmoplegia often missed. It is common for strabismus to remain unnoticed for several months and then discounted as transitory esotropia. Therefore, consider congenital ophthalmoplegia even when a history of ophthalmoplegia at birth is lacking.

Oculomotor Nerve Palsy/III Cranial Nerve

Clinical Features. Congenital oculomotor nerve palsy usually is unilateral and complete. Pupillary reflex paralysis is variable. Other cranial nerve palsies, especially abducens, may be associated. The palsy is often unrecognized at birth. Most oculomotor nerve palsies are idiopathic, but some are genetic or caused by orbital trauma. The affected eye is exotropic and usually amblyopic. Lid retraction on attempted adduction or downward gaze may be evidence of aberrant regeneration.

Diagnosis. Magnetic resonance imaging (MRI) excludes the possibility of an intracranial mass compressing the nerve. Exophthalmos suggests an orbital tumor. An unreactive, dilated pupil excludes the diagnosis of myasthenia gravis, but a normal pupil requires testing for myasthenia.

Management. Extraocular muscle surgery may improve the cosmetic appearance but rarely improves ocular motility or visual function.

TABLE 15-1 **The Extraocular Muscles**

Ocular muscles	Innervation	Functions
Lateral rectus	Abducens	Abduction
Medial rectus	Oculomotor	Adduction
Superior rectus	Oculomotor	Elevation, intorsion, adduction
Inferior rectus	Oculomotor	Depression, extorsion, adduction
Inferior oblique	Oculomotor	Extorsion, elevation, abduction
Superior oblique	Trochlear	Intorsion, depression, abduction

Trochlear Nerve Palsy/IV Cranial Nerve

Clinical Features. Congenital superior oblique palsy is usually unilateral. Birth trauma is usually the suspected cause, but the actual cause is rarely established. Most congenital cases are idiopathic. The head tilts away from the paralyzed side to keep the eyes in alignment and avoid diplopia. The major ocular features are hypertropia, greatest in the field of action of the involved superior oblique muscle; underaction of the paretic superior oblique muscle and overaction of the inferior oblique muscle; and increased hypertropia when the head tilts to the paralyzed side (positive *Bielschowsky test*).

Diagnosis. Head tilt, or *torticollis* (see Chapter 14), is not a constant feature. Once examination confirms a superior oblique palsy, important etiological considerations other than congenital include trauma, myasthenia gravis, and brainstem glioma.

Management. Prisms are effective for small angle deviations; otherwise patients require surgery.

Abducens Nerve Palsy/VI Cranial Nerve

Clinical Features. Congenital abducens nerve palsy may be unilateral or bilateral and is sometimes associated with other cranial nerve palsies. Lateral movement of the affected eye(s) is limited partially or completely. Most infants use cross-fixation and thereby retain vision in both eyes. In the few reported cases of congenital palsy with pathological correlation, the abducens nerve is absent and its nucleus is hypoplastic.

Möbius syndrome is the association of congenital facial diplegia and bilateral abducens nerve palsies (see Chapter 17). *Duane syndrome* is aplasia of one or both nuclei of the abducens nerve with innervation of the atrophic lateral rectus by fibers of the oculomotor nerve (Chung et al, 2000). Ten percent of cases are genetic; the gene locus is on chromosome 8. The characteristic features are lateral rectus palsy, some limitation of adduction, and narrowing of the palpebral fissure because of globe retraction on attempted adduction. *Möbius* and *Duane syndromes* are rhombencephalic maldevelopment often associated with lingual, palatal, respiratory or long track motor and coordination deficits (Verzijl et al, 2003).

Diagnosis. MRI excludes the possibility of an intracranial mass lesion and hearing testing is required.

Management. Surgical procedures may be useful to correct head turn and to provide binocular single vision, but they do not restore ocular motility.

Brown Syndrome

Brown syndrome results from congenital shortening of the superior oblique muscle or tendon. The result is mechanical limitation of elevation in adduction. Usually, only one eye is involved.

Clinical Features. Elevation is limited in adduction but is relatively normal in abduction. Passive elevation (forced duction) is also restricted. Other features include widening of the palpebral fissure on adduction and backward head tilt.

Diagnosis. The diagnosis of Brown syndrome requires the exclusion of acquired shortening of the superior oblique muscle. The causes of acquired shortening of the superior oblique muscle include juvenile rheumatoid arthritis, trauma, and inflammatory processes affecting the top of the orbit (see section on Orbital Inflammatory Disease later in this chapter).

Management. Surgical procedures that extend the superior oblique muscle can be useful in congenital cases.

Congenital Fibrosis of the Extraocular Muscles

Inheritance of congenital fibrosis of the extraocular muscles (CFEOM) is by autosomal dominant inheritance and the abnormal gene maps to chromosome 12p (OMIM, 2011). If all affected members of a family have typical CFEOM, the phenotypic classification is CFEOM1. CFEOM2 is associated with bilateral ptosis with the eyes fixed in an exotropic position. Genetic transmission is as an autosomal recessive trait. A CFEOM3 caused by TUBB3, R262C, and D417N amino acid substitutions has been described and is associated with abnormalities of extraocular muscle innervation and function. CFEOM3 has subarachnoid CN3 hypoplasia, occasional abducens nerve hypoplasia, and subclinical cranial nerve II hypoplasia that can resemble CFEOM1. Clinical and MRI findings in CFEOM3 are more variable than those in CFEOM1 and are often asymmetrical. Lateral rectus innervation by the inferior rectus motor nerve is an overlapping feature of Duane retraction syndrome and CFEOM1. These findings suggest that CFEOM3 is an asymmetrical, variably penetrant, congenital cranial dysinnervation disorder leading to secondary EOM atrophy (Demer et al, 2010)

Clinical Features. Affected children have congenital bilateral ptosis and restrictive ophthalmoplegia, with their eyes partially or completely fixed in a downward position. CFEOM is a relatively static disorder that is phenotypically homogeneous when completely penetrant. Some children have mild delay in achieving milestones during infancy, and some have a mild facial diplegia. The head is tilted back to allow vision, and diplopia is not associated despite the severe misalignment of the eyes.

Diagnosis. The clinical findings and the family history are the basis for diagnosis. Laboratory studies are useful only to exclude other possibilities.

Management. The goal of treatment is improvement of vision by correcting ptosis.

Congenital Myasthenia Gravis

Several clinical syndromes of myasthenia gravis occur in the newborn (see Chapter 6). Congenital myasthenic syndromes (CMS) are genetic disorders of the neuromuscular junction. They are classified as presynaptic, synaptic, or postsynaptic. Postsynaptic disorders are divisible by the kinetic defects into fast channel and slow channel and a third disorder of acetylcholine receptor (AChR) deficiency. Approximately 10 % of CMS cases are presynaptic, 15 % are synaptic, and 75 % are postsynaptic.

Primary AChR deficiency with or without minor kinetic defect, primary kinetic defect with or without AChR deficiency, endplate acetylcholinesterase (AChE) deficiency, rapsyn deficiency, Dok-7 myasthenia, choline acetyltransferase (ChAT) deficiency, congenital Lambert–Eaton-like and other presynaptic defects, plectin deficiency, sodium channel myasthenia, paucity of synaptic vesicles, and reduced quantal release have been identified as causes of congenital myasthenia (Engel et al, 2010). AChR deficiency causes most postsynaptic cases (Engel et al, 2003, 2010). Genetic transmission is by autosomal recessive inheritance. Other underlying defects include abnormal acetylcholine resynthesis or immobilization, reduced endplate acetylcholinesterase, and impaired function of the AChR. In 25% of patients with AChR deficiency, AChR mutations are undetectable. Among these patients, rapsyn (*receptor-associated protein at the synapse*) deficiency is an important causative factor (Burke et al, 2003).

Clinical Features. Although transmission of these disorders is by autosomal recessive inheritance, a male-to-female bias of 2:1 exists. Symmetric ptosis and ophthalmoplegia are present at birth or shortly thereafter. Mild facial weakness may be present but is not severe enough to impair feeding. If partial at birth, the ophthalmoplegia becomes complete during infancy or childhood. Generalized weakness sometimes develops. Electrophysiological studies in patients suffering from sudden apnea suggest a defect in acetylcholine resynthesis and choline acetyltransferase (ChAT). Refractoriness to anticholinesterase medications and partial or complete absence of AChE from the endplates suggest a mutation in COLQ (Engel et al, 2010).

Diagnosis. Suspect the diagnosis in any newborn with bilateral ptosis or limitation of eye movement. Intramuscular injection of edrophonium chloride produces a transitory improvement in ocular motility. Repetitive nerve stimulation of the limbs at a frequency of 3 Hz may evoke a decremental response after 5 to 10 minute stimulation that is reversible with edrophonium chloride. The 50 Hz repetitive stimulation may also show a 10% decrease in CMAP between the first and fifth stimulation. This suggests that the underlying defect, although producing symptoms only in the eyes, causes generalized weakness at birth. Commercial testing is available for rapsyn mutations.

Management. No evidence of an immunopathy exists and immunosuppressive therapy is not a recommendation. Thymectomy and corticosteroids are ineffective. Anticholinesterases may decrease facial paralysis but have little or no effect on ophthalmoplegia. The weakness, in some children, responds to 3,4-diaminopyridine (DAP), an agent that releases acetylcholine (Harper & Engel, 2000) combined with anticholinesterases. DAP is now commercially available in the United States. The FDA granted DAP an orphan designation for Lambert-Eaton myasthenic syndrome.

BOX 15-1 Causes of Ptosis

CONGENITAL

- Congenital fibrosis of extraocular muscles
- Horner syndrome*
- Myasthenia*
- Oculomotor nerve palsy*

ACQUIRED

- Horner syndrome*
- Lid inflammation
- Mitochondrial myopathies (see Chapter 8)
- Myasthenia gravis*
- Oculomotor nerve palsy*
- Oculopharyngeal dystrophy (see Chapter 17)
- Ophthalmoplegic migraine
- Orbital cellulitis
- Trauma

*Denotes the most common conditions and the ones with disease modifying treatments

Congenital Ptosis

Congenital drooping of one or both lids is relatively common, and the drooping is unilateral in 70% of cases. The cause is unknown, but the condition rarely occurs in other family members. The three forms of hereditary congenital ptosis are simple, with external ophthalmoplegia, and with blepharophimosis. Genetic transmission of the simple form is either by autosomal dominant (Pavone et al, 2005) or X-linked inheritance.

Clinical Features. Congenital ptosis is often unnoticed until early childhood or even adult life and then diagnosed as an "acquired" ptosis. Miosis is sometimes an associated feature and suggests the possibility of a Horner syndrome, except that the pupil responds normally to pharmacological agents. Some patients have a synkinesis between the oculomotor and trigeminal nerves; jaw movements produce opening of the eye (*Marcus-Gunn phenomenon*).

Diagnosis. Box 15.1 lists the differential diagnosis of ptosis. Distinguishing congenital ptosis from acquired ptosis is essential. The examination of baby pictures is more cost-effective than MRI to make the distinction. If miosis is present, test the eye with pharmacological agents (Paredrine® and cocaine test for denervation) to determine whether denervation rather than sympathetic hypersensitivity is present indicating a Horner syndrome. Concurrent paralysis of extraocular motility is evidence against congenital ptosis.

Management. Early corrective surgery to elevate the lid improves appearance and vision.

Acute Unilateral Ophthalmoplegia

Box 15.2 summarizes the causes of acquired ophthalmoplegia. The discussion of many of these conditions is in other chapters.

BOX 15-2 Causes of Acquired Ophthalmoplegia

BRAINSTEM

- Brainstem encephalitis* (see Chapter 10)
- Intoxication
- Multiple sclerosis* (see Chapter 10)
- Subacute necrotizing encephalopathy (see Chapter 10)
- Tumor
  - Brainstem glioma*
  - Craniopharyngioma (see Chapter 16)
  - Leukemia
  - Lymphoma
  - Metastases
  - Pineal region tumors
- Vascular
  - Arteriovenous malformation
  - Hemorrhage
  - Infarction
  - Migraine*
  - Vasculitis

NERVE

- Familial recurrent cranial neuropathies (see Chapter 17)
- Increased intracranial pressure (see Chapter 4)
- Infectious
  - Diphtheria
  - Gradenigo syndrome
  - Meningitis (see Chapter 4)
  - Orbital cellulitis
- Inflammatory
  - Sarcoid
- Postinfectious
  - Idiopathic* (postviral)
  - Miller Fisher syndrome* (see Chapter 10)
  - Polyradiculoneuropathy (see Chapter 7)
- Trauma
  - Head
  - Orbital
- Tumor
  - Cavernous sinus hemangioma
  - Orbital tumors
  - Sellar and parasellar tumors (see Chapter 16)
  - Sphenoid sinus tumors
- Vascular
  - Aneurysm
  - Carotid-cavernous fistula
  - Cavernous sinus thrombosis
  - Migraine

NEUROMUSCULAR TRANSMISSION

- Botulism* (see Chapter 7)
- Myasthenia gravis*
- Tic paralysis

MYOPATHIES

- Fiber-type disproportion myopathies (see Chapter 6)
- Kearns-Sayres syndrome
- Mitochondrial myopathies (see Chapter 8)
- Oculopharyngeal dystrophy (see Chapter 17)
- Orbital inflammatory disease
- Thyroid disease
- Vitamin E deficiency

*Denotes the most common conditions and the ones with disease modifying treatments

The definition of acute ophthalmoplegia is reaching maximum intensity within 1 week of onset. It may be partial or complete (Box 15-3). Generalized increased intracranial pressure is always an important consideration in patients with unilateral or bilateral abducens palsy (see Chapter 4).

Aneurysm

The full discussion of arterial aneurysms is in Chapter 4, because the important clinical feature in children is hemorrhage rather than nerve compression. This section deals only with possible ophthalmoplegic features.

Clinical Features. Aneurysms at the junction of the internal carotid and posterior communicating arteries are an important cause of unilateral oculomotor palsy in adults but are a rare cause in children. Compression of the nerve by expansion of the aneurysm causes the palsy. Intense pain in and around the eye is frequently experienced at the time of hemorrhage. Because the parasympathetic fibers are at the periphery of the nerve, mydriasis is an almost constant feature of ophthalmoplegia caused by aneurysms of the posterior communicating artery. However, pupillary involvement may develop several days after onset of an incomplete external ophthalmoplegia. A normal pupil with complete external ophthalmoplegia effectively excludes the possibility of aneurysm.

Sometimes, aneurysms affect the superior branch of the oculomotor nerve earlier and more severely than the inferior branch. Ptosis may precede the development of other signs by hours or days.

Diagnosis. Contrast-enhanced MRI and magnetic resonance angiography (MRA) or CT angiogram identify most aneurysms.

Management. Surgical clipping is the treatment of choice whenever technically feasible. Oculomotor function often returns to normal after the procedure.

BOX 15-3 Causes of Acute Unilateral Ophthalmoplegia

- Aneurysm*†
- Brain tumors
  - Brainstem glioma
  - Parasellar tumors (see Chapter 16)
  - Tumors of pineal region (see Chapter 4)
- Brainstem stroke*
- Cavernous sinus fistula
- Cavernous sinus thrombosis
- Gradenigo syndrome
- Idiopathic ocular motor nerve palsy*
- Increased intracranial pressure (see Chapter 4)
- Multiple sclerosis* (see Chapter 10)
- Myasthenia gravis*
- Ophthalmoplegic migraine*†
- Orbital inflammatory disease*†
- Orbital tumor†
- Recurrent familial* (see Chapter 17)
- Trauma
  - Head
  - Orbital

*May be recurrent
†May be associated with pain

Brainstem Glioma

Clinical Features. Symptoms begin between 2 and 13 years of age, with a peak between ages 5 and 8 years. The period from onset of symptoms to diagnosis is less than 6 months. Cranial nerve palsies, usually abducens and facial, are the initial features in most cases. Later, contralateral hemiplegia and ataxia, dysphagia, and hoarseness develop. Hemiplegia at onset is associated with a more rapid course. With time, cranial nerve and corticospinal tract involvement may become bilateral. Increased intracranial pressure is not an early feature, but direct irritation of the brainstem emetic center may cause vomiting rather than increased pressure. Intractable hiccup, facial spasm, personality change, and headache are early symptoms in occasional patients.

Brainstem gliomas carry the worst prognosis of any childhood tumor due to their location. The course is one of steady progression, with median survival times of 9 to 12 months.

Diagnosis. MRI delineates the tumor well and differentiates tumor from inflammatory and vascular disorders (Figure 15-1).

Management. Radiation therapy is the treatment of choice. Several chemotherapeutic programs are undergoing experimental trials, but none has established benefit.

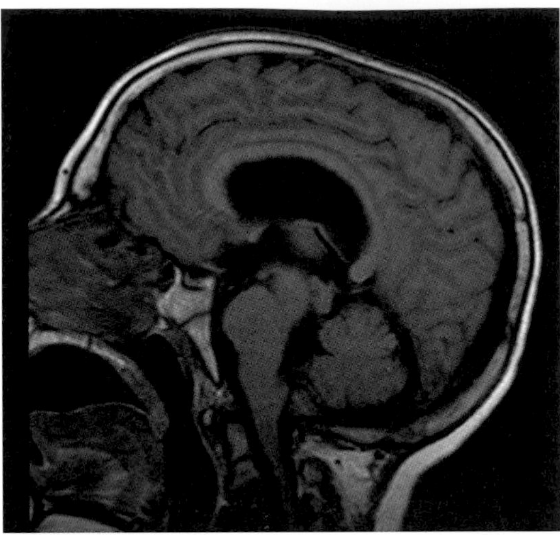

FIGURE 15-1 ■ Brainstem glioma. T_1 sagittal MRI shows a distorted and homogeneous pons.

Brainstem Stroke

Box 11.2 summarizes the causes of stroke in children. Small brainstem hemorrhages resulting from emboli, leukemia, or blood dyscrasias have the potential to cause isolated ocular motor palsies, but this is not the rule. Other cranial nerves are also involved, and hemiparesis, ataxia, and decreased consciousness are often associated features.

Carotid-Cavernous Sinus Fistula

Clinical Features. Arteriovenous communications between the carotid artery and the cavernous sinus may be congenital but trauma is the usual cause in children. The injury may be closed or penetrating. The carotid artery or one of its branches ruptures into the cavernous sinus, increasing pressure in the venous system. The results are a pulsating proptosis, redness and swelling of the conjunctiva, increased intraocular pressure, and ophthalmoplegia. If a bruit is present over the eye, compression of the ipsilateral carotid artery reduces the volume.

Diagnosis. Carotid arteriography reveals rapid cavernous sinus filling, poor filling of the distal intracranial branches, and engorgement of and retrograde flow within venous drainage pathways.

Management. Transarterial balloon embolization or coiling of the affected cavernous sinus is the mainstay of treatment.

Cavernous Sinus Thrombosis

Cavernous sinus thrombosis may produce either unilateral or bilateral ophthalmoplegia. The cause is usually the anterograde spread of infection from the mouth, face, nose, or paranasal sinuses.

Clinical Features. The development of fever, malaise, and frontal headache following dental infection is the typical history. Proptosis, orbital congestion, ptosis, external ophthalmoplegia, pupillary paralysis, and blindness may follow the initial symptoms. The infection begins in one cavernous sinus and spreads to the other. If untreated, it may extend to the meninges. Even with vigorous antibiotic treatment, the mortality rate is 15 %.

Diagnosis. The ocular signs may suggest orbital cellulitis or orbital pseudotumor. The cerebrospinal fluid is normal early in the course. A mixed leukocytosis develops, and the protein concentration is moderately elevated even in the absence of meningitis. Once the meninges are involved, the pressure becomes elevated, the leukocytosis increases, and the glucose concentration falls.

Cranial CT may show clouding of infected paranasal sinuses. MRA shows decreased or absent flow in the cavernous portion of the carotid artery.

Management. Intravenous antibiotic therapy is similar to the course used to treat meningitis. Surgical drainage of infected paranasal sinuses is sometimes necessary.

Gradenigo Syndrome

Clinical Features. The abducens nerve lies adjacent to the medial aspect of the petrous bone before entering the cavernous sinus. Infections of the middle ear sometimes extend to the petrous bone and cause thrombophlebitis of the inferior petrosal sinus. The infection involves not only the abducens nerve but also the facial nerve and the trigeminal ganglion. The resulting syndrome consists of ipsilateral paralysis of abduction, facial palsy, and facial pain.

Diagnosis. The combination of unilateral abducens and facial palsy also occurs after closed head injuries. The diagnosis of Gradenigo syndrome requires the demonstration of middle-ear infection. CT of the mastoid bone shows the infection. Lumbar puncture reveals a cellular response and an elevation of protein content.

Management. Prompt antibiotic therapy prevents permanent nerve damage.

Idiopathic Cranial Nerve Palsy

The sudden onset of a single, otherwise unexplained, cranial neuropathy is usually attributed to an immune-mediated reaction to a prior viral infection. However, a cause-and-effect relationship between viral infection and ocular motor palsies is not established. Abducens nerve palsy is more common than either oculomotor or trochlear nerve palsies. Bilateral involvement is unusual.

Clinical Features. The chief complaint is a painless diplopia. Examination reveals a paralytic strabismus. Girls are more often affected than are boys and the left eye more often than the right. Restoration of full motility is within 6 months, but shorter-duration recurrences occur in half of children.

Diagnosis. Examination of the cerebrospinal fluid and MRI of the head and orbit exclude tumor and infection. Tumors in and around the orbit are sometimes difficult to demonstrate, and, if ophthalmoplegia persists, a repeat MRI may be necessary. Myasthenia gravis is a diagnostic consideration. An edrophonium chloride test may be useful, but myasthenia gravis is unlikely when there is a fixed single nerve deficit.

Management. Isolated cranial nerve palsies are not an indication for corticosteroid therapy. In children less than 9 years of age, intermittent patching of the normal eye may be necessary if the affected eye never fixates.

Myasthenia Gravis

The discussion of some neonatal forms of myasthenia is in Chapter 6; congenital myasthenia is included in the section on Congenital Ophthalmoplegia earlier in this chapter, and limb-girdle myasthenia in Chapter 7. This section describes the immune-mediated form of myasthenia encountered from late infancy through adult life. The two clinical forms are *ocular myasthenia,* which primarily or exclusively affects the eye muscles (but facial and limb muscles may be mildly involved), and *generalized myasthenia,* in which weakness of bulbar and limb muscles is moderate to severe. The term *juvenile myasthenia* to denote immune-mediated myasthenia gravis in children has no special meaning. The disease is similar in children and adults.

Clinical Features. The initial symptoms do not appear until after 6 months of age; 75 % of children first have symptoms after age 10 years. Prepubertal onset is associated with a male preference, only ocular symptoms, and seronegativity for acetylcholine receptor antibodies, whereas postpubertal onset is associated with a strong female preference, generalized myasthenia, and seropositivity. In general, the disease is less severe in boys than in girls.

The initial features of both the ocular and the generalized form are usually ptosis, diplopia, or both. Myasthenia is the most common cause of acquired unilateral or bilateral ptosis. Pupillary function is normal. Between 40 % and 50 % of patients have weakness of other bulbar or limb muscles at the onset of ocular symptoms. Ocular motor weakness is generally not constant initially, and the specific muscles affected may change from examination to examination. Usually both eyes are affected, but one is more affected than is the other.

Children with ocular myasthenia may have mild facial weakness and easy fatigability of the limbs. However, they do not have respiratory distress or difficulty speaking or swallowing. The subsequent courses of ocular myasthenia may be one of steady progression to complete ophthalmoplegia or by relapses and remissions. The relapses are of varying severity and last for weeks to years. At least 20 % of patients have permanent remissions. Prepubertal onset is more commonly associated with spontaneous remission than postpubertal onset.

Children with generalized myasthenia have generalized weakness within 1 year of the initial ocular symptoms. The symptoms include dysarthria, dysphagia, difficulty chewing, and limb muscle fatigability. Spontaneous remissions are unusual. Respiratory insufficiency (*myasthenic crisis*) occurs in one-third of untreated children.

Children with generalized myasthenia, but not those with ocular myasthenia, have a higher than expected incidence of other autoimmune disorders, especially thyroiditis and collagen vascular diseases. Thymoma is present in 15 % of adults with generalized myasthenia but occurs in less than 5 % of children. When thymoma occurs in children, it is likely to be malignant.

Diagnosis. The edrophonium chloride test is often set as a standard of diagnosis for both the ocular and generalized forms of myasthenia gravis, but it has limitations and dangers. Edrophonium chloride is a short-acting anticholinesterase administered intravenously at a dose of 0.15 mg/kg. Before initiating the test, an endpoint for the study must be determined. The best endpoint is the resolution of ptosis or the restoration of ocular motility, and test results are difficult to evaluate in their absence. Ptosis generally responds better than ocular motor paralysis to edrophonium chloride.

Some patients with myasthenia are supersensitive to edrophonium chloride. Fasciculations and respiratory arrest may develop following administration. For this reason, first inject a test dose of one-tenth the full dose. Unfortunately, respiratory embarrassment sometimes develops in response to the test dose, and a hand ventilator should be readily available before any drug is given. Atropine is an effective antidote to the muscarinic side effects of edrophonium chloride but does not counteract the nicotinic effects on the motor endplate that result in paralysis of the skeletal muscles.

After the test dose is given, the remainder should be injected one-third at a time (approximately 0.05 mg/kg), allowing up to 1 minute after each injection to test the response. Interpretation may be difficult. The judgment of improved strength is always subjective and influenced by examiner bias. The test becomes more objective when combined with electrophysiological studies. We do not use the edrophonium test for diagnosis because of its inherent dangers and rely more on the clinical features, the serum antibody concentrations, and electrophysiological studies.

Some physicians now use the *ice-pack test* instead. Place a very cold compress on the ptotic lid for 2 minutes. Partial opening of the lid suggests myasthenia. Five minutes of resting with the eye closed may accomplish the same result without the ice pack.

Results of repetitive nerve stimulation studies are abnormal in 66 % of children when proximal nerves are stimulated but in only 33 % when distal nerves are studied. Abnormal repetitive nerve study findings are unusual in children with ocular myasthenia but are the rule in children with generalized myasthenia. Patients with mild myasthenia show a decremental response at low rates of stimulation (2 to 5 per second) but not at high rates (50 per second). In severe myasthenia, both low and high rates of stimulation produce a decremental response. Single fiber EMG of the frontalis or orbicularis oculi is very sensitive for the diagnosis of myasthenia.

Eight-five percent of patients with generalized immune-mediated myasthenia have elevated serum concentrations of antibodies against the acetylcholine receptor (>10 nmol/L). Patients with ocular myasthenia may be seronegative or have low antibody concentrations. Among those children who are seronegative, many have a genetic disorder secondary to rapsyn mutations and others have antibodies directed against muscle-specific tyrosine kinase (*MuSK*). The distinction between early-onset, seronegative immune-mediated and genetic myasthenia is important: one responds to immunotherapy and the other does not. MuSK antibody concentration testing is commercially available; rapsyn mutation analysis is not.

Management. The basis for managing nongenetic myasthenia in children is experience and retrospective studies, primarily done in adults (Richman & Agius, 2003). Children with ocular myasthenia, but not those with generalized myasthenia, have a reasonable hope of spontaneous remission. Anticholinesterase therapy is the treatment of choice for ocular myasthenia. The initial dose of neostigmine is 0.5 mg/kg every 4 hours in children younger than 5 years of age and 0.25 mg/kg in older children, not to exceed 15 mg per dose in any child. The equivalent dose of pyridostigmine is four times greater. After initiating treatment, the dose slowly increases as needed and tolerated. Diarrhea and gastrointestinal cramps are the usual limiting factors. Do not administer edrophonium chloride to determine whether the child would benefit from higher oral doses of anticholinesterases. It is not an accurate guide and may cause cholinergic crisis in children with generalized myasthenia.

Several retrospective studies in adults suggest that early immunotherapy (Kuppersmith, 2003; Mee et al, 2003) and thymectomy reduce the conversion of ocular myasthenia to generalized myasthenia. *The evidence is not convincing and not applicable to children.*

Ocular myasthenia can be difficult to treat and evaluating the efficacy of treatment is especially difficult. The response to anticholinesterase is often transitory, and the addition of corticosteroids is often without benefit. The efficacy of any drug regimen in ocular myasthenia is difficult to assess because of the fluctuating course of the disease.

The place of thymectomy in the management of myasthenia is not established. Experience indicates that most children who undergo thymectomy early in the course will be in remission within 3 years. However, corticosteroids accomplish the same result, and prior thymectomy does not reduce the need for long-term corticosteroid treatment.

The starting dose of prednisone is 1.5 mg/kg/day, not to exceed 100 mg/day. High-dose corticosteroids may make the patient weaker at first. After 5 days of daily treatment, switch to alternate-day therapy for the remainder of the month. The prednisone dose then tapers by 10 % each month until reaching a dose that keeps the patient symptom free. The usual maintenance dose is 10–20 mg every other day. We have been unsuccessful in eventually stopping prednisone. Concurrent anticholinesterase medication is unnecessary with corticosteroids but is useful if the patient weakens on the alternate days when corticosteroids are not used.

The clinical characteristics and response to treatment of individuals with nongenetic, generalized myasthenia who are seronegative do not differ from the characteristics and response of those who are seropositive, except that seronegative patients are unlikely to show thymic abnormalities and are unlikely to benefit from thymectomy. Plasmapheresis, intravenous immunoglobulin, and high-dose intravenous corticosteroids are useful for acute intervention in patients who have respiratory insufficiency.

Ophthalmoplegic Migraine

The mechanism of ophthalmoplegia in migraine is not established. Although migraine is hereditary, the tendency for ophthalmoplegia is not.

Clinical Features. Transitory ocular motor palsy, lasting as long as 4 weeks, may occur as part of a migraine attack in children and adults. The palsy affects the oculomotor nerve alone in 83 % of cases and affects all three nerves in the remainder. Ptosis usually precedes ophthalmoplegia. Partial or complete pupillary involvement is present in 60 % of cases. The average age at onset is 15 years, but the onset may be as early as infancy. In infants, recurrent painless ophthalmoplegia or ptosis may be the only feature of the migraine attack. In older children, ophthalmoplegia usually occurs during the headache phase and is ipsilateral to the headache.

Diagnosis. The diagnosis is obvious when ophthalmoplegia occurs during a typical migraine attack in a child previously known to have migraine. Diagnostic uncertainty is greatest when an infant has transitory strabismus or ptosis as an isolated sign. In such cases, a family history of migraine is essential for diagnosis. Even so, MRI studies of the head and orbit are appropriate in most infants with a first episode of ophthalmoplegia.

Management. The management of ophthalmoplegic migraine is the same as other forms of migraine (see Chapter 3). In addition, a short course of steroids may shorten the attack.

Orbital Inflammatory Disease

The term *orbital inflammatory disease* encompasses a group of nonspecific inflammatory conditions involving the orbit. Inflammation may be diffuse or localized to specific tissues within the orbit. The differential diagnosis includes idiopathic inflammatory orbit disease, orbital myositis, dacryoadenitis, sarcoidosis, Graves disease, histiocytosis, orbital pseudotumor, lymphoproliferative disease, Wegener granulomatosis, rhabdomyosarcoma, retinoblastoma, and neuroblastoma (Belanger et al, 2010).

Clinical Features. The disorder is unusual before age 20 years but may occur as early as 3 months of age. Males and females are equally affected. Acute and chronic forms exist. The main features are pain, ophthalmoplegia, proptosis, and lid edema evolving over several days or weeks. One or both eyes may be involved. Ocular motility is disturbed in part by the proptosis but mainly by myositis. Some patients have only myositis, whereas others have inflammation in other orbital structures. Vision is initially preserved, but loss of vision is a threat if the condition remains untreated.

Diagnosis. The development of unilateral pain and proptosis in a child suggests an orbital tumor. Bilateral proptosis suggests thyroid myopathy. MRI shows a soft tissue mass without sinus involvement or bone erosion. Orbital involvement by lymphoma or leukemia produces a similar imaging appearance. The extraocular muscles may appear enlarged. Biopsy should be considered in cases where refractory or rebound inflammation is noted during or after steroid treatment (Belanger et al, 2010).

Management. Orbital inflammatory disease has a self-limited course but treatment is required to prevent vision loss or permanent ophthalmoplegia. Administer prednisone, 1 mg/kg/day, for at least 1 month before tapering. Reinitiate the full dose if the disorder recurs during the taper.

Orbital Tumors

Clinical Features. The initial feature of intraorbital tumors is proptosis, ophthalmoplegia, or ptosis. When the globe displaces forward, the palpebral fissure widens and closing the eye fully may not be possible. The exposed portion of the eye becomes dry and erythematous and may suffer exposure keratitis. The direction of displacement of the globe is the best clue to the tumor's position. Ophthalmoplegia may occur because of forward displacement of the globe, causing direct pressure on one or more ocular muscles.

Diagnosis. The differential diagnosis of proptosis in children includes infection and inflammation, hemorrhage and other vascular disorders, orbital tumors, hyperthyroidism and other metabolic disorders, developmental anomalies, and Hand-Schüller-Christian disease and related disorders; some are idiopathic. The most common orbital tumors are dermoid cyst, hemangioma, metastatic neuroblastoma, anterior visual pathway glioma, and rhabdomyosarcoma. Orbit CT and MRI, and biopsy are necessary for the diagnosis and selection of treatment.

Management. Treatment varies with the tumor type. Many require surgical resection.

Trauma

Trauma accounts for 40% of isolated acquired ocular motor nerve palsies and 55% of multiple nerve palsies in children. Hemorrhage and edema into the nerves or muscles may occur from closed head injuries even in the absence of direct orbital injury. In the presence of orbital fractures, the nerves and muscles are vulnerable to laceration, avulsion, or entrapment by bone fragments.

Clinical Features. Superior oblique palsy, caused by trochlear nerve damage, is a relatively common consequence of closed head injuries. Usually the trauma is severe, often causing loss of consciousness, but it may be mild. The palsy is more often unilateral than bilateral. Patients with unilateral superior oblique palsy have a marked hypertropia in the primary position and a compensatory head tilt to preserve fusion; 65 % of cases resolve spontaneously. When bilateral involvement is present, the hypertropia is milder and alternates between the two eyes; spontaneous recovery occurs in only 25 % of cases.

Transitory lateral rectus palsy is rare in newborns and the cause attributed to birth trauma. The palsy is unilateral and clears completely within 6 weeks.

Diagnosis. Direct injuries to the orbit with associated hemorrhage and swelling do not pose a diagnostic dilemma. CT of the head with orbital views shows the extent of fracture so that the need for surgical intervention can be determined. CT may also show a lateral midbrain hemorrhage as the cause of trochlear nerve palsy.

A delay between the time of injury and the onset of ophthalmoplegia makes diagnosis more problematic. The possible mechanisms of delayed ophthalmoplegia following trauma to the head include progressive local edema in the orbit; progressive brainstem edema; progressive increased intracranial pressure; development of meningitis, mastoiditis, or petrous osteomyelitis; venous sinus or carotid artery thrombosis; and carotid cavernous fistula.

Management. Local trauma and fracture of the orbit may require surgical repair. Surgery directed at rebalancing the extraocular muscles sometimes improves vision after permanent paralysis of ocular motor nerves following head injury. Botulinum toxin is another treatment option for bilateral sixth nerve palsies.

Acute Bilateral Ophthalmoplegia

Many of the conditions that cause acute unilateral ophthalmoplegia (see Box 15-3) may also cause acute bilateral ophthalmoplegia. The conditions listed in Box 15-4 often have a high incidence of bilateral involvement. The discussion of thyroid orbitopathy is with the chronic conditions because progression of ophthalmoplegia usually occurs over a period greater than 1 week.

BOX 15-4 Causes of Acute Bilateral Ophthalmoplegia

Basilar meningitis (see Chapter 4)
Brainstem encephalitis* (see Chapter 10)
Carotid-cavernous fistula
Cavernous sinus thrombosis
Diphtheria
Intoxication
Miller Fisher syndrome* (see Chapter 10)
Myasthenia gravis*
Polyradiculoneuropathy (see Chapter 7)
Subacute necrotizing encephalomyelopathy (see Chapter 5)
Tick paralysis (see Chapter 7)

*Denotes the most common conditions and the ones with disease modifying treatments

Botulism

Several strains of the bacterium *Clostridium botulinum* elaborate a toxin that disturbs neuromuscular transmission. The discussion of the infantile form of botulism, which causes ptosis but not ophthalmoplegia, is in Chapter 6. This section deals with late-onset cases.

Clinical Features. The cause of botulism is most often the ingestion of toxin in home-canned food. This is most likely when canning at high altitudes, where the boiling temperature is too low to destroy spores. Because *C. botulinum* spores are ubiquitous in soil, infection may also follow burns, wounds, and the sharing of needles among drug addicts. Blurred vision, diplopia, dizziness, dysarthria, and dysphagia begin 12 to 36 hours after ingestion of toxin. The pupillary response is usually normal. An ascending paralysis similar to the Guillain-Barré syndrome follows the early symptoms and may lead to death from respiratory paralysis. Patients remain conscious and alert throughout. Most patients make a complete recovery within 2 to 3 months, but those with severe involvement may not return to normal for a year.

Diagnosis. The presence of ophthalmoplegia and the EMG findings distinguishes botulism from the Guillain-Barré syndrome. The motor and sensory nerve conduction velocities are normal, the amplitude of evoked muscle action potentials reduced, and a decremental response is not ordinarily present at low rates of stimulation, although facilitation may be present at high rates of stimulation. Showing the organism or the toxin in food, stool, or a wound establishes the diagnosis.

Management. Antitoxin administration, 20 000 to 40 000 units two or three times a day, is the recommended treatment. Empty the stomach and intestines of their contents. DAP is effective in some patients and should be used for those with potential respiratory failure. Assure the availability of mechanical respiratory support when the diagnosis is suspect.

BOX 15-5 Causes of Chronic Bilateral Ophthalmoplegia

Brainstem glioma
Chronic meningitis (see Chapter 4)
Chronic orbital inflammation
Kearns-Sayre syndrome
Myasthenia gravis*
- Thyroid orbitopathy*
- Congenital
- Juvenile

Myopathies
- Fiber-type disproportion myopathy (see Chapter 6)
- Mitochondrial myopathies (see Chapter 8)
- Myotubular myopathy (see Chapter 6)
- Oculopharyngeal muscular dystrophy (see Chapter 17)

Subacute necrotizing encephalomyelopathy (see Chapter 5)
Thyroid disease*
Vitamin E deficiency

*Denotes the most common conditions and the ones with disease modifying treatments

Intoxications

Clinical Features. Anticonvulsants, tricyclic antidepressants, and many other psychoactive drugs selectively impair ocular motility at toxic blood concentrations. Overdose may be accidental or intentional. A child, found unconscious, arrives at the emergency department. The state of consciousness varies from obtundation to stupor, but the eyes do not move, either by rapidly rotating the head laterally or with ice water irrigation of the ears. Complete ophthalmoplegia is expected in a comatose child if brainstem function is otherwise impaired (see Chapter 2), but in a noncomatose child with otherwise intact brainstem function, ingestion of a drug that selectively impairs ocular motility should be suspected.

Diagnosis. Question the family about drugs available in the household, and screen the blood and urine for toxic substances.

Management. Specific treatment depends on the drug ingested; in most cases, supportive care is sufficient.

Chronic Bilateral Ophthalmoplegia

Box 15-5 lists the conditions responsible for bilateral ophthalmoplegia developing over a period longer than 1 week. The discussion of most conditions is in previous sections of this chapter or in other chapters.

Thyroid Ophthalmopathy

The association of ophthalmopathy with hyperthyroidism is not causal. The two conditions are associated autoimmune diseases. One hypothesis suggests the presence of a cross-reacting antigen in thyroid and orbital tissues. Myasthenia gravis may be associated as well.

Clinical Features. Disorders of ocular motility are sometimes present in most patients with hyperthyroidism and may precede systemic features of nervousness, heat intolerance, diaphoresis, weight loss, tachycardia, tremulousness, and weakness. The main orbital pathology is a myopathy of the extraocular muscles. They become inflamed, swollen with interstitial edema, and finally fibrotic. If the two eyes are equally affected, the patient may not complain of diplopia despite considerable limitation of ocular motility. Staring or lid retraction (*Dalrymple sign*) occurs in more than 50% of cases, lid lag on downward gaze (*von Graefe sign*) in 30–50%, and proptosis (exophthalmos) in almost 90%. Severe exophthalmos is due to edema and infiltration of all orbital structures.

Diagnosis. Thyroid disease is a consideration in any child with evolving ophthalmoplegia. CT of the orbit shows enlargement of the extraocular muscles. Thyroid function tests are often normal, but a thyroid-releasing hormone stimulation test and a measure of the concentration of thyroid-stimulating immunoglobulin may confirm the diagnosis.

Management. Meticulous control of hyperthyroidism does not necessarily cure the ophthalmopathy. While treating hyperthyroidism, avoid over-treatment causing hypothyroidism. If the exophthalmos progresses, even after the patient is euthyroid, corticosteroids may prevent further proptosis, but persistent optic nerve compression requires surgical decompression.

Kearns-Sayre Syndrome

Nearly all cases of Kearns-Sayre syndrome (KSS) are sporadic and caused by a single large deletion or duplication of the mtDNA, arising either in the maternal oocyte or in early embryonic life (DiMauro & Hirano, 2011).

Clinical Features. The defining features of KSS are the triad of progressive external ophthalmoplegia, onset before age 20 years, and at least one of the following: short stature, pigmentary retinopathy, cerebellar ataxia, heart block, and elevated cerebrospinal fluid protein (>100mg/dL). The onset of KSS is so insidious that patients do not complain of diplopia. The clinical course is progressive, and most patients with associated mental retardation die in the third or fourth decade.

Diagnosis. The basis for diagnosis are the major clinical criteria. Electrocardiographic monitoring for cardiac arrhythmia and cerebrospinal fluid examination are essential.

Management. Treatment with vitamins or coenzyme Q, depending on the specific respiratory complex defect, is common but of unproven benefit. This mitochondrial cocktail includes riboflavin 100mg/day, pyridoxine 20mg/kg/day, coenzyme Q 10–20mg/kg/day, biotin 5–20mg/day, and carnitine 50–100mg/kg/day. A cardiac pacemaker may be lifesaving.

Gaze Palsies

This section deals with supranuclear palsies. The examiner must show that the eyes move normally in response to brainstem gaze center reflexes (doll's head maneuver, caloric testing, and Bell's phenomenon) to verify supranuclear palsy. Box 15-6 gives the differential diagnosis of gaze palsies.

Apraxia of Horizontal Gaze

Ocular motor apraxia is a deficiency in voluntary, horizontal, lateral, fast eye movements (saccades) with retention of slow pursuit movements. Bringing the eyes to a desired position requires jerking movements of the head. The rapid phases of optokinetic nystagmus are absent.

Congenital Ocular Motor Apraxia

Clinical Features. Although ocular motor apraxia is present at birth, detection is not until late infancy. Failure of fixation raises questions concerning visual impairment. Refixation requires overshooting head thrusts, often accompanied by blinking of the eyes. With the head held immobile, the child makes no effort to initiate horizontal eye movements.

Many children with ocular motor apraxia have other signs of cerebral abnormality, such as psychomotor retardation, learning disabilities, and clumsiness. When hypotonia is present, the child may have difficulty making the head movements needed for refixation. Agenesis of the corpus callosum and agenesis of the cerebellar vermis are comorbidities in some children. The association does not indicate that the malformations are responsible for ocular motor apraxia.

Diagnosis. Consider the possibility of ocular motor apraxia in any infant referred for

BOX 15-6 Gaze Palsies

APRAXIA OF HORIZONTAL GAZE
- Ataxia-telangiectasia (see Chapter 10)
- Ataxia-ocular motor apraxia (see Chapter 10)
- Brainstem glioma
- Congenital ocular motor apraxia
- Huntington disease (see Chapter 5)

INTERNUCLEAR OPHTHALMOPLEGIA
- Brainstem stroke
- Brainstem tumor
- Exotropia (pseudo-internuclear ophthalmoplegia [INO])
- Multiple sclerosis
- Myasthenia gravis (pseudo-INO)
- Toxic-metabolic

VERTICAL GAZE PALSY
- Aqueductal stenosis (see Chapter 18)
- Congenital vertical ocular motor apraxia
- Gaucher's disease (see Chapter 5)
- Hydrocephalus (see Chapters 4 and 18)
- Miller Fisher syndrome (see Chapter 10)
- Niemann-Pick disease type C (see Chapter 5)
- Tumor (see Chapter 4)
  - Midbrain
  - Pineal region
  - Third ventricle

HORIZONTAL GAZE PALSY
- Adversive seizures (see Chapter 1)
- Brainstem tumors
- Destructive lesions of the frontal lobe (see Chapter 11)
- Familial horizontal gaze palsy

CONVERGENCE PARALYSIS
- Head trauma
- Idiopathic
- Multiple sclerosis (see Chapter 10)
- Pineal region tumors (see Chapter 4)

evaluation of visual impairment. Children with ocular motor apraxia require brain MRI to search for other cerebral malformations, and tests for ataxia-telangiectasia (see Chapter 10) and lysosomal storage diseases (see Chapter 5).

Management. Management depends on the underlying condition.

Internuclear Ophthalmoplegia

The medial longitudinal fasciculus (MLF) contains fibers that connect the abducens nucleus to the contralateral oculomotor nucleus to perform horizontal conjugate lateral gaze. Unilateral lesions in the MLF disconnect the two nuclei, so that, when the patient attempts lateral gaze, the adducting eye ipsilateral to the abnormal MLF is unable to move medially but the abducting eye is able to move laterally. Nystagmus (actually *overshoot dysmetria*) is often present in the abducting eye. This symptom complex, which may be unilateral or bilateral, is *internuclear ophthalmoplegia* (INO). The usual cause of unilateral INO is vascular occlusive disease, and of bilateral INO is either demyelinating disease or rarely toxic-metabolic causes.

Patients with myasthenia gravis sometimes have ocular motility dysfunction that resembles an INO except that nystagmus is usually lacking. The disorder is a *pseudo-INO* because the MLF is intact. Exotropia is another cause of pseudo-INO. When the normal eye is fixating in full abduction, there is no visual stimulus to bring the paretic eye into full adduction. Nystagmus is not present in the abducting eye.

The combination of an INO in one direction of lateral gaze and complete gaze palsy in the other is a *one-and-a-half syndrome*. The underlying pathology is a unilateral lesion in the dorsal pontine tegmentum that affects the pontine lateral gaze center and the adjacent MLF. Multiple sclerosis is the usual cause. Other causes include brainstem glioma, infraction, or myasthenia gravis.

Toxic-Metabolic Disorders

Clinical Features. Toxic doses of several drugs may produce the clinical syndrome of INO. Usually, the patient is comatose and may have complete ophthalmoplegia that evolves into a bilateral INO. The drugs reported to produce INO include amitriptyline, barbiturates, carbamazepine, doxepin, phenothiazine, and phenytoin. INO may also occur during hepatic coma.

Diagnosis. Drug intoxication is always a consideration in children with decreased consciousness who were previously well. The presence of INO following drug ingestion suggests the possibility of anticonvulsant or psychotropic drug ingestion.

Management. The INO resolves as the blood concentration of the drug falls.

Vertical Gaze Palsy

Children with supranuclear vertical gaze palsies are unable to look upward or downward fully, but they retain reflex eye movements such as the doll's eye reflex and the Bell phenomenon. Disorders of upward gaze in children generally are due to damage to the dorsal midbrain; the usual cause is a tumor in the pineal region. *Parinaud's syndrome* is the combination of paralysis of upgaze, a dilated pupil unresponsive to light but becoming smaller when focusing on a near object (light near dissociation or *Argyll Robertson pupil*), convergence retraction nystagmus (the eyes pull in and retract with attempt to look upward), eyelid retraction (*Collier's sign*), and a tendency to look down in primary gaze position. Isolated paralysis of upward gaze may be the initial feature of the Miller Fisher syndrome and of vitamin B1 deficiency.

Bilateral lesions in the midbrain reticular formation cause isolated disturbances of downward gaze. They are rare in children but may occur in neurovisceral lipid storage disease.

Congenital Vertical Ocular Motor Apraxia

Clinical Features. Congenital vertical ocular motor apraxia is a rare syndrome similar to congenital horizontal ocular motor apraxia, except for the direction of gaze palsy. At rest, the eyes are fixated in either an upward or a downward position, with little random movement. Initially, the child uses head flexion or extension to fixate in the vertical plane; later, the child learns to use head thrusts. The Bell phenomenon is present.

Diagnosis. Vertical gaze palsy suggests intracranial tumor, and head MRI is required. However, gaze palsies present from birth without the later development of other neurological signs usually indicate a nonprogressive process. Bilateral restriction of upward eye movement resulting from muscle fibrosis is a consideration. In children with ocular motor apraxia, the eyes can move upward reflexively or by forced ductions; in children with muscle fibrosis, the eyes will not move upward by any means.

Management. Specific treatment is not available.

Horizontal Gaze Palsy

The usual cause of inability to look to one side is a lesion in the contralateral frontal or ipsilateral pontine gaze center. Immediately after developing a frontal lobe lesion, the eyes are tonically deviated toward the side of the lesion and contralateral hemiplegia is often present. The eyes move horizontally reflexively by stimulation of the brainstem gaze center with ice water caloric techniques. In contrast, an irritative frontal lobe lesion, such as one causing an epileptic seizure, generally causes the eyes to deviate in a direction opposite to the side with the seizure focus. When the focus is parietal, the eye deviation may be ipsilateral. Movements of the head and eyes during a seizure are *adversive seizures* (see Chapter 1). The initial direction of eye deviation reliably predicts a contralateral focus, especially if the movement is forced and sustained in a unilateral direction. Later movements that are mild and unsustained are not predictive.

Convergence Paralysis

Convergence paralysis, inability to adduct the eyes to focus on a near object in the absence of medial rectus palsies, can be caused by a pineal region tumor; in such cases, however, other signs of midbrain compression are usually present. Convergence paralysis is sometimes factitious or due to lack of motivation or attention. The absence of pupillary constriction when convergence is attempted identifies factitious convergence paralysis.

Convergence insufficiency is common after closed head injuries. The head injury need not be severe. Patient complaints may include diplopia, headache, or eyestrain while reading or other close work. Convergence insufficiency also occurs in the absence of prior head injury. The onset often follows a change in study time or intensity, poor lighting in the workplace, or the use of new contact lenses or eyeglasses. Treatment consists of convergence exercises.

NYSTAGMUS

Nystagmus is an involuntary, rhythmic ocular oscillation in which at least one phase is slow. With *pendular nystagmus*, both phases are slow. The oscillations of congenital pendular nystagmus are in the horizontal plane, even with the eyes in vertical gaze. On lateral gaze, the oscillations may change to jerk nystagmus.

Movements of unequal speed characterize *jerk nystagmus*. Following an initial slow component in one direction is a fast component with saccadic velocity in the other direction. Oscillation may be horizontal or vertical. The direction of jerk nystagmus is named for the fast (saccadic) component. Nystagmus intensity increases in the horizontal plane when gaze is in the direction of the fast phase.

Table 15-2 describes other eye movements that cannot be classified as nystagmus but that have diagnostic significance. *Opsoclonus* consists of conjugate, rapid, chaotic movements in all directions of gaze, often referred to as "dancing eyes." It occurs in infants with neuroblastoma (see Chapter 10). *Ocular flutter* is a brief burst of conjugate horizontal saccadic eye movements that interrupt fixation. It occurs in the recovery

TABLE 15-2 **Abnormal Eye Movements**

Movement	Appearance	Pathology
Nystagmus	Rhythmic oscillation	Variable
Opsoclonus	Nonrhythmic, chaotic conjugate movements	Neuroblastoma
Ocular flutter	Intermittent bursts of rapid horizontal oscillations during fixation	Cerebellar/brainstem disease
Ocular dysmetria	Overshooting, undershooting, or oscillation on refixation	Cerebellar disease
Ocular bobbing	Intermittent, rapid downward movement	Pontine lesions
Periodic alternating gaze	Cyclic conjugate lateral eye deviations, alternating from side to side	Posterior fossa

phase of opsoclonus or in association with cerebellar disease. *Ocular dysmetria* is overshooting or undershooting of the eyes during refixation or an oscillation before the eyes come to rest on a new fixation target. *Ocular bobbing* is not downbeat nystagmus, but is a sudden downward movement of both eyes with a slow drift back to midposition. It most often occurs in comatose patients with pontine dysfunction. The discussions of congenital and acquired nystagmus are separate because their differential diagnoses are different (Box 15-7).

Physiological Nystagmus

A high frequency (1–3 Hz), low-amplitude oscillation of the eyes occurs normally when sustaining lateral gaze to the point of fatigue. A jerk nystagmus, present at the endpoint of lateral gaze, is also normal. A few beats are usual, but even sustained nystagmus occurring at the endpoint is normal unless associated with other signs of neurological dysfunction or is distinctly asymmetric.

Congenital Nystagmus

Although congenital nystagmus is present at birth, it may be unnoticed until infancy or childhood and then misdiagnosed as acquired nystagmus. One reason that congenital nystagmus may remain unnoticed is that the *null point*, the angle of ocular movement at which the nystagmus is minimal, may be very wide. Often, nystagmus is mistaken for normal movement.

BOX 15-7 Differential Diagnosis of Nystagmus

PHYSIOLOGICAL

CONGENITAL

- Albinism
- Associated with blindness
- Familial
- Idiopathic

SPASMUS NUTANS

- Idiopathic
- Tumors of optic nerve and chiasm (see Chapter 16)

ACQUIRED NYSTAGMUS

- Dissociated
- Divergence
- Jerk
  - Horizontal
    - Drug-induced
    - Ictal nystagmus
    - Vestibular nystagmus
  - Vertical
    - Downbeat
    - Upbeat
- Pendular
  - Brainstem infarction
  - Multiple sclerosis (see Chapter 10)
  - Oculopalatal syndrome
    - Brainstem infarction
    - Spinocerebellar degeneration
- Monocular
- See-saw

A defect in the gaze-holding mechanism, secondary to loss of visual acuity before 2 years of age, was once the accepted mechanism of congenital nystagmus. The present belief is that the visual defect is not causal, but associated. When congenital nystagmus is genetic, transmission may occur as an autosomal recessive, autosomal dominant, or X-linked trait.

Clinical Features. Congenital nystagmus is usually in a horizontal in plane but may be either pendular or jerk in character. Convergence generally diminishes and fixation increases the intensity of nystagmus. Because a null zone exists where nystagmus is minimal, the head may be held to one side, or tilted, or both to improve vision. Periodic head turning may accompany periodic alternating nystagmus.

Two forms of head oscillation are associated with congenital nystagmus. One is involuntary and does not improve vision. The other, also seen in spasmus nutans, is opposite in direction to the nystagmus but not phase locked and improves vision. Many children have impaired vision from the nystagmus in the absence of a primary disturbance in visual acuity.

Diagnosis. Determination that the nystagmus was present at birth is important but not always possible. Carefully examine the eyes for abnormalities in the sensory visual system that may accentuate nystagmus. If the neurological findings are otherwise normal, MRI is unnecessary.

Management. Nystagmus may reduce after correcting a visual defect, particularly with contact lenses rather than eyeglasses, and by the use of prisms or surgery to move the eyes into the null zone without the head turning. In a double-blind, placebo-controlled study, memantine and gabapentin improved visual acuity, reduced nystagmus intensity, and improved foveation in patients with congenital nystagmus (Mclean et al, 2007).

ACQUIRED NYSTAGMUS

Spasmus Nutans

Spasmus nutans is an acquired nystagmus with onset in early infancy. Nystagmus, head nodding, and abnormal head positioning are the clinical features of spasmus nutans.

Clinical Features. Onset typically occurs between 6 and 12 months of age. Nystagmus is characteristically binocular (but may be monocular), has high frequency and low amplitude, is often dysconjugate, and can be horizontal, vertical, or rotatory in direction. The head is held in a tilted position and titubates in a manner that resembles nodding. Head tilt and movement may be more prominent than nystagmus, and torticollis is often the first complaint (see Chapter 14). The rotatory nystagmus may be difficult to see in children with dark irises and detected by the rotational movements of the blood vessels in a fundoscopic exam. The syndrome usually lasts for 1 to 2 years, rarely as long as 5 years, and then resolves spontaneously.

Diagnosis. Spasmus nutans is ordinarily a transitory, benign disorder of unknown cause. On rare occasions, a glioma of the anterior visual pathways or subacute necrotizing encephalopathy (see Chapter 10) mimics the syndrome. Tumor is a consideration if the nystagmus is monocular, the optic nerve is pale, or the onset is after 1 year of age. Typical cases do not require imaging studies of the head and orbit.

Management. Treatment is not required.

Pendular Nystagmus

Pendular nystagmus may be either congenital or acquired. In adults, the usual causes of acquired pendular nystagmus are brainstem infarction and multiple sclerosis. In children, pendular nystagmus in the absence of other neurological signs is either congenital or the first sign of spasmus nutans. However, the development of optic atrophy in a child with pendular nystagmus indicates a glioma of the anterior visual pathway.

Vertical pendular nystagmus is unusual and sometimes occurs in association with rhythmic vertical oscillations of the palate (*palatal myoclonus or tremor*). One encounters the syndrome of oculopalatal oscillation in some spinocerebellar degenerations and in ischemic disorders of the deep cerebellar nuclei and central tegmental tract.

Jerk Nystagmus

Drug-Induced Nystagmus

Clinical Features. Many psychoactive drugs, including tranquilizers, antidepressants, anticonvulsants, and alcohol, produce nystagmus at high therapeutic or toxic blood concentrations. The nystagmus evoked by lateral gaze is either horizontal or horizontal-rotary. Vertical nystagmus may be present on upward, but rarely on downward, gaze. Toxic dosages of most antiepileptic drugs and lithium produce primary-position downbeat nystagmus as well.

Diagnosis. Suspect drug overdose in patients with nystagmus and decreased consciousness. Request a quantitative and qualitative drug screen.

Management. Nystagmus resolves when the blood concentration of the drug falls.

Ictal Nystagmus

Clinical Features. Nystagmus as a seizure manifestation is binocular. It may occur alone or in association with other ictal manifestations. Sometimes, pupillary oscillations synchronous with nystagmus are present. As a rule, concurrent epileptiform discharges are focal, contralateral to the fast phase of nystagmus in frontal foci (saccades center) and ipsilateral to the fast phase of nystagmus in parieto-occipital foci (pursuit center). However, individual cases exist of nystagmus accompanying generalized 3 Hz spike-wave discharges, and periodic lateralized epileptiform discharges.

Diagnosis. Other seizure manifestations that identify the nature of the nystagmus are usually present. The electroencephalogram (EEG) confirms the diagnosis by the presence of epileptiform activity concurrent with nystagmus.

Management. Ictal nystagmus responds to anticonvulsant drug therapy (see Chapter 1).

Vestibular Nystagmus

Vestibular nystagmus occurs with disorders of the labyrinth, vestibular nerve, vestibular nuclei of the brainstem, or vestibulocerebellum.

Clinical Features. Labyrinthine disease (especially labyrinthitis) is usually associated with severe vertigo, nausea, vomiting, and autonomic features such as tachycardia and diaphoresis (see Chapter 17). Deafness, tinnitus, or both may be present as well. Movement of the head enhances the nystagmus and is more critical to the mechanism of nystagmus than the position obtained. Nystagmus is usually horizontal and torsional, with an initial slow phase followed by a rapid return. It is worse when gaze is in the direction of the fast phase. Fixation reduces nystagmus and vertigo.

Vertigo and nausea are mild when nystagmus is of central origin. Nystagmus is constantly present and not affected by head position. It may be horizontal or vertical and not affected by fixation. Other neurological disturbances referable to the brainstem or cerebellum are frequently associated features.

Diagnosis. Observation alone readily identifies vestibular nystagmus. It is identical to the nystagmus provoked by caloric stimulation or rotation. Labyrinthine disorders in children are usually infectious, sometimes viral, and sometimes a result of otitis media. Central causes of vestibular nystagmus include spinocerebellar degeneration, brainstem glioma or infarction, subacute necrotizing encephalomyelitis, periodic ataxias, and demyelinating disorders.

Management. Several different classes of drugs appreciably reduce the vertigo and nausea associated with labyrinthine disease. Diazepam is especially effective. Other useful drugs include scopolamine, antihistamines, and tranquilizers.

Downbeat Nystagmus

Clinical Features. In primary position, the eyes drift slowly upward and then reflexly beat downward. The intensity of the nystagmus is usually greatest when directing the eyes slightly downward and laterally. Downbeat nystagmus is distinguishable from *downward-beating nystagmus*, in which the nystagmus is present only on downward gaze. The cause of downward-beating nystagmus is toxic doses of anticonvulsant and sedative drugs, whereas downbeat nystagmus often indicates a structural abnormality of the brainstem, especially the cervicomedullary junction or cerebellum. Patient complaints include dizziness, oscillopsia, blurred vision, and difficulty reading. Approximately one-third of patients are asymptomatic. Cerebellar ataxia is present in about half of patients and usually is the only associated neurological sign.

Diagnosis. Cerebellar degenerations, both congenital and acquired, are the most common identifiable cause. The Chiari malformation is another consideration. Metabolic disturbances include phenytoin toxicity, thiamine deficiency, and hypomagnesemia resulting from either dietary depletion or the use of lithium salts.

A mother and her son had a congenital hereditary downbeat nystagmus. The condition was present in the boy at birth. By infancy, he needed to keep his chin down to look at people. He had no other neurological abnormalities, but the nystagmus caused difficulty in learning to read. His mother had a subclinical downbeat nystagmus evident only in oblique downward gaze.

Management. Clonazepam, baclofen, gabapentin, or DAP improves oscillopsia and acuity in some individuals. First, try a single test dose to determine whether long-term therapy will be useful. Prisms that increase convergence are rarely useful.

Upbeat Nystagmus

Clinical Features. In primary position, the eyes drift slowly downward and then spontaneously beat upward. Upward gaze accentuates the nystagmus. A large- and a small-amplitude type occur. Large-amplitude nystagmus increases in intensity during upward gaze and indicates a lesion in the anterior vermis of the cerebellum or an abnormality in the anterior visual pathway. Anterior visual pathway abnormalities include Leber congenital amaurosis, bilateral optic nerve hypoplasia, and congenital cataract (see Chapter 16). Small-amplitude nystagmus decreases in intensity during upward gaze and, when present, suggests an intrinsic lesion of the medulla.

Diagnosis. Upbeat nystagmus is usually an acquired disorder caused by vascular lesions or tumors of the brainstem or cerebellar vermis. Therefore, every child with a normal anterior visual pathway requires a head MRI. Upbeat nystagmus also occurs with impairment of smooth pursuit movements in dominantly inherited cerebellar vermian atrophy.

Management. Specific treatment is not available. Sometimes, gabapentin or DAP are useful.

Dissociated Nystagmus

Divergence Nystagmus

Divergence nystagmus is a rare condition in which both eyes beat outward simultaneously. The mechanism, while poorly understood, suggests a posterior fossa abnormality and occurs with spinocerebellar degenerations.

Monocular Nystagmus

Monocular nystagmus may be congenital or acquired. The most important diagnostic considerations in children are spasmus nutans and chiasmal tumors. Although no clinical feature consistently differentiates the two groups, optic nerve abnormalities, especially optic hypoplasia, sometimes occur in children with tumors but not in those with spasmus nutans.

A coarse pendular vertical nystagmus may develop in an amblyopic eye years after the visual loss. The nystagmus occurs in the blind eye when attempting distance fixation with the sighted eye and inhibited by convergence.

See-Saw Nystagmus

See-saw nystagmus is the result of two different oscillations. One is a pendular vertical oscillation. The other is a torsional movement in which one eye rises and intorts while the other falls and extorts. It may be congenital or acquired. The congenital form is sometimes associated with absence of the chiasm and a horizontal pendular nystagmus. Acquired cases are usually due to tumors of the sellar and parasellar regions and are associated with bitemporal hemianopia.

REFERENCES

Belanger C, Zhang KS, Reddy AK, et al. Inflammatory disorders of the orbit in childhood: A case series. American Journal of Ophthalmology 2010;150:460–3.

Burke G, Cossins J, Maxwell S, et al. Rapsyn mutations in hereditary myasthenia. Distinct early- and late-onset phenotypes. Neurology 2003;61:826–8.

Chung M, Stout JT, Borchert MS. Clinical diversity of hereditary Duane's retraction syndrome. Ophthalmology 2000;107:500–3.

Demer JL, Clark RA, Tischfield MA, et al. Evidence of an asymmetrical endophenotype in congenital fibrosis of extraocular muscles type 3 resulting from TUBB3 mutations. Investigative Ophthalmology and Visual Science 2010;51:4600–11.

DiMauro S and Hirano H. Mitochondrial deletion syndromes. In: GeneReviews at GeneTests: Medical Genetics Information Resource [database online]. Seattle: University of Washington. Available at http://www.genetests.org. PMID: 20301382. Last updated May 3, 2011.

Engel AG, Ohno K, Shen X-M, et al. Congenital myasthenic syndromes: multiple molecular targets at the neuromuscular junction. Annals of the New York Academy of Sciences 2003;998:138–60.

Engel AG, Shen XM, Selcen D, et al. What have we learned from the congenital myasthenic syndrome. Journal of Molecular Neuroscience 2010;40:143–53.

Harper CM, Engel AG. Treatment of 31 congenital myasthenic syndrome patients with 3,4-diaminopyridine. Neurology 2000;54(Suppl 3):A395.

Kuppersmith MJ. Does early immunotherapy reduce the conversion of ocular myasthenia gravis to generalized myasthenia gravis. Journal of Neuro-Ophthalmology 2003;23:249–50.

McLean R, Proudlock F, Thomas S, et al. Congenital nystagmus: Randomized, controlled, double-masked trial of memantine/gabapentin. Annals of Neurology 2007;61:130–8.

Mee J, Paine M, Byrne E, et al. Immunotherapy of ocular myasthenia gravis reduces conversion to generalized myasthenia gravis. Journal of Neuro-Ophthalmology 2003;23:251–5.

Online Mendelian Inheritance in Man, OMIM. Baltimore, MD: Johns Hopkins University. Available at http://www.ncbi.nlm.nih.gov/omim/. MIM 135700. Last edited 01/04/2011.

Pavone P, Barbagalio M, Parano E, et al. Clinical heterogeneity in familial congenital ptosis: Analysis of fourteen cases in one family over five generations. Pediatric Neurology 2005;33:251–4.

Richman DP, Agius MA. Treatment of autoimmune myasthenia gravis. Neurology 2003;61:1652–61.

Verzijl HT, van der Zwaag B, Cruysberg JR, Padberg GW. Möbius syndrome redefined. A syndrome of rhombencephalic maldevelopment. Neurology 2003;61:327–33.

CHAPTER 16

Disorders of the Visual System

Both congenital and acquired visual impairments in children are often associated with neurological disorders. The most common visual disorders are uncorrected refractive errors, amblyopia, strabismus, cataracts, and genetic disorders.

ASSESSMENT OF VISUAL ACUITY

The assessment of visual acuity in preverbal children relies mainly on assessing fixation and tracking as the infant or young child interacts with the environment.

Clinical Assessment

The pupillary light reflex is a test of the functional integrity of the subcortical afferent and efferent pathways and is reliably present after 31 weeks, gestation. A blink response to light develops at about the same time, and the lid may remain closed for as long as light is present (the dazzle reflex). The blink response to threat may not be present until 5 months of age. These responses are integrated in the brainstem and do not provide information on the cognitive (cortical) aspects of vision.

Observing fixation and following behavior is the principal means to assess visual function in newborns and infants. The human face, at a distance of approximately 30 cm, is the best target for fixation. Ninety percent of infants fixate on faces by 9 weeks of age. After obtaining fixation, the examiner slowly moves from side to side to test *tracking*. Visually directed grasping is present in normal children by 3 months of age but is difficult to test before 6 months of age. Absence of visually directed grasping may indicate a motor rather than a visual disturbance.

The *refixation reflex* evaluates the visual fields in infants and young children by moving an interesting stimulus in the peripheral field. Clues to visual impairment are structural abnormalities (e.g., microphthalmia, cloudy cornea), an absent or asymmetric pupillary response to light, dysconjugate gaze, nystagmus, and failure to fixate or track. Staring at a bright light source and oculodigital stimulation indicate severe visual impairment.

Visual Evoked Response

The visual evoked response to strobe light demonstrates the anatomical integrity of visual pathways without patient cooperation. At 30 weeks, gestation, a positive "cortical" wave with a peak latency of 300 ms is first demonstrable. The latency linearly declines at a rate of 10 ms each week throughout the last 10 weeks of gestation. In the newborn, the morphology of the visual evoked response is variable during wakefulness and active sleep and easiest to obtain just after the child goes to sleep. By 3 months of age, the morphology and latency of the visual evoked response are mature.

CONGENITAL BLINDNESS

Cortical blindness is the most common cause of congenital visual impairment among children referred to a neurologist. Ophthalmologists are more likely to see ocular abnormalities. The causes of congenital visual impairment are numerous and include prenatal and perinatal disturbances. Optic nerve hypoplasia, with or without other ocular malformations, is the most common ocular abnormality, followed by congenital cataracts and corneal opacities. Corneal abnormalities usually do not cause visual loss unless clouding is extensive. Such extensive clouding may develop in the mucopolysaccharidoses and Fabry disease. Box 16-1 lists conditions with corneal clouding present during childhood.

Congenital Cataract

For the purpose of this discussion, congenital cataract includes cataracts discovered within the first 3 months. Box 16-2 lists the differential diagnosis. Approximately one-third are hereditary, one-third syndromic, and one-third idiopathic.

In previous studies, intrauterine infection accounted for one-third of congenital cataracts. That percentage has declined with prevention of rubella embryopathy by immunization. Genetic and chromosomal disorders account for at least

BOX 16-1 Corneal Clouding in Childhood

- Cerebrohepatorenal syndrome (Zellweger syndrome)
- Congenital syphilis*
- Fabry disease (ceramide trihexosidosis)
- Familial high-density lipoprotein deficiency (Tangier island disease)
- Fetal alcohol syndrome
- Glaucoma*
- Infantile GM_1 gangliosidosis
- Juvenile metachromatic dystrophy
- Marinesco-Sjögren disease
- Mucolipidosis
- Mucopolysaccharidoses
- Multiple sulfatase deficiency
- Pelizaeus-Merzbacher disease
- Trauma (forceps at birth)

*Denotes the most common conditions and the ones with disease modifying treatments

BOX 16-2 Cataract Etiology

CONGENITAL CATARACT

- Chromosomal aberrations
  - Trisomy 13
  - Trisomy 18
  - Trisomy 21*
  - Turner syndrome*
- Drug exposure during pregnancy
  - Chlorpromazine
  - Corticosteroids
  - Sulfonamides
- Galactokinase deficiency
- Galactose-1-phosphate uridyltransferase deficiency
- Galactosemia
- Genetic
  - Autosomal dominant inheritance
    - Hereditary spherocytosis*
    - Incontinentia pigmenti*
    - Marshall syndrome*
    - Myotonic dystrophy*
    - Schäfer syndrome*
    - Without other anomalies
  - Autosomal recessive inheritance
    - Congenital ichthyosis*
    - Congenital stippled epiphyses (Conradi disease)
    - Marinesco-Sjögren syndrome*
    - Siemens syndrome*
    - Smith-Lemli-Opitz syndrome
  - X-linked inheritance (oculocerebrorenal syndrome)*
- Idiopathic
  - Intrauterine infection*
  - Mumps
  - Rubella
  - Syphilis
- Maternal factors
  - Diabetes
  - Malnutrition
  - Radiation
  - Prematurity
- Syndromes of uncertain etiology
  - Hallerman-Streiff syndrome
  - Pseudo-Turner syndrome*
  - With oxycephaly
  - With polydactyly

ACQUIRED CATARACT

- Drug-induced
  - Corticosteroids
  - Long-acting miotics
- Genetic
  - Autosomal dominant inheritance (Alport syndrome)
  - Autosomal recessive inheritance
    - Cockayne disease
    - Hepatolenticular degeneration (Wilson disease)
    - Rothmund-Thompson syndrome
    - Werner syndrome
  - X-linked inheritance (pseudo-pseudohypoparathyroidism)
- Chromosomal (Prader-Willi syndrome)
- Metabolic
  - Cretinism
  - Hypocalcemia
  - Hypoparathyroidism
  - Juvenile diabetes
  - Pseudohypoparathyroidism
- Trauma
- Varicella (postnatal)

DISLOCATED LENS

- Crouzon syndrome
- Ehlers-Danlos syndrome
- Homocystinuria
- Hyperlysinemia
- Marfan syndrome
- Sturge-Weber syndrome
- Sulfite oxidase deficiency

*Cataracts may not be noted until infancy or childhood

one-third, and the cause cannot be determined in half of the cases. Nonsyndromic, solitary, congenital cataracts are usually transmitted by autosomal dominant inheritance. The mode of transmission of syndromic congenital cataracts varies. In many hereditary syndromes, cataracts can be either congenital or delayed in appearance until infancy, childhood, or even adulthood. Several of these syndromes are associated with dermatoses: incontinentia pigmenti (irregular skin pigmentation), *Marshall syndrome* (anhidrotic ectodermal dysplasia), *Schäfer syndrome* (follicular hyperkeratosis), congenital ichthyosis, and *Siemens syndrome* (cutaneous atrophy).

Congenital cataracts occur in approximately 10 % of children with trisomy 13 and trisomy 18 and many children with trisomy 21. The association of congenital cataract and lactic acidosis or cardiomyopathy suggests a mitochondrial disorder.

Clinical Features. Small cataracts may impair vision and may be difficult to detect by direct ophthalmoscopy. Large cataracts appear as a white mass in the pupil and, if left in place, quickly cause deprivation amblyopia. The initial size of a cataract does not predict its course; congenital cataracts may remain stationary or increase in density but never improve spontaneously. Other congenital ocular abnormalities, aniridia, coloboma, and microphthalmos occur in 40–50 % of newborns with congenital cataracts.

Diagnosis. Large cataracts are obvious on inspection. Smaller cataracts distort the normal red reflex when the direct ophthalmoscope is at arm's length distance from the eye and a +12 to +20 lens is used.

Genetic disorders and maternal drug exposure are important considerations when cataracts are the only abnormality. Intrauterine disturbances, such as maternal illness and fetal infection, are usually associated with growth retardation and other malformations. Dysmorphic features are always an indication for ordering chromosome analysis. Galactosemia is suspected in children with hepatomegaly and milk intolerance (see Chapter 5), but cataracts may be present even before the development of systemic features.

Management. Developmental amblyopia is preventable by recognizing and removing cataracts before age 3 months. Urgent referral to a pediatric ophthalmologist is the standard of care.

Congenital Optic Nerve Hypoplasia

Optic nerve hypoplasia is a developmental defect in the number of optic nerve fibers and may result from excessive regression of retinal ganglion cell axons. Hypoplasia may be bilateral or unilateral and varies in severity. It may occur as an isolated defect or be associated with intracranial anomalies. The most common association is with midline defects of the septum pellucidum and hypothalamus (septo-optic dysplasia). Septo-optic dysplasia (*DeMorsier syndrome*) is familial in some cases and transmitted as an autosomal recessive trait.

Clinical Features. The phenotype is highly variable; 62 % of affected children have isolated hypopituitarism and 30 % have the complete phenotype of pituitary hypoplasia, optic nerve hypoplasia, and agenesis of midline structures (Thomas et al, 2001). In one study group of 55 patients with optic nerve hypoplasia (Birkebaek et al, 2003), 49 % had an abnormal septum pellucidum on magnetic resonance imaging (MRI), and 64 % had a hypothalamic-pituitary axis abnormality. Twenty-seven patients (49 %) had endocrine dysfunction, and 23 of these had hypothalamic-pituitary axis abnormality. The frequency of endocrinopathy was higher in patients with an abnormal septum pellucidum (56 %) than a normal septum pellucidum (39 %) and the appearance of the septum pellucidum predicts the likely spectrum of endocrinopathy.

When hypoplasia is severe, the child is severely visually impaired and the eyes draw attention because of strabismus and nystagmus. Ophthalmoscopic examination reveals a small, pale nerve head (Figure 16-1). A pigmented area surrounded by a yellowish mottled halo is sometimes present at the edge of the disk margin, giving the appearance of a double ring. The degree of hypothalamic-pituitary involvement varies. Possible symptoms include neonatal hypoglycemia and seizures, recurrent hypoglycemia in childhood, growth retardation, diabetes insipidus, and sexual infantilism. Some combination of mental retardation, cerebral palsy, and epilepsy is often present and indicates malformations in other portions of the brain.

Diagnosis. All infants with ophthalmoscopic evidence of optic nerve hypoplasia require cranial MRI and an assessment of endocrine status. The common findings on MRI are cavum septum pellucidum, hypoplasia of the cerebellum, aplasia of the corpus callosum, aplasia of the fornix, and an empty sella. Absence of the pituitary infundibulum with posterior pituitary ectopia indicates congenital hypopituitarism. Endocrine studies should include assays of growth hormone, antidiuretic hormone, and the integrity of hypothalamic-pituitary control of the thyroid, adrenal, and gonadal systems. Infants with hypoglycemia usually have growth hormone deficiency.

Superior segmental optic nerve hypoplasia is associated with congenital inferior visual field defects and occurs in children born to mothers with insulin-dependent diabetes.

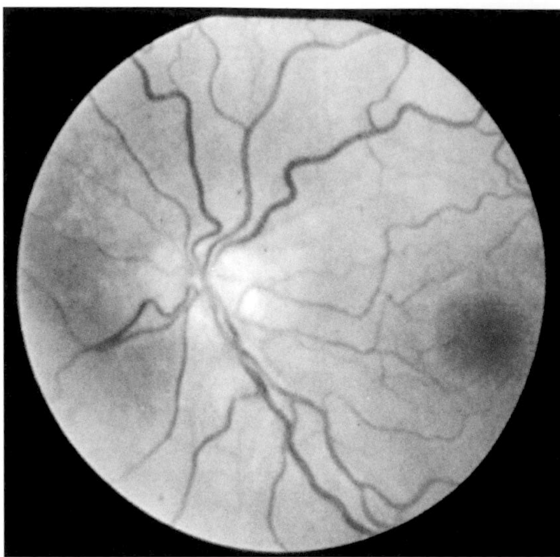

FIGURE 16-1 ■ Optic nerve hypoplasia. The optic nerve is small and pale, but the vessels are of normal size.

Management. No treatment is available for optic nerve hypoplasia, but endocrine abnormalities respond to replacement therapy. Children with corticotrophin deficiency may experience sudden death. Children with visual impairment may benefit from visual aids.

Coloboma

Coloboma is a defect in embryogenesis that may affect only the disk or may include the retina, iris, ciliary body, and choroid. Colobomas isolated to the nerve head appear as deep excavations, deeper inferiorly. They may be unilateral or bilateral. The causes of congenital coloboma are genetic (monogenic and chromosomal) and intrauterine disease (toxic and infectious). Retinochoroidal colobomas are glistening white or yellow defects inferior or inferior nasal to the disk. The margins are distinct and surrounded by pigment. *Morning glory disk* is not a form of coloboma; it is an enlarged dysplastic disk with a white excavated center surrounded by an elevated annulus of pigmentary change. Retinal vessels enter and leave at the margin of the disk, giving the appearance of a morning glory flower. The morning glory syndrome is associated with transsphenoidal encephaloceles. Affected children are dysmorphic with midline facial anomalies.

ACUTE MONOCULAR OR BINOCULAR BLINDNESS

The differential diagnoses of acute and progressive blindness show considerable overlap. Although older children recognize sudden visual loss, slowly progressive ocular disturbances may produce an asymptomatic decline until vision is severely disturbed, especially if unilateral. When finally noticed, the child's loss of visual acuity seems acute. Teachers or parents are often the first to recognize a slowly progressive visual disturbance. Box 16-3 lists conditions in which visual acuity is normal and then suddenly lost. Box 16-4 lists disorders in which the underlying pathological process is progressive. The patient first perceives the condition. Therefore, consult both lists in the differential diagnosis of acute blindness. The duration of a transitory monocular visual loss suggests the underlying cause: seconds indicate optic disk disorders such as papilledema or drusen, minutes indicate emboli, hours indicate migraine, and days indicate optic neuropathy, most commonly optic neuritis.

BOX 16-3 Causes of Acute Loss of Vision

Carotid dissection* (see Chapter 11)
Cortical blindness
- Anoxic encephalopathy (see Chapter 2)
- Benign occipital epilepsy* (see Chapter 1)
- Hydrocephalus*
- Hypoglycemia*
- Hypertension* (malignant or accelerated)
- Hyperviscosity
- Hypotension
- Migraine* (see Chapter 3)
- Occipital metastatic disease
- Posttraumatic transient cerebral blindness
- Systemic lupus erythematosus
- Toxic* (cyclosporine, etc.)
- Trauma

Psychogenic blindness
Optic neuropathy*
- Demyelinating
  - Idiopathic optic neuritis
  - Multiple sclerosis (see Chapter 10)
  - Neuromyelitis optica (see Chapter 12)
- Ischemic
- Toxic
- Traumatic
- Pituitary apoplexy
- Pseudotumor cerebri* (see Chapter 4)

Retinal disease
- Central retinal artery occlusion
- Migraine*

*Denotes the most common conditions and the ones with disease modifying treatments

Cortical Blindness

Cortical blindness in children may be permanent or transitory, depending on the cause. The causes of transitory cortical blindness in childhood include migraine (see Chapter 3), mild

BOX 16-4 Causes of Progressive Loss of Vision

COMPRESSIVE OPTIC NEUROPATHIES

- Aneurysm* (see Chapters 4 and 15)
- Arteriovenous malformations* (see Chapters 4, 10, and 11)
- Craniopharyngioma*
- Hypothalamic and optic tumors
- Pituitary adenoma*
- Pseudotumor cerebri* (see Chapter 4)

DISORDERS OF THE LENS (SEE BOX 16-3)

- Cataract
- Dislocation of the lens

HEREDITARY OPTIC ATROPHY

- Leber hereditary optic neuropathy
- Wolfram syndrome

INTRAOCULAR TUMORS

TAPETORETINAL DEGENERATIONS

- Abnormal carbohydrate metabolism
  - Mucopolysaccharidosis (see Chapter 5)
  - Primary hyperoxaluria
- Abnormal lipid metabolism
  - Abetalipoproteinemia (see Chapter 10)
  - Hypobetalipoproteinemia (see Chapter 10)
  - Multiple sulfatase deficiency (see Chapter 5)
  - Neuronal ceroid lipofuscinosis (see Chapter 5)
  - Niemann-Pick disease (see Chapter 5)
  - Refsum disease (see Chapter 7)
- Other syndromes of unknown etiology
  - Bardet-Biedl syndrome
  - Cockayne syndrome
  - Laurence-Moon syndrome
  - Refsum disease (see Chapter 7)
  - Usher syndrome (see Chapter 17)

*Denotes the most common conditions and the ones with disease modifying treatments

head trauma, brief episodes of hypoglycemia or hypotension, and benign occipital epilepsy (see Chapter 1). Acute and sometimes permanent blindness may occur following anoxia; secondary to massive infarction of, or hemorrhage into, the visual cortex; and when multifocal metastatic tumors or abscesses are located in the occipital lobes. The main feature of cortical blindness is loss of vision with preservation of the pupillary light reflex. Fundoscopic examination is normal.

Hypoglycemia

Repeated episodes of acute cortical blindness may occur at the time of mild hypoglycemia in children with glycogen storage diseases and following insulin overdose in diabetic children.

Clinical Features. Sudden blindness is associated with clinical evidence of hypoglycemia (sweating and confusion). Ophthalmoscopic and neurological findings are normal. Recovery is complete in 2 to 3 hours.

Diagnosis. During an episode of cortical blindness caused by hypoglycemia, electroencephalography (EEG) shows high-voltage slowing over both occipital lobes. Afterward the EEG returns to normal. Brain MRI shows diffuse edema in the occipital lobes.

Management. Recovery occurs when blood glucose concentration normalizes.

Transitory Posttraumatic Cerebral Blindness

Clinical Features. Transitory posttraumatic cerebral blindness is a benign syndrome that most often occurs in children with a history of migraine or epilepsy. The spectrum of visual disturbance is broad, but a juvenile and an adolescent pattern exist. In children younger than 8 years, the precipitating trauma is usually associated with either a brief loss of consciousness or a report that the child was "stunned." The child claims blindness almost immediately on regaining consciousness, which lasts for an hour or less. During the episode, the child may be lethargic and irritable but is usually coherent. Recovery is complete, and the child may not recall the event.

In older children, a syndrome of blindness, confusion, and agitation begins several minutes or hours after trivial head trauma. Consciousness is not lost. All symptoms resolve after several hours, and the child has complete amnesia for the event. These episodes share many features with acute confusional migraine and are probably a variant of that disorder (see Chapter 2).

Diagnosis. Head computed tomography (CT) is invariable in children with any neurological abnormality following head trauma, but is probably unnecessary if the blindness has cleared. Those with persistent blindness require MRI to exclude injury to the occipital lobes. Occipital intermittent rhythmic delta on EEG suggests migraine or epilepsy as the underlying cause. Recognition of the syndrome can avoid the trouble and expense of other studies. Scrutinize the family history for the possibility of migraine or epilepsy. The rapid and complete resolution of all symptoms confirms the diagnosis.

Management. Treatment is unnecessary if the symptoms resolve spontaneously.

Psychogenic Blindness

A spurious claim of complete binocular blindness is easy to identify. A pupillary response to light indicates that the anterior pathway is intact and only cortical blindness is a possibility. Simply observing the child's visual behavior such as making eye contact, avoiding obstructions in the waiting room and following nonverbal instructions, confirms effective visual capability. Otherwise, assess visual function by using a full-field optokinetic stimulus tape or by moving a large mirror in front of the patient to stimulate matching eye movements. In the case of psychogenic monocular blindness, perform the same tests with a patch covering the normal eye.

Spurious claims of partial visual impairment are more difficult to challenge. Helpful tests include observing visual behavior, failure of acuity to improve linearly with increasing test size, inappropriate ability to detect small test objects on a tangent screen, and constricted (tunnel) visual fields to confrontation.

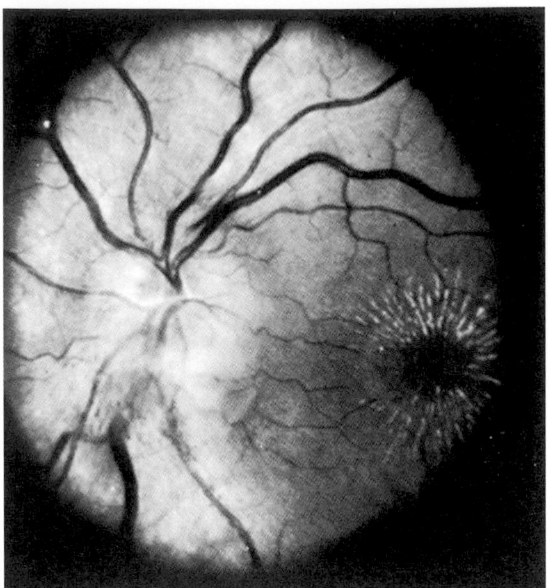

FIGURE 16-2 ■ Neuroretinitis. The optic disk is swollen and the peripapillary nerve fiber layer opacificied. Exudates surround the macula in a star pattern. (Courtesy of Patrick Lavin, MD.)

Optic Neuropathies

Demyelinating Optic Neuropathy

Demyelination of the optic nerve (optic neuritis) may occur as an isolated finding affecting one or both eyes, or it may be associated with demyelination in other portions of the nervous system. Discussion of neuromyelitis optica (NMO, *Devic syndrome*), the syndrome combining optic neuritis and transverse myelitis, is in Chapter 12, and multiple sclerosis in Chapter 10. MRI is a useful technique for surveying the central nervous system for demyelinating lesions (see Figure 10-1). The incidence of later multiple sclerosis among children with optic neuritis is 15 % or less if the child has no evidence of more diffuse involvement when brought to medical attention. The incidence is much higher when diffuse involvement is present or when optic neuritis recurs within 1 year. Unilateral optic neuritis, and retrobulbar as opposed to papillitis, has a higher incidence of later multiple sclerosis than bilateral optic neuritis.

Clinical Features. Monocular involvement is characteristic of optic neuritis in adults, but binocular involvement occurs in more than half of children. Binocular involvement may be concurrent or sequential, sometimes occurring over a period of weeks. The initial feature in some children is pain in the eye, but for most it is blurred vision, progressing within hours or days to partial or complete blindness. Visual acuity reduces to less than 20/200 in almost all affected children within 1 week. A history of a preceding "viral" infection or immunization is common, but a cause-and-effect relationship between optic neuritis and these events is not established.

Results of ophthalmoscopic examination may be normal at the onset of symptoms if neuritis is primarily retrobulbar. Visual loss readily distinguishes papillitis from papilledema. In optic neuritis, visual loss occurs early; in papilledema, visual loss is a late feature.

Neuroretinitis is the association of swelling of the optic nerve head with macular edema or a macular star. Ophthalmoscopic examination shows disk swelling, peripapillary retinal detachment, and a macular star (Figure 16-2). Neuroretinitis suggests the possibility of conditions other than idiopathic optic neuritis.

In the absence of myelitis, the prognosis in children with bilateral optic neuritis is good. Complete recovery occurs in the majority of those affected.

Diagnosis. Optic neuritis is a consideration whenever monocular or binocular blindness develops suddenly in a child. Ophthalmoscopic or slit-lamp examination confirms the diagnosis. Visual evoked response testing further confirms the diagnosis. MRI of the orbit may reveal swelling and demyelination of the optic nerve. Examination of the cerebrospinal fluid may be helpful to check for markers of demyelinating disease, such as oligoclonal bands, IgG index, and anti-NMO antibodies. Such examination sometimes shows a leukocytosis and an increased concentration of protein. Accelerated hypertension causes bilateral swelling of the optic nerves and recording blood pressure is an essential part of the evaluation.

Management. In adults, intravenous methylprednisolone, 250 mg every 6 hours for 3 days, followed by oral prednisone, 1 mg/kg/day for 11 days then tapering over 4 days, speeds the recovery of vision and reduces recurrence of neuritis in the first 2 years according to the results of the optic neuritis treatment trial. The long-term outcome from optic neuritis is not significantly changed by the treatment (Balcer, 2006). In children, we use intravenous methylprednisolone 3.5 mg/kg/dose q 6 hours for 3 days followed by 11 days of oral prednisone 1 mg/kg/day and then a tapering over 4 days.

Ischemic Optic Neuropathy

Infarction of the anterior portion of the optic nerve is rare in children and is usually associated with systemic vascular disease or hypotension.

Clinical Features. Ischemic optic neuropathy usually occurs as a sudden segmental loss of vision in one eye, but slow or stepwise progression over several days is possible. Recurrent episodes are unusual except with migraine and some idiopathic cases.

Diagnosis. Altitudinal visual field defects are present in 70–80 % of patients. Color vision loss is roughly equivalent in severity to visual acuity loss, whereas in demyelinating optic neuritis the disturbance of color vision is greater than that of visual acuity. Ophthalmoscopic examination reveals diffuse or partial swelling of the optic disk. When swelling is diffuse, it gives the appearance of papilledema and flame-shaped hemorrhages appear adjacent to the disk margin. After acute swelling subsides, optic atrophy follows.

Management. Treatment depends on the underlying cause of ischemia.

Toxic-Nutritional Optic Neuropathies

Drugs, toxins, and nutritional deficiencies alone or in combination may cause an acute or progressive optic neuropathy. These factors may cause optic neuropathy by inducing mitochondrial changes, perhaps in susceptible populations with mitochondrial DNA (mtDNA) mutations.

Clinical Features. Implicated drugs include barbiturates, antibiotics (chloramphenicol, isoniazid, streptomycin, and sulfonamides), chemotherapeutic agents, chlorpropamide, digitalis, ergot, halogenated hydroxyquinolines, penicillamine, and quinine. Nutritional deficiencies that may cause such optic neuropathies include folic acid and vitamins B1, B2, B6, and B12.

Symptoms vary with the specific drug, but progressive loss of central vision is typical. In some cases, visual loss is rapid and develops as acute binocular blindness that may be asymmetric at onset, suggesting monocular involvement. Many of the drugs produce optic neuropathy by interfering with the action of folic acid or vitamin B12 and thereby causing a nutritional deficiency.

Diagnosis. Drug toxicity is suspect whenever central and paracentral scotomas develop during the course of drug treatment. Optic nerve hyperemia with small paracentral hemorrhages may be an early feature. Later the disk becomes pale.

Management. Drug-induced optic neuropathy is dose-related. Dosage reduction may be satisfactory in some cases, especially if concurrent treatment with folic acid or vitamin B12 reverses the process. Some drugs require complete cessation of therapy.

Traumatic Optic Neuropathies

Trauma to the head may cause an indirect optic neuropathy in one or both eyes. The optic nerve, tethered along its course, is subject to shearing forces when the skull suddenly accelerates or decelerates. Possible consequences include acute swelling, hemorrhage, or tear. This is particularly common in children who sustain bicycle injuries when not wearing a helmet.

Clinical Features. Loss of vision is usually immediate. Delayed visual loss caused by a hematoma or edema may respond to corticosteroids and has a better prognosis. The distinction between traumatic optic neuropathy and cortical blindness is easy because the pupillary response in optic neuropathy diminishes. The prognosis for recovery is best if there is a brief delay between the time of injury and the onset of blindness.

Diagnosis. The loss of vision and pupillary light response immediately following a head injury should suggest the diagnosis. Ophthalmological examination may reveal peripapillary hemorrhages.

Management. Suggested treatments consist of corticosteroids and surgical decompression of the nerve.

Pituitary Apoplexy

Pituitary apoplexy in children is a very rare, life-threatening condition caused by hemorrhagic infarction of the pituitary gland.

Clinical Features. Pituitary infarction occurs most often when there is a preexisting pituitary tumor but may also occur in the absence of tumor. Several different clinical features are possible, depending on the structures affected by the swollen gland, including monocular or binocular blindness, visual field defects, ophthalmoplegia, chemical meningitis, cerebrospinal fluid rhinorrhea, and shock from hypopituitarism. Leakage of blood and necrotic material into the subarachnoid space causes chemical meningitis associated with headache, meningismus, and loss of consciousness.

Diagnosis. MRI of the head with views of the pituitary gland establishes the diagnosis. Endocrine testing may show a deficiency of all pituitary hormones.

Management. Patients deteriorate rapidly and may die within a few days without prompt administration of corticosteroids. Replacement of other hormones is required but is not lifesaving. In patients who continue to do poorly, as evidenced by loss of consciousness, hypothalamic instability, or loss of vision, urgent surgical decompression of the expanding pituitary mass is required. In patients that develop acute secondary adrenal crisis, intravenous hydrocortisone at 1–1.5 mg/kg followed by 1.5–2.5 mg/kg over 24 hours and continuous infusion of intravenous fluids with continuous cardiovascular monitoring is required to decrease fatalities (Arlt & Alloli, 2003).

Retinal Disease

Central Retinal Artery Occlusion

The most common risk factors for central retinal artery occlusion are congenital heart disease, mitral valve prolapse, sickle cell disease, migraine, vasculitis, and pregnancy.

Clinical Features. Most affected children have an abrupt loss of monocular vision of variable intensity without premonitory symptoms. Some describe spots, a shadow, or a descending veil before the loss of vision. Bilateral retinal artery occlusion is very rare in children.

Diagnosis. The clinical history and ophthalmoscopic examination are the basis for the diagnosis of retinal artery obstruction. The posterior pole of the retina becomes opacified except in the foveal region, which contains a cherry-red spot. The peripheral retina appears normal. Visual field examination and fluorescein angiography help confirm the diagnosis in some cases. One must seek the underlying cause once the diagnosis is established. Evaluation should include cranial MRI and MR angiography or CT angiography, auscultation of the heart, radiographs of the chest, echocardiography in selected cases, complete blood cell count with sedimentation rate, cholesterol and triglyceride screening, coagulation studies, hemoglobin electrophoresis, and lupus anticoagulant and antiphospholipid antibodies.

Management. Acute treatment requires immediate ophthalmological consultation. The management of idiopathic occlusion of the retinal artery in adults is controversial, with some authorities recommending the use of corticosteroids. In children, steroids should be considered only in suspected vasculitis. Visual acuity is more likely to improve when the obstruction is in a branch artery rather than in the central retinal artery.

Retinal ischemia lasting longer than 240 minutes may lead to irreversible loss of vision. Restoration of blood flow within 100 minutes may preserve vision, so timely therapy is critical. Spontaneous recovery is rare. Visual acuity at presentation is a predictive of eventual acuity after the event. Although several treatment modalities are available, none has been prospectively shown to have more than a limited or marginal benefit. Therapies include ocular massage to dislodge the embolus, decreasing intraocular pressure through anterior chamber paracentesis or administering intravenous diuretics. The use of vasodilators or inhaling carbogen (95 % oxygen and 5 % carbon dioxide) has also been tried. A more aggressive approach involves using thrombolytics similar to their use in acute myocardial infarction and ischemic stroke. For patients with sickle cell disease, exchange transfusion, used similarly in other vaso-occlusive crises, may be employed but the evidence is unclear (Kalpesh & Patel, 2010).

Retinal Migraine

Clinical Features. Visual symptoms are relatively common during an attack of migraine with aura (see Chapter 3). The typical scintillating scotomas, or "fortification spectra," are field defects caused by altered neuronal function in the occipital cortex. The affected field is usually contralateral to the headache.

Transitory monocular blindness is an unusual feature of migraine. Careful questioning differentiates a field defect from a monocular defect. Migraine is the main cause of transitory monocular blindness in children. The visual loss is sudden in most cases, may be partial or complete, and often precedes and is ipsilateral to the headache. Recurrences are usually in the same eye, and attacks may occur without headache. One parent, usually the mother, has a history of migraine.

Typical patients have a long personal history of migraine with aura in which both field defects and monocular blindness occur separately or together. A mosaic or jigsaw pattern of scotomas that clear within minutes is experienced. The International Headache Society Classification requires the blindness to be fully reversible and associated with headache and the patient to have a normal neuro-ophthalmologic exam between attacks (Headache Classification Subcommittee of the International Headache Society, 2004). When permanent monocular blindness occurs, particularly in the setting of vascular risk factors or the use of oral contraceptives, stroke or vasculitis are more likely etiologies.

Diagnosis. Consider the diagnosis in children with a history of migraine with aura. Ophthalmoscopic findings may be normal initially and then include retinal edema with scattered hemorrhages. Fluorescein angiography reveals several patterns of retinal vaso-occlusive disease involving the branch retinal artery, the central retinal artery, the central retinal vein, and the cilioretinal artery.

Management. Children who have retinal ischemia during migraine attacks require prophylaxis with pharmaceutical agents that prevent further episodes. The use of a baby aspirin may be considered if not contraindicated.

Retinal Trauma

Direct blunt injury to the orbit causes visual impairment by retinal contusion, tear, or detachment. A diminished pupillary response characterizes all three. Contusion is associated with retinal edema. Although visual loss is immediate, the retina appears normal for the first few hours and only later becomes white and opaque. The severity of visual loss varies, but complete recovery is the rule.

Retinal tear is often associated with vitreous hemorrhage. Visual loss is usually immediate and easily diagnosed by its ophthalmoscopic appearance. Recovery is spontaneous unless there is detachment, for which cryotherapy is required.

PROGRESSIVE LOSS OF VISION

Compressive Optic Neuropathy

Compression of one or both optic nerves often occurs in the region of the chiasm. The visual loss may involve one eye or one visual field. In children with tumors in and around the diencephalon, the most constant feature is growth failure, which may be unrecognized until other symptoms develop.

Craniopharyngioma

Clinical Features. Craniopharyngiomas are the most common nonglial tumors in children. The peak age range for diagnosis of this tumor is 6 to 14 years. The typical onset is insidious, and a 1- to 2-year history of slowly progressive symptoms is common. These symptoms may include progressive visual loss, delayed sexual maturation, growth failure, weight gain, and diabetes insipidus. Field defects are frequently asymmetric or unilateral. Bitemporal hemianopia is present in 50 % of children with craniopharyngioma, and homonymous hemianopia in 10–20 %. Diminished visual acuity in one or both eyes and optic atrophy are constant features.

Approximately 25 % of children have hydrocephalus that causes headache and papilledema. Hypothalamic involvement may produce diabetes insipidus or the hypodipsia-hyponatremia syndrome, characterized by lethargy, confusion, and hypotension. Other features depend on the direction of tumor growth. Anterior extension may compress the olfactory tract, causing anosmia, whereas lateral extension may compress the third and fifth nerves.

Diagnosis. MRI is diagnostic. The important feature is a multicystic and solid enhancing suprasellar mass, which causes hydrocephalus and stretches the optic nerves and chiasm (Brunel et al, 2002).

Management. Surgical removal of the tumor is the most effective treatment. Recurrences occur in 30 % of cases after "complete" resection, 57 % after incomplete resection, and 30 % when radiation follows subtotal resection. The 5- and 10-year survival rates after postoperative radiotherapy are 84 % and 72 %, respectively, for children. Most long-term survivors experience panhypopituitarism, cognitive impairment, and obesity.

Optic Pathway and Diencephalic Gliomas

Sixty percent of optic pathway gliomas are pilocytic astrocytomas and the remaining 40 % are fibrillary astrocytomas. Optic gliomas represent 3–5 % of childhood brain tumors. They may involve any part of the optic pathway from the optic nerves to the optic radiations. They also infiltrate the adjacent hypothalamus and temporal lobes. More than 50 % of children with optic gliomas have neurofibromatosis type 1 (NF1). Precocious puberty is a common initial feature in children with NF1. The rate of tumor growth is slower in children with NF1 than when NF1 is not present. Some patients with NF1 exhibit static lesions or even regression in tumor volume.

Clinical Features. Initial symptoms depend on the location, but hypothalamic tumors eventually affect the optic chiasm and optic chiasm tumors affect the hypothalamus. In children younger than 3 years, tumors of the hypothalamus may produce *the diencephalic syndrome*, characterized by marked loss of subcutaneous fat and total body weight with maintenance or acceleration of long bone growth. Despite the appearance of cachexia, the infant is mentally alert and does not seem as sick as the appearance suggests. Pendular or see-saw nystagmus may be associated. The precise endocrine mechanism that leads to the diencephalic syndrome is unknown. Hamartomas of the tuber cinereum, optic pathway gliomas that compress the hypothalamus, and craniopharyngiomas are also associated with the diencephalic syndrome. Precocious puberty, rather than the diencephalic syndrome, can be the initial feature of hypothalamic tumors in infants and children.

Age is an important prognostic factor for optic gliomas. Children less than 5 years of age have a more aggressive course. The presenting features of unilateral optic nerve gliomas are visual loss, proptosis, and optic atrophy. Chiasmatic tumors in infants present as very large suprasellar masses that may also extend into the hypothalamus and third ventricle producing hydrocephalus and endocrine abnormalities. Binocular involvement suggests involvement of the optic chiasm or tract. Visual field deficits vary. Increased intracranial pressure suggests extension of tumor from the chiasm to the hypothalamus.

Although the tumor is usually benign, their location results in serious morbidity. Children with NF1 have a better progression-free survival, while age less than 1 year is associated with a higher risk of tumor progression (Opocher et al, 2006).

Diagnosis. MRI of the hypothalamus identifies gliomas as high-density signals on T_2-weighted studies. MRI permits visualization of the hypothalamus in several different planes and identification of brainstem extension of tumor (Figure 16-3).

MRI with enhancement identifies optic pathway gliomas as an enlarged tubular appearance of the nerve and chiasm. Examine the entire visual pathway in all children with optic nerve gliomas because many tumors involve the chiasm and retrochiasmal pathways. Routine MRI screening for optic pathway gliomas in asymptomatic children with NF1 does not affect the outcome (Listernick et al, 1997). Regular ophthalmological examinations are the preferred method for surveillance.

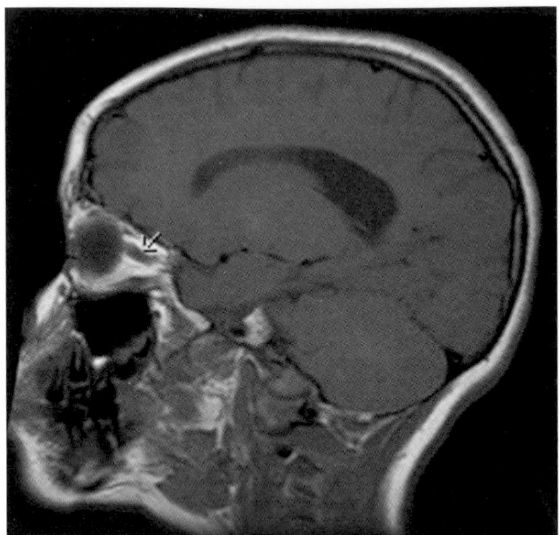

FIGURE 16-3 ■ Optic nerve glioma. Sagittal T_1 MRI shows an enlarged optic nerve in a patient with neurofibromatosis.

Management. Several factors influence management decisions. The indications for early intervention are younger age, progressive symptoms, and extensive central nervous system involvement. Chemotherapy, the initial treatment, may provide stabilization or regression (Silva et al, 2000). Older children and those who fail chemotherapy receive radiation therapy, which provides 5-year survival rates up to 30%. Stereotaxic-guided biopsy of hypothalamic tumors is often dangerous and provides no greater diagnostic information than imaging. Tumors located in the floor of the fourth ventricle, lateral recesses, cerebellar pontine angle, or cervical medullary junction may be surgically accessible and have a more benign course. Resection of intrinsic optic nerve or chiasmal gliomas should be avoided unless the child is already blind and the tumor is impinging on adjacent structures.

Optic pathway gliomas associated with NF1 rarely progress significantly after the time of diagnosis. Biopsy or removal of tumor from a sighted eye is only a consideration when the tumor is malignant, progressively enlarging or causing severe proptosis, and likely to cause blindness or death.

Pituitary Adenoma

Pituitary adenomas represent only 1–2% of intracranial tumors of childhood. Visual field defects may be unilateral temporal, bitemporal, or occasionally homonymous. Optic atrophy is present in 10–20% of cases.

Clinical Features. The onset of symptoms is usually during adolescence. The presenting features relate to the hormone secreted by the tumor. Approximately one-third of adenomas secrete prolactin, one-third are nonfunctioning, and many of the rest secrete growth hormone or adrenocorticotropic hormone (ACTH). Amenorrhea is usually the first symptom in girls with prolactin-secreting tumors. Galactorrhea may also be present. In boys, the initial features are growth retardation, delayed puberty, and headache.

Gigantism results when increased concentrations of growth hormone circulate before the epiphyses close. After closure, growth hormone causes acromegaly. Increased concentrations of ACTH cause Cushing syndrome.

Diagnosis. MRI provides excellent visualization of the tumor and identification of its extrasellar extent. Measurement of hormone production is useful in distinguishing the tumor type.

Management. Surgical resection is the preferred treatment for tumors that compress the optic pathways. Medical treatment may suffice for small tumors. Perform an endocrine evaluation, as hormone replacement may be needed.

Hereditary Optic Neuropathy

Hereditary optic neuropathies may affect only the visual system, or the visual system and central nervous system, or multiple systems. The underlying abnormality may lie in the nuclear or the mt DNA. These disorders can cause acute, subacute, or chronic visual decline.

Leber Congenital Amaurosis

Leber congenital amaurosis (LCA), a group of autosomal recessive retinal dystrophies, is the most common genetic cause of congenital visual impairment (Weleber et al, 2010). Eight different gene mutations cause one-third of cases. The common feature is disturbance of the retinal pigmentary epithelium.

Clinical Features. The clinical characteristics of LCA are moderate to severe visual impairment at or within a few months of birth, nystagmus, and sluggish pupillary responses. Additional features include symmetric midfacial hypoplasia with enophthalmos and hypermetropic refractive errors. While substantial variation between families exists, the phenotype is relatively constant within families. Ophthalmoscopy of the retina shows no abnormality in infancy and early childhood, but, with time, progressive retinal stippling and pallor of the disk appear. Mental retardation and other neurological disturbances may be associated. Visual acuity is rarely better than 20/400. A characteristic finding is *Franceschetti's oculodigital sign*, comprising eye poking, pressing, and rubbing.

Diagnosis. The retinal appearance and abnormal electroretinogram establish the diagnosis in infants. Neuroimaging shows cerebellar atrophy in children with mental slowing. Other disorders that may be mistaken for LCA are peroxisomal disorders and several varieties of infantile-onset progressive retinal degeneration.

Management. The retinopathy is not reversible.

Wolfram Syndrome

Wolfram syndrome is the combination of diabetes insipidus and mellitus with optic atrophy and bilateral neurosensory hearing loss. A mutation in a gene in the 4p16 region predisposes to multiple mt DNA deletions in families with Wolfram syndrome (OMIM, 2012). A second form, Wolfram syndrome 2, linking to a different site, is less common.

Clinical Features. The onset of diabetes is usually in the first decade. Insulin therapy is required soon after diagnosis. Visual loss progresses rapidly in the second decade but does not lead to complete blindness. Diabetes does not cause optic atrophy, rather all clinical features result from a progressive neurodegenerative process. The sensorineural hearing loss affects high frequencies first. The hearing loss is progressive but rarely leads to severe hearing loss. Features reported in some patients include anosmia, autonomic dysfunction, ptosis, external ophthalmoplegia, tremor, ataxia, nystagmus, seizures, central diabetes insipidus, and endocrinopathies. Psychiatric illness occurs in most cases of Wolfram syndrome, and heterozygous carriers have a predisposition for psychiatric disorders.

Diagnosis. Diagnosis depends on the combination of the preceding list of clinical features. mtDNA analysis confirms the clinical suspicion.

Management. Symptomatic treatment is required for each of the clinical features.

Retinoblastoma

Although retro-orbital tumors generally cause strabismus and proptosis, intraocular tumors always diminish vision. Retinoblastoma is the only malignant intraocular tumor of childhood. Its prompt recognition can be life-saving.

The typical features of retinoblastoma in a young child are an abnormal appearance of the eye, loss of vision, and strabismus. Monocular blindness is usually unrecognized by parents.

Older children may complain of visual blurring and floaters. Ocular pain is uncommon.

Leukocoria, a white pupillary reflex, is the initial feature in most children with retinoblastoma. In bright sunlight or in a flash photograph, the pupil does not constrict and has a white color. Strabismus occurs when visual acuity is impaired. The sighted eye fixates and the other remains deviated outward in all directions of gaze.

Refer all children with intraocular tumors to an ophthalmologist. A neurologist may be the primary consulting physician when the tumor is part of a larger syndrome that includes mental retardation. Such syndromes include retinoblastoma associated with deletion of the long arm of chromosome 13, retinal astrocytoma associated with tuberous sclerosis, choroidal hemangioma associated with Sturge-Weber disease, and optic nerve glioma in children with neurofibromatosis.

Tapetoretinal Degenerations

Most tapetoretinal degenerations are hereditary and due to inborn errors of lipid or carbohydrate metabolism. These disorders cause dementia, peripheral neuropathy, and ataxia as initial features and are discussed in several chapters. The conditions discussed here are less common, but other neurological features are not prominent initial complaints.

Bardet-Biedl Syndrome

The Bardet-Biedl syndrome is a genetically heterogeneous disorder (Ross & Beales, 2011). The common features of all types are mental retardation, pigmentary retinopathy, polydactyly, obesity, and hypogenitalism.

Clinical Features. Cone-rod dystrophy is usually manifest in the second decade. Its characteristic features may be salt-and-pepper retinopathy, macular pigmentation, or macular degeneration. In some patients, the retina appears normal, but the electroretinogram always shows abnormalities. Other features include truncal obesity, postaxial polydactyly, cognitive impairment, male hypogonadotropic hypogonadism, complex female genitourinary malformations, and renal dysfunction. Heterozygotes have an increased frequency of obesity, hypertension, diabetes mellitus, and renal disease.

Diagnosis. Diagnosis depends on recognition of the clinical constellation of symptoms and signs.

Management. Treatment is symptomatic.

Cockayne Syndrome

Cockayne syndrome, like xeroderma pigmentosum (see Chapter 5), is a disorder of DNA repair (Nance, 2006). It has several types: CS types I, II, III, and xeroderma pigmentosum-Cockayne syndrome (XP-CS). Inheritance is autosomal recessive.

Clinical Features. In CS type I, prenatal growth is normal. Growth and developmental failure begins in the first 2 years. Height, weight, and head circumference will be below the 5th percentile. Progressive impairment of vision, hearing, and central and peripheral nervous system function lead to severe disability. Death typically occurs in the first or second decade.

The characteristic features of CS type II are growth failure at birth, with little or no postnatal neurological development. Congenital cataracts or other structural anomalies of the eye may be present. Contractures develop in the spine and joints. Patients typically die by age 7 years. CS type III is rare and has late onset. XP-CS includes facial freckling and early skin cancers typical of XP and some features typical of CS, such as mental retardation, spasticity, short stature, and hypogonadism. Approximately 55 % of affected children develop a pigmentary retinopathy and 60 % develop a sensorineural hearing loss.

Diagnosis. The diagnosis is by the clinical features and by molecular genetic testing.

Management. Treatment is symptomatic.

Laurence-Moon Syndrome

The Laurence-Moon syndrome is a distinct disorder with mental retardation, pigmentary retinopathy, hypogenitalism, and spastic paraplegia without polydactyly and obesity. Its highest prevalence is in the Arab population of Kuwait.

DISORDERS OF THE PUPIL

When the person is awake, the size of the pupil is constantly changing in response to light and autonomic input. This pupillary unrest is *hippus*. An isolated disturbance of pupillary size is not evidence of intracranial disease.

Aniridia

Hypoplasia of the iris may occur as a solitary abnormality or may be associated with mental retardation, genitourinary abnormalities, and

Wilms tumor. About two-thirds of cases are genetic and transmitted as an autosomal dominant trait. One-third of sporadic cases are associated with Wilms tumor. In some cases, the short arm of chromosome 11 is abnormal.

Benign Essential Anisocoria

Between 20% and 30% of healthy people have an observable difference in pupillary size. Like congenital ptosis, it may go unnoticed until late childhood or adult life and is then thought to be a new finding. The size difference is constant at all levels of illumination but may be greater in darkness. The absence of other pupillary dysfunction or disturbed ocular motility suggests essential anisocoria, but old photographs are invaluable to confirm the diagnosis.

Fixed, Dilated Pupil

Clinical Features. A fixed, dilated pupil is an ominous sign in unconscious patients because it suggests transtentorial herniation (see Chapter 4). However, a dilated pupil that does not respond to light or accommodation in a child who is otherwise well and has no evidence of ocular motor dysfunction or ptosis can result only from the application of a pharmacological agent or from a damaged iris sphincter. The application may be accidental, as when inadvertently wiping a drug or chemical from the hand to the eye. Many cosmetics, particularly hair sprays, contain chemicals that can induce mydriasis. A careful history is essential to diagnosis.

Factitious application of mydriatics is a relatively common attention-seeking device, and convincing parents that the problem is self-inflicted may be difficult. Occasionally, a parent is the responsible party.

Diagnosis. Instill 1% pilocarpine in both eyes using the normal eye as a control. Parasympathetic denervation produces prompt constriction. A slow or incomplete response indicates pharmacological dilation.

Management. Pharmacologically induced mydriasis is often long lasting, but eventually resolves.

Horner Syndrome

Horner syndrome results from sympathetic denervation; it may be congenital or acquired. When acquired, it may occur at birth as part of a brachial plexus injury, during infancy from neuroblastoma, or in childhood from tumors or injuries affecting the superior cervical ganglion or the carotid artery.

Clinical Features. Unilateral Horner syndrome consists of the following ipsilateral features: mild to moderate ptosis (ptosis of the lower lid in one-third); miosis, which is best appreciated in dim light so that the normal pupil dilates; and anhidrosis of the face, heterochromia, and apparent enophthalmos when the syndrome is congenital.

Diagnosis. Disruption of the sympathetic system, anywhere from the hypothalamus to the eye, causes a Horner syndrome. Brainstem disturbances from stroke are common in adults, but peripheral lesions are more common in children. Topical instillation of 1% hydroxyamphetamine usually produces pupillary dilation after 30 minutes when postganglionic denervation is present. However, false-negative results can occur during the first week after injury (Donahue et al, 1996). Ten percent cocaine solution produces little or no dilation, regardless of the site of abnormality.

Management. Treatment depends on the underlying cause.

Tonic Pupil Syndrome (Adie Syndrome)

Clinical Features. The cause of tonic pupil syndrome is a defect in the orbital ciliary ganglion. The onset usually occurs after childhood but may occur as early as 5 years. Women are more often affected than are men.

The defect is usually monocular and manifests as anisocoria or photophobia. The abnormal pupil is slightly larger in bright light but changes little, if at all, with alteration in illumination. In a dark room, the normal pupil dilates and then is larger than is the tonic pupil. With attempted accommodation, which may also be affected, the pupil constricts slowly and incompletely and redilates slowly afterward. Binocular tonic pupils occur in children with dysautonomia and in association with diminished tendon reflexes (Holmes-Adie syndrome).

Diagnosis. The tonic pupil is supersensitive to parasympathomimetic agents; 0.125% pilocarpine achieves constriction.

Management. The condition is benign and seldom needs treatment.

REFERENCES

Arlt W, Alloli B. Adrenal insufficiency. Lancet 2003; 361:1881–93.

Balcer LJ. Optic neuritis. New England Journal of Medicine 2006;354:1273–8.

Brunel H, Raybaud C, Peretti-Viton P, et al. Craniopharyngioma in children: MRI study of 43 cases. Neurochirurgie 2002;48:309–18.

Birkebaek NH, Patel L, Wright NB, et al. Endocrine status in patients with optic nerve hypoplasia: relationship to midline central nervous system abnormalities and appearance of the hypothalamic-pituitary axis on magnetic resonance imaging. Journal of Clinical Endocrinology and Metabolism 2003;88:5281–6.

Donahue SP, Lavin PJM, Digre K. False-negative hydroxyamphetamine (Paredrine) test in acute Horner's syndrome. American Journal of Ophthalmology 1996;122:900–1.

Headache Classification Subcommittee of the International Headache Society. The International Classification of Headache Disorders, 2nd edition. Cephalalgia 2004;24(Suppl 1):1–6.

Kalpesh N, Patel M. Acute visual loss. Clinical Pediatric Emergency Medicine 2010;11(2):137–42.

Listernick R, Louis DN, Packer RJ, et al. Optic pathway gliomas in children with neurofibromatosis 1: Consensus statement from the NF1 optic pathway glioma task force. Annals of Neurology 1997;41:143–9.

Nance MA. Cockayne syndrome. In: GeneReviews at GeneTests: Medical Genetics Information Resource [database online]. Seattle: University of Washington. Available at http://www.genetests.org. PMID: 20301516. Last updated March 7, 2006.

Opocher E, Kremer LCM, Da Dalt L, et al. Prognostic factors for progression of childhood optic pathway glioma: a systematic review. European Journal of Cancer 2006;42:1807–16.

Ross AJ, Beales PI. Bardet-Biedl syndrome. In: GeneReviews at GeneTests: Medical Genetics Information Resource [database online]. Seattle: University of Washington. Available at http://www.genetests.org. PMID: 20301537. Last updated September 29, 2011.

Silva MM, Goldman S, Keating G, et al. Optic pathway hypothalamic gliomas in children under three years of age: the role of chemotherapy. Pediatric Neurosurgery 2000;33(3):151–8.

Thomas PQ, Dattani MT, Brickman JM, et al. Heterozygous HESX1 mutations associated with isolated congenital pituitary hypoplasia and septo-optic dysplasia. Human Molecular Genetics 2001;10:39–45.

Online Mendelian Inheritance in Man, OMIM. Wolfram syndrome. Available at http://www.ncbi.nlm.nih.gov/omim/ . OMIM 222300. Last edited 02/13/2012.

Weleber RG, Francis PJ, Trzupek KM. Leber congenital amaurosis. In: GeneReviews at GeneTests: Medical Genetics Information Resource [database Online]. Seattle: University of Washington. Available at http://www.genetests.org. PMID: 20301475. Last updated March 30, 2010.

CHAPTER 17

LOWER BRAINSTEM AND CRANIAL NERVE DYSFUNCTION

This chapter will review disorders causing dysfunction of the VII through XII cranial nerves. Many such disorders also disturb ocular motility and the discussion of these is in Chapter 15. The basis for chapter assignment is by the most usual initial clinical feature. For example, the discussion of myasthenia gravis is in Chapter 15 because diplopia is a more common initial complaint than dysphagia.

An acute isolated cranial neuropathy, such as facial palsy, is usually a less ominous sign than multiple cranial neuropathies and is likely to have a self-limited course. However, an isolated cranial neuropathy may be the first sign of progressive cranial nerve dysfunction. Therefore, the discussion of conditions causing isolated and multiple cranial neuropathies are together because they may not be separable at onset.

FACIAL WEAKNESS AND DYSPHAGIA

Anatomical Considerations

Facial Movement

The motor nucleus of the facial nerve is a column of cells in the ventrolateral tegmentum of the pons. Nerve fibers leaving the nucleus take a circuitous path in the brainstem before emerging close to the pontomedullary junction. The fibers then enter the internal auditory meatus with the acoustic nerve. Fibers for voluntary and reflexive facial movements separate rostral to the lower pons. After bending forward and downward around the inner ear, the facial nerve traverses the temporal bone in the facial canal and exits the skull at the stylomastoid foramen. Extracranially, the facial nerve passes into the parotid gland where it divides into several branches, which innervate all muscles of facial expression except the levator palpebrae superioris, which is innervated by cranial nerve III.

Sucking and Swallowing

The sucking reflex requires the integrity of the trigeminal, facial, and hypoglossal nerves. Stimulation of the lips produces coordinated movements of the face, jaw, and tongue. The automatic aspect of the reflex disappears after infancy but may return with bilateral dysfunction of the cerebral hemispheres.

Fibers of the trigeminal and glossopharyngeal nerves ending in the nucleus solitarius form the afferent arc of the swallowing reflex. The motor roots of the trigeminal nerve, the glossopharyngeal and vagus fibers from the nucleus ambiguous, and the hypoglossal nerves form the efferent arc. A swallowing center that coordinates the reflex is located in the lower pons and upper medulla. A bolus of food stimulates the pharyngeal wall or back of the tongue, and the combined action of the tongue, palatine arches, soft palate, and pharynx move the food into the esophagus.

Approach to Diagnosis

The causes of facial muscle weakness may be supranuclear palsy (pseudobulbar palsy), intrinsic brainstem disease, or disorders of the motor unit: facial nerve, neuromuscular junction, and facial muscles (Boxes 17-1 and 17-2). The differential diagnosis of dysphagia is similar (Box 17–3), except that isolated dysfunction of the nerves that enable swallowing is very uncommon.

Pseudobulbar Palsy

Because the corticobulbar innervation of most cranial nerves is bilateral, pseudobulbar palsy

BOX 17-1 Causes of Congenital Facial Weakness

- Aplasia of facial muscles
- Birth injury
- Congenital myotonic dystrophy (see Chapter 6)
- Congenital bilateral perisylvian syndrome
- Fiber-type disproportion myopathies (see Chapter 6)
- Myasthenic syndromes*
  - Congenital myasthenia (see Chapter 15)
  - Familial infantile myasthenia (see Chapter 6)
  - Transitory neonatal myasthenia (see Chapter 6)

*Denotes the most common conditions and the ones with disease modifying treatments

BOX 17-2 Causes of Postnatal Facial Weakness

AUTOIMMUNE AND POSTINFECTIOUS

Bell's palsy*
Idiopathic cranial polyneuropathy
Miller Fisher syndrome* (see Chapter 10)
Myasthenia gravis* (see Chapter 15)

GENETIC

Juvenile progressive bulbar palsy (Fazio-Londe disease)
Muscular disorders
Facioscapulohumeral syndrome (see Chapter 7)
Facioscapulohumeral syndrome, infantile form
Fiber-type disproportion myopathies (see Chapter 6)
Melkersson syndrome
Myotonic dystrophy (see Chapter 7)
Oculopharyngeal dystrophy
Myasthenic syndromes*
Congenital myasthenia* (see Chapter 15)
Familial infantile myasthenia* (see Chapter 6)
Osteopetrosis (Albers-Schönberg disease)
Recurrent facial palsy

HYPERTENSION

INFECTIOUS

Diphtheria
Herpes zoster oticus*
Infectious mononucleosis
Lyme disease* (see Chapter 2)
Otitis media*
Sarcoidosis*
Tuberculosis*

METABOLIC DISORDERS

Hyperparathyroidism*
Hypothyroidism*

MULTIPLE SCLEROSIS (SEE CHAPTER 10)

SYRINGOBULBIA*

TOXINS

TRAUMA

Delayed
Immediate

TUMOR

Glioma of brainstem (see Chapter 15)
Histiocytosis X
Leukemia
Meningeal carcinoma
Neurofibromatosis

*Denotes the most common conditions and the ones with disease modifying treatments

BOX 17-3 Neurological Causes of Dysphagia

AUTOIMMUNE/POSTINFECTIOUS

Dermatomyositis (see Chapter 7)
Guillain-Barré syndrome (see Chapter 7)
Idiopathic cranial polyneuropathy
Myasthenia gravis* (see Chapter 15)
Transitory neonatal myasthenia gravis* (see Chapter 6)

CONGENITAL OR PERINATAL

Aplasia of brainstem nuclei
Cerebral palsy (see Chapter 5)
Chiari malformation* (see Chapter 10)
Congenital bilateral perisylvian syndrome
Syringobulbia*

GENETIC

Degenerative disorders (see Chapter 5)
Familial dysautonomia (see Chapter 6)
Familial infantile myasthenia (see Chapter 6)
Fiber-type disproportion myopathies (see Chapter 6)
Myotonic dystrophy (see Chapters 6 and 7)
Oculopharyngeal dystrophy

GLIOMA OF BRAINSTEM

INFECTIOUS

Botulism* (see Chapters 6 and 7)
Diphtheria
Poliomyelitis (see Chapter 7)

JUVENILE PROGRESSIVE BULBAR PALSY

*Denotes the most common conditions and the ones with disease modifying treatments

occurs only when hemispheric disease is bilateral. Many children with pseudobulbar palsy have a progressive degenerative disorder of gray or white matter. The discussion of most of these disorders is in Chapter 5 because dementia is usually the initial feature. Bilateral strokes, simultaneous or in sequence, cause pseudobulbar palsy in children; the usual causes are coagulation defects, leukemia, and trauma (see Chapter 11). Pseudobulbar palsy is the main feature of the congenital bilateral perisylvian syndrome, discussed in this chapter. Episodic pseudobulbar palsy (oral apraxia, dysarthria, and drooling) may indicate the acquired epileptiform opercular syndrome (see Chapter 1).

The characteristic feature of pseudobulbar palsy is an inability to use bulbar muscles in voluntary effort, while reflex movements, initiated at a brainstem level, are normal. Extraocular motility is unaffected. The child can suck, chew, and swallow but cannot coordinate these reflexes for eating; movement of a food bolus from the front of the mouth to the back has a volitional component.

Emotionally derived facial expression occurs, but voluntary facial movements do not. Severe dysarthria is often present. Affected muscles do not show atrophy or fasciculations. The gag reflex and jaw jerk are usually exaggerated, and emotional volatility is often an associated feature.

Newborns with familial dysautonomia have difficulty feeding, despite normal sucking and swallowing, because they fail to coordinate the two reflexes (see Chapter 6). Box 6-7 summarizes the differential diagnosis of feeding difficulty in an alert newborn. Children with cerebral palsy often have a similar disturbance in the coordination of chewing and swallowing that impairs feeding.

Motor Unit Disorders

Disorders of the facial nuclei and nerves always cause ipsilateral facial weakness and atrophy, but associated features vary with the site of abnormality:

1. Motor nucleus: Hyperacusis is present, but taste, lacrimation, and salivation are normal.
2. Facial nerve between the pons and the internal auditory meatus: Taste sensation is spared, but lacrimation and salivation are impaired and hyperacusis is present.
3. Geniculate ganglion: Taste, lacrimation, and salivation are impaired, and hyperacusis is present.
4. Facial nerve from the geniculate ganglion to the stapedius nerve: Taste and salivation are impaired and hyperacusis is present, but lacrimation is normal.
5. Facial nerve from the stapedius nerve to the chorda tympani: Taste and salivation are impaired, hyperacusis is not present, and lacrimation is normal.
6. Facial nerve below the exit of the chorda tympani nerve: Only facial weakness is present.

Disturbances of cranial nerve nuclei seldom occur in isolation; they are often associated with other features of brainstem dysfunction (bulbar palsy). Usually some combination of dysarthria, dysphagia, and diplopia is present. Examination may show strabismus, facial diplegia, loss of the gag reflex, atrophy of bulbar muscles, and fasciculations of the tongue.

The facial weakness associated with myasthenia gravis and facial myopathies is usually bilateral. In contrast, brainstem disorders usually begin on one side and eventually progress to bilateral impairment. Facial nerve palsies are usually unilateral. The differential diagnosis of recurrent facial palsy or dysphagia is limited to disorders of the facial nerve and neuromuscular junction (Box 17-4).

Congenital Syndromes

Congenital Bilateral Perisylvian Syndrome

This syndrome results from a disturbance in neuronal migration that results in pachygyria of the sylvian and rolandic regions. Most cases are sporadic. The transmission of familial cases is by X-linked inheritance; such cases are more severe in males than in females (Villard et al, 2002).

Clinical Features. All affected children have a pseudobulbar palsy that causes failure of speech development (apraxia) and dysphagia. Cognitive impairment and seizures are present in approximately 85 % of cases. The cognitive deficit varies from mild to severe, and the seizures, which begin between 4 and 12 years, may be atypical absence, atonic/tonic, partial, or generalized tonic-clonic.

Diagnosis. Magnetic resonance imaging (MRI) shows bilateral perisylvian gyral dysgenesis including pachygyria, and polymicrogyria (Figure 17-1). Postmortem studies have confirmed the MRI impression.

Management. The seizures are usually difficult to control, and corpus callosotomy has been useful in some cases with intractable drop attacks. Speech therapy does not overcome the speech disorder, and instruction in sign language is the better alternative for children of near-normal intelligence. Drooling is very disruptive and may benefit from the use of glycopyrolate, excision of the submandibular glands, ligation of parotid gland ducts, or botulinum toxin injections to the parotid glands.

Congenital Dysphagia

Congenital dysphagia is usually associated with infantile hypotonia and therefore discussed in Chapter 6. Because the neuroanatomical substrates of swallowing and breathing are contiguous, congenital dysphagia and dyspnea are often concurrent. Isolated aplasia of the cranial

BOX 17-4 Causes of Recurrent Cranial Neuropathies/Palsies

Familial
- Isolated facial palsy
- Melkersson syndrome

Hypertensive Facial Palsy*

Myasthenia Gravis*

Sporadic Multiple Cranial Neuropathies

Toxins

*Denotes the most common conditions and the ones with disease modifying treatments

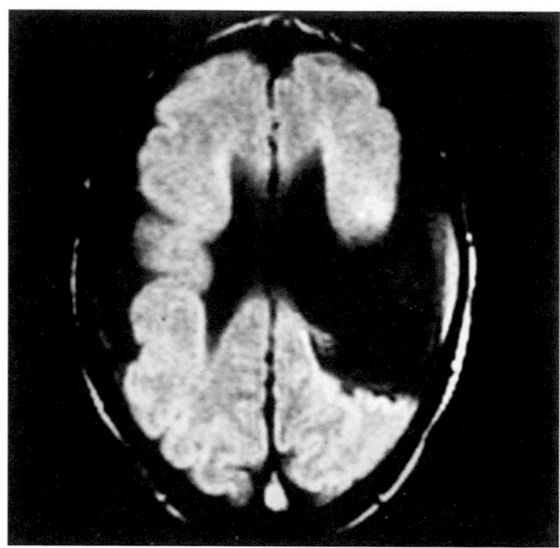

FIGURE 17-1 ■ MRI of congenital bilateral perisylvian syndrome. This child has lissencephaly and schizencephaly. Bilateral disturbances in the perisylvian region caused a pseudobulbar palsy.

nerve nuclei subserving swallowing is not established.

Congenital Facial Asymmetry

The cause of most facial asymmetries at birth is congenital aplasia of muscle and not trauma to the facial nerve. Facial diplegia, whether complete or incomplete, suggests the Möbius syndrome or other congenital muscle aplasia. Complete unilateral palsies are likely to be traumatic in origin, whereas partial unilateral palsies may be either traumatic or aplastic. The term neonatal facial asymmetry is probably more accurate than facial nerve palsy to denote partial or complete unilateral facial weakness in the newborn and emphasizes the difficulty in differentiating traumatic nerve palsies from congenital aplasias. A common cause of asymmetry of the lower face/mouth is the unilateral absence of the depressor anguli oris.

Aplasia of Facial Muscles

Clinical Features. The Möbius syndrome is the best-known congenital aplasia of facial nerve nuclei and facial muscles. The site of pathology is usually the facial nerve nuclei and their internuclear connections. Facial diplegia may occur alone, with bilateral abducens palsies, or with involvement of several cranial nerves (Harriette et al, 2003). Congenital malformations elsewhere in the body (dextrocardia, talipes equinovarus, absent pectoral muscle, and limb deformities) are sometimes associated features. Most cases are sporadic, but familial recurrence occurs. Autosomal dominant, autosomal recessive, and X-linked recessive modes of inheritance are proposed. Identified loci are on chromosomes 13, 3, and 10.

Other developmental causes of unilateral facial palsy are *Goldenhar syndrome*, the *Poland anomaly*, *DiGeorge syndrome*, osteopetrosis, and trisomy 13 and 18.

Diagnosis. Congenital facial diplegia is by definition a Möbius syndrome. All such cases require MRI of the brain to determine if other cerebral malformations are present. Causes other than primary malformations include intrauterine toxins (e.g., thalidomide), vascular malformations, or infarction.

Electromyography (EMG) can help determine the timing of injury. Denervation potentials are only present if injury to the facial nuclei or nerve occurred 2 to 6 weeks before the study. Facial muscles that are aplastic, as in the Möbius syndrome, or nerve injury occurring early in gestation, do not show active denervation.

Management. Surgical procedures may provide partial facial movement.

Depressor Anguli Oris Muscle Aplasia

Clinical Features. Isolated unilateral weakness of the depressor anguli oris muscle (DAOM) is the most common cause of facial asymmetry at birth. One corner of the mouth fails to move downward when the child cries. All other facial movements are symmetrical. The lower lip on the paralyzed side feels thinner to palpation, even at birth, suggesting antepartum hypoplasia.

Diagnosis. Traumatic lesions of the facial nerve would not selectively injure nerve fibers to the DAOM and spare all other facial muscles. Electrodiagnostic studies aid in differentiating aplasia of the DAOM from traumatic injury. In aplasia, the conduction velocity and latency of the facial nerve are normal. Fibrillations are not present at the site of the DAOM. Instead, motor unit potentials are absent or decreased in number. The pulling of the mouth in the direction of the healthy DAOM when crying often causes the referring physician to believe that this is the abnormal side.

Management. No treatment is available or needed. The DAOM is not a significant component of facial expression in older children and adults, and absence of the muscle is difficult to notice.

Birth Injury. Perinatal traumatic facial palsy is a disorder of large term newborns delivered vaginally after a prolonged labor. Nerve compression against the sacrum during labor is more often the cause than is the misapplication of forceps. Children with forceps injuries, an unusual event, have forceps marks on the cheeks.

Clinical Features. The clinical expression of complete unilateral facial palsy in the newborn can be subtle and may not be apparent immediately after birth. Failure of eye closure on the affected side is the first noticeable evidence of weakness. Only when the child cries does flaccid paralysis of all facial muscles become obvious. The eyeball rolls up behind the open lid, the nasolabial fold remains flat, and the corner of the mouth droops during crying. The normal side appears paralyzed because it pulls and distorts the face; the paralyzed side appears to be normal. When paralysis of the facial nerve is partial, the orbicularis oculi is the muscle most frequently spared. In these injuries, the compression site is usually over the parotid gland, with sparing of nerve fibers that course upward just after leaving the stylomastoid foramen.

Diagnosis. The diagnosis of facial asymmetry is by observing the face of the crying newborn. Carefully examine the facial skin for laceration. Otoscopic examination is useful to establish the presence of hemotympanum. EMG does not alter the management of the palsy.

Management. Prospective studies regarding the natural outcome of perinatal facial nerve injuries are not available. Most authors are optimistic and indicate a high rate of spontaneous recovery. Such optimism may be appropriate, but its basis is only anecdotal experience. In the absence of data on long-term outcome, one cannot evaluate the efficacy of any suggested therapeutic intervention. Most newborns are not candidates for surgical intervention unless the nerve laceration occurs at delivery. In that event, the best response is to reconstitute the nerve if possible or at least to allow the proximal stump a clear pathway toward regeneration by debridement of the wound.

Immune-Mediated and Infectious Disorders

Postinfectious demyelination of the VII nerve is the cause of most cases of acute unilateral facial neuritis (Bell's palsy) or bilateral facial neuritis. The basis for distinguishing a bilateral Bell palsy from the Guillain-Barré syndrome (acute inflammatory demyelinating polyneuropathy) is the preservation of limb tendon reflexes in Bell palsy. Discussion of the Guillain-Barré syndrome is in Chapter 7.

Bell Palsy

Bell palsy is an acute, idiopathic, self-limited, typically monophasic, paralysis of the face caused by dysfunction of the facial nerve. The pathogenesis is believed to be viral (most often herpes simplex) but may also be postviral, immune-mediated, demyelination. The annual incidence is approximately 3/100,000 in the first decade, 10/100,000 in the second decade, and 25/100,000 in adults. Only 1 % of cases have clinical evidence of bilateral involvement, but many have electrophysiological abnormalities on the unaffected side.

Clinical Features. A history of viral infection, usually upper respiratory, is recorded in many cases, but the frequency is not significantly greater than expected by chance. The initial feature of neuritis is often pain or tingling in the ear canal ipsilateral to the subsequent facial palsy. Pain accompanies facial weakness in 60 % of patients, impaired lacrimation in 60 %, taste changes in 30–50 %, and hyperacusis in 15–30 %.

Ipsilateral facial sensory symptoms are usually mild and explained by extension of inflammation from the facial nerve to the trigeminal nerve via the greater superficial petrosal nerve (Vanopdenbosch et al, 2005). The palsy has an explosive onset and becomes maximal within hours. Either the child or the parents may first notice the palsy, which affects all muscles on one side of the face. Half of the face sags, enlarging the palpebral fissure. Weakness of the orbicularis muscle prevents closure of the lid. Efforts to use muscles of expression cause the face to pull to the normal side. Eating and drinking become difficult, and dribbling of liquids from the weak corner of the mouth causes embarrassment.

The most commonly affected portion of the nerve is within the temporal bone; taste, lacrimation, and salivation are impaired, and hyperacusis is present. However, examination of all facial nerve functions in small children is difficult, and precise localization is not critical to diagnosis or prognosis. The muscles remain weak for 2 to 4 weeks, and then strength returns spontaneously. The natural history of Bell palsy in children is not established, but experience indicates that almost all patients recover completely.

Diagnosis. Complete neurological examination is required in every child with acute unilateral facial weakness to determine whether the palsy is an isolated abnormality. Mild facial weakness on the other side or the absence of tendon reflexes in the limbs suggests the possibility of Guillain-Barré syndrome. Such children require observation for the development of progressive limb weakness.

Exclude possible underlying causes (e.g., hypertension, infection, and trauma) of facial nerve palsy before considering the diagnosis of Bell palsy. Examine the ear ipsilateral to the facial palsy for herpetic lesions (see the later discussion of Herpes Zoster Oticus). MRI shows contrast enhancement of the involved nerve, but acute, isolated facial palsy is not an indication for MRI in every child. A more reasonable approach is to watch the child and recommend an imaging study if other neurological disturbances develop or if the palsy does not begin to resolve within 1 month.

Management. Always protect the cornea if the blink reflex is absent and especially if the palpebral fissure remains open while sleeping. This may result in corneal ulcers due to prolonged ocular exposure and dryness. Ophthalmologic ointments are needed to prevent this complication. Patch the eye when the child is outside the home or at play, and apply artificial tears several times a day to keep the cornea moist. The use of corticosteroids has shown modest benefits in some reports; however, it is difficult to assess in children because their prognosis for complete spontaneous recovery is excellent. The clinician who elects to use corticosteroid therapy must first exclude hypertension or infection as an underlying cause.

Idiopathic Cranial Polyneuropathy

As the name implies, idiopathic cranial neuropathy is of uncertain nosology. The presumed mechanism is postinfectious, and many consider the syndrome an abortive form of the Guillain-Barré syndrome.

Clinical Features. Onset is usually in adults, and most childhood cases occur in adolescence. Similar cases described in infants subsequently developed limb weakness, and infantile botulism was the more likely diagnosis (see Chapter 6).

Constant, aching facial pain usually precedes weakness by hours or days. The pain is often localized to the temple or frontal region but can be anywhere in the face. Weakness may develop within 1 day or may evolve over several weeks. Extraocular motility is usually affected. Facial and trigeminal nerve disturbances occur in half of cases, but lower cranial nerve involvement is uncommon. Occasional patients have transitory visual disturbances, ptosis, pupillary abnormalities, and tinnitus. Tendon reflexes in the limbs remain active. Recurrent idiopathic cranial neuropathies occur as sporadic cases in adults but usually occur on a familial basis in children.

Diagnosis. The differential diagnosis includes the Guillain-Barré syndrome, infant and childhood forms of botulism, brainstem glioma, juvenile progressive bulbar palsy, pontobulbar palsy with deafness, and the Tolosa-Hunt syndrome. Preservation of tendon reflexes in idiopathic cranial polyneuropathy is the main feature distinguishing it from the Guillain-Barré syndrome. Prominent autonomic dysfunction and limb weakness separates botulism from idiopathic cranial polyneuropathy (see Chapters 6 and 7). Cranial nerve dysfunction in patients with brainstem glioma, juvenile progressive bulbar palsy, and pontobulbar palsy with deafness usually evolves over a longer period. The Tolosa-Hunt syndrome of painful ophthalmoplegia and idiopathic cranial polyneuropathy shares many features and may be a variant of the same disease process (see Chapter 15).

All laboratory findings are normal. The possibility of a brainstem glioma requires MRI of the brainstem in all cases. Examination of the cerebrospinal fluid occasionally reveals a mild elevation of protein concentration and a lymphocyte count of 5–6/mm^3.

Management. The disease is self-limited, and full recovery is the expected outcome 2 to 4 months after onset. The use of corticosteroids is routine and believed to ease facial pain and shorten the course. The relief of pain may be dramatic, but evidence documenting a shortened course is lacking.

Genetic Disorders

Facioscapulohumeral Dystrophy

Facioscapulohumeral dystrophy (FSHD) sometimes begins during infancy as bilateral facial weakness (facial diplegia). Inheritance is by autosomal dominant transmission (Lemmers, 2009). Approximately 70–90% of individuals have inherited the disease-causing deletion from a parent, and the rest are de novo deletions. Offspring of an affected individual have a 50% chance of inheriting the deletion. Prenatal testing is available.

Clinical Features. The onset of infantile FSHD is usually no later than age 5 years. Facial diplegia is the initial feature. When onset is early in infancy, the common misdiagnosis is congenital aplasia of facial muscles. Later, nasal speech and sometimes ptosis develop. Progressive proximal weakness begins 1 to 2 years after onset, first affecting the shoulders and then the pelvis. Pseudohypertrophy of the calves may be present. Tendon reflexes are depressed and then absent in weak muscle. Progression of weakness is often rapid and unrelenting, leading to disability and death from respiratory insufficiency before age 20 years. Typical features are a striking asymmetry of muscle involvement from side to side and sparing of bulbar extraocular and respiratory muscles. The weakness may also stabilize for long intervals and not cause severe disability until adult life.

Retinal telangiectasia and high-frequency hearing loss occurs in about half of affected families (Padberg et al, 1995). Both conditions are progressive and may not be symptomatic in early childhood.

Diagnosis. The diagnosis of FSHD is a possibility in every child with progressive facial diplegia. A family history of FSHD syndrome is not always obtainable because the affected parent may show only minimal expression of the phenotype. Molecular-based testing is reliable for diagnosis.

Myasthenia gravis and brainstem glioma are a consideration in infants with progressive facial diplegia. The serum concentration of creatine kinase is helpful in differentiating these disorders. It is usually elevated in the infantile FSHD syndrome and normal in myasthenia gravis and brainstem glioma. Electrophysiological studies show brief, small-amplitude polyphasic potentials in weak muscles, and a normal response to repetitive nerve stimulation.

Management. Treatment is supportive.

Juvenile Progressive Bulbar Palsy

Juvenile progressive bulbar palsy, also known as *Fazio-Londe disease*, is a motor neuron disease limited to bulbar muscles. Most cases are sporadic; autosomal recessive inheritance is the suspected means of transmission, but a rare autosomal dominant subtype may occur.

Clinical Features. Age at onset separates two clinical patterns. Stridor is the initial feature in early-onset cases (age 1 to 5 years). Progressive bulbar palsy follows, and respiratory compromise causes death within 2 years of onset. Respiratory symptoms are less common in later-onset cases (age 6 to 20 years). The initial feature may be facial weakness, dysphagia, or dysarthria. Eventually, the disorder affects all lower motor cranial nerve nuclei except the ocular motor nerve nuclei. Some children show fasciculations and atrophy of the arms, but limb strength and tendon reflexes usually remain strong despite severe bulbar palsy.

Diagnosis. The major diagnostic considerations are myasthenia gravis and brainstem glioma. MRI of the brainstem excludes brainstem tumors. EMG is useful to show active denervation of facial muscles, with sparing of the limbs and normal repetitive stimulation of nerves. Children with rapidly progressive motor neuron disease affecting the face and limbs may represent a childhood form of amyotrophic lateral sclerosis.

Pontobulbar palsy with deafness (*Brown-Vialetto-Van Laere syndrome*), a distinct disorder with phenotypic overlap, is characterized by a mixed upper and lower motor neuron bulbar palsy and deafness (Dipti et al, 2005).

Management. The disorder is often devastating. A previously normal child is no longer able to speak intelligibly or swallow. Feeding gastrostomy and a communication device are soon required. The child needs considerable psychological support. Treatment is not available for the underlying disease.

Oculopharyngeal Muscular Dystrophy

Autosomal dominant inheritance is the usual means of genetic transmission. The incidence is highest in families of French Canadian descent but the disorder is not restricted to any ethnic group. Mitochondrial myopathies account for cases with similar features not transmitted by autosomal dominant inheritance.

Clinical Features. Onset is usually in the fourth decade but may be as early as adolescence. The initial features are ptosis and dysphagia, followed by proximal weakness in the legs and external ophthalmoplegia. Eventually the disease affects all skeletal muscle, but spares smooth and cardiac muscle.

Many patients with oculopharyngeal muscular dystrophy also have EMG or biopsy evidence of denervation in the limbs. The neurogenic features may be attributable to neuronopathy rather than neuropathy, suggesting that this disorder is actually a spinal (bulbar) muscular atrophy.

Diagnosis. Definitive diagnosis relies on DNA testing. Muscle biopsy reveals a random variation in the size of the fibers, necrotic fibers, some fibrosis, and occasional internal nuclei. Autophagic vacuoles (rimmed vacuoles) and intranuclear fibrillary inclusion bodies are features common to OCPD, inclusion body myositis, and several hereditary distal myopathies/dystrophies. The presence of ragged-red fibers on histological examination of muscle indicates an underlying mitochondrial myopathy.

Management. The goal of therapy is symptom relief. Dietary changes help early dysphagia but gastrostomy is eventually required. Levator palpebral shortening may correct ptosis.

Osteopetrosis (Albers-Schönberg Disease)

The term osteopetrosis encompasses at least three hereditary skeletal disorders of increased bone density. Transmission of the most common form is by autosomal recessive inheritance (chromosome 11q). The features are macrocephaly, progressive deafness and blindness, hepatosplenomegaly, and severe anemia beginning in fetal life or early infancy. The calvarium thickens, and cranial nerves are compressed and compromised as they pass through the bone. The thickened calvarium may also impair venous return and cause increased intracranial pressure.

The main clinical features of the dominant form (1p) are fractures and osteomyelitis, especially of the mandible. Treatment with high-dose calcitrol reduces the sclerosis and prevents many neurological complications.

Melkersson Syndrome

Seven percent of facial palsies are recurrent. Autosomal dominant inheritance with variable expression is the suspected means of transmission in many cases. Some kindred members may have only recurrent facial nerve palsy, whereas others have recurrent neuropathies of the facial and ocular motor nerves. The Melkersson syndrome may be genetically distinct from other recurrent facial palsies with a gene locus at chromosome 9p11.

Clinical Features. Melkersson syndrome is a rare disorder characterized by the triad of recurrent facial palsy, lingua plicata, and facial edema. Attacks of facial palsy usually begin in the second decade, but the deeply furrowed tongue is present from birth.

The first attack of facial weakness is indistinguishable from Bell palsy except that a migraine-like headache may precede the attack. Subsequent attacks are associated with eyelid edema, which is soft, painless, nonerythematous, and nonpruritic. The edema is most often asymmetric, involving only the upper lip on the paralyzed side, but it may affect the cheek and eyelid of one or both sides. Cold weather or emotional stress may precipitate an attack of facial swelling. Lingua plicata is present in 30–50 % of cases. Furrowing and deep grooving on the dorsal surface of the tongue are permanent from birth. The transmission of this feature is by autosomal dominant inheritance but occurs as an isolated finding in some families.

Diagnosis. The diagnosis of Melkersson syndrome is established when two features of the triad are present. It is a consideration in any child with a personal or family history of recurrent facial palsy or recurrent facial edema. The presence of lingua plicata in any member of the kindred confirms the diagnosis. Histopathology of the affected eyelid reveals a granulomatous lymphangitis unique to the disease (Cockerham et al, 2000).

Management. This disease has no established treatment.

Hypertension

Unilateral facial palsy may be a feature of malignant hypertension in children. The cause of the palsy is swelling and hemorrhage into the facial canal.

Clinical Features. The course of the facial paralysis is indistinguishable from that in Bell palsy. Nerve compression occurs in its proximal segment, impairing lacrimation, salivation, and taste. The onset coincides with a rise in diastolic blood pressure to greater than 120 mmHg, and recovery begins when the pressure reduces. The duration of palsy varies from days to weeks. Recurrences are associated with repeated episodes of hypertension.

Diagnosis. The occurrence of facial palsy in a child with known hypertension suggests that the hypertension is out of control.

Management. Control of hypertension is the only effective treatment.

Infection

The facial nerve is sometimes involved when bacterial infection spreads from the middle ear to the mastoid. External otitis may lead to facial nerve involvement by spread of infection from the tympanic membrane to the chorda tympani.

Diphtheria may cause single or multiple cranial neuropathies from a direct effect of its toxin. Facial palsy, dysarthria, and dysphagia are potential complications. Basilar meningitis, from tuberculosis or other bacterial infections, causes inflammation of cranial nerves as they leave the brain and enter the skull. Multiple and bilateral cranial nerve involvement is usually progressive.

Herpes Zoster Oticus (Ramsay Hunt Syndrome)

Herpes zoster infection of the geniculate ganglion causes herpes zoster oticus.

Clinical Features. The initial feature is pain in and behind the ear. This pain is often more severe and persistent than that expected with other causes of Bell palsy. Unilateral facial palsy, indistinguishable from Bell palsy by appearance, follows. However, examination of the ipsilateral ear, especially in the fossa of the helix and behind the lobule, shows a vesicular eruption characteristic of herpes zoster. Hearing loss is associated in 25 % of cases.

Diagnosis. The only historical feature distinguishing herpes zoster oticus from Bell palsy is the severity of ear pain. Examination of the ear for vesicles is critical to the diagnosis.

Management. Herpes zoster infections are usually self-limited but painful. A combination of oral acyclovir, 800 mg five times a day for 7 days, and oral prednisone, 1 mg/kg for 5 days and then tapered, improves the outcome for facial nerve function in people 15 years and older (Murakami et al, 1997). Complete recovery occurs in 75 % of those treated within 7 days of onset and in 30 % treated after 7 days. The varicella vaccine may reduce the incidence of new cases and decrease the severity of symptoms (Hato et al, 2000).

Sarcoidosis

Cranial nerve dysfunction is the most common neurological complication of sarcoidosis. Basilar granulomatous meningitis is the usual cause (Figure 17-2), but the facial nerve may also be involved when parotitis is present.

Clinical Features. Onset is usually in the third decade but may be as early as adolescence. Neurological complications occur in only 5 % of patients with sarcoidosis but, when present, they are often an early feature of the disease. Facial nerve palsy, unilateral or bilateral, is the single most common feature. Visual impairment or deafness is next in frequency. Single cranial neuropathies are present in 73 % and multiple cranial neuropathies in 58 %. Any cranial nerve except the accessory nerve may be involved. Systemic features of sarcoidosis occur in almost every case: intrathoracic involvement is present in 81 % and ocular involvement in 50 %. Uveoparotitis is an uncommon manifestation of sarcoidosis. The patient ordinarily comes to medical attention because of visual impairment and a painful eye. The mouth is dry and the parotid gland swollen. Facial nerve compression and palsy are present in 40 % of cases.

Diagnosis. Sarcoidosis is a consideration in any patient with single or multiple cranial neuropathies. Documentation of multisystem disease confirms the diagnosis. Radiographs of the chest either establish or are compatible with the diagnosis in almost all patients with neurological manifestations.

Increased serum concentrations of angiotensin-converting enzyme (ACE) are detectable in 75 % of patients with active pulmonary disease, and patients with neurosarcoidosis may have elevated cerebrospinal fluid concentrations of ACE. Biopsy of lymph nodes or other affected tissues provides histological confirmation.

Management. Prednisone therapy, 0.5–1 mg/kg/day, is maintained until a clinical response is evident and then slowly tapered at a rate that prevents relapse. The prognosis for neurological complications of sarcoidosis is good without treatment, but corticosteroids appear to hasten recovery.

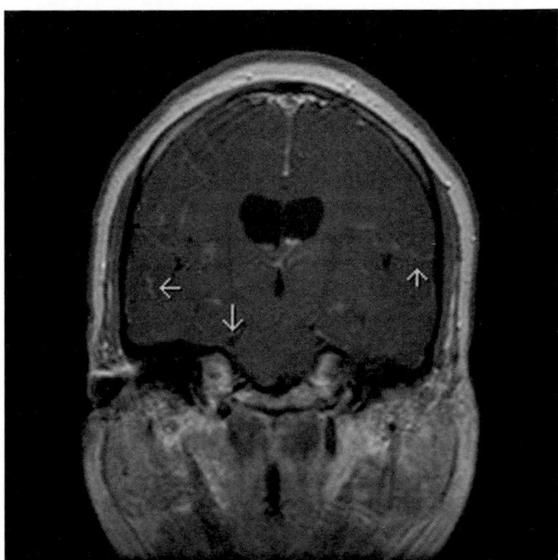

FIGURE 17-2 ■ Neurosarcoidosis. T_1 coronal MRI with contrast shows enhancing leptomeninges (arrows).

Metabolic Disorders

Hyperparathyroidism

The most common neurological features of primary hyperparathyroidism are headache and confusion (see Chapter 2). Occasionally, hyperparathyroidism is associated with a syndrome that is similar to amyotrophic lateral sclerosis and includes ataxia and internuclear ophthalmoplegia. Dysarthria and dysphagia are prominent features.

Hypothyroidism

Cranial nerve abnormalities are unusual in hypothyroidism. Deafness is the most common feature, but acute facial nerve palsy resembling Bell palsy also occurs.

Syringobulbia

Syringobulbia is usually the medullary extension of a cervical syrinx (see Chapter 12) but may also originate in the medulla. The syrinx usually involves the nucleus ambiguous and the spinal tract and motor nucleus of the trigeminal nerve. Symptoms in order of frequency are headache, vertigo, dysarthria, facial paresthesias, dysphagia, diplopia, tinnitus, and palatal palsy.

Toxins

Most neurotoxins produce either diffuse encephalopathy or peripheral neuropathy. Only ethylene glycol, trichlorethylene, and chlorocresol exposure cause selective cranial nerve toxicity. Ethylene glycol is antifreeze. Ingestion causes facial diplegia, hearing impairment, and dysphagia. Trichlorethylene intoxication can cause multiple cranial neuropathies but has a predilection for the trigeminal nerve. It was once a treatment for tic douloureux. Chlorocresol, a compound used in the industrial production of heparin, caused recurrent unilateral facial palsy in one exposed worker. Inhalation of the compound caused tingling of one side of the face followed by weakness of the muscles. The neurological disturbance was brief, relieved by exposure to fresh air, and could be reproduced experimentally.

Trauma

Facial palsy following closed head injury is usually associated with bleeding from the ear and fracture of the petrous bone.

Clinical Features. The onset of palsy may be immediate or delayed for as long as 3 weeks after injury. In most cases, the interval is between 2 and 7 days. The mechanism of delay is unknown.

Diagnosis. Electrophysiological studies are helpful in prognosis. If the nerve is intact but shows a conduction block, recovery usually begins within 5 days and is complete. Most patients with partial denervation recover full facial movement but have evidence of aberrant reinnervation. Full recovery is not an expected outcome when denervation is complete.

Management. The management of traumatic facial palsy is controversial. Some authors have recommended surgical decompression and corticosteroids, but no evidence supporting either mode of therapy is available.

Tumors

Tumors of the facial nerve are rare in children. The major neoplastic cause of facial palsy is brainstem glioma (see Chapter 15), followed by tumors that infiltrate the meninges, such as leukemia, meningeal carcinoma, and histiocytosis X. Acoustic neuromas are unusual in childhood and are limited to children with neurofibromatosis type 2. These neuromas cause hearing impairment before facial palsy and are discussed in the next section.

HEARING IMPAIRMENT AND DEAFNESS

Anatomical Considerations

Sound, mechanically funneled through the external auditory canal, causes the tympanic membrane to vibrate. Ossicles transmit the vibrations to the oval window of the cochlea, the sensory organ of hearing. The air-filled space extending from the tympanic membrane to the cochlea comprises *the middle ear*. The membranous labyrinth within the osseous labyrinth is the principal structure of *the inner ear*. It contains the cochlea, the semicircular canals, and the vestibule. The semicircular canals and vestibule are the sensory organs of vestibular function. The cochlea consists of three fluid-filled canals wound into a snail-like configuration.

The organ of Corti is the transducer within the cochlea that converts mechanical to electrical energy. The auditory portion of the eighth nerve transmits impulses to the ipsilateral cochlear nuclei of the medulla. The transmission of information from the cochlear nuclei on each side is to both superior olivary nuclei, causing bilateral representation of hearing throughout the remainder of the central pathways. From the superior olivary nuclei, transmission is by the lateral lemniscus to the inferior colliculus. Further cross-connections occur in collicular synapses. Rostrally directed fibers from the inferior colliculi ascend to the medial geniculate and auditory cortex of the temporal lobe.

Symptoms of Auditory Dysfunction

The major symptoms of disturbance in the auditory pathways are hearing impairment, tinnitus, and hyperacusis. The characteristic feature of hearing impairment in infants is failure to develop speech (see Chapter 5) and in older children inattentiveness and poor school performance. Fifty percent of infants use words with meaning by 12 months and join words into sentences by 24 months. Failure to accomplish these tasks by 21 months and 3 years, respectively, is always abnormal. A hearing loss of 25–30 dB is sufficient to interfere with normal acquisition of speech.

Hearing Impairment

Hearing impairment is classified as conductive, sensorineural (perceptive), or central. The cause of conductive hearing impairment is a disturbance in the external or middle ear. Faithful delivery of the mechanical vibrations that make up the sensory input of hearing to the inner ear does not occur because the external canal is blocked or the tympanic membrane or ossicles are abnormal. The major defect in conductive hearing loss is sound amplification. Patients with conductive hearing impairment are better able to hear loud speech in a noisy background than soft speech in a quiet background. Tinnitus may be associated.

Sensorineural hearing impairment may be congenital or acquired and a disturbance of the cochlea or auditory nerve is the cause. The frequency content of sound is improperly analyzed and transduced. High frequencies may be selectively lost. Individuals with sensorineural hearing impairment have difficulty discriminating speech when there is background noise. Central hearing impairment results from disturbance of the cochlear nuclei or their projections to the cortex. Brainstem lesions usually cause bilateral hearing impairment. Cortical lesions lead to difficulty in processing information. Pure-tone audiometry is normal, but background noise or competing messages impair speech discrimination. The cause of approximately one-third of childhood deafness is genetic, one-third acquired, and one-third idiopathic. Many of the idiopathic cases are probably genetic as well.

Tinnitus

Tinnitus is the illusion of noise in the ear. The noise is usually high-pitched and constant. In most cases, the cause of tinnitus is a disturbance of the auditory nerve, but it may also occur as a simple partial seizure originating from the primary auditory cortex. Sounds generated by the cardiovascular system (heartbeat and bruit) are sometimes audible, especially while a person is lying down, but should not be confused with tinnitus.

Hyperacusis

The cause of hyperacusis is failure of the stapedius muscle to dampen sound by its effect on the ossicles. This occurs with damage to the chorda tympani branch of the facial nerve (see the discussion of Bell palsy earlier in this chapter).

Tests of Hearing

Office Testing

Hearing assessment in the office is satisfactory for severe hearing impairment but is unsatisfactory for detecting loss of specific frequency bands. The speech and hearing handicap generated by a high-frequency hearing impairment should not be underestimated. When testing an infant, the physician should stand behind the patient and provide interesting sounds to each ear. Bells, chimes, rattles, or a tuning fork is useful for that purpose. Dropping a large object and watching the infant and parents startle from the noise is not a test of hearing. Once the infant sees the source of the interesting sound or hears it several times, interest is lost. Therefore, the use of different high- and low-frequency sounds is required for each ear. The normal responses of the infant are to become alert and to attempt to localize the source of the sound.

In older children, observing their response to spoken words at different intensities and with tuning forks that provide pure tones of different frequencies tests hearing. The *Rinne test* compares air conduction (conductive plus sensorineural hearing) with bone conduction (sensorineural hearing). Hold a tuning fork against the mastoid process until the sound fades and is then held 1 inch from the ear. Normal children hear the vibration produced by air conduction twice as long as that produced by bone conduction. Impaired air conduction with normal bone conduction indicates a conductive hearing loss.

The *Weber test* compares bone conduction in the two ears. Localization of the signals transmitted by bone conduction is to the better-hearing ear or the ear with the greater conductive deficit. With a tuning fork placed at the center of the forehead, inquire whether the perception of sound is equal in both ears. A normal response is to hear the sound in the center of the head. If bone conduction is normal in both ears, sound localization is to the ear with impaired air conduction because the normal blocking response of air conduction is lacking. If a sensorineural hearing impairment is present in one ear, the perception of bone conduction is in the good ear. Otoscopic examination is imperative in every child with hearing problems or tinnitus. The cause seen through the speculum may be impacted wax, otitis media, perforated tympanic membrane, or cholesteatoma.

Specialized Testing

The usual battery of auditory tests includes pure-tone air and bone conduction testing, and measures of speech threshold and word discrimination.

Pure-Tone Audiometry. With selected frequencies presented by earphones (air conduction) or by a vibrator applied to the mastoid (bone conduction), the minimum level perceived for each frequency is determined. International standards define the normal hearing levels. The test can be performed adequately only in children old enough to cooperate. With conductive hearing impairment, air conduction is abnormal and bone conduction is normal;

with sensorineural hearing impairment, both are abnormal; and with central hearing impairment, both are normal.

Speech Tests. The speech reception threshold measures the intensity at which a subject can repeat 50% of presented words. The speech discrimination test measures the subject's ability to understand speech at normal conversational levels. Both tests are abnormal out of proportion to pure-tone loss with auditory nerve disease, abnormal in proportion to pure-tone loss with cochlear disease, and normal with conductive and central hearing loss.

Special Tests. Cochlear lesions may cause diplacusis and recruitment. Auditory nerve lesions produce tone decay. Diplacusis is a distortion of pure tones so that the subject perceives a mixture of tones. With recruitment, the sensation of loudness increases at an abnormally rapid rate as the intensity of sound is increased. Tone decay is diminished perception of a suprathreshold tone with time.

Brainstem Auditory Evoked Response

The brainstem auditory evoked response (BAER) is a useful test of hearing and the integrity of the brainstem auditory pathways in infants and small children. No cooperation is required, and sedation improves the accuracy of results.

When each ear is stimulated with repetitive clicks, an electrode over the ipsilateral mastoid referenced to the forehead records five waves. Wave I is generated by the acoustic nerve, wave II by the cochlear nerve, wave III by the superior olivary complex, wave IV by the lateral lemniscus, and wave V by the inferior colliculus. The BAER first appears at a conceptional age of 26 to 27 weeks. The absolute latencies of waves I and V and the V-I interpeak interval decline progressively with advancing conceptional age. The latency of wave V bears an inverse relationship to the intensity of the stimulus and tests hearing.

An initial test uses a stimulus intensity of 70 dB. Failure to produce wave V indicates a hearing impairment. Repeated tests at higher intensities find the response threshold. If wave V is present, the repeated tests at sequential reductions of 10 dB establish the lowest intensity capable of producing wave V, the *hearing threshold*. Because the latency of wave V is proportional to the intensity of the stimulus, a latency-intensity curve is drawn. In normal newborns, the latency of wave V will decrease by 0.24 to 0.44 ms for each 10 dB in sound intensity between 70 and 110 dB.

In children with conductive hearing impairment, prolonged time is required to transmit sound across the middle ear and activate the cochlea. This reduces the total amount of sound energy, prolongs the latency of wave I, and shifts the latency-intensity curve of wave V to the right. The amount of shift is equivalent to the hearing impairment, without altering the slope of the curve.

In children with sensorineural hearing impairment, the latency-intensity curve of wave V shifts to the right because of the hearing impairment. In addition, the slope of the curve becomes steeper, exceeding 0.55 ms/dB.

Congenital Deafness

The diagnosis of congenital deafness in newborns is rarely entertained in the absence of an external ear deformity or a family history of genetic hearing loss. Congenital ear malformations are present in approximately 2% of newborns with congenital deafness. Genetic factors account for one-third of all congenital deafness and half of profound deafness. Between 1/2000 (0.05%) and 1/1000 (0.1%) children are born with profound hearing loss; one-half of prelingual deafness is genetic, most often autosomal recessive and nonsyndromic. Mutations in the genes that encodes the protein connexin 26 and 30, account for half of autosomal recessive nonsyndromic hearing loss. The carrier rate is 3/100. Only a small percentage of prelingual deafness is syndromic or autosomal dominant nonsyndromic (Smith & Van Camp, 2007).

Aplasia of Inner Ear

Inner ear aplasia is always associated with auditory nerve abnormalities. The three main types are the *Michel defect*, complete absence of the otic capsule and eighth cranial nerve; the *Mondini defect*, incomplete development of the bony and membranous labyrinths and dysgenesis of the spiral ganglion; and the *Scheibe defect*, dysplasia of the membranous labyrinth and atrophy of the eighth nerve.

Chromosome Disorders

Hearing impairment is relatively uncommon in children with chromosomal disorders. Abnormalities of chromosome 18 are often associated with profound sensorineural hearing loss and malformations of the external ear.

Genetic Disorders

Several hundred gene abnormalities are associated with hereditary hearing loss and deafness.

The hearing loss may be conductive, sensorineural, or mixed. Some are congenital and some develop later in childhood.

Infantile Refsum Disease. Infantile Refsum disease is part of the Zellweger spectrum of disorders (ZSS) of peroxisome biogenesis. It differs from later-onset Refsum disease (see Chapter 7), a single-enzyme peroxisomal disorder. The gene locus is on chromosome 7q21–q22 and transmission of the disorder is by autosomal recessive inheritance (Steinberg et al, 2012).

Clinical Features. Features include early-onset, cognitive impairment, minor facial dysmorphism, retinitis pigmentosa, sensorineural hearing deficit, hepatomegaly, osteoporosis, failure to thrive, and hypocholesterolemia.

Diagnosis. The concentration of protein in the spinal fluid is elevated, and electroencephalography (EEG) may show epileptiform activity. Liver transaminase levels are elevated, as is the serum concentration of bile acids. An elevated plasma concentration of very-long-chain fatty acids is essential to the diagnosis.

Management. No curative therapy is presently available for ZSS. Symptomatic therapy includes evaluation of feeding, hearing, vision, liver function, and neurological function. All affected children benefit from appropriate educational placement and the use of hearing aids.

Isolated Deafness. Isolated deafness in newborns and infants is usually genetic and transmission may be by autosomal dominant, autosomal recessive, or X-linked inheritance. In many sporadic cases, transmission is by autosomal recessive inheritance. Genetic disorders transmitted by autosomal dominant inheritance are often causative of congenital deafness associated with external ear deformities, but chromosomal disorders and fetal exposure to drugs and toxins are considerations. Maternal use of heparin during pregnancy produces an embryopathy characterized by skeletal deformities, flattening of the nose, cerebral dysgenesis, and deafness.

In the absence of an external malformation or family history, deafness often goes unnoticed until the infant fails to develop speech. Intrauterine infection with cytomegalovirus is an important cause of congenital deafness (see Chapter 5). Ten percent of newborns infected in utero with cytomegalovirus develop a sensorineural hearing loss. Mass immunization has now almost eliminated rubella embryopathy, once a significant cause of childhood deafness in the United States.

Pendred Syndrome. Pendred syndrome, the second most common type of autosomal recessive syndromic hearing loss, is a genetic defect in thyroxine synthesis. Transmission is by autosomal recessive inheritance. Goiter and sensorineural hearing impairment are the characteristic features. The hearing impairment is profound. Goiter is not present at birth and develops in early puberty (40 %) or adulthood (60 %).

Clinical Features. Sensorineural hearing impairment is present at birth and is severe in 50 % of cases. Milder hearing impairment may not be detectable until the child is 2 years of age. Vestibular function may also be impaired. A diffuse, nonnodular goiter becomes apparent during the first decade, often in infancy. No clinical signs of hypothyroidism are present. Growth and intelligence are usually normal.

Diagnosis. A perchlorate discharge test documents delayed organification of iodine by the thyroid. The deafness is associated with an abnormality of the bony labyrinth (Mondini dysplasia or dilated vestibular aqueduct) diagnosed by CT examination of the temporal bones. Vestibular function is abnormal in the most affected persons. Molecular genetic testing of the *SLC26A4* gene (chromosomal locus 7q22-q31) is available clinically. Seventy-five percent of cases show recognized mutations in the chromosomal locus 7q22–q31.

Thin-section high-resolution MRI in the axial and sagittal planes shows enlargement of the endolymphatic sac and duct in association with a large vestibular aqueduct (Phelps et al, 1998).

Management. Medical rather than surgical treatment is better for managing goiter. Exogenous hormone decreases production of thyroid-stimulating hormone, with subsequent reduction in goiter size. The hearing loss is irreversible.

Usher Syndrome. Usher syndrome is the most common type of autosomal syndromic hearing loss. Affected individuals are born with sensorineural hearing loss. Later, they develop retinitis pigmentosa. Usher syndrome affects over 50 % of the deaf-blind in the United States. The visual impairment, caused by retinitis pigmentosa, is usually not apparent in the first decade. During the second decade, night blindness and loss of peripheral vision become evident and inexorably progress.

Clinical Features. Three types of Usher syndrome are recognized. Severe-to-profound sensorineural hearing loss and abnormal vestibular dysfunction characterize type 1. The vestibular deficit delays developmental motor milestones for sitting and walking.

Mild-to-severe sensorineural hearing loss and normal vestibular function characterize type 2. Hearing aids provide effective amplification and oral communication is possible. Characteristic features of type 3 are progressive hearing loss and progressive deterioration of vestibular function.

Vestibular responses to caloric testing are absent, and mild ataxia may be present. Mental retardation is present in 25 % of cases.

Diagnosis. Molecular genetic testing is available for some subtypes of Usher syndrome types 2 and 3. The combination of retinitis pigmentosa and hearing impairment is also present in other syndromes. Usher syndrome is the only one in which profound deafness is present at birth.

Management. Deafness type 1 is not correctable with hearing aids.

Waardenburg Syndrome. Waardenburg syndrome (WS) is the most common type of autosomal dominant syndromic hearing loss. It consists of sensorineural hearing loss and pigmentary abnormalities of the skin, hair (white forelock), and eyes (heterochromia iridis). Several clinical forms exist (Smith & Van Camp, 2007). The gene map locus is chromosome 2q35.

Clinical Features. WS is relatively easy to recognize because of its cutaneous features: a white forelock, eyes of different colors (usually different shades of blue), hypertelorism, and depigmented dermal patches. Hearing loss is not a constant feature. An additional feature is a wide bridge of the nose owing to lateral displacement of the inner canthus of each eye.

The presence of other abnormalities differentiates four subtypes. Lateral displacement of the inner canthus of the eye, a characteristic feature of WS I, is not present in WS II. In WS III, arm abnormalities are present, and Hirschsprung disease is part of WS IV.

Diagnosis. The family history and the cutaneous features establish the diagnosis. Molecular genetic testing is available for WS I and III.

Management. Treatment is symptomatic.

Later-Onset Genetic Disorders

The discussion of several of the disorders listed in Box 17-5 is in other chapters. Sensorineural hearing impairment occurs as part of several spinocerebellar degenerations, hereditary motor sensory neuropathies, and sensory autonomic neuropathies. It is a major feature of Refsum disease (hereditary motor sensory neuropathy type IV); dietary measures reduce the serum concentrations of phytanic acid.

Deafness-Dystonia-Optic Neuronopathy Syndrome

Inheritance of this disorder is as an X-linked trait. Carrier females are unaffected (Blesa et al, 2007).

Clinical Features. Progressive deafness begins before age 2 years and progresses to profound hearing loss by age 10 years. Dystonia and/or ataxia develop in the second decade followed by decreased vision from optic neuropathy in the third decade, and dementia at age 40 years.

Diagnosis. The clinical features are diagnostic. The serum IgG is <200 mg/dL and the IgM and IgA are <20 mg/dL. Molecular genetic testing is available.

Management. Treatment is symptomatic.

Pontobulbar Palsy with Deafness

Pontobulbar palsy (*the Brown-Vialetto-Van Laere syndrome*) with deafness is a rare hereditary motor neuron disorder. The mode of transmission is autosomal recessive (Megarbane et al, 2000).

Clinical Features. Bilateral nerve deafness and a variety of cranial nerve disorders, usually involving the motor components of the VII and IX to XII (more rarely the III, V, and VI) cranial nerves characterize the disorder. Spinal motor nerves and, less commonly, upper motor neurons are sometimes affected. Onset most often occurs during the second decade. Progressive sensorineural hearing loss is the initial symptom and may affect first one ear and then the other. Facial weakness and dysphagia accompany or quickly follow deafness. Tongue atrophy occurs in most cases, but masseter and ocular motor palsies are uncommon.

Approximately half of patients have evidence of pyramidal tract dysfunction, such as extensor plantar responses, and half have atrophy and fasciculations of limb muscle. Loss of tendon reflexes is an early feature of most cases. Respiratory insufficiency is a common feature and a frequent cause of death.

Diagnosis. The presence of deafness and areflexia distinguishes pontobulbar palsy from juvenile progressive bulbar palsy but can also suggest a hereditary motor sensory neuropathy if symptoms of bulbar palsy are delayed. The diagnosis depends on the clinical features. MRI of the brainstem excludes the possibility of tumor.

Management. Most patients require a feeding gastrostomy. Treatment is not available for the underlying disease.

BOX 17-5 Hearing Impairment and Deafness

CONGENITAL
- Aplasia of inner ear
- Michel defect
- Mondini defect
- Scheibe defect

CHROMOSOME DISORDERS
- Trisomy 13
- Trisomy 18
- 18q syndrome

GENETIC DISORDERS
- Isolated deafness
- Pendred syndrome
- Usher syndrome
- Waardenburg syndrome

INTRAUTERINE VIRAL INFECTION (SEE CHAPTER 5)

MATERNAL DRUG USE
- Drugs
- Antibiotics
- β-Blockers
- Chemotherapy

GENETIC NEUROLOGICAL DISORDERS
- Familial spastic paraplegia (see Chapter 12)
- Hereditary motor sensory neuropathies (see Chapter 7)
- Hereditary sensory autonomic neuropathies (see Chapter 9)
- Infantile Refsum disease
- Neurofibromatosis type 2 (see Acoustic Neuroma)
- Pontobulbar palsy with deafness
- Mitochondrial disorders (see Chapter 8)
- Spinocerebellar degenerations (see Chapter 10)
- Wolfram syndrome (see Chapter 16)
- Xeroderma pigmentosum (see Chapter 5)

INFECTIOUS DISEASES
- Bacterial meningitis*
- Otitis media* (see Vertigo)
- Sarcoidosis* (see Facial Weakness)
- Viral encephalitis (see Chapter 2)
- Viral exanthemas

METABOLIC DISORDERS
- Hypothyroidism*
- Menière disease (see Vertigo)

SKELETAL DISORDERS
- Apert acrocephalosyndactyly
- Cleidocranial dysostosis
- Craniofacial dysostosis (Crouzon disease)
- Craniometaphyseal dysplasia (Pyle disease)
- Klippel-Feil syndrome
- Mandibulofacial dysostosis (Treacher-Collins syndrome)
- Osteogenesis imperfecta
- Osteopetrosis (Albers-Schönberg disease)

SUSAC SYNDROME (SEE CHAPTER 2)

TRAUMA (SEE VERTIGO)

TUMOR
- Acoustic neuroma*
- Cholesteatoma* (see Vertigo)

*Denotes the most common conditions and the ones with disease modifying treatments

Acquired Hearing Impairment

Drug-Induced Impairment

Antibiotics are the most commonly used class of drugs with potential ototoxicity in children. The incidence of toxic reactions is greatest with amikacin, furosemide, and vancomycin and only a little less with kanamycin and neomycin. Permanent damage is unusual with any of these drugs. The characteristic syndrome consists of tinnitus and high-frequency hearing impairment. Vancomycin produces hearing loss only when blood concentrations exceed 45 μg/mL. By contrast, aminoglycosides may cause irreversible cochlear toxicity, which begins as tinnitus, progresses to vertigo and high-frequency hearing impairment, and finally impairs all frequencies. This is of special concern in sick preterm newborns given aminoglycosides for periods of 15 days or longer.

β-Adrenoceptor blocking drugs are a rare cause of hearing impairment and tinnitus. Cessation of therapy reverses symptoms. Cisplatin, an anticancer drug, has ototoxic effects in 30% of recipients. Tinnitus is the major feature. The hearing impairment is at frequencies above those used for speech.

Salicylates tend to concentrate in the perilymph of the labyrinth and are ototoxic. Tinnitus and high-frequency hearing impairment result from long-term exposure to high doses.

Infectious Diseases

Otitis media is a common cause of reversible conductive hearing impairment in children, but only rarely does infection spread to the inner ear (see section on Vertigo later in this chapter). Hearing impairment is a relatively common symptom of viral encephalitis (see Chapter 2) and may be an early feature. Sudden hearing loss may also accompany childhood exanthemas (chickenpox, mumps, and measles), and in such cases virus can be isolated from the cochlear and auditory nerves.

The overall incidence of persistent unilateral or bilateral hearing loss in children with acute bacterial meningitis is 10 %. Early treatment with dexamethasone reduces the risk (see Chapter 4). *Streptococcus pneumoniae* meningitis is also associated with a 20 % incidence of persistent dizziness, gait ataxia, and other neurological deficits.

The site of disease is probably the inner ear or auditory nerve. Organisms may gain access to the inner ear from the subarachnoid space. Otitis media is the source of meningitis in many children and produces a transitory conductive hearing loss but does not cause a permanent sensorineural hearing loss. It is common in many centers to screen all children hospitalized for treatment of acute bacterial meningitis with BAER audiometry prior to discharge.

Metabolic Disorders

Menière disease is characterized by vertigo, tinnitus, and hearing impairment. Vertigo is often the presenting feature (see the later discussion of Vertigo). Tinnitus and decreased hearing are common features of hypothyroidism and are reversible by thyroid replacement therapy.

Skeletal Disorders

The combination of hearing impairment and skeletal deformities almost always indicates a genetic disease. Skeletal disorders may be limited, usually to the face and digits, or generalized. The partial list in Box 17-6 highlights the more common syndromes. Genetic transmission for almost all is autosomal dominant inheritance with variable expression. The exceptions are osteopetrosis, which is an autosomal recessive inheritance trait; craniometaphyseal dysplasia, which has both a dominant and a recessive form; and the Klippel-Feil anomaly, for which the pattern of transmission is uncertain.

Trauma

Acute auditory and vestibular injuries occur with fractures of the petrous portion of the temporal bone. Vestibular function is more likely to be impaired than auditory function (see section on Vertigo later in this chapter).

Tumor

Acoustic neuroma and cholesteatoma are the tumors most likely to impair children's hearing. Other cerebellopontine angle tumors are extremely rare before the third or fourth decade. The discussion of cholesteatoma is in the section on Vertigo.

Acoustic Neuroma. Acoustic neuromas are actually schwannomas of the eighth nerve. Only 6 % of acoustic neuromas come to medical attention in the second decade, and even fewer in the first decade. Children with acoustic neuroma usually have neurofibromatosis type 2 (NF2), a genetic disease distinct from neurofibromatosis type 1 (see Chapter 5). Genetic transmission of NF2 is by autosomal dominant inheritance, with the gene locus on chromosome 22. Acoustic neuromas are the most constant feature of the phenotype. Later, other cerebral tumors such as meningioma, glioma, schwannoma, and juvenile posterior subcapsular lenticular opacity may develop. Café au lait spots may be present on the skin but are fewer than five in number.

Clinical Features. Deafness or tinnitus is the usual initial complaint. Approximately one-third of patients have nonaudiological symptoms, such as facial numbness or paresthesia, vertigo, headache, and ataxia. Hearing impairment is present in almost every patient; ipsilateral diminished corneal reflex occurs in half; and ataxia, facial hypoesthesia or weakness, and nystagmus in 30–40 %. Large tumors cause obstructive hydrocephalus with symptoms of increased intracranial pressure and brainstem compression.

Diagnosis. Molecular-based testing is available. Several schemes for the clinical diagnosis of NF2 are available (Baser et al, 2002). One commonly used scheme includes bilateral vestibular

BOX 17-6 Causes of Vertigo

DRUGS AND TOXINS

EPILEPSY

- Complex partial seizures
- Simple partial seizures

INFECTIONS

- Otitis media
- Vestibular neuronitis

MENIÈRE DISEASE

MIGRAINE

- Basilar migraine (see Chapter 10)
- Benign paroxysmal vertigo (see Chapter 10)

MOTION SICKNESS

MULTIPLE SCLEROSIS (SEE CHAPTER 10)

PSYCHOGENIC

- Hyperventilation syndrome (see Chapter 1)
- Panic attacks

TRAUMA

- Migraine
- Posttraumatic neurosis
- Temporal bone fracture
- Vestibular concussion
- Whiplash injury

schwannomas or a family history of NF2 in one or more first degree relative(s) plus (1) unilateral vestibular schwannomas at age less than 30 years or (2) any two of the following: meningioma, glioma, schwannoma, or juvenile posterior subcapsular lenticular opacities/juvenile cortical cataract. Every child with progressive hearing impairment or tinnitus requires careful examination for café au lait spots. Exploration of the family history for acoustic neuroma or other neurological disturbance is also required.

Abnormalities in pure-tone audiometry and in the BAER are present in almost every patient, but are not necessary for diagnosis. Gadolinium-enhanced MRI is the test of choice to visualize tumors in the cerebellopontine angle (Figure 17-3).

Management. Both surgery and the photon (gamma ray) knife are useful for tumor resection. Surgery often sacrifices residual hearing and sometimes causes a facial palsy. The superiority of the photon knife to standard surgery is not yet established.

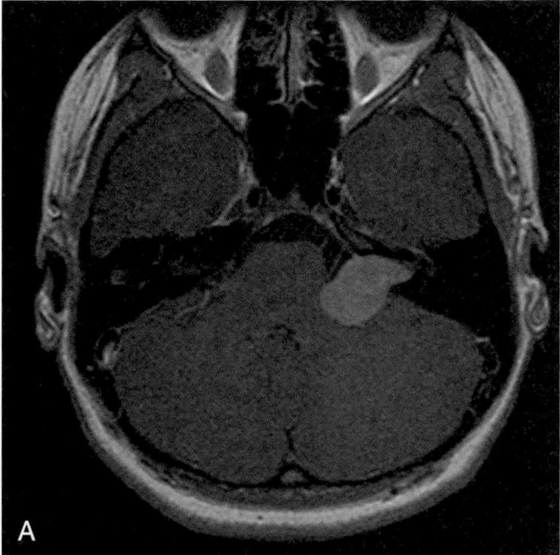

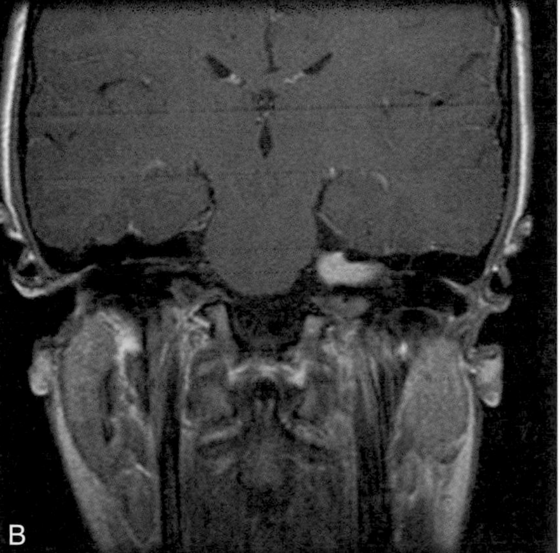

FIGURE 17-3 ■ Acoustic neuroma. (A) T_1 coronal and (B) axial MIR of a left acoustic neuroma.

VERTIGO

Vertigo is the sensation of rotation or spinning. It terrifies small children. Balance is lost and posture is difficult to maintain, giving the appearance of ataxia (see Chapter 10). Nausea and nystagmus are often associated features. When nystagmus is present, the fast phase is in the same direction as the perceived rotation. Movement of the head exacerbates all symptoms.

Anatomical Considerations

The semicircular canals and the vestibule, within the labyrinth, are the sensory organs of the vestibular system. The stimulus for excitation of the semicircular canals is rotary motion of the head; for the vestibule, it is gravity. The vestibular portion of the VIII cranial nerve transmits information from the sensory organs to the vestibular nuclei in the brainstem and the cerebellum. The vestibular nuclei have extensive connections with the cerebellum and medial longitudinal fasciculus. Cortical projections terminate in the superior temporal gyrus and frontal lobe.

Approach to Vertigo

History and Physical Examination

Children often complain of dizziness or lightheadedness but rarely complain of vertigo. Carefully question those who complain of dizziness or lightheadedness about the sensation of rotation. Whether the subject or the environment rotates is irrelevant. The illusion of rotation separates vertigo from presyncope, ataxia and other disturbances of balance and localizes the disturbance to the vestibular system. Vertigo implies dysfunction of the labyrinth or vestibular nerve (peripheral vertigo) or the brainstem or temporal lobe (central vertigo).

Important historical points to document include the course of vertigo (acute, recurrent, or chronic), precipitating events (trauma, infection, or position change), association of hearing impairment and tinnitus, drug exposure, cardiovascular disease, and family history of migraine. Migraine and epilepsy are the usual causes of acute, episodic attacks of vertigo, not induced by motion, with migraine as the more common of the two. The usual cause of a single, prolonged attack of vertigo, especially in combination with nausea and vomiting, is infection of the labyrinth or vestibular nerve. Chronic vertigo often waxes and wanes, and may seem intermittent rather than chronic. Both central and peripheral causes of vertigo are considerations (Box 17-6), but the clinical and laboratory features readily distinguish central from peripheral vertigo (Table 17-1).

Special Tests

Not every child who complains of dizziness requires caloric and audiometric testing (Fife et al, 2000). A description of caloric testing is in this section and audiometric testing in the section on Hearing Impairment and Deafness. The Nylan-Hallpike test is useful to define position-induced vertigo.

Caloric Testing. The simplest method of caloric testing is to instill small quantities of cool water into the external auditory canal with a rubber-tipped syringe. Before instilling the water, inspect the canal to determine whether there is clear passage to an intact tympanic membrane. Use a sufficient quantity of water, depending on the child's size, to keep the tympanic membrane cooled for 20 seconds. A normal response is slow deviation of the eyes to the side stimulated, followed by a fast component to the opposite side. If stimulation with cool water fails to produce a response, repeat the procedure with ice water. Absence of nystagmus indicates absence of peripheral vestibular function. Partial dysfunction of one vestibular apparatus results in asymmetry of response (directional preponderance).

Nylan-Hallpike Test. The Nylan-Hallpike test requires tilting the patient backward from the sitting position to the supine position so that the head hangs down below the level of the examining table. Observe the eyes for position-induced nystagmus after turning the head 45 degrees to the right and then to the left.

Causes of Vertigo

Drugs

Many drugs that disturb vestibular function also disturb auditory function. This section deals only with drugs affecting vestibular function more than auditory function. Toxic doses of anticonvulsant and neuroleptic medications produce ataxia, incoordination, and measurable disturbances of vestibular function, but patients do not ordinarily complain of vertigo.

Antibiotics are the main class of drugs with vestibular toxicity. Streptomycin, minocycline, and aminoglycosides have a high incidence of toxic reactions, and sulfonamides have a low incidence.

Streptomycin disturbs vestibular function but has little effect on hearing. Variation in individual susceptibility prevents the establishment of a toxic milligram-per-kilogram dose. However, the vestibular toxicity of streptomycin is so predictable that high dosages of the drug are therapeutic to destroy vestibular function in patients with severe Menière disease.

Minocycline produces nausea, vomiting, dizziness, and ataxia at standard therapeutic doses. Onset of symptoms is 2 to 3 days after starting treatment and cease 2 days after cessation. Gentamicin and other aminoglycosides have an adverse effect on both vestibular and auditory function. Some disturbance occurs in 2% of patients treated with gentamicin. Vestibular

TABLE 17-1 **Distinguishing Peripheral and Central Vertigo**

	Clinical features	Laboratory features
Peripheral vertigo	Hearing loss, tinnitus, and otalgia may be associated features Past pointing and falling in the direction of unilateral disease occur Ataxia occurs with the eyes closed in bilateral disease Vestibular and positional nystagmus is present	Caloric testing reveals vestibular paresis directional preponderance, or both Pure-tone audiometry reveals sensorineural hearing loss Recruitment is present with end-organ disease and tone decay with nerve disease
Central vertigo	Cerebellar and cranial nerve dysfunction are frequently associated Hearing is intact Loss of consciousness may be associated	Pure-tone audiometry and speech discrimination are normal Comprehension of competing messages is impaired Caloric testing may reveal directional preponderance but not vestibular paresis Brainstem evoked response, EEG, CT, or MRI may be abnormal

dysfunction, either alone or in combination with auditory dysfunction, occurs in 84% of cases, whereas auditory dysfunction alone occurs in only 16%. Ototoxic effects develop when the total dose exceeds 17.5 mg/kg.

Epilepsy

Vertigo can be the only feature of a simple partial seizure or the initial feature of a complex partial seizure. The experience of vertigo is an aura in 10–20% of patients with complex partial seizures.

Clinical Features. The recognition of vertigo as an aura is simple when a complex, partial seizure follows. Diagnosis is more problematic when vertigo is the only feature of a simple partial seizure. The child ceases activity, becomes pale, appears frightened, and then recovers. Unsteadiness and nausea may be associated features.

Diagnosis. All children with unexplained brief attacks of vertigo, especially when vestibular and auditory function is normal between attacks, require EEG. Ambulatory EEG or 24-hour video monitoring is required to capture an attack if interictal EEG is normal.

Management. Discussion of the management of simple and complex partial seizures is in Chapter 2.

Infections

Bacterial Infection. Otitis media and meningitis are leading causes of vestibular and auditory impairment in children. Acute suppurative labyrinthitis resulting from extension of bacterial infection from the middle ear has become uncommon since the introduction of antibiotics. However, even without direct bacterial invasion, bacterial toxins may cause serous labyrinthitis.

Chronic otitic infections cause labyrinthine damage by the development of cholesteatoma. A cholesteatoma is a sac containing keratin, silvery-white debris shed by squamous epithelial cells. Such cells are not normal constituents of the middle ear but gain access from the external canal after infection repeatedly perforates the eardrum. Cholesteatomas erode surrounding tissues, including bone, and produce a fistula between the perilymph and the middle ear.

Clinical Features. The characteristics of acute suppurative or serous labyrinthitis are the sudden onset of severe vertigo, nausea, vomiting, and unilateral hearing loss. Meningismus may also be present. Chronic otitis causes similar symptoms. Severe vertigo that is provoked by sneezing, coughing, or merely applying pressure on the external canal indicates fistula formation. Otoscopic examination reveals evidence of otitis media and tympanic membrane perforation and allows visualization of cholesteatoma.

Diagnosis. When vestibular dysfunction develops in children with otitis media, order radiographs or computed tomography (CT) of the skull to visualize erosion of bone or mastoiditis. The presence of meningismus or increased intracranial pressure (see Chapter 4) necessitates CT to exclude the possibility of abscess and then examination of cerebrospinal fluid to exclude meningitis.

Management. Vigorous antibiotic therapy and drainage of the infected area are required in every case. Myringotomy and mastoidectomy provide drainage when needed. Cholesteatomas are progressive and require surgical excision.

Viral Infections. Viral infections may affect the labyrinth or vestibular nerve. The two are difficult to differentiate by clinical features, and the terms *vestibular neuritis* or *neuronitis* describe acute peripheral vestibulopathies. Vestibular neuritis may be part of a systemic viral infection, such as mumps, measles, and infectious mononucleosis, or it may occur in epidemics without an identifiable viral agent, or as part of a postinfectious cranial polyneuritis. The incidence in children is low, accounting for less than 7% of all cases.

Clinical Features. The main feature is the acute onset of vertigo. Any attempt to move the head results in a severe exacerbation of vertigo, nausea, and vomiting. Nystagmus is present on fixation and increased by head movement. The patient is unable to maintain posture and lies motionless in bed. Recovery begins during the first 48 hours. Spontaneous nausea diminishes, and nystagmus on fixation ceases. With each day, vertigo decreases in severity but positional nystagmus is still present. Recovery is usually complete within 3 weeks.

Diagnosis. The clinical features are the basis for establishing the diagnosis. Brain imaging is unnecessary when acute-onset vertigo is an isolated symptom and begins improving within 48 hours (Hotson & Baloh, 1998).

Management. During the acute phase, keep the child in bed and provide vestibular sedation. Diazepam is very effective in dampening the labyrinth and relieving the symptoms. Children should not use transdermal scopolamine. As recovery progresses, activity is gradually increased and sedation reduced.

Menière Disease

Menière disease is uncommon in children. An overaccumulation of endolymph that results in rupture of the labyrinth is the mechanism of disease.

Clinical Features. Rupture of the labyrinth causes the clinical features, hearing impairment, tinnitus, and vertigo. Hearing impairment fluctuates and may temporarily return to normal when the rupture heals. Tinnitus is ignorable, but vertigo demands attention and is often the complaint that brings the disorder to attention. A typical attack consists of disabling vertigo and tinnitus lasting for 1 to 3 hours. Tinnitus, fullness in the ear, or increased loss of hearing may precede the vertigo. Tinnitus becomes worse during the attack. Pallor, sweating, nausea, and vomiting are often associated features. Afterward, the patient is tired and sleeps. Attacks occur at unpredictable intervals for years and then subside, leaving the patient with permanent hearing loss. Bilateral involvement is present in 20 % of cases. Nystagmus is present during an attack. At first, the fast component is toward the abnormal ear (irritative); later, as the attack subsides, the fast component is away (paralytic). Between attacks, the results of examination are normal, with the exception of unilateral hearing impairment.

Diagnosis. Pure-tone audiometry shows threshold fluctuation. Speech discrimination is preserved, and recruitment is present on the abnormal side. Caloric stimulation demonstrates unilateral vestibular paresis or directional preponderance.

Management. The underlying disease is not reversible. Management of the acute attack and increasing the interval between attacks is the goal of therapy. Bed rest, sedation, and antiemetic drugs are the treatment of acute attacks. Maintenance therapy usually consists of a low-salt diet and diuretics; neither provides substantial benefit.

Migraine

Seventeen percent of migraineurs report vertigo at the time of an attack. Such individuals have no difficulty in recognizing vertigo as a symptom of migraine. Another 10 % experience vertigo in the interval between attacks and may have difficulty relating vertigo to migraine. Brief (minutes), recurrent episodes of vertigo in infants and small children are usually a migraine equivalent, despite the absence of headache. The attacks later evolve into classic migraine. Affected children appear ataxic; discussion of the syndrome is therefore in Chapter 10 (see the section on Benign Paroxysmal Vertigo).

Motion Sickness

Unfamiliar body accelerations or a mismatch in information provided to the brain by the visual and vestibular systems during acceleration of the body induces motion sickness. Motion in the visual field opposed to actual body movement induces motion sickness. Therefore, allowing a child to look out of the window while riding in a car reduces the incidence of motion sickness. Small children in the back seat, where the only visual input is the car interior, are at the greatest risk for motion sickness. A minivan may reduce the incidence of motion sickness by allowing children access to a window.

The prevalence of motion sickness depends on how violent the movement is and approaches 100 % in the worst case. Twenty-five percent of a ship's passengers become sick during a 2- to 3-day Atlantic crossing, and 0.5 % of commercial airline passengers are affected. The first symptom is pallor, which is followed by nausea and vomiting. Because nausea usually precedes vomiting, there is time to prevent vomiting in some situations. Stopping the motion is the best way to abort an attack. Watching the environment move opposite the direction of body movement may inhibit early attacks. Individuals with known susceptibility to motion sickness should take an antihistamine, diazepam, or scopolamine before travel.

Trauma

Fifty percent of children complain of dizziness and headache during the first 3 days after a closed head injury, with or without loss of consciousness. One-third have persistent vertigo without hearing loss. This group is separable into patients with direct trauma to the labyrinth (vestibular concussion) and those in whom the vestibular apparatus is not injured.

Vestibular Concussion

Clinical Features. Vestibular concussion follows blows to the parieto-occipital or temporoparietal region of the skull. Severe vertigo is present immediately after injury. The child is unsteady and sways toward the affected side. Symptoms persist for several days and then resolve completely, but specific movements of the head (paroxysmal positional vertigo) precipitate recurrent episodes of vertigo and nausea lasting for 5 to 10 seconds.

Diagnosis. All children with vertigo following a head injury require head CT. Fractures through the petrous pyramid require special attention. Bleeding from the ear or a facial palsy should raise suspicion of such a skull fracture. Moving the injured ear downward induces positional nystagmus by the Nylan-Hallpike technique. Caloric testing or electronystagmography shows a reduced response from the injured ear.

Management. Immediately after injury, treat with an antihistamine and diazepam until the acute phase is over. Fatigue therapy treats individuals with paroxysmal positional vertigo. Tilt the patient to a position that reproduces symptoms and maintain the position until the vertigo subsides for at least 30 seconds. The patient then sits up for 30 seconds. Repeat the procedure four times. Repeat this exercise several times each day until the patient is no longer sensitive to positional change.

Whiplash Injury. Whiplash injuries are frequently associated with vestibular and auditory dysfunction. Basilar artery spasm probably causes the symptoms.

Clinical Features. Vertigo may be present immediately after injury and subsides within a few days. Brief attacks of vertigo and tinnitus, sometimes associated with headache or nausea, may develop months later in children who appear fully recovered from the injury. Many features of the attacks suggest basilar artery migraine (see Chapter 10) and probably represent a posttraumatic migraine.

Diagnosis. During the acute phase, the Nylan-Hallpike technique induces vertigo and caloric testing documents unilateral dysfunction. Vestibular function may also be abnormal in children who are experiencing basilar artery migraine, especially at the time of an attack. EEG often shows occipital intermittent rhythmic delta activity (see Figure 10-2).

Management. Treatment is symptomatic.

REFERENCES

Baser ME, Friedman JM, Wallace AJ, et al. Evaluation of clinical diagnostic criteria for neurofibromatosis 2. Neurology 2002;59:1759–65.

Blesa JR, Solano A, Briones P, et al. Molecular genetics of a patient with Mohr-Tranebjaer syndrome due to a new mutation in the DDP1 gene. Molecular Medicine 2007;9(4):285–91.

Cockerham KP, Hidayat AA, Cockerham GC, et al. Melkersson-Rosenthal syndrome: new clinicopathologic findings in 4 cases. Archives of Ophthalmology 2000; 118:227–32.

Dipti S, Childs A-M, Livingston JH, et al. Brown-Vialetto-Von Laere syndrome: Variability in age at onset and disease progression highlighting the phenotypic overlap with Fazio-Londe disease. Brain and Development 2005;27:443–6.

Fife TD, Tusa RJ, Furman JM, et al. Assessment: Vestibular testing techniques in adults and children. Report of the Therapeutics and Technology Assessment Subcommittee of the American Academy of Neurology. Neurology 2000;55:1431–41.

Harriette TFM, van der Zwaag B, Cruysberg JRM, et al. Mobius syndrome redefined. A syndrome of rhombencephalic maldevelopment. Neurology 2003;61:327–33.

Hato N, Kisaki H, Honda N, et al. Ramsay-Hunt syndrome in children. Archives of Neurology 2000;48:254–6.

Hotson JR, Baloh RW. Acute vestibular syndrome. New England Journal of Medicine 1998;333:680–6.

Lemmers RJLF, van der Maarel SM. Facioscapulohumeral muscular dystrophy. In: GeneClinics: Medical Genetics Knowledge Base [database online]. Seattle: University of Washington. Available at http://www.geneclinic.org. Last updated July 9, 2009.

Murakami S, Hato N, Horiuchi J, et al. Treatment of Ramsay Hunt syndrome with acyclovir-prednisone: Significance of early diagnosis and treatment. Annals of Neurology 1997;41:353–7.

Megarbane A, Desguerres I, Rizkallah E, et al. Brown-Vialetto-Van Laere syndrome in a large inbred Lebanese family: confirmation of autosomal recessive inheritance? American Journal of Medical Genetics 2000;92:117–21.

Padberg GW, Brouwer OF, de Keizer RJW, et al. On the significance of retinal vascular disease and hearing loss in facioscapulohumeral muscular dystrophy. Muscle and Nerve 1995;2(Suppl):S73–80.

Phelps PD, Coffey RA, Trembath RC, et al. Radiological malformations of the ear in Pendred syndrome. Clinical Radiology 1998;53:268–73.

Smith RJH, Van Camp G. Deafness and Hereditary Hearing Loss Overview. In: Pagon RA, Bird TD, Dolan CR, et al., eds. GeneReviews™ [Internet]. Seattle: University of Washington. Available at http://www.geneclinics.org. Last updated January 30, 2007.

Steinberg, SJ, Raymond GV, Braverman, NE. Peroxisome biogenesis disorders, Zellweger syndrome spectrum. In: Pagon RA, Bird TD, Dolan CR, et al., eds. GeneReviews™ [Internet]. Seattle: University of Washington. Available at http://www.geneclinics.org. Last revision May 10, 2012.

Vanopdenbosch LJ, Verhoeven K, Casselman JW. Bell's palsy with ipsilateral numbness. Journal of Neurology, Neurosurgery and Psychiatry 2005;76:1017–8.

Villard L, Nguyen K, Cardoso C, et al. A locus for bilateral perisylvian polymicrogyria maps to Xq28. American Journal of Human Genetics 2002;70:1003–8.

CHAPTER 18

DISORDERS OF CRANIAL VOLUME AND SHAPE

The brain, cerebrospinal fluid (CSF), and blood are the three intracranial compartments that determine the size of the skull during infancy. Expansion of one compartment comes at the expense of another in order to maintain volume and pressure (see Chapter 4). The epidural, subdural, and subarachnoid spaces may expand with blood or CSF fluid and significantly affect cranial volume and the other intracranial compartments. Less important factors contributing to head size are the thickness of the skull bones and the rate of their fusion.

The intracranial content, the fusion of the sutures, and external forces on the skull determine its shape. Infants left supine all the time tend to develop flat occiputs. Premature infants resting on one side of the head all the time develop heads with large occipitofrontal diameter (dolichocephaly).

MEASURING HEAD SIZE

Head circumference is determined by measuring the greatest occipitofrontal circumference. Influencing the accuracy of the measurement is the head shape and fluid in and beneath the scalp. Following a prolonged and difficult delivery, edema or blood may thicken the scalp and a cephalohematoma may be present as well. Fluid that infiltrates from a scalp infusion can markedly increase head circumference.

A round head has a larger intracranial volume than an oval head of equal circumference. A head with a relatively large occipitofrontal diameter has a larger volume than a head with a relatively large biparietal diameter.

Head circumference measurements are most informative when plotted over time (head growth). The head sizes of male and female infants are different, and one should not rely on head growth charts that provide median values for both genders. The rate of head growth in premature infants is considerably faster than in full-term newborns (Figure 18-1). For this reason, the charting of head circumference is always by conceptional age and not by postnatal age.

MACROCEPHALY

Macrocephaly means a large head, larger than two standard deviations from the normal distribution. Thus, 2% of the "normal" population has macrocephaly. Investigation of such individuals may show an abnormality causing macrocephaly, but many are normal, often with a familial tendency for a large head. When asked to evaluate a large head in an otherwise normal child, first measure and plot the parents' heads.

The causes of a large head include hydrocephalus (an excessive volume of CSF intracranially), megalencephaly (enlargement of the brain), thickening of the skull, and hemorrhage into the subdural or epidural spaces. Hydrocephalus is traditionally communicating (nonobstructive) or noncommunicating (obstructive), depending on whether CSF communicates or not between the ventricles and subarachnoid space (Box 18-1). Hydrocephalus is the main cause of macrocephaly at birth in which intracranial pressure is increased.

The causes of megalencephaly are anatomical and metabolic. The anatomical disorders are primary megalencephaly and neurocutaneous disorders (Box 18-2). Children with anatomical megalencephaly are often macrocephalic at birth but have normal intracranial pressure. Children with metabolic megalencephaly are usually normocephalic at birth and develop megalencephaly from cerebral edema during the neonatal period.

Increased thickness of the skull bones does not cause macrocephaly at birth or in the newborn period. Macrocephaly develops during infancy. Box 18-3 lists the conditions associated with increased skull growth. The text does not contain a separate discussion. The discussion of intracranial hemorrhage in the newborn is in Chapter 1, and intracranial hemorrhage in older children is in Chapter 2.

Communicating Hydrocephalus

The usual cause of communicating hydrocephalus is impaired absorption of CSF secondary to meningitis or subarachnoid hemorrhage.

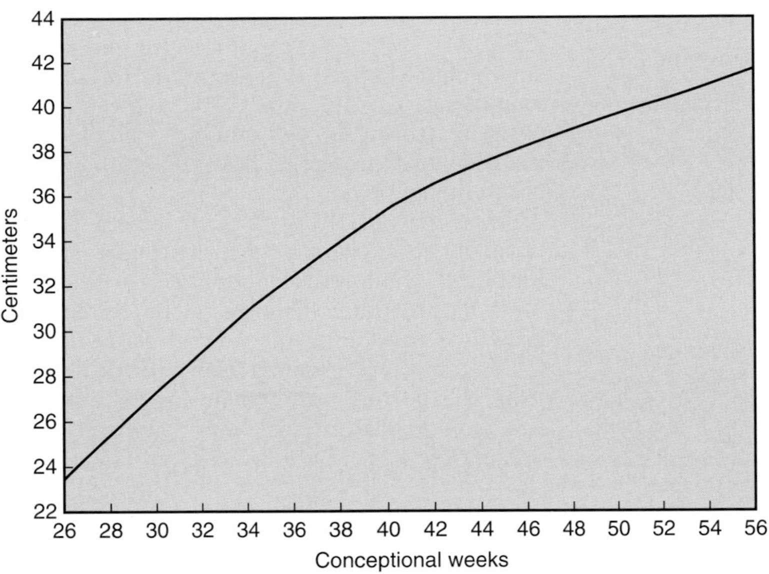

FIGURE 18-1 ■ Normal growth of head circumference in boys. The rate of growth in premature infants is greater than in full-term infants.

BOX 18-1 Causes of Hydrocephalus

COMMUNICATING

- Achondroplasia
- Basilar impression (see Chapter 10)
- Choroid plexus papilloma* (see Chapter 4)
- Meningeal malignancy
- Meningitis* (see Chapter 4)
- Posthemorrhagic (see Chapter 4)

NONCOMMUNICATING

- Abscess* (see Chapter 4)
- Aqueductal stenosis*
- Chiari malformation (see Chapter 10)
- Dandy-Walker malformation
- Hematoma* (see Chapters 1 and 2)
- Infectious*
- Klippel-Feil syndrome
- Mass lesions*
- Tumors and neurocutaneous disorders
- Vein of Galen malformation*
- Walker-Warburg syndrome
- X-linked

OTHER CAUSES OF INCREASED INTRACRANIAL CSF

- Benign enlargement of subarachnoid space
- Holoprosencephaly
- Hydranencephaly
- Porencephaly

*Denotes the most common conditions and the ones with disease modifying treatments

BOX 18-2 Causes of Megalencephaly

ANATOMICAL MEGALENCEPHALY

- Genetic megalencephaly
- Megalencephaly with achondroplasia
- Megalencephaly with gigantism (Sotos syndrome)
- Megalencephaly with a neurological abnormality
- Neurocutaneous disorders
  - Epidermal nevus syndrome
  - Hypomelanosis of Ito
  - Incontinentia pigmenti (see Chapter 1)
  - Neurofibromatosis (see Chapter 5)
  - Tuberous sclerosis (see Chapter 5)

METABOLIC MEGALENCEPHALY

- Alexander disease (see Chapter 5)
- Canavan disease (see Chapter 5)
- Galactosemia: transferase deficiency (see Chapter 5)
- Gangliosidosis (see Chapter 5)
- Globoid leukodystrophy (see Chapter 5)
- Glutaric aciduria type I (see Chapter 14)
- Maple syrup urine disease* (see Chapter 1)
- Megalencephalic leukoencephalopathy with subcortical cysts
- Metachromatic leukodystrophy (see Chapter 5)
- Mucopolysaccharidoses (see Chapter 5)

*Denotes the most common conditions and the ones with disease modifying treatments

Meningeal malignancy, usually by leukemia or primary brain tumor, is a less common cause. Any of these processes may cause arachnoiditis or arachnoid infiltration and decrease reabsorption of CSF by the arachnoid villi. The excessive production of CSF by a choroid plexus papilloma rarely causes communicating hydrocephalus because the potential rate of CSF reabsorption far exceeds the productive capacity of the choroid plexus (see Chapter 4). Such tumors more

BOX 18-3 Conditions with a Thickened Skull Causing Macrocephaly

Anemia*
Cleidocranial dysostosis
Craniometaphyseal dysplasia of Pyle
Epiphyseal dysplasia
Hyperphosphatemia
Leontiasis ossea
Orodigitofacial dysostosis
Osteogenesis imperfecta
Osteopetrosis
Pyknodysostosis
Rickets*
Russell dwarf

*Denotes the most common conditions and the ones with disease modifying treatments

commonly cause hydrocephalus by obstructing one or more ventricles.

Benign Enlargement of Subarachnoid Space

The terms used to describe benign enlargement of the subarachnoid space include external hydrocephalus, extraventricular hydrocephalus, benign subdural effusions, and benign extracerebral fluid collections. It is a relatively common cause of macrocephaly in infants, a fact not fully appreciated before the widespread use of computed tomography (CT) to investigate large head size. A genetic cause is likely in some cases, with the infant's father often having a large head.

Clinical Features. The condition occurs more commonly in males than females. A large head circumference is the only feature. An otherwise normal infant is brought to medical attention because serial head circumference measurements show an enlarging head size. The circumference is usually above the 90th percentile at birth, grows to exceed the 98th percentile, and then parallels the normal curve (Figure 18-2). The anterior fontanelle is large but soft. Neurological findings are normal, but motor development is often slower. Head control is one of the earliest achievements in motor development for an infant. Macrocephalic infants take longer to control their heads and this delays other milestones such as sitting and standing; however, the ultimate development is normal in these children.

Diagnosis. Cranial CT shows an enlarged frontal subarachnoid space, widening of the sylvian fissures and other sulci, and normal or minimally enlarged ventricular size (Figure 18-3). Normal ventricular size distinguishes this condition from cerebral atrophy. In infants, the upper limit of normal size for the frontal subarachnoid space is 5.7 mm and for the sylvian fissure 7.6 mm. The CT scan often is read as brain atrophy as the brain looks smaller than the container; however, both the brain and the cranium are large.

Management. Most affected infants develop normally and do not require ventricular shunts. Plot head circumference measurements monthly for 6 months after diagnosis to be certain that growth is paralleling the normal curve. Repeat CT is unnecessary unless head growth deviates from the normal curve, neurological examination is abnormal, or social and language development are slow.

Meningeal Malignancy

Tumors that infiltrate the meninges and subarachnoid space impair the reabsorption of CSF and cause communicating hydrocephalus. Meningeal spread usually occurs from a known primary tumor site. Diffuse meningeal gliomatosis is the exception where the initial feature may be hydrocephalus.

Clinical Features. Tumors that infiltrate the meninges are usually aggressive and cause rapid progression of symptoms. Headache and vomiting are the initial features and lethargy and personality change follow. Meningismus and papilledema are common features and may suggest bacterial meningitis. Multifocal neurological disturbances may be present.

Diagnosis. Magnetic resonance imaging (MRI) shows dilatation of the entire ventricular system but not of the subarachnoid space, which may appear obliterated except for a layer of enhancement. The pressure of the CSF and its protein concentration are increased. The glucose concentration may be depressed or normal. Tumor cell identification in the CSF is rarely successful and meningeal biopsy is usually required for tissue diagnosis.

Management. Ventricular shunt relieves symptoms of increased intracranial pressure. Radiation therapy and chemotherapy provide palliation and extend life in some cases, but the outcome is generally poor.

Noncommunicating Hydrocephalus

Complete obstruction of the flow of CSF from the ventricles to the subarachnoid space causes increased pressure and dilation of all ventricles proximal to the obstruction. The incidence of congenital hydrocephalus is 1 in 1500 live births. The best estimate is that 40 % of the cases of

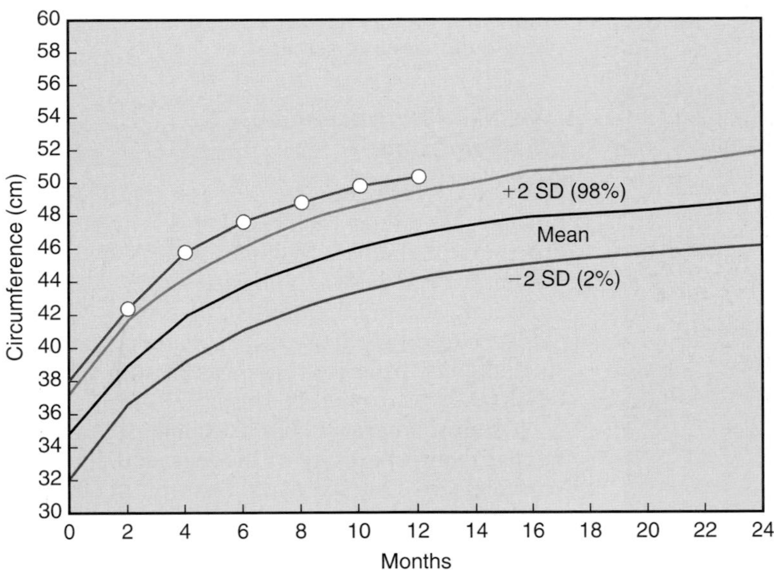

FIGURE 18-2 ■ Benign enlargement of the subarachnoid space. Head circumference is already large at birth, grows to exceed the 98th percentile, and then parallels the curve.

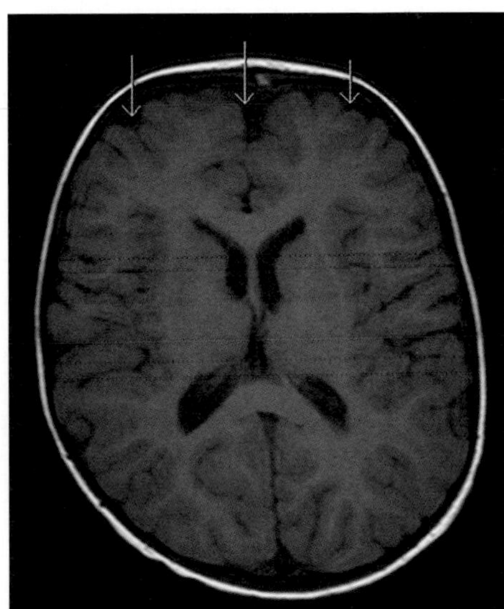

FIGURE 18-3 ■ Benign enlargement of the subarachnoid space. T_1 axial MRI showing enlargement of the subarachnoid space (arrows) in a child with macrocephaly and normal development.

congenital hydrocephalus have a genetic basis. X-linked hydrocephalus accounts for 5–15 % of all cases. The responsible gene is at Xq28 encoding for L1CAM. Other environmental factors that may lead to congenital hydrocephalus are exposure to radiation, alcohol or infections in utero (Zhang et al, 2006).

Noncommunicating hydrocephalus is the most common form of hydrocephalus in fetuses. Aqueductal stenosis is the usual cause of congenital hydrocephalus in the absence of other associated cerebral malformations. Aqueductal stenosis is less common during infancy but its frequency increases during childhood. Mass lesions are the most common cause of aqueductal obstruction during childhood. Children with congenital hydrocephalus who have seizures usually have other cerebral malformations. Such children have a higher incidence of cognitive impairment.

Congenital Aqueductal Stenosis

At birth, the mean length of the cerebral aqueduct is 12.8 mm and its smallest cross-sectional diameter is usually 0.5 mm. The small lumen of the cerebral aqueduct, in relation to its length, makes it especially vulnerable to internal compromise from infection and hemorrhage, and to external compression by tumors and venous malformations. Congenital atresia or stenosis of the cerebral aqueduct can occur as a solitary malformation or can occur as part of a spectrum of abnormalities associated with the *L1 syndrome* described below.

Clinical Features. Hydrocephalus is present at birth. Head circumference ranges from 40–50 cm and may cause cephalopelvic disproportion and poor progress of labor requiring cesarean section. The forehead is bowed, the scalp veins dilated, the skull sutures widely separated, and the fontanelles large and tense. These signs exaggerate when the child cries but also are present in the quiet state. The eyes are deviated downward so that the sclera shows above the iris (*setting-sun sign*), and abducens palsies may be present.

Diagnosis. Intrauterine sonography is diagnostic after 20 weeks when the ventricles expand. Sonograms performed earlier are misleading. When macrocephaly is present in the fetus, amniotic fluid assay of α-fetoprotein is useful for

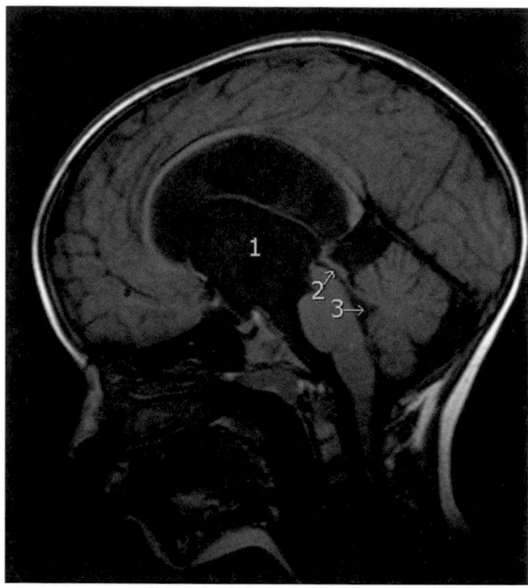

FIGURE 18-4 ■ Aqueduct stenosis. T_1 sagittal MRI shows (1) dilated third ventricle; (2) stenosis of aqueduct; and (3) normal size fourth ventricle.

the detection of neural tube defects (see Chapter 12). Chromosomal analysis provides further information concerning the integrity of the fetal nervous system to develop a management plan.

CT readily provides the postpartum diagnosis of aqueductal stenosis. Marked enlargement of the lateral ventricle, the third ventricle, and the cephalic end of the cerebral aqueduct is easily visualized. The remainder of the cerebral aqueduct and the fourth ventricle cannot be seen (Figure 18-4).

Management. Congenital hydrocephalus caused by aqueductal stenosis is severe, does not respond to medical therapy directed at decreasing the volume of CSF, and progresses to a stage that harms the brain. Diversion of the CSF from the ventricular system to an extracranial site is the only effective method of management.

The management of fetal hydrocephalus depends on the presence of other malformations. Three-quarters of affected fetuses have other abnormalities, usually spina bifida.

Ventriculoperitoneal shunt is the procedure of choice for newborns and small infants with aqueductal stenosis. It is easier to revise and is better tolerated than ventriculoatrial shunt. Mechanical obstruction and infection are the most common complications of shunt placement in infancy (see Chapter 4).

The relief of hydrocephalus increases the potential for normal development, even when the cerebral mantle appears very thin preoperatively, but does not necessarily result in a normal child. The growth of intelligence is often uneven, with better development of verbal skills than of nonverbal skills. Associated anomalies may cause motor deficits and seizures.

X-Linked Hydrocephalus (L1 Syndrome)

The L1 syndrome encompasses HSAS syndrome (X-linked hydrocephalus with stenosis of the aqueduct of Sylvius), MASA syndrome (mental retardation, aphasia, spastic paraplegia, and adducted thumbs), X-linked complicated hereditary spastic paraplegia type 1, and X-linked complicated corpus callosum agenesis (Schrander-Stumpel & Vos, 2010).

Clinical Features. Hydrocephalus, cognitive impairment, spasticity of the legs, and adducted thumbs are characteristic features in affected males. The spectrum of severity is wide depending on the nature of the mutation. Mental retardation ranges from mild to severe, and the gait abnormality from shuffling gait to spastic paraplegia. Adducted thumbs are characteristic of several phenotypes.

Diagnosis. Molecular genetic testing is commercially available.

Management. Most affected infants require early ventriculoperitoneal shunt placement.

Dandy-Walker Malformation

The Dandy-Walker malformation consists of a ballooning of the posterior half of the fourth ventricle, often associated with failure of the foramen of Magendie to open, aplasia of the posterior cerebellar vermis, heterotopia of the inferior olivary nuclei, pachygyria of the cerebral cortex, and other cerebral and sometimes visceral anomalies. Hydrocephalus may not be present at birth but develops during childhood or later. The size of the lateral ventricles does not correlate with the size of the cyst in the fourth ventricle. Other malformations are present in two-thirds of children. The most common associated malformation is agenesis of the corpus callosum. Other malformations are heterotopia, abnormal gyrus formation, dysraphic states, aqueductal stenosis, and congenital tumors.

The responsible gene is on chromosome 3, but the mode of inheritance is uncertain (Grinberg et al, 2004).

Clinical Features. Diagnosis at birth occurs in only a quarter of affected newborns and in three-quarters by 1 year of age. Macrocephaly is the usual initial feature. Bulging of the skull, when present, is more prominent in the occipital than in the frontal region. The speed of head growth is considerably slower than with aqueductal stenosis. Compression of posterior fossa structures

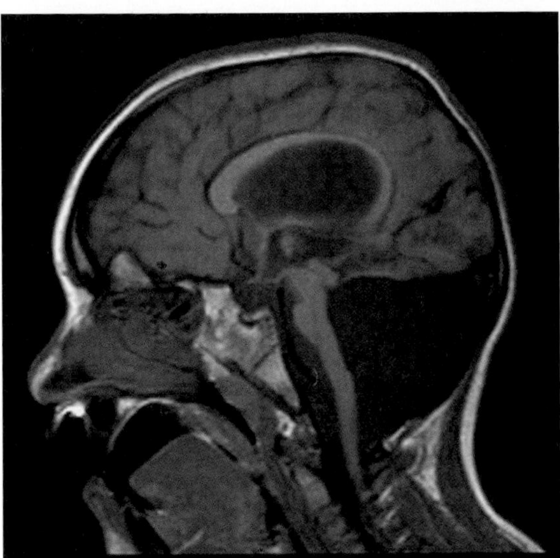

FIGURE 18-5 ■ Dandy-Walker syndrome. T_1 sagittal MRI shows a large cystic area in the posterior fossa with narrowing and elongation of the brainstem.

leads to neurological dysfunction, including apneic spells, nystagmus, truncal ataxia, cranial nerve palsies, and hyperreflexia in the legs.

Diagnosis. Macrocephaly or ataxia is the indication for CT or MRI. Both studies show cystic dilatation of the posterior fossa and partial or complete agenesis of the cerebellar vermis (Figure 18-5). MRI is more useful because it also identifies other cerebral abnormalities such as heterotopia. Incomplete vermian agenesis may be difficult to differentiate from an enlarged cisterna magna. The Dandy-Walker malformation is part of the spectrum of anomalies associated with trisomy 9 and with mutations on the X chromosome.

Management. Decompression of the cyst alone provides immediate relief of symptoms; however, hydrocephalus recurs and ventricular shunting is required in two–thirds of affected children. Shunting of the lateral ventricle alone provides immediate relief of hydrocephalus but fails to relieve brainstem compression. The procedure of choice is a dural shunt of both the lateral ventricle and the posterior fossa cyst.

Even after successful shunt placement, many children have transitory episodes of lethargy, personality change, and vomiting that falsely suggest shunt failure. The mechanism of such episodes, which may prove fatal, is unknown.

Klippel-Feil Syndrome

Klippel-Feil syndrome is a malformation of the craniocervical skeleton that may be associated with the Chiari malformation and with basilar impression. It involves the congenital fusion of at least two cervical vertebrae. The incidence is about 1 in 40 000–42 000 live births. Obstruction of the flow of CSF from the fourth ventricle to the subarachnoid space causes hydrocephalus. Several different entities comprise the syndrome. One or more are recessive, one is dominant, and some may have no genetic basis. There are three types of Klippel-Feil syndrome: type I is the single fusion of two cervical vertebrae; type II is the fusion of multiple non-contiguous cervical vertebrae; and type III is the fusion of multiple contiguous cervical vertebrae. Scoliosis occurs in about 50 % of the cases and occurs more often with involvement of the lower cervical vertebrae, with multiple fusions, and with hemivertebrae (Samartiz et al, 2011).

Clinical Features. The essential features of the Klippel-Feil syndrome are a low posterior hairline, a short neck, and limitation of neck movement. Head asymmetry, facial asymmetry, scoliosis, and mirror movements of the hands are common. Unilateral or bilateral failure of downward migration of the scapula (*Sprengel deformity*) is present in 25–35 % of patients. Malformations of the genitourinary system and deafness are associated features. The deafness may be of the sensorineural, conductive, or mixed type. Hydrocephalus affects the fourth ventricle first and then the lateral ventricles. The resulting symptoms are those of posterior fossa compression: ataxia, apnea, and cranial nerve dysfunction.

Diagnosis. Radiographs of the spine reveal the characteristic fusion and malformations of vertebrae. MRI may show an associated Chiari malformation and dilatation of the ventricles.

Management. Children with unstable cervical vertebrae require cervical fusion to prevent myelopathy. Those with symptoms of obstructive hydrocephalus require a ventriculoperitoneal shunt to relieve pressure in the posterior fossa.

Congenital Brain Tumors

Congenital brain tumors and congenital brain malformations are both disorders of cellular proliferation. A noxious agent active during early embryogenesis might stimulate either or both abnormalities. The relative oncogenicity or teratogenicity depends on the virulence of the agent, the timing of the insult, the duration of exposure, and the genetic background and health of the fetus. The most common tumors of infancy are astrocytoma, medulloblastoma, teratoma, and choroid plexus papilloma.

Clinical Features. Congenital tumors are more often supratentorial than infratentorial and more often in the midline than situated laterally. Newborns with hemispheric gliomas and teratomas may develop hydrocephalus in utero or in the first days or weeks postpartum. The point of obstruction is usually at the cerebral aqueduct (see Chapter 4). Choroid plexus papillomas are usually located in one lateral ventricle and become symptomatic during infancy rather than in the perinatal period. They produce hydrocephalus either by obstruction of the foramen of Monro or less likely by excessive production of CSF (see Chapter 4). Medulloblastomas are located in the posterior fossa and obstruct the fourth ventricle and cerebral aqueduct (see Chapter 10).

The clinical features of all congenital tumors are those of increasing intracranial pressure: enlarging head size, separation of the sutures, lethargy, irritability, difficult feeding, and vomiting. Seizures are unusual. Because of its posterior fossa location, medulloblastoma also produces nystagmus, downward deviation of the eyes, opisthotonus, and apnea.

Diagnosis. CT or MRI, performed to investigate hydrocephalus, readily visualizes all congenital tumors. Intrauterine sonography identifies some tumors.

Management. Complete resection of congenital brain tumors is unusual, with the exception of choroid plexus papilloma. Discussion of individual tumor management is in Chapters 4 and 10.

Vein of Galen Malformation

Arteriovenous malformations of the cerebral circulation may become symptomatic during infancy and childhood (see Chapters 4 and 10), but the malformation associated with congenital hydrocephalus is the vein of Galen malformation. Vein of Galen vascular malformations are not aneurysms and do not involve the vein of Galen. Instead, the normal vein of Galen does not develop and the median prosencephalic vein of Markowsky persists, dilates, and drains to the superior sagittal sinus. Multiple arteriovenous fistulas are associated.

Clinical Features. Eighty percent of newborns with vein of Galen malformations are male. The usual initial feature is either high-output cardiac failure or an enlarging head size. Hemorrhage almost never occurs early in the course. A cranial bruit is invariably present. Some affected children experience unexplained persistent hypoglycemia.

Large midline arteriovenous malformations produce a hemodynamic stress in the newborn because of the large quantities of blood shunted from the arterial to the venous system. The heart enlarges in an effort to keep up with the demands of the shunt, but high-output cardiac failure ensues. Affected newborns often come first to the attention of a pediatric cardiologist because of the suspicion of congenital heart disease. Then, the initial diagnosis of an intracranial malformation is during cardiac catheterization.

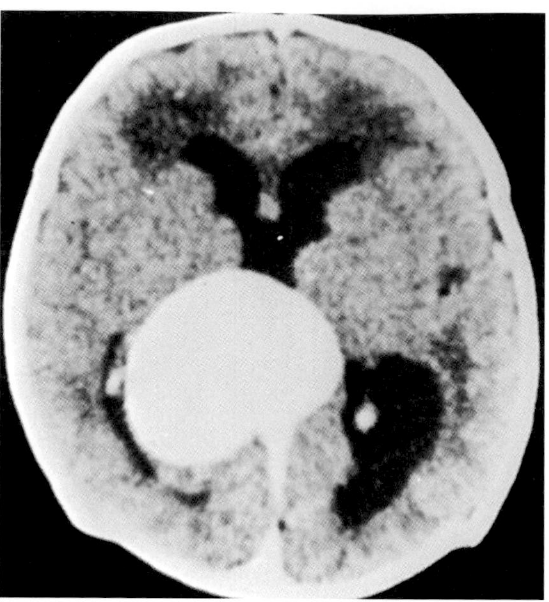

FIGURE 18-6 ■ Vein of Galen malformation. The malformation is visible on contrast-enhanced CT as a large aneurysmal sac compressing the midbrain and producing obstructive hydrocephalus.

When the hemodynamic stress is not severe and cardiac compensation is possible, the initial symptoms are in infancy or early childhood. In such a case, obstructive hydrocephalus results from compression of the tegmentum and aqueduct. Symptoms usually begin before age 5 and always before age 10. The lateral ventricles enlarge, causing headache, lethargy, and vomiting. In infants, the head enlarges and the fontanelle feels full.

Diagnosis. Contrast-enhanced CT (Figure 18-6) or MRI readily visualizes the vein of Galen malformation. The lateral and third ventricles dilate behind the compressed cerebral aqueduct. Radiographs of the chest in newborns with high-output cardiac failure show an enlarged heart with a normal shape.

Management. The overall results of direct surgical approaches are poor; the mortality rate is high, as is neurological morbidity in survivors. Embolization has become the treatment of choice, but the long-term results are not established.

Walker-Warburg Syndrome

Walker-Warburg syndrome (WWS) is caused by mutation in the genes encoding protein O-mannosyltransferase-1 (POMT1) and -2 (POMT2). In addition, a phenotype consistent with WWS occurs with mutation in the fukutin gene (*FKTN*), the same gene causing Fukuyama congenital muscular dystrophy (see Chapter 6). This is a rare disease and the incidence is about 1 in 100 000.

WWS is an autosomal recessive muscular dystrophy associated with lissencephaly type II and ocular abnormalities. Hydrocephalus is a constant feature. The syndrome, also known as the *HARD ± E* syndrome, consists of hydrocephalus (H), agyria (A), and retinal dysplasia (RD), with or without encephalocele (+/-E). The condition is usually lethal within the first few months of life.

Clinical Features. Hydrocephalus is usually present at birth. The cause may be aqueductal stenosis or the Dandy-Walker malformation. Most children with both a Dandy-Walker malformation and ocular abnormalities have the WWS. Some children are born with microcephaly yet have enlarged ventricles. Severe neurological abnormalities are caused by partial or total agyria (lissencephaly) resulting from failure of neuronal migration. The pattern of architectural abnormalities throughout the neuraxis suggests a disruption of cerebral maturation in the fourth conceptional month.

Several ocular abnormalities may be present, usually in combination: hypoplasia of the iris, abnormal anterior chamber, microphthalmos, cataracts, persistence of primary vitreous, optic disk coloboma, retinal detachment, retinal dysplasia, hypoplasia of the optic nerve, glaucoma or buphthalmos. In addition to having hydrocephalus and blindness, affected infants are hypotonic and have difficulty feeding. Seizures are uncommon. Most affected children die during the neonatal period or early infancy.

Diagnosis. The basis for diagnosis is the characteristic combination of cerebral and ocular abnormalities. Congenital infections may produce similar disturbances, but multisystem disease (visceromegaly and disturbed hematopoesis), an expected feature of most intrauterine infections, is lacking in the Warburg syndrome.

Cerebro-ocular abnormalities at birth are also encountered in septo-optic dysplasia (see Chapter 16) and the oculocerebrorenal syndrome (see Chapter 6), but hydrocephalus is not a component of either syndrome.

Management. The management of hydrocephalus is by ventricular shunt, but the outcome is poor because of the concomitant severe cerebral malformations.

Hydranencephaly

The term hydranencephaly encompasses several conditions that result in the extensive replacement of brain by CSF. The cause of hydranencephaly may be failure of normal brain development or an intrauterine disorder that destroys the brain parenchyma. Progressive obstructive hydrocephalus, if left untreated, may cause a clinical picture very similar to hydranencephaly. Excessive pressure within the lateral ventricles destroys the midline structures and reduces the cerebral mantle to a thin membrane. However, pure hydrancencephaly lacks any cerebral mantle.

Head circumference at birth is large in cases of severe hydrocephalus. Hydranencephaly is associated with microcephaly when the condition is due to intrauterine diseases, and may be associated with any head size when caused by primary malformations.

Porencephaly

Porencephaly is a term used loosely in the literature. Originally, the term described hemispheric cysts that communicated with both the subarachnoid space and the lateral ventricle secondary to defects in the final stages of prosencephalization. The present use of the term is broader and includes any hemispheric cyst; the usual causes are intrauterine or perinatal infarction or trauma. The injured immature brain loses neurons, glia, and supporting structures. A fluid-filled cyst is formed in the injured area and may not communicate with either the ventricular system or the subarachnoid space. Pressure within the cyst often becomes excessive, causing compression of adjacent structures and macrocrania.

Congenital Midline Porencephaly. Congenital midline porencephaly is a distinct malformation characterized by congenital hydrocephalus, alopecia, or encephalocele in the parietal midline, and a midline defect in the posterior cerebral mantle. Midline porencephaly differs from holoprosencephaly, because the forebrain divides into two separate hemispheres. The cause may be early hydrocephalus with upward outpouching and destruction of adjacent structures, including the corpus callosum, cerebral mantle, skull, and scalp. The syndromes of giant interhemispheric cyst and dygenesis of the corpus callosum are probably the same (Griebel et al, 1995).

Clinical Features. The head is large in utero and may cause cephalopelvic disproportion at delivery. Possible defects in the parietal midline range from a small, round area of alopecia to an encephalocele. Affected children are severely retarded and blind. Most die during infancy or early childhood.

Diagnosis. CT or MRI shows a large dorsal cyst that has destroyed the septum pellucidum and corpus callosum. The cyst communicates with enlarged lateral ventricles and extends through a skull defect to produce an encephalocele.

Management. Shunting the cyst may ease care by reducing the size of the head or encephalocele, but it does not prevent severe neurological impairment from the underlying cerebral malformation.

Anatomical Megalencephaly

Anatomical megalencephaly includes conditions in which the brain enlarges because the number or size of cells increases in the absence of a metabolic disease or an acute encephalopathy.

Achondroplasia

Achondroplasia is a genetic disorder, transmitted as an autosomal dominant trait (4p16.3). New mutations account for more than 80 % of cases. It is the most frequent form of short-limbed dwarfism (Pauli, 2012).

Clinical Features. The main features are short stature caused by rhizomelic shortening of the limbs (the proximal portion of the limbs is shorter than the distal portion), large head with frontal bossing and midface hypoplasia, lumbar lordosis, and limitation of elbow extension. Stunted formation of enchondral bone causes the typical recessed facial appearance.

Affected newborns have true megalencephaly. Increased intracranial pressure occurs at times secondary to stenosis of the sigmoid sinus at the level of the jugular foramina. Despite considerable, and sometimes alarming, enlargement of head circumference, achondroplastic dwarfs seldom show clinical evidence of increased intracranial pressure or progressive dementia. Respiratory disturbances are common. Dyspnea may result from cervicomedullary compression. Other features of cervicomedullary compression are hyperreflexia, spasticity, and sensory disturbances of the limbs.

Diagnosis. Clinical examination and radiological features establish the diagnosis. Accurate molecular diagnosis is available. CT shows a small posterior fossa and enlargement of the sphenoid sinuses. Basilar impression is sometimes present. Ventricular size varies from normal in newborns and young infants to moderate or severe dilatation in older children and adults.

Management. Ventricular size, after initial dilatation, usually remains stable and rarely is surgical diversion of CSF needed. Decompressive surgery is required in children with evidence of progressive cervicomedullary compromise.

Benign Familial Macrocephaly

Clinical Features. The term describes a familial condition in which neurological and mental function is normal but head circumference is larger than the 98th percentile. The suspected mechanism of transmission is autosomal dominant inheritance, but the genetic basis for nonsyndromic macrocephaly is probably multifactorial, with a polymorphic genetic basis. Head circumference may not be large at birth but increases during infancy, usually to between 2 cm and 4 cm above the 98th percentile. Body size is normal, and no physical deformities are present.

Diagnosis. The enlargement is indistinguishable by physical examination from benign enlargement of the subarachnoid space, but CT distinguishes the two. CT is normal in benign familial macrocephaly.

Management. Treatment is not required.

Megalencephaly with a Neurological Disorder

The term megalencephaly with a neurological disorder encompasses all disorders, other than neurocutaneous syndromes, in which the head is large and the child is neurologically abnormal.

Clinical Features. Head circumference may be large at birth or may become large during infancy. It is generally 2–4 cm greater than the 98th percentile. Results of neurological tests are normal, but the children have learning disabilities, mental deficiency, or seizures. Neurological status remains stable.

Diagnosis. Excluding the possibility of a neurocutaneous disorder requires careful examination of the skin and retina of other family members. Results of CT or MRI may be normal or may show mild dilatation of the ventricular system. Agenesis of the corpus callosum is the only abnormality found in some families with macrocrania and borderline intelligence.

Management. Seizures often respond to anticonvulsant drugs. Special education is usually required. Treatment is not available for the underlying disorder.

Megalencephaly with Gigantism

Megalencephaly with gigantism, termed *cerebral gigantism* or *Sotos syndrome* (Tatton-Brown et al, 2012), probably encompasses several disorders; most are sporadic and some clearly genetic, transmitted by autosomal dominant inheritance (5q35). Chromosome studies are usually normal. Some show a translocation.

Clinical Features. Affected children are in the 75th to 90th percentile at birth and grow at an excessive rate in height, weight, head circumference, and bone age up to the age of 3. Afterward, the rate of growth is normal. A prominent forehead, high-arched palate, and hypertelorism are present in almost every case. Small numbers of other patients may have other dysmorphic features. Many have mild learning problems that are less apparent as they become adults. All children with the syndrome are large as adults, but not gigantic. Indeed, many appear normal as adults.

Diagnosis. Cranial CT is usually normal except for mild ventricular widening. Extensive studies of endocrine function have failed to show a consistent abnormality other than glucose intolerance. Plasma somatomedin levels are elevated during the first year in some infants and fall below normal during early childhood.

Management. Treatment is neither available nor required.

Neurocutaneous Disorders

Neurocutaneous syndromes are often associated with seizures (see Box 1-8) and cognitive impairment (see Chapter 5). The skin manifestations may be present at birth (incontinentia pigmenti) or during infancy (neurofibromatosis, tuberous sclerosis). The cause of macrocephaly is either hydrocephalus or megalencephaly. Hemimegalencephaly, hemihypertrophy of the body, or hypertrophy of a single limb should always suggest the possibility of a neurocutaneous disorder.

Hypomelanosis of Ito. Hypomelanosis of Ito, also called *incontinentia pigmenti achromians*, does not represent a distinct entity but rather a symptom of many different states of mosaicism. Most cases are sporadic, and several different chromosomal anomalies are associated. The X chromosome often is involved.

Clinical Features. The cutaneous feature is a large, hypopigmented area that has a whorled or streaked appearance. It appears in the first year and is a negative image of the hyperpigmented lesions of incontinentia pigmenti (see Chapter 1). Other cutaneous features are café au lait spots, angiomatous nevi, heterochromia of the iris or hair, and other nevi. Seizures and cognitive impairment are the most common neurological abnormalities. IQ scores are below 70 in more than half of patients, but approximately 20% have IQ scores above 90. Approximately half of patients have seizures, usually with onset in the first year. Focal seizures are most common, although occasional patients have infantile spasms and epilepsies refractory to treatment evolving into the spectrum of epileptic encephalopathy/Lennox-Gastaut syndrome. Spastic diplegia may also be present. Disturbances of neuronal migration cause these symptoms. Megalencephaly occurs in approximately 25% of cases.

One-third of patients have skeletal and eye anomalies, including limb hypertrophy or atrophy, facial hemiatrophy, poorly formed ears, dysplastic teeth, hypertelorism, strabismus, and corneal opacities.

Diagnosis. The characteristic skin lesions are critical to the diagnosis, and all family members, as well as the child, require careful examination. Chromosome studies may be useful in the child and parents. MRI usually shows generalized cerebral or cerebellar hypoplasia, severe cortical neuronal migration anomalies, and hemimegalencephaly and lissencephaly. Hemimegalencephaly may be ipsilateral or contralateral to the cutaneous hypopigmentation.

Management. Treatment is symptom directed. Special education and anticonvulsants are often necessary.

Epidermal Nevus Syndrome. Epidermal nevus syndrome, also called the linear nevus sebaceous syndrome, refers to several disorders that have in common an epidermal nevus and neurological manifestations such as seizures or hemimegalencephaly.

Clinical Features. A unilateral linear nevus is present on the skin of the face or scalp. It may not be visible at birth but darkens during infancy and becomes verrucous. Hemihypertrophy of the face, head, and limbs ipsilateral to the nevus may be present at birth or may develop during infancy.

The spectrum of neurological disability is considerable. Developmental delay and seizures are expected. Head enlargement may be generalized or unilateral. Focal neurological deficits, such as hemiplegia and hemianopia, contralateral to the nevus are relatively common. Eye abnormalities, such as microphthalmia and coloboma, occur in one-third of children.

Diagnosis. Diagnosis relies on recognition of the linear nevus. Electroencephalography (EEG) usually shows unilateral slowing and epileptiform discharges ipsilateral to the nevus. EEG shows hypsarrhythmia when infantile spasms are the initial feature (see Chapter 1). Hemihypsarrhythmia may also occur.

Megalencephaly ipsilateral to the epidermal nevus is the most frequent finding on MRI. Several types of cerebral dysplasia may be associated, usually ipsilateral to the epidermal nevus. Focal pachygyria is the most common.

Management. Seizures may respond to standard anticonvulsant therapy (see Chapter 1), but treatment is not available for the underlying cerebral malformation.

Metabolic Megalencephaly

Several inborn errors of metabolism produce megalencephaly by storage of abnormal substances or by producing cerebral edema (see Box 18-2). Their discussion is elsewhere in the text because the initial features are usually developmental regression (see Chapter 5) or seizures (see Chapter 1). Two exceptions are glutaric aciduria type I (see Chapter 14) and metabolic leukoencephalopathy with subcortical cysts. Infants with glutaric aciduria type I are normal up to 3 years, except for macrocephaly, and then develop an acute encephalitic illness that resembles encephalitis. Most infants with metabolic megalencephaly have a normal head circumference at birth. Head enlargement parallels neurological regression and clinical evidence of increased intracranial pressure. The ventricles are often small.

Megalencephalic Leukoencephalopathy with Subcortical Cysts (MLC)

The metabolic defect in MLC is unknown, but the presence of affected sibling pairs and instances of parental consanguinity establish autosomal recessive inheritance (van der Knaap & Scheper, 2011).

Clinical Features. Early-onset macrocephaly combined with mild developmental delay and seizures are characteristic. The gradual development of ataxia and spasticity follow. Extrapyramidal findings may develop and mild mental deterioration occurs late in life. The degree of macrocephaly is variable and can be as much as 4–6 standard deviations above the mean in some individuals. After the first year of life, head growth rate normalizes and growth follows a line several centimeters above the 98th percentile. Mental deterioration is late and mild. Motor impairment ranges from independent walking only during early childhood to independent walking in the fifth decade. Some individuals have died in their teens or twenties; others are alive in their forties.

Diagnosis. MRI shows a severe leukoencephalopathy that suggests a demyelinating white matter disorder. The hemispheres appear swollen, with cyst-like spaces in the frontoparietal and anterior temporal areas, but with relative sparing of the occipital white matter. Sequence analysis, available commercially, reveals mutations in *MLC1* in approximately 60–70% of affected individuals.

Management. Treatment is symptomatic.

MICROCEPHALY

Microcephaly means a head circumference that is smaller than two standard deviations below the normal distribution. The standard for head circumference varies among different ethnic groups. A small head circumference indicates a small brain. Most full-term newborns whose head circumferences are smaller than two standard deviations, but who are neurologically normal, will have normal intelligence at age 7 years, but a head circumference smaller than three standard deviations usually indicates later cognitive impairment.

A small head circumference at birth suggests a prenatal brain insult, but does not distinguish primary from secondary microcephaly (Box 18-4). Primary microcephaly encompasses conditions in which the brain is small and has never formed properly because of genetic or chromosomal abnormalities. Secondary microcephaly implies that the brain was forming normally but a disease process impaired further growth. Normal head circumference at birth, followed by failure of normal head growth, usually indicates a secondary microcephaly. Chromosomal disorders are an exception to that rule unless they cause defective prosencephalization or cellular migration.

Perinatal brain insult does not cause a recognizable decrease of head circumference until 3 to 6 months postpartum. Failure of normal brain growth removes the force keeping the cranial bones separated, and they fuse prematurely. A primary disorder of the skull (craniostenosis) may cause premature closure of the cranial sutures even though the brain is attempting to grow normally. The distinction between the two is relatively simple: craniostenosis is always associated with an abnormal skull shape and heaping up of bone along the cranial sutures; failure of brain growth produces a relatively normal-shaped skull with some overlapping of skull bones.

Cranial MRI may be informative in distinguishing primary from secondary microcephaly. In most children with primary microcephaly, either MRI results are normal or a recognizable pattern of cerebral malformation is present. In those with secondary microcephaly, the brain

BOX 18-4 Conditions Causing Microcephaly

PRIMARY MICROCEPHALY
- Chromosomal disorders
- Defective neurulation
  - Anencephaly
  - Encephalocele
- Defective prosencephalization
  - Agenesis of the corpus callosum
  - Holoprosencephaly (arhinencephaly)
- Defective cellular migration
- Microcephaly vera (genetic)

SECONDARY MICROCEPHALY
- Intrauterine disorders
  - Infection
  - Toxins
  - Vascular
- Perinatal brain injuries
  - Hypoxic-ischemic encephalopathy*
  - Intracranial hemorrhage
  - Meningitis and encephalitis*
  - Stroke
- Postnatal systemic diseases
  - Chronic cardiopulmonary disease
  - Chronic renal disease
  - Malnutrition

*Denotes the most common conditions and the ones with disease modifying treatments

image is usually abnormal, characterized by one or more of the following features: ventricular enlargement, cerebral atrophy, and porencephaly.

Primary Microcephaly

Many cerebral malformations are of uncertain cause, and classification as primary or secondary is not possible. Morphogenetic errors, although lacking in the traditional stigmata of tissue injury, could result from exposure of the embryo to a noxious agent during the first weeks after conception. At this early stage, disorganization of the delicate sequencing of neuronal development could occur when the brain is incapable of generating a cellular response.

Microcephaly Vera (Genetic)

The term microcephaly vera encompasses genetic defects that decrease bulk growth of the brain. Transmission of the defect is as an autosomal recessive trait. Chromosomes 8, 15, and 19 have identifiable gene loci responsible for primary microcephaly in different families.

Clinical Features. Children with microcephaly vera are usually short and have a characteristic disproportion in size between the face and the skull. The forehead slants backward, and the reduced size of the skull causes the scalp to wrinkle in the occipital region. The chin is small, and the ears and nose are prominent. Cognitive impairment is moderate to severe, and other neurological abnormalities, such as spastic diplegia and seizures, may be present.

Diagnosis. Results of brain imaging are normal other than the size.

Management. Treatment is symptomatic.

Chromosomal Disorders

Chromosomal disorders are not usually a cause of microcephaly at birth unless cerebral aplasia, such as holoprosencephaly, is part of the syndrome. Hypotonia and dysmorphism are the prominent features of chromosomal disorders in the newborn (see Chapter 5), and microcephaly becomes evident during infancy.

Defective Neurulation

At the end of the first week, a rostrocaudal axis appears on the dorsal aspect of the embryo. This axis is responsible for the subsequent induction of a neural plate, the anlage of the nervous system. The neural plate changes into a closed neural tube during the third and fourth weeks. Defects in closure are *dysraphic states*. The most rostral portion of the neural tube, the anterior neuropore, closes at about the 24th day.

Anencephaly

Anencephaly is the result of defective closure of the anterior neuropore and myelomeningocele is the result of defective closure of the posterior neuropore (see Chapter 12). The rate of each is declining. Folic acid supplementation from 400 micrograms to 4 milligrams a day has reduced the incidence of spinal dysraphism.

Clinical Features. Less than half of anencephalic children are born alive, and those who are rarely survive the first month. The scalp is absent, and the skull is open from the vertex to the foramen magnum. The exposed brain appears hemorrhagic and fibrotic. It consists mainly of the hindbrain and parts of the diencephalon; the forebrain is completely lacking. The orbits are shallow, and the eyes protrude. The neck is in retroflexion, and the proximal portions of the arms seem overgrown compared with the legs. The overall appearance of the anencephalic newborn is grotesque.

Diagnosis. Following the birth of a child with a neural tube defect, the chance of anencephaly or myelomeningocele in subsequent pregnancies increases 2-fold to 5-fold. After two affected children have been born, the chance of having another affected child doubles again. The section on myelomeningocele (Chapter 12) contains the discussion of prenatal diagnosis of dysraphic states.

Management. Support to the family. Do not recommend interventions that prolong life.

Encephalocele

An encephalocele is a protrusion of brain and meninges, covered by skin, through a defect in the skull. An encephalocele may occur in any location; however, most are midline-occipital, except in Asians, in whom the defects are usually midline-frontal.

Clinical Features. The size of the encephalocele may range from a small protrusion to a cyst as big as the skull. When the protrusion is large, the skull is likely to be microcephalic. The size of the mass does not predict its contents, but an encephalocele with a sessile base is more likely to contain cerebral tissue than is one with a pedunculated base. Encephaloceles rarely occur as a solitary cerebral malformation and are usually associated with abnormalities of the cerebral hemispheres, cerebellum, and midbrain.

Diagnosis. Head MRI is reasonably accurate in defining the contents of the encephalocele. Despite its midline location, the derivation of the protruded material is usually from the one hemisphere that is smaller than the other is and displaced across the midline by the larger hemisphere.

Management. The surgical treatment of meningoceles has an excellent prognosis as the protrusion includes only meninges and CSF. The prognosis for surgical resection of encephalocele depends on the size and the location of the protruding brain. The extent of comorbid malformations should also influence any decision to remove the encephalocele surgically. Children with protruded brain material and associated malformations usually die during infancy.

Defective Prosencephalization

The forebrain develops between 25 and 30 days' gestation from a midline vesicle generated from the closed anterior neuropore. Between 30 and 40 days' gestation, bilateral cerebral vesicles are formed by the cleavage and outpouching of the midline vesicle. The midline vesicle is the primordium of the third ventricle, and the bilateral cerebral vesicles are the primordia of the lateral ventricles.

Holoprosencephaly

Defective cleavage of the embryonic forebrain leads to a spectrum of malformations. Use of the term arhinencephaly to refer to the full spectrum of abnormalities is common, but holoprosencephaly (HPE) is a more accurate term.

Total failure of cleavage produces a small brain with a midline vesicle covered by a horseshoe of limbic cortex. With less severe defects, the third ventricle and diencephalon differentiate, and partial cleavage of the occipital hemispheres occurs. The corpus callosum is hypoplastic or absent. The minimal defect (arhinencephaly) is the unilateral or bilateral absence of the olfactory bulbs and tracts associated with some degree of rhinic lobe aplasia. Hemispheric cleavage is complete, the ventricles are normal, and the corpus callosum is present in part or in total.

Almost half of patients with HPE have an abnormal numerical or structural chromosomal abnormality. Less than a quarter of children with monogenic HPE have a recognizable syndrome and the remainder have nonsyndromic HPE (Solomon et al, 2011). An autosomal dominant form maps to the chromosome 7p36.2 locus, and a defect at the same locus results in sacral agenesis. Abnormalities of chromosome 13 account for most chromosomal abnormalities that cause HPE.

Clinical Features. Craniofacial dysplasia is usually associated, and malformations in other organs are common. The facial deformities are primarily in the midline (cyclopia or ocular hypotelorism, flat nose, cleft lip, and cleft palate), and their severity is often predictive of the severity of the brain malformation. Associated malformations include congenital heart defects, clubbing of the hands or feet, polydactyly and syndactyly, hypoplasia of the genitourinary system, an accessory spleen, and liver, and malrotation of the intestine.

Most children with severe defects in cleavage of the forebrain are stillborn or die in the neonatal period. Microcephaly, hypotonia, apnea, and seizures are prominent features. Hypotonia is especially severe when the defect is associated with a chromosomal abnormality. Infants who survive have severe intellectual, motor, and sensory impairment. Children with only arhinencephaly may appear physically normal and may display minor disturbances in neurological function such as learning disabilities and seizures.

Diagnosis. Suspect HPE in every child with midline facial deformities, especially when malformations are present in other organs. MRI provides excellent visualization of the malformation.

Molecular genetic testing is available for many forms.

Management. The management is symptomatic. The appearance of the ventricles is often confused with hydrocephalus but the pathogenesis is different and shunting is not essential. The extent of supportive care depends on the severity of the defect. In many cases, palliative care should be an option for families.

Agenesis of the Corpus Callosum

Anomalous development of the three telencephalic commissures (the corpus callosum and the anterior and hippocampal commissures) is an almost constant feature of defective prosencephalization. The incidence of callosal abnormalities (complete or partial agenesis or hypoplasia of corpus callosum) detected by MRI obtained for all reasons was reported to be about 0.25 % (Hetts et al, 2006). However, a study population in Hungary found the prevalence in newborns to be about 0.018 % in a group of subjects with agenesis of corpus callosum as an isolated finding (Szabó et al, 2011). Agenesis also occurs in association with other prosencephalic dysplasias and with some metabolic defects (see the section on Glycine Encephalopathy in Chapter 1) and as a solitary genetic defect. When only the corpus callosum is absent, the anterior and hippocampal commissures may be normal or enlarged. Callosal agenesis is part of the Aicardi syndrome (see Chapter 1), the Andermann syndrome (autosomal recessive callosal agenesis, mental deficiency, and peripheral neuropathy), and trisomies 8, 11, and 13.

Clinical Features. Solitary agenesis of the corpus callosum is clinically silent except for subtle disturbances in the interhemispheric transfer of information, for which special testing is needed. Cognitive impairment or learning disabilities occur in most cases, and epilepsy usually indicates concurrent additional brain dysgenesis (focal heterotopias, cortical dysplasia, etc).

Diagnosis. Neuroimaging shows lateral displacement of the lateral ventricles and upward displacement of the third ventricle. Intraventricular pressure is normal.

Management. Treatment is symptomatic.

Defective Cellular Migration

Lissencephaly is a failure of cerebral cortical development because of defective neuroblast migration (Hehr et al, 2011). When neurons that should form the superficial layers of the cerebral cortex are unable to pass through the already established deeper layers of neurons, the cortical convolution pattern is lacking (agyria) and neurons accumulate in the white matter (*heterotopia*). Complete absence of gyri causes a smooth cerebral surface (*lissencephaly-1*), whereas incomplete gyral formation reduces the number and enlarges the size of the existing convolutions (*pachygyria*). Neurons that come close to their cortical position form a subcortical band (*band heterotopia*).

The migrations of the cerebellum and the brainstem also are usually involved, but the embryonic corpus gangliothalamicus pathway is not disturbed, so the thalamus and basal ganglia form properly. Structural and metabolic abnormalities of the fetal ependyma may be important factors in disturbing the normal development of radial glial cells. Decreased brain size leads to microcephaly, with widened ventricles representing a fetal stage rather than pressure from hydrocephalus and an uncovered sylvian fossa representing lack of operculation.

The second form of cortical architectural abnormality in lissencephaly is disorganized clusters of neurons with haphazard orientation, forming no definite layers or predictable pattern (*lissencephaly-2*). Lissencephaly-2 is associated with several closely related genetic syndromes: Walker-Warburg syndrome, Fukuyama muscular dystrophy, muscle-eye-brain disease of Santavuori, and Meckel-Gruber syndrome. Microcephaly and a peculiar facies that includes micrognathia, high forehead, thin upper lip, short nose with anteverted nares, and low-set ears characterize the *Miller-Dieker syndrome*. A microdeletion at the 17p13.3 locus occurs in most patients with Miller-Dieker syndrome, and deletions on chromosome 17 occur in many other lissencephaly syndromes.

Genetic transmission of lissencephaly also occurs as an X-linked dominant trait with two different phenotypes; males show classical lissencephaly, while females show bilateral periventricular nodular heterotopia (BPNH) (Figure 18-7).

Clinical Features. Referral of most children with lissencephaly is for evaluation of developmental delay or intractable myoclonic seizures. Many initially exhibit muscular hypotonia that later evolves into spasticity and opisthotonus. Microcephaly is not always present, but all children have severe cognitive impairment, epilepsy, and cerebral palsy. BPNH usually presents with sporadic or familial epilepsy and normal intelligence. Small, isolated heterotopic cortical nodules are an important cause of intractable epilepsy in an otherwise normal child (see Chapter 1).

Diagnosis. MRI abnormalities establish the diagnosis. A smooth cortical surface except for rudimentary sulci (agyria) may be limited to

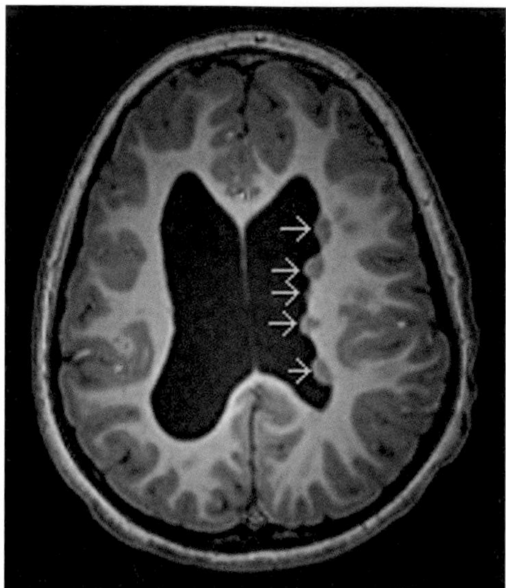

FIGURE 18-7 ■ Nodular heterotopias. T_1 axial MRI shows (arrows) multiple nodular heterotopias protruding into a dilated ventricular system.

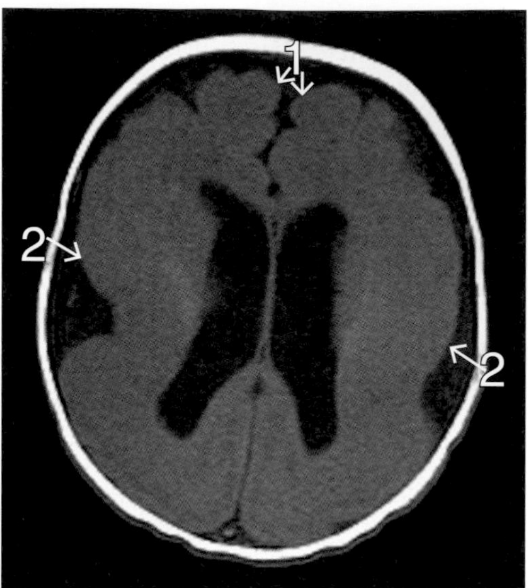

FIGURE 18-8 ■ Lissencephaly and pachygyria. T_1 axial MRI shows (1) frontal pachygyria and (2) posterior lissencephaly.

the parietal or frontal regions or encompass the whole brain (Figure 18-8). The sylvian fissure is broad and triangular, the interhemispheric fissure widened, and nests of gray matter are present within the white matter. The ventricles may be enlarged and the corpus callosum absent. Molecular genetic testing is available for several specific syndromes.

Management. Seizures are usually intractable, but standard drugs for the management of infantile spasms or myoclonic seizures may provide partial relief (see Chapter 1). Death often occurs during infancy, but long survival is possible.

Secondary Microcephaly

Intrauterine Disorders

Intrauterine infection is an established cause of microcephaly. Cytomegalovirus infection (see Chapter 5) can be manifest as microcephaly, without any features of systemic disease. Because maternal infection is asymptomatic, such cases are difficult to identify as caused by cytomegalovirus disease. However, surveys of cytomegalovirus antibody demonstrate a higher rate of seropositive individuals among microcephalic than normocephalic children. This suggests that such cases do exist.

Efforts to identify environmental toxins that produce cerebral malformation have had only limited success. Drugs of abuse and several pharmaceutical agents are suspects, but the evidence is rarely compelling. The only absolute conclusion derived from an abundance of studies is that a negative impact occurs on fetuses of women whose lifestyle includes some combination of heavy alcohol or drug use, poor nutrition, and inadequate health care. The expression of the negative impact includes intrauterine growth retardation, dysmorphic features, and microcephaly.

Aplasia of major cerebral vessels is a rare malformation of unknown cause. Brain tissue that the aplastic vessels should have supplied with blood either never forms or is infarcted and replaced by calcified cystic cavities. The cavities are present at birth, and the CT appearance suggests an intrauterine infection except that the cysts conform to a vascular distribution.

Perinatal Brain Injuries

Perinatal brain injuries are an important cause of failure of brain growth during infancy when head circumference is normal at birth. The initial features of this group of disorders are neonatal encephalopathy and seizures (see Chapter 1). Children with microcephaly and cognitive impairment from perinatal brain injuries always have cerebral palsy and often have epilepsy. Microcephaly and cognitive impairment in the absence of motor impairment are always of prenatal origin.

Postnatal Systemic Disease

Infants who are chronically ill and malnourished fail to thrive. All growth is retarded, but usually head growth maintains itself better than length and weight. If body size is below the 3rd percentile, head circumference might be at the 5th or

10th percentile. Failure to correct the systemic disturbance usually causes brain injury, brain growth slows, and head circumference falls into the microcephalic range.

ABNORMAL HEAD SHAPE

Whereas skull content almost exclusively determines skull size, skull shape results from forces acting from within and without, and of the time of closure of the cranial sutures.

Intracranial Forces

The shape of the brain contributes to the shape of the skull by influencing the time of closure of cranial sutures. Temporal lobe agenesis results in a narrower calvarium, and cerebellar agenesis results in a small posterior fossa. Hydrocephalus produces characteristic changes in skull shape. Large lateral ventricles cause bowing of the forehead, and the Dandy-Walker malformation causes bowing of the occiput. In infants with subdural hematomas, separation of the sagittal suture may cause bitemporal widening.

Extracranial Forces

Constricting forces in utero, such as a bicornuate uterus or multiple fetuses, may influence head shape. Physical constraint of the skull in utero may contribute to premature closure of a cranial suture, but perinatal and postnatal constraints do not. Molding of the skull is common during a prolonged vaginal delivery, but the closure of cranial sutures is unaffected. Molding does not influence eventual head shape.

In premature infants, *scaphocephaly* (Table 18-1) often develops because the poorly mineralized skull flattens on one side and then the other with turning of the child from side-to-side. The shape of the skull becomes normal with maturity.

Plagiocephaly or occipital flattening is the rule in normal infants who always sleep on their backs, and especially frequent in hypotonic infants who constantly lay in the same position. The hair over the flattened portion of skull is usually sparse from rubbing against the bed surface. A normal head shape resumes by changing the infant's position.

TABLE 18-1 Terms that Describe Head Shapes

Term	Description
Acrocephaly	High, tower-like head with vertical forehead
Brachycephaly	Broad head with recessed lower forehead
Oxycephaly	Pointed head
Plagiocephaly	Flattening of one side of head
Scaphocephaly (dolichocephaly)	Abnormally long, narrow head
Trigonocephaly	Triangular head with prominent vertical ridge in the midforehead

Craniostenosis

Craniostenosis and craniosynostosis are terms for premature closure of one or more cranial sutures; the result is always an abnormal skull shape. These terms are only applicable to infants in whom the sutures close while the brain is growing. Early closure of sutures in infants with microcephaly is not premature because the intracranial pressure required to keep sutures apart is lacking.

Most cases of craniostenosis are sporadic and of uncertain etiology. Autosomal dominant and recessive forms of single-suture closure occur. Autosomal dominant inheritance is more common than autosomal recessive inheritance but is also more easily identifiable as hereditary. Many sporadic cases could represent autosomal recessive inheritance.

Craniostenosis may be one feature of a larger recognized syndrome of chromosomal or genetic abnormality. Many of the genetic disorders are secondary to mutations of *fiber growth factor receptor* (FGFR). Table 18-2 summarizes these disorders (Robin et al, 2011). FGFR disorders are often associated with syndactyly or polydactyly (see the section on Acrocephalosyndactyly later in this chapter), whereas chromosomal disorders are usually characterized by other limb malformations and growth retardation.

Craniostenosis is also associated with other disorders. Some of these associations are coincidental, but a cause-and-effect relationship probably does exist with metabolic disorders of bone.

Clinical Features. In nonsyndromic craniostenosis, the only clinical feature is an abnormal head shape. Normal bone growth is impaired in a plane perpendicular to the fused sutures but is able to occur in a parallel plane. The cause of scaphocephaly is premature fusion of the sagittal suture, brachycephaly is premature fusion of both coronal sutures, plagiocephaly is premature fusion of one coronal or one lambdoid suture, trigonocephaly is premature fusion of the metopic suture, and oxycephaly is premature fusion of all sutures. When several sutures close prematurely, the growing brain is constricted

TABLE 18-2 **Distinguishing Clinical Features in the FGFR-Related Craniosynostosis Syndromes**

Disorder	Thumbs	Hands	Great toes	Feet
Muenke syndrome	Normal	± Carpal fusion	± Broad	± Tarsal fusion
Crouzon syndrome	Normal	Normal	Normal	Normal
Crouzon syndrome with acanthosis nigricans	Normal	Normal	Normal	Normal
Jackson-Weiss syndrome	Normal	Variable	Broad, medially deviated	Abnormal tarsals
Apert syndrome	Occasionally fused to fingers	Bone syndactyly	Occasionally fused to toes	Bone syndactyly
Pfeiffer syndrome	Broad, medially deviated	Variable brachydactyly	Broad, medially deviated	Variable brachydactyly
Beare-Stevenson syndrome	Normal	Normal	Normal	Normal
FGFR2-related isolated coronal synostosis	Normal	Normal	Normal	Normal

(Data from Robin NH, Falk MJ, Haldeman-Englert CR. FGFR-related craniosynostosis syndromes. In: GeneClinics: Medical Genetic Knowledge Base [database online]. Seattle: University of Washington. Available at http://www.geneclinics.org. PMID: 20301628. Last updated June 7, 2011.)

and symptoms of increased intracranial pressure develop. Communicating and noncommunicating hydrocephalus occur more frequently in children with craniostenosis than in normal children. It is more likely that a common underlying factor causes both rather than one causing the other. Two-suture craniostenosis is common. The sagittal suture is usually involved, in combination with either the metopic or the coronal suture.

Diagnosis. Visual inspection of the skull and palpation of the sutures are sufficient for diagnosis in most cases of one- or two-suture craniostenosis. Radiography of the skull shows a band of increased density at the site of the prematurely closed sutures. All children with craniostenosis of multiple sutures and children with craniostenosis of a single suture and suspected hydrocephalus require an imaging study of the head.

Management. The two indications for surgery to correct craniostenosis are to improve the appearance of the head and to relieve increased intracranial pressure. The cosmetic indication should be used sparingly and only to make severe deformities less noticeable. The early use of a helmet may be beneficial in reshaping the head in early cases of partial craniostenosis.

Acrocephalosyndactyly

The combination of craniostenosis and fusion of fingers and toes characterizes acrocephalosyndactyly. Some degree of cognitive impairment is often present.

Apert syndrome is syndactyly and premature closure of the coronal suture resulting in brachycephaly. The gene abnormality, inherited as a dominant trait, is a mutation in the gene encoding fibroblast growth factor receptor-2 (FGFR2) (10q26). The forehead is high and prominent, and the face is similar to but less severely deformed than the face in Crouzon disease. Agenesis of the corpus callosum and limbic structures may be an associated feature. The IQ is greater than 70 in 50 % of the children who have a skull decompression before 1 year of age versus only 7% in those operated on later in life (Reiner et al, 1996).

Carpenter syndrome differs from Apert syndrome because transmission is by autosomal recessive inheritance, and polydactyly as well as syndactyly are associated with premature closure of all sutures, obesity, and hypogonadism. Approximately 75 % of patients are retarded secondary to cerebral malformations that are demonstrable on MRI.

Crouzon Disease (Craniofacial Dysostosis)

Crouzon disease is the combination of premature closure of any or all cranial sutures and maldevelopment of facial bones. Transmission is by autosomal dominant inheritance.

Clinical Features. The facial deformity is present at birth and becomes worse during infancy. The skull is usually widened anteriorly secondary to premature closure of the coronal suture. The eyes are widely separated and prominent, but the lower face appears recessed because of maxillary hypoplasia and prognathism. Adding to the deformity are a beak-like nose and a large, protuberant tongue. Intracranial pressure often increases because several cranial sutures are usually involved.

Diagnosis. The typical facies and genetic pattern of inheritance are diagnostic. Head CT or MRI is useful to follow the progression of cerebral compression.

Management. A sequential neurosurgical and plastic surgical approach has been successful in opening the sutures to relieve intracranial pressure and in advancing the facial bones forward to improve the cosmetic appearance.

REFERENCES

Griebel ML, Williams JP, Russell SS, et al. Clinical and developmental findings in children with giant interhemispheric cysts and dysgenesis of the corpus callosum. Pediatric Neurology 1995;13:119–24.

Grinberg I, Northrup H, Ardinger H, et al. Heterozygous deletion of the linked genes ZIC1 and ZIC4 is involved in Dandy-Walker malformation. Nature Genetics 2004;36:1053–5.

Hehr U, Uyanik G, Aigner L, et al. DCX-related disorders (includes: DCX-related lissencephaly, DCX-related subcortical band heterotopia). In: GeneClinics: Medical Genetic Knowledge Base [database online]. Seattle: University of Washington. Available at http://www.geneclinics.org. PMID: 20301364. Last updated March 24, 2011.

Hetts SW, Sherr EH, Chao S, et al. Anomalies of the corpus callosum: An MR analysis of the phenotypic spectrum of associated malformations. American Journal of Roentgenology 2006;187:1343–8.

Pauli RM. Achondroplasia. In: GeneClinics: Medical Genetic Knowledge Base [database online]. Seattle: University of Washington. Available at http://www.geneclinics.org. PMID: 20301331. Last updated February 16, 2012.

Reiner D, Arnaud E, Cinalli G, et al. Prognosis for mental function in Apert's syndrome. Journal of Neurosurgery 1996;85:66–72.

Robin NH, Falk MJ, Haldeman-Englert CR. FGFR-related craniosynostosis syndromes. In: GeneClinics: Medical Genetic Knowledge Base [database online]. Seattle: University of Washington. Available at http://www.geneclinics.org. PMID: 20301628. Last updated June 7, 2011.

Samartzis D, Kalluri P, Herman J, et al. Cervical scoliosis in the Klippel-Feil patient. Spine 2011;36:E1501–8.

Schrander-Stumpel C, Vos, YJ. L1 syndrome. In: GeneClinics: Medical Genetic Knowledge Base [database online]. Seattle: University of Washington. Available at http://www.geneclinics.org. PMID: 20301657. Last updated December 23, 2010.

Solomon BD, Gropman A, Muenke M. Holoprosencephaly overview. In: GeneClinics: Medical Genetic Knowledge Base [database online]. Seattle: University of Washington. Available at http://www.geneclinics.org. PMID: 20301702. Last updated November 3, 2011.

Szabó N, Gergev G, Kóbor J, et al. Corpus callosum anomalies: Birth prevalence and clinical spectrum in Hungary. Pediatric Neurology 2011;44:420–6.

Tatton-Brown K, Cole TRP, Rahman N. Sotos syndrome. In: GeneClinics: Medical Genetic Knowledge Base [database online]. Seattle: University of Washington. Available at http://www.geneclinics.org. PMID: 20301652. Last updated March 8, 2012.

van der Knaap MS, Scheper GC. Megancephalic leukoencephalopathy with subcortical cysts. In: GeneClinics: Medical Genetic Knowledge Base [database online]. Seattle: University of Washington. Available at http://www.geneclinics.org. PMID: 20301707. Last updated November 3, 2011.

Zhang J, Williams MA, Rigamonti D. Genetics of human hydrocephalus. Journal of Neurology 2006;253:1255–66.

INDEX

Page numbers ending in 'b', 'f' and 't' refer to Boxes, Figures and Tables respectively.

B

C

F

G

I

M

N

Q

R

S

T

U

V

W

X

Y

Z